www.harcourt-international.com

Bringing you products from all Harcourt Health Sciences companies including Baillière Tindall, Churchill Livingstone, Mosby and W.B. Saunders

- **Browse** for latest information on new books, journals and electronic products

- **Search** for information on over 20 000 published titles with full product information including tables of contents and sample chapters

- **Keep up to date** with our extensive publishing programme in your field by registering with **eAlert** or requesting postal updates

- **Secure online ordering** with prompt delivery, as well as full contact details to order by phone, fax or post

- **News** of special features and promotions

If you are based in the following countries, please visit the country-specific site to receive full details of product availability and local ordering information

USA: www.harcourthealth.com

Canada: www.harcourtcanada.com

Australia: www.harcourt.com.au

Baillière Tindall   CHURCHILL LIVINGSTONE   Mosby   W.B. SAUNDERS

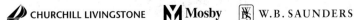

Publisher: Richard Furn
Project Development Manager: Fiona Conn
Project Manager: Frances Affleck
Designer: Judith Wright
Page Make-up: Kate Walshaw
Illustration Manager: Bruce Hogarth
Illustrations: Marion Tasker (first edition),
   MTG (second edition)

Second Edition
ILLUSTRATED TEXTBOOK OF
PAEDIATRICS

Dr Tom Lissauer
MB BChir FRCP FRCPCH
Consultant Paediatrician
St Mary's Hospital
London, UK

Dr Graham Clayden
MD FRCP FRCPCH
Reader in Paediatrics
The Guy's, Kings & St Thomas' School of Medicine
(Kings College London)
London, UK

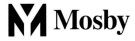

EDINBURGH LONDON NEW YORK PHILADELPHIA ST LOUIS SYDNEY TORONTO 2001

MOSBY
An imprint of Harcourt Publishers Limited

© Mosby International Limited 2001

M is a registered trademark of Harcourt Publishers Limited

The right of Tom Lissauer and Graham Clayden to be identified as editors
of this work has been asserted by them in accordance with the Copyright,
Designs and Patents Act 1988

First edition 1997
Second edition 2001

ISBN 0 723 43178 7
International edition ISBN 0 723 43243 0

British Library Cataloguing in Publication Data
A catalogue record for this book is available from the British Library

Library of Congress Cataloging in Publication Data
A catalog record for this book is available from the Library of Congress

Note
Medical knowledge is constantly changing. As new information becomes
available, changes in treatment, procedures, equipment and the use of
drugs become necessary. The editors and the publishers have taken care
to ensure that the information given in this text is accurate and up-to-date.
However, readers are strongly advised to confirm that the information,
especially with regard to drug usage, complies with the latest legislation
and standards of practice.

The
publisher's
policy is to use
**paper manufactured
from sustainable forests**

Printed in Spain

Contents

Foreword to the second edition

The publication of the first edition of this book has proved to be an important milestone in paediatric undergraduate education. It immediately became enormously popular with medical students, its distinctive cover the hallmark of students on their paediatric clinical attachment. The authors, both well known for their contribution to undergraduate and postgraduate medical education and examinations, have produced an outstanding book, covering core information for paediatrics and child health in a concise but informative manner, without overburdening the reader with more obscure conditions. The large number of colour photographs and drawings which enliven most pages of the book both hold the reader's attention and help to guide one to the most fundamental points described in the text. Furthermore, the book successfully captures the fundamental elements of humanity, sensitivity and emotional understanding required by all professionals who care for children and their families. It was not surprising that the book received awards for innovation and excellence in the British Medical Association and Royal Society of Medicine Book Competitions and has been translated into several languages.

Medical students beginning clinical paediatrics face a daunting task. Children are affected by the full range of medical and surgical conditions which affect adults but in addition suffer from a large number of inherited or acquired disorders which occur uniquely in the early years of life. In the few weeks allocated to paediatrics in the crowded medical school curriculum the student must acquire knowledge not only of the diagnosis and management of common paediatric disorders but of the complex social developmental, educational and emotional problems faced by them. Meticulous care has been taken in this book to distill to essentials the information required for paediatric undergraduate training, highlighting the important differences between paediatrics and adult medicine.

This second edition has enabled the authors to keep the information up to date and to incorporate some extra material to reflect the current ethos of paediatric medicine.

Professor Michael Levin
Professor of Paediatrics,
Imperial College School of Medicine, London
2001

Foreword to the first edition

You are about to read a textbook unlike any you have ever read before. It is unique in its presentation, organization, graphics and design. I predict that the *Illustrated Textbook of Paediatrics* will become a standard by which all other medical textbooks will be judged. The plethora of information which every medical student is expected to absorb and integrate is unending. Therefore, it is incumbent on teachers and texts to be innovative and creatively selective in their presentation of information and wisdom. The editors, Tom Lissauer and Graham Clayden, have been successful in achieving this.

The information is presented in a clear, concise fashion and has been supplemented by original illustrations and colourful, easy-to-read charts and graphs.

Each section of the book deserves praise. The chapter on genetics is noteworthy because it does not present overwhelming details of biochemical/molecular biology but presents a comprehensive compendium of the subject, the importance of which is undisputed in the 20th century. Perinatology and nutrition offer the student important information that has occasionally been slighted in older texts.

The reader will find both enjoyment and instruction in this new introduction to clinical paediatrics. The text is practical and the information is easily accessible.

In conclusion, I salute the authors and editors. I wish I had written this book.

The late Frank A Oski, MD
Distinguished Service Professor,
The John Hopkins University School of Medicine,
Baltimore, Maryland
1997

Preface

This textbook has been written for undergraduates. Our aim has been to provide the core information required by students for the 6–10 weeks assigned to paediatrics in the curriculum of most undergraduate medical schools. It will also be of assistance to those preparing for postgraduate examinations such as the Diploma of Child Health (DCH) and Membership of the Royal College of Paediatrics and Child Health (MRCPCH).

The huge amount of positive feedback we have received on the first edition from medical students in the UK and abroad has spurred us on to produce this new edition. We have updated the text and added three new topics which have become important in paediatrics. These are an introductory chapter 'The child in society' which discusses wider issues of social paediatrics that affect children's health both in the UK and elsewhere; and coverage of ethics in paediatrics and evidence-based medicine. We have also added extra photographs and diagrams to this edition. We have, though, kept any additional text to a minimum. In consideration of the pressure of exams, an innovation in this edition has been the identification of 'key topics' with a ⌖ highlighting the areas which should be focused on during revision.

In order to make learning from this book easier we have followed a lecture-note style using short sentences and lists of important features. Illustrations have been used to help the student recognise important signs or clinical features and to make the book more attractive and interesting to use. Key learning points have been identified for most topics. Case histories have been chosen to highlight points within their clinical context.

A new self-assessment book, *Illustrated Self Assessment in Paediatrics*, based on the contents of this book, has also been produced to assist students in their learning and revision. This companion book contains case scenarios, including clinical photographs and images, and uses a number of different methods of assessment. We hope this variety will make the book more instructive and enjoyable.

The male gender for children has been used throughout the book for stylistic simplicity alone.

We would like to thank all our contributors and Richard Furn, Publisher, and Fiona Conn, Project Development Manager, for their assistance in producing this new edition. Thanks also to Ann, Rachel and David Lissauer for their ideas and assistance, and for their understanding of the time taken away from the family in the preparation of this new edition.

We welcome any comments about the book.

Tom Lissauer and Graham Clayden
2001

Acknowledgements

We would like to acknowledge the major contribution made to the first edition by the following contributors: Lynn Ball (Haematological disorders), Gill Du Mont (Skin), Tony Hulse (Growth and puberty; and Endocrine and metabolic disorders), Nigel Klein (Paediatric emergencies), Nicholas Madden (Genitalia), Angus Nicoll (Development, language, hearing and vision), Jo Sibert (Environment), Karen Simmer (Perinatal medicine; and neonatal medicine), Elizabeth Thompson (Genetics).

The contributors to the second edition have extensively drawn on the material that they prepared for the first edition.

Contributors

Dr Paula Bolton-Maggs
Consultant Paediatric Haematologist
Royal Liverpool Children's Hospital, Liverpool, UK
Ch. 20: Haematological disorders

Professor Ian Booth
Institute of Child Health, Birmingham, UK
Ch. 11: Nutrition
Ch. 12: Gastroenterology

Dr Graham Clayden
Reader in Paediatrics
The Guy's, Kings & St Thomas' School of Medicine,
(Kings College London),
London, UK
Ch. 4: Care of the sick child

Dr Jon Couriel
Consultant in Paediatric Respiratory Medicine
Royal Liverpool Children's Hospital, Liverpool, UK
Ch. 14: Respiratory disorders

Dr Ruth Gilbert
Senior Lecturer in Clinical Epidemiology
Centre for Evidence-Based Child Health, Institute of
Child Health, University College London Medical
School, London, UK
Ch. 4: Care of the sick child (evidence-based medicine)

Professor Denis Gill
Consultant Paediatrician/Paediatric Nephrologist
Children's Hospital, Dublin, Republic of Ireland
Ch. 2: History and examination

Professor Raanan Gillon
Emeritus Professor of Medical Ethics
Imperial College School of Medicine, Southside,
Prince's Gardens, London, UK
Ch. 4: Care of the sick child (ethics)

Professor Peter Hill
Great Ormond Street Hospital for Children,
London, UK
Ch. 21: Emotions and behaviour

Dr Helen Jenkinson
Lecture in Paediatric Oncology
The Birmingham Children's Hospital,
Birmingham, UK
Ch. 19: Malignant disease

Dr Deirdre Kelly
Reader in Paediatric Hepatology
Birmingham Children's Hospital, Birmingham, UK
Ch. 18: Liver disorders

Dr Helen Kingston
Consultant Clinical Geneticist
St Mary's Hospital, Manchester, UK
Ch. 7: Genetics

Dr Nigel Klein
Senior Lecturer and Consultant in Immunology
and Infectious diseases
Great Ormond Street Hospital for Children and
Institute of Child Health, London, UK
Ch. 13: Infection and immunity

Mr Anthony Lander
Senior Lecturer in Paediatric Surgery
Institute of Child Health, Birmingham, UK
Ch. 12: Gastroenterology

Dr Tom Lissauer
Consultant Paediatrician
St Mary's Hospital, London, UK
Ch. 1: The child in society
Ch. 4: Care of the sick child
Ch. 8: Perinatal medicine
Ch. 9: Neonatal medicine

Dr Hermione Lyall
Senior Lecturer in Paediatric Infectious Diseases
St Mary's Hospital, London, UK
Ch. 13: Infection and immunity

Dr Maud Meates
Consultant Paediatrician
North Middlesex Hospital, London, UK
Ch. 4: Care of the sick child (evidence-based medicine)

Dr Simon Nadel
Consultant in Paediatric Intensive Care
St Mary's Hospital, London, UK
Ch. 5: Paediatric emergencies

Dr Richard Newton
Consultant Paediatric Neurologist
Royal Manchester Children's Hospital, Manchester, UK
Ch. 25: Neurological disorders
Ch. 26: The child with special needs

Dr Barbara Phillips
Consultant in Paediatric Emergency Medicine
Royal Liverpool Children's Hospital, Liverpool, UK
Ch. 6: Environment

Professor Andrew Redington
Professor of Paediatric Cardiology
Great Ormond Street Hospital, London, UK
Ch. 15: Cardiac disorders

Dr Lesley Rees
Consultant Paediatric Nephrologist
Great Ormond Street Hospital, London, UK
Ch. 16: Kidney and urinary tract

Dr John Sills
Consultant Paediatrician
Royal Liverpool Children's Hospital, Liverpool, UK
Ch. 24: Bones and joints

Dr Diane Smyth
Consultant in Paediatric Neurology and
Neurodisability,
St Mary's Hospital, London, UK
Ch. 3: Child development, hearing and vision

Dr Mike Stevens
Consultant Paediatric Oncologist
The Birmingham Children's Hospital, Birmingham, UK
Ch. 19: Malignant disease

Mr Mark Stringer
Consultant Paediatric Surgeon
Leeds Teaching Hospitals Trust, Leeds, UK
Ch. 17: Genitalia

Dr Rashmin Tamhne
Consultant Community Paediatrician
Fosse Health Trust, Leicester, UK
Ch. 1: The child in society

Professor Julian Verbov
Consultant Paediatric Dermatologist
Royal Liverpool Children's Hospital, Liverpool, UK
Ch. 22: Skin

Dr Jerry Wales
Senior Lecturer in Paediatric Endocrinology
University of Sheffield, Sheffield Children's Hospital,
Sheffield, UK
Ch. 10: Growth and puberty
Ch. 23: Endocrine and metabolic disorders

Professor Michael Weindling
Consultant Neonatologist
Liverpool Women's Hospital, Liverpool, UK
Ch. 8: Perinatal medicine
Ch. 9: Neonatal medicine

1

The child in society

Most medical encounters with children involve an individual child presenting to a doctor with a symptom, such as diarrhoea. After taking a history, examining the child and performing any necessary investigations, the doctor arrives at a diagnosis or differential diagnosis and makes a management plan. This disease-oriented approach plays an important part in ensuring the immediate and long-term well-being of an individual. However, the nature of the child's illness needs to be seen within the wider context of the society in which he lives. This will affect the likely cause (if the diarrhoea is likely to be from a contaminated water supply), the severity of the child's illness (the organism likely to be responsible and the child's nutritional status) and management options (who will take care of the child when ill, what medications are available, if hospital treatment is possible, and what facilities it can offer). In order to be a truly effective clinician, the doctor must be able to place the child's clinical problems within the context of the family and of the society in which they live.

The way in which the environment impacts on a child is exemplified by the contrast between the major child health problems in developing and developed countries (Fig. 1.1). In developing countries, the predominant problems are infection (Fig. 1.2) and malnutrition, whereas in developed countries they are a range of complex, often previously fatal, chronic disorders and behavioural, emotional or developmental problems.

THE CHILD'S WORLD

The life of any child is profoundly influenced by their social, cultural, psychological and physical environment. This can be considered in terms of the child himself, his family and immediate social environment, the local social fabric and, directly and indirectly, national and international affairs (Fig. 1.3).

Fig. 1.1 Contrast between main child health problems in developed and developing countries.

Developing countries

Infection – respiratory tract, diarrhoea, malaria, tuberculosis and, recently, HIV

Malnutrition – marasmus, kwashiorkor, severe iron deficiency anaemia

Developmental and learning problems of organic pathology – Down's syndrome, congenital anomalies

Sanitation, water supply, food hygiene, housing and education

Poverty and unemployment

Health care – not available or poor quality

High birth rate – children constitute high proportion of population

Developed countries

Severe, often previously fatal chronic disorders – malignant disease, cystic fibrosis, postneonatal and paediatric intensive care, organ transplantation

Behavioural and emotional disorders – attention deficit disorder, anorexia nervosa

Neurodevelopmental disorders – language delay, reading difficulties, clumsiness

Reduction in morbidity and mortality from road traffic and other accidents

Lack of family cohesion

Socioeconomic disadvantage among the 'have-nots' – from lack of money, unemployment, inadequate housing and education

Inequality of access to health services

Excessive consumption – obesity

Drug abuse, smoking, teenage pregnancies

Fig. 1.2 Infectious diseases in children in developing countries.

Each year, 8 million children die before 5 years of age from the following infections:

Pneumonia
Risk factors – low birthweight, young age, not breast-fed, vitamin A deficiency, overcrowding
Predominantly bacterial
Mortality reduced by WHO guidelines for community health workers for diagnosis (tachypnoea, cough, fever, head nodding and chest recession) and treatment with an antibiotic

Diarrhoea
Most < 2 years old
Often bacterial
Results in undernutrition, poor growth, death
Usually treated with oral rehydration solution, continuing to breast-feed
Antibiotics only for cholera, dysentery, giardiasis, amoebiasis

Measles
Preventable by immunisation

Malaria
Deaths mostly in children from cerebral malaria from *Plasmodium falciparum* in sub-Saharan Africa
Antimalarial therapy must be started promptly, on clinical suspicion
Drug resistance is problematic

HIV Infection
> 1 million children infected
> 5 million children orphaned through infection of parents

Tuberculosis
Increasing incidence, especially with HIV infection
> 150 000 deaths/year, from meningitis and disseminated miliary tuberculosis
Usually acquired from infected adult in household

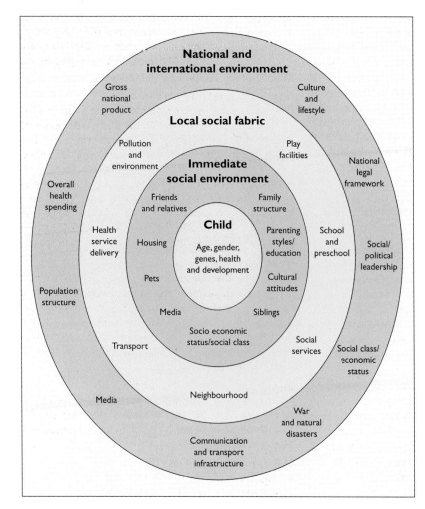

Fig. 1.3 A child's world consists of overlapping, interconnected and expanding socio-environmental layers, which influence children's health and development. (After Bronfenbrenner U, Contexts of child rearing – problems and prospects. *American Psychologist* 34: 844–850, 1979.)

The child

The child's world will be affected by gender, genes, physical health, temperament and development. It will also vary markedly with age; the life of an infant or toddler is mainly determined by the home environment, and that of the young child by school and friends, whereas the teenager will be aware of and influenced by events not only nationally but also internationally, e.g. in music, sport, fashion or politics.

Immediate social environment

Family structure

Although the 'two biological parent family' remains the norm, there are many variations in family structure. Nearly one-third of all children in the UK live in a single-parent household. This also varies with ethnicity. In the UK, about 50% of Afro-Caribbean children live with a single parent, compared with 15% of white children and less than 10% of those from the Indian subcontinent. Disadvantages of single parenthood include a higher level of unemployment, poor housing and financial hardship (Fig. 1.4). An increased incidence of long-term emotional and behavioural problems amongst the children has been reported.

The increase in the number of parents who change partners and the accompanying rise in reconstituted families mean that children are having to cope with a range of new and complex parental and sibling relationships. This may result in emotional, behavioural and social difficulties.

The trend towards smaller families provides an increased standard of living. However, it may also result in an increased expectation that each child will have optimal health and development and achievement. With many parents now leaving home in order to work, there is a greater demand for professional child care. This may be in the form of child-minding or day-care nurseries. Increasing attention is being paid to the quality of day-care facilities in terms of supervision of the children and improving the opportunities they provide for social interaction and learning.

Approximately 3% of children under 16 years old in the UK live away from a permanent home; 50,000 of these are 'looked after' by social services, and the remainder live in temporary housing.

Refugees are often placed in temporary housing and may be moved repeatedly into areas unfamiliar to them. They may encounter additional problems from communication difficulties, poverty, fragmentation of families, loss of family members and not knowing if friends and family members are safe. Raising children under these circumstances is fraught with difficulties.

Parenting styles

Parenting that is warm and receptive to the child, whilst imposing reasonable and consistent boundaries, will promote the development of an autonomous and self-reliant adult. Some parents are either excessively authoritarian or permissive. Children's emotional development may be damaged by parents who neglect or abuse their children.

The child's temperament is also important, especially when there is a mismatch with the parenting style of the parents; for example, a child with a very determined temperament may be in constant conflict with an authoritarian parent and this may result in tantrums and other behavioural problems.

Siblings have a marked influence on the family dynamics. The arrival of a new baby may engender a feeling of insecurity in older brothers and sisters and result in attention-seeking behaviour. How siblings affect each other appears to be determined by the emotional quality of the relationships between each other and also with other members of the family, including their parents. The role of grandparents and other family members varies widely and is influenced by the family's culture; in some, they are the main caregivers, while in others they play only a peripheral role, exacerbated by geographical separation.

Cultural attitudes to child-rearing

The way in which children are brought up evolves within a community over generations. An example is the use of physical punishment by parents to discipline their children. This is seen as acceptable or even desirable by a high proportion of parents in the UK and the USA, where there is strong public opinion against making physical punishment by parents illegal. However, such legislative measures have been adopted in countries such as Sweden, where they have been largely successful in changing cultural practice.

Peers

Peers exert a major influence on children. Peer relationships and activities provide a 'sense of group belonging' and have potentially long-term benefits for the child. Relationships can also go wrong, e.g. persistent bullying, which may result in or contribute to psychosomatic symptoms, misery and even, in extreme cases, suicide.

Socioeconomic status/social class

Poverty is a key determinant of health and well-being of children. Health care problems in which the UK prevalence rates are increased by poverty and deprivation include:

- low-birthweight infants
- injuries
- hospital admissions

Fig. 1.4 Percentage of families on low gross weekly household income in UK (Office for National Statistics General Household Survey 1996).

	£<100	£100–£500	£>500
Married couple	3	49	48
Lone parent	33	61	6

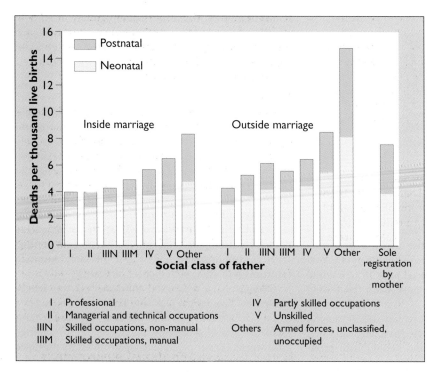

Fig. 1.5 Effect of social class of father and marital status on infant mortality (England & Wales, 1998). (Source: Office for National Statistics, Mortalitiy statistics, Series DH3.)

I	Professional
II	Managerial and technical occupations
IIIN	Skilled occupations, non-manual
IIIM	Skilled occupations, manual
IV	Partly skilled occupations
V	Unskilled
Others	Armed forces, unclassified, unoccupied

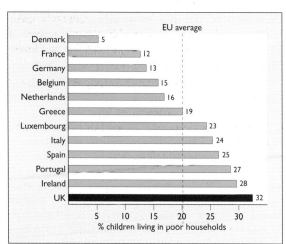

Fig. 1.6 Percentage of children living in poor households, 1993. (Source: Eurostat.)

- asthma
- behavioural problems
- special educational needs
- child abuse.

The increase in infant mortality with social class is shown in Figure 1.5.

Socioeconomic status is usually described by a comparison between the family income and the national average income. For example, taking poverty as below half the national mean household income (as defined by the European Union) shows that the UK has the highest proportion of children living in poverty (Fig. 1.6). Locally, socioeconomic deprivation may be based on area of residence or on a composite score of a number of markers. Low socioeconomic status is often associated with multiple disadvantages, e.g. food of inadequate quantity and poor in nutrition, inadequate housing or homelessness, lack of 'good enough' parenting and an inadequate access to health care and educational facilities. Poor housing may restrict opportunities for play and this may adversely affect the child's development. In general, higher levels of maternal education benefit children's development; maternal low intelligence and mental illness have an adverse effect.

Local social fabric

Neighbourhood

Cohesive communities and amicable neighbourhoods are positive influences on children. Racial tension and other social adversities, such as gang violence and drugs, will adversely affect the emotional and social development of children, as well as their physical health. Parental concern about safety may create tensions in balancing their children's freedom with overprotection and restriction of their lifestyles.

Lifestyle issues concerning children include:
- *teenage pregnancies* – in England and Wales, around 2 per 1000 girls aged 15 or less become pregnant each year, the highest incidence in developed countries
- *smoking and alcohol* – around 30% of children smoke regularly and over 40% of 15-year-olds consume alcohol
- *drug abuse* – nearly 30% of 15-year-olds have had personal experience of using drugs in England and Wales

- *poor nutrition* – the National Diet and Nutrition Survey in 2000 in the UK found that four out of five teenagers ate a diet predominantly consisting of chips, white bread, crisps, biscuits, ketchup and fizzy drinks; 16% of 15- to 18-year-old females were on a diet and 1 in 5 ate no fruit at all, with some living in inner city estates saying that they had easier access to illegal drugs than fresh fruit and vegetables
- *obesity* – a survey of 3–4 year old children in the UK showed that the proportion who were overweight (BMI >85th centile) rose from 15% to 24% over 10 years (1989–98). There has also been a marked increase in the proportion of overweight teenagers, mainly attributed to a reduction in exercise rather than an increase in calorie intake.

These lifestyle issues follow a complex interaction between attitudes and practices in the home and in the community. Their prevalence is greater in deprived communities.

Health service delivery

The variation in the quality of health care is an important component in preventing morbidity and mortality in children. In all countries, health services for children are increasingly provided within primary care. Some aspects of specialist paediatric care are also increasingly provided within the child's home, local community or local hospital through shared care arrangements and specialist community nursing and medical teams. However, access to and the range of these services varies widely.

Schools

Schools provide a powerful influence on children's emotional and intellectual development and their subsequent lives. Differences in the quality of schools in different areas can accentuate inequalities already present in society. Good education also provides the opportunity for children brought up in poverty to improve their social circumstances.

Travel

The increasing ease of travel can broaden children's horizons and opportunities. Especially in rural areas, the ease and availability of transport allow greater access to medical care and influence the pattern of provision of both primary and specialist medical services. However, a consequence of the increasing use of motor vehicles is the large number of injuries sustained by children from road traffic accidents, mainly as pedestrians. Attention to accident prevention, such as calming traffic in residential areas and separating cars from pedestrians and cyclists, is helping to reduce the number of children injured. The widespread use of cars also contributes to a reduction in children's levels of exercise. Whereas 80% of children in the UK went to school by foot or bicycle in 1971, this had dropped to 9% in 1990.

National and international environment

Gross national product

There is a relationship between a country's gross national product and child health; some examples of this are shown in Figure 1.7. It shows that the lower the gross national product:

- the greater the proportion of the population who are children
- the higher the childhood mortality
- the higher the proportion of newborn infants with low birthweight
- the lower the immunisation rate.

Fig. 1.7 National socioeconomic conditions and child health. (Based on the UNICEF report *State of the World's Children*, 1996.)

Category of countries	Health indicators					
	Gross national product (average, in US$ per person)	% of world population (6.2 bn)	Under 5 years (% of population)	Mortality rate under 5 years (per 1000 live births)	Nutrition (low birthweight) (% of births <2.5 kg)	Immunisation (DPT at 1 year) (%)
Developed or industrialised, e.g. USA, UK	23195	13	6.5	9	6	88
Countries in transition, e.g. Poland	2000	7	7	36	Not available	78
Developing countries, e.g. Brazil	987	71	12.5	101	19	80
Least developed countries, e.g. Haiti	237	9	17	170	24	60

However, even in countries with a high gross national product, many children live in financially deprived circumstances.

Worldwide, there has been an enormous improvement in children's health. It is estimated that the proportion of children who die before reaching 5 years of age is now less than half the level of 1960. Even in developed countries, there has been a dramatic reduction in childhood mortality over the last century (Fig. 1.8), although the reduction in childhood mortality rates is now much smaller than previously.

Media

The media has a powerful influence on children. It can be positive and educational. The negative impact of television, video and film is largely through reduced opportunities for social interaction and active learning, lack of physical exercise as well as exposure to undesirable influences, such as violence, sex and cultural stereotypes, e.g. an expectation that teenage girls should be slim. The extent to which the aggressive tendencies of children may be exacerbated or encouraged by exposure to violence in films and television is an unresolved issue of widely held concern.

The internet is enabling parents and children to become better informed about their children's medical problems. This is especially beneficial for the many rare conditions encountered in paediatrics. Parents and children can now access the latest information from around the world and can also communicate directly with other affected children or families. A disadvantage that is already apparent is that it has already led to the dissemination of information which is incorrect or presented from a biased viewpoint, requests for inappropriate investigations or treatment and demands for 'new interventions', even before their safety and efficacy have been established.

New technology

The phenomenal technological advances in the delivery of health care have benefited children enormously. However, their cost forces difficult decisions about how to spend scarce resources. There is a conflict between high-technology care or expensive drugs – which are often of proven efficacy but of benefit to only a small number of children – and preventative measures, which could benefit a larger number of children but are often of poorly established efficacy. An example is neonatal intensive care at the extreme of viability. The cost of these infants' care is high and a significant proportion of the survivors have long-term developmental disabilities. In many developing countries, such treatment is rationed, e.g. by instituting a minimum birthweight at which mechanical ventilation can be provided or by limiting the quantity of expensive drugs, such as surfactant, that can be prescribed. Difficult choices are also being faced in developed countries in deciding the affordability of very expensive procedures, such as heart or liver transplantation, and certain drugs, such as the genetically engineered enzyme replacement therapy for Gaucher's disease.

War and natural disasters

Children are especially vulnerable when there is war, civil unrest or natural disasters (Fig. 1.9). Not only are they at greater risk from infectious diseases and malnutrition, but they may lose their care-givers and other members of their families and are likely to have been exposed to highly traumatic events. Their lives will have been uprooted, socially and culturally, especially if they are forced to flee from their homes and become refugees.

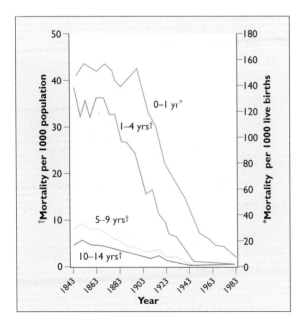

Fig. 1.8 Marked reduction in mortality of children aged 0–14 years between 1843 and 1993. In 1900, 15% of babies born in England died by 1 year of age and 23% by 14 years of age; the figures are now 0.6 and 0.8%, respectively.

> **Fig. 1.9** Children and war: worldwide, devastating effect of war on children, 1986–96. (Source: *State of World's Children*, UNICEF, 1996.)
>
> ---
>
> Mortality – 2 million children died
> Morbidity – 4.5 million children disabled, mainly paraplegia and sensory deficits
> Loss of home and refugee status – 12 million people homeless
> Orphans – 1 million children orphaned
> Psychological trauma – 10 million children estimated to have post-traumatic stress syndrome
> Children as soldiers – escalation of use of children as soldiers with the availability of lighter weapons
> Disruption of health care system – immunisation and child health surveillance programmes interrupted or disbanded
> Anti-personnel mines – major ongoing cause of childhood injury and disability

Children may also be harmed as a result of gun use outside areas of conflict. In the USA, where guns are widely kept in homes for self-defence, for every death occurring as a result of self-defence, there are 1.3 unintentional deaths of children or adults, as well as 4.6 homicides and 37 suicides.

INTERNATIONAL RIGHTS

Children are now recognised as having their own human rights. These are laid down in the United Nations Convention on The Rights of the Child, which has been ratified by all members of the United Nations, including the UK, but excluding the USA and Somalia (Fig. 1.10). Implications of the convention include the involvement of children in clinical decision-making and in issues of consent.

THE NEW PAEDIATRICS AND CHILD HEALTH

In developed countries, there has been a marked shift in emphasis of paediatric practice from children with acute infections, which are now mostly prevented by immunisation or easily treated, to complex, multi-system physical disorders and disabilities and emotional and behavioural problems. This necessitates a more holistic approach to their care (Fig. 1.11). Instead of care being decided by doctors, the child and family are increasingly involved in a partnership determining the pattern of this care, based on the information provided to them. Other services are often involved, including the primary health care team, paediatric community nurses, the playschool/nursery or school, social services, religious community, the voluntary services and complementary health practitioners. Specialist services may be from secondary or tertiary

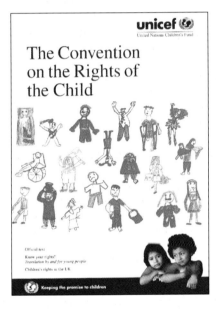

Fig. 1.10a United Nations Convention on the Rights of the Child (1989).

Fig. 1.10b Summary of the United Nations Convention on the Rights of the Child (1989).

1. Survival rights
The child's right to life and to the most basic needs – food, shelter and access to health care

2. Developmental rights
To achieve their full potential – education, play, freedom of thought, conscience and religion. Those with disabilities to receive special services

3. Protection rights
Against all forms of abuse, neglect, exploitation and discrimination

4. Participation rights
To take an active role in their communities and nations

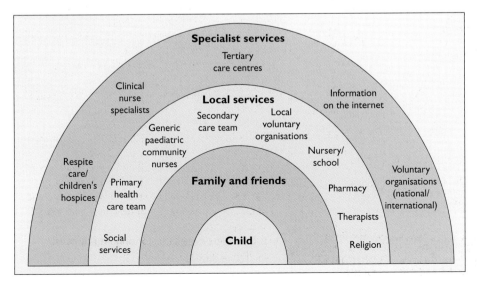

Fig. 1.11 Health care is now centred around the child and family. It is adapted according to the child's condition. Good communication and co-operation between professionals is crucial. A key worker is often appointed to assist the family with this. (Courtesy of Dr Ann Goldman.)

care paediatric centres. Good communication and close cooperation is required between all the parties involved. A designated key worker is often chosen to help families with this. Information may also be obtained from professional or voluntary organisations or parent support groups, which may be national or, increasingly, international.

Doctors can also play an important role in the population-based approach to improving child health. This also requires consideration not only of health care issues but also of social welfare, education and the local community, the voluntary sector and the general public as well as parents and children. Doctors can also help children by advocacy, when public awareness is raised about children's issues and information is provided to inform public debate. Examples of this are child labour, gun control and tobacco advertising.

FURTHER READING

Kohler L 1995 New child public health. In: Spencer N J (ed) Progress in community child health. Churchill Livingstone, Edinburgh, p 1–10
Spencer N J 1996 Poverty and child health. Radcliffe Medical Press, Oxford
United Nations Children's Fund 1995 The convention on the rights of the child. UNICEF, London
Waterson T 2000 Giving guidance on child discipline. British Medical Journal 320: 261–262

Internet
www.unicef.org
www.who.int

2

History and examination

The cornerstone of clinical practice continues to be history-taking and clinical examination. Good doctors will continue to be admired for their ability to distil the important information from the history, for their clinical skills, for their attitude towards patients, and for their knowledge of diseases, disorders and disturbed behaviours.

Parents are acutely interested in and anxious about their children. They will quickly recognise doctors who demonstrate interest, empathy and concern. They will seek out doctors who possess the appropriate skills and attitudes towards their children.

In approaching clinical history and examination of children, it is helpful to visualise some common clinical scenarios in which children are seen by doctors:

- an acute illness, e.g. respiratory tract infection, meningitis, appendicitis
- a chronic problem, e.g. failure to thrive, chronic cough
- a newborn infant with a congenital malformation or abnormality, e.g. developmental dysplasia of the hip, Down's syndrome
- suspected delay in development, e.g. slow to walk, talk or acquire skills
- behaviour problems, e.g. temper tantrums, hyperactivity, eating disorders.

The aims and objectives are:
- to establish the relevant facts of the history; this is always the most fruitful source of diagnostic information
- to elicit all relevant clinical findings
- to collate the findings from the history and examination
- to formulate a working diagnosis or differential diagnosis on the basis of logical deduction
- to assemble a problem list and management plan.

The above can be summarised by the acronym HELP:
H = history
E = examination
L = logical deduction
P = plan of management

Key points in paediatric history and examination are:
- The child's age is always a key feature in the history and examination (Fig. 2.1) as it determines:
  — the nature and presentation of illnesses, developmental or behaviour problems
  — the way in which the history-taking (Fig. 2.2) and examination are conducted
  — the way in which any subsequent management is organised.
- Parents are astute observers of their children. Never ignore or dismiss what they say.

TAKING A HISTORY

Introduction

- Make sure you have read any referral letter and scanned the notes *before* the start of the interview.
- When you welcome the child, parents and siblings, check that you know the child's first name and gender. Ask how the child prefers to be addressed.
- Introduce yourself.
- Determine the relationship of the adults to the child.
- Establish eye contact and rapport with the family. Infants and some toddlers are most secure in parents' arms or laps. Young children may need some time to get to know you.
- Ensure that the interview environment is as welcoming and unthreatening as possible. Avoid having desks or beds between you and the family.
- Have toys available. Observe how the child separates, plays and interacts with any siblings present.
- Don't forget to address questions to the child, when appropriate.
- There will be occasions when the parents will not want the child present or when the child should be seen alone. This is usually to avoid embarrassing older children or teenagers or to impart sensitive information. It must be handled tactfully, often by negotiating to talk separately to each in turn.

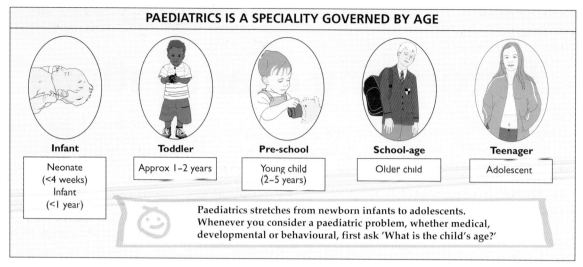

PAEDIATRICS IS A SPECIALITY GOVERNED BY AGE

Infant	Toddler	Pre-school	School-age	Teenager
Neonate (<4 weeks) Infant (<1 year)	Approx 1–2 years	Young child (2–5 years)	Older child	Adolescent

Paediatrics stretches from newborn infants to adolescents. Whenever you consider a paediatric problem, whether medical, developmental or behavioural, first ask 'What is the child's age?'

Fig. 2.1 The illnesses and problems children encounter are highly age-dependent. The child's age will determine the questions you ask on history-taking, how you conduct the examination, the diagnosis or differential diagnosis and your management plan.

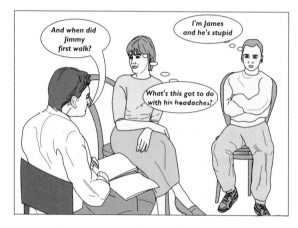

Fig. 2.2 The history must be adapted to the child's age. The age when a child first walks is highly relevant when taking the history of a toddler but irrelevant for a teenager with headaches.

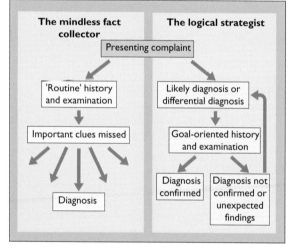

Fig. 2.3 The history and examination should be goal-oriented, based on the presenting complaint. Comprehensive history-taking is best reserved for training or for complex, multi-system disorders. (Adapted from Hutson J M, Beasley SW, *The Surgical Examination of Children*, Heinemann Medical Books, London, 1988.)

Presenting symptoms

Full details are required of the presenting symptoms. Let the parents and child recount the presenting complaints in their own words and at their own pace. Note the parent's words verbatim about the presenting complaint: onset, duration, previous episodes, what relieves/aggravates them, time course of the problem, if getting worse and any associated symptoms. Has the child's or the family's lifestyle been affected? What has the family done about it?

Make sure you know:
- what prompted referral to a doctor
- what the parents think or fear is the matter.

The scope and detail of further history-taking are determined by the nature and severity of the presenting complaint and the child's age. Whilst the comprehensive assessment listed here is sometimes required, usually a selective approach is more appropriate (Fig. 2.3). This is not an excuse for a short, slipshod history, but instead allows one to focus on the areas where a thorough, detailed history is required.

General enquiry

Check:
- general health – how active and lively?
- normal growth
- pubertal development (if appropriate)
- feeding/drinking/appetite
- any recent change in behaviour or personality.

Systems review

Selected, as appropriate:
- general rashes, fever (and if measured)
- respiratory – cough, wheeze, breathing problems
- ENT – throat infections, snoring, noisy breathing (stridor)
- cardiovascular – heart murmur, cyanosis, exercise tolerance
- gastrointestinal – vomiting, diarrhoea/constipation, abdominal pain
- genitourinary – dysuria, frequency, wetting, toilet-trained
- neurological – seizures, headaches, abnormal movements.

Past medical history

Check:
- maternal obstetric problems, delivery
- birthweight and gestation
- perinatal problems, whether admitted to special care baby unit
- immunisations (ideally from the personal child health record)
- past illnesses, hospital admissions and operations, accidents and injuries.

Medication

Check:
- past and present medications
- known allergies.

Family history

Families share houses, genes and diseases!
- Have any members of the family or friends had similar problems or any serious disorder?
- Draw a family tree. If there is a positive family history, extend family pedigree over several generations.
- Is there consanguinity?

Social history

Check:
- Relevant information about the family and its community – parental occupation, economic status, housing, relationships, parental smoking, marital stresses.
- Is the child happy at home?
- Is the child happy at nursery/school?

This 'social snapshot' is crucial since many childhood illnesses or conditions are permeated by adult problems, e.g.:

- alcohol and drug abuse
- long-term unemployment/poverty
- poor, damp, cramped housing
- parental psychiatric disorders
- unstable partnership.

Development

Check:
- parental worries about vision, hearing, development
- key developmental milestones (Fig. 2.4)
- previous child health surveillance developmental checks
- bladder and bowel control
- child's temperament, behaviour
- sleeping problems
- concerns and progress at nursery/school?

Look through the personal child health record.

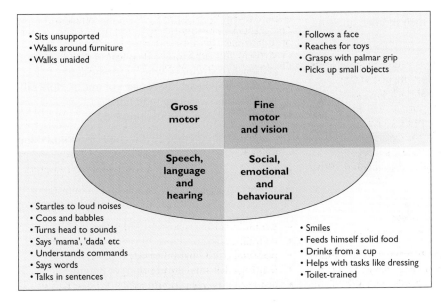

- Sits unsupported
- Walks around furniture
- Walks unaided

- Follows a face
- Reaches for toys
- Grasps with palmar grip
- Picks up small objects

Gross motor

Fine motor and vision

Speech, language and hearing

Social, emotional and behavioural

- Startles to loud noises
- Coos and babbles
- Turns head to sounds
- Says 'mama', 'dada' etc
- Understands commands
- Says words
- Talks in sentences

- Smiles
- Feeds himself solid food
- Drinks from a cup
- Helps with tasks like dressing
- Toilet-trained

Fig. 2.4 Some key developmental milestones in young children. These are considered in detail in Chapter 3.

AN APPROACH TO EXAMINING CHILDREN

Obtaining the child's cooperation

- Make friends with the child.
- Be confident but gentle.
- Avoid dominating the child.
- Short mock examinations, e.g. auscultating a teddy or the mother's hand, may allay a young child's fears.
- When first examining a young child, start at a non-threatening area, such as a hand or knee.
- Explain what you are about to do and what you want him to do, in language he can understand. As the examination is essential, not optional, it is best not to ask his permission, as it may well be refused!
- A smiling, talking doctor appears less threatening, but this should not be overdone as it can interfere with one's relationship with the parents.
- Leave unpleasant procedures until last.

Adapting to the child's age

Adapt the examination to suit the child's age. Whilst it may be difficult to examine some toddlers and young children fully, it is usually possible with resourcefulness and imagination on the doctor's part.

- Babies in the first few months are best examined on an examination couch with a parent next to them.
- A toddler is best initially examined on his mother's lap or occasionally over a parent's shoulder. Parents are reassuring for the child and helpful in facilitating the examination if guided as to what to do (Fig. 2.5).
- Pre-school children may initially be examined whilst they are playing.
- Older children and teenagers are often concerned about privacy. Teenage girls should normally be examined in the presence of their mother, nurse or

suitable chaperone. Be aware of cultural sensitivities in different ethnic groups.

Undressing children

Be sensitive to children's modesty. The area to be examined must be inspected fully, but this is best done in stages, redressing the child when each stage has been completed. It is easiest and kindest to ask the child or parent to do the undressing.

Warm, clean hands

Hands must be washed before (and after) examining a child. Warm smile, warm hands and a warm stethoscope all help!

Developmental skills

A good overview of developmental skills can be obtained by watching the child play. A few simple toys, such as some bricks, a car, doll, ball, pencil and paper, are all that is required, as they can be adapted for any age. If developmental assessment (see Ch. 3) is the focus of the examination, it is advisable to assess this before the physical examination, as cooperation may then be lost.

EXAMINATION

Initial observations

Careful observation is usually the key to success in examining children. Look before touching the child. Inspection will provide information on:

- severity of illness
- growth and nutrition
- behaviour and social responsiveness
- level of hygiene and care.

Severity of illness

Is the child sick or well? If sick, how sick? For the acutely ill infant or child, perform the '60 second rapid assessment':

- Airway and Breathing – respiration rate and effort, presence of stridor or wheeze, cyanosis.
- Circulation – heart rate, pulse volume, peripheral temperature, capillary refill time.
- Disability – level of consciousness.

The care of the seriously ill child is described in Chapter 4.

Measurements

As abnormal growth may be the first manifestation of illness in children, always measure and plot growth on centile charts for:

- weight, noting previous measurements from personal child health record
- length (in infants, if indicated) or height
- head circumference in infants.

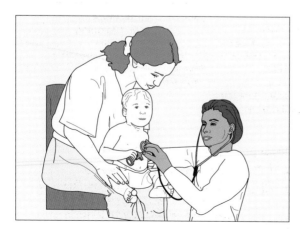

Fig. 2.5 Distracting a toddler with a toy allows auscultation of the heart.

As appropriate:

- temperature
- blood pressure
- peak expiratory flow rate.

General appearance

The face, head and neck, and hands are examined. The general morphological appearance may suggest a chromosomal or dysmorphic syndrome. In infants, palpate the fontanelle and sutures.

Respiratory system

Cyanosis

Central cyanosis is best observed on the tongue.

Clubbing of the fingers and/or toes

Clubbing (Fig. 2.6a) is usually associated with chronic suppurative lung disease, e.g. cystic fibrosis, or cyanotic congenital heart disease. It is occasionally seen in inflammatory bowel disease or cirrhosis.

Tachypnoea

Rate of respiration is age-dependent (Fig. 2.6b)

Dyspnoea

Laboured breathing. Increased work of breathing is judged by:

- nasal flaring
- expiratory grunting – to increase positive end-expiratory pressure
- use of accessory muscles, especially sternomastoids
- retraction (recession) of the chest wall, from use of suprasternal, intercostal and subcostal muscles
- difficulty speaking (or feeding).

Chest shape

- hyperexpansion or barrel shape (Fig. 2.6c), e.g. asthma
- pectus excavatum (hollow chest) or pectus carinatum (pigeon chest)
- Harrison's sulcus (from diaphragmatic tug), e.g. from poorly controlled asthma
- asymmetry of chest movements.

RESPIRATORY SYSTEM

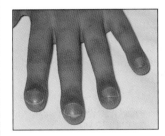

Fig. 2.6a Clubbing of the fingers. There is increased curvature, loss of nail angle and fluctuation. This child had cystic fibrosis.

Fig. 2.6b Respiratory rate in children (breaths/min).

Age	Normal	Tachypnoea
Neonate	30–50	>60
Infants	20–30	>50
Young children	20–30	>40
Older children	15–20	>30

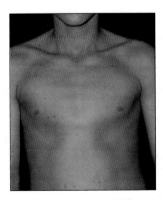

Fig. 2.6c Hyperexpanded chest from chronic obstructive airways disease. This boy had severe asthma.

Fig. 2.6d Chest signs of some common chest disorders of children.

	Chest movement	Percussion	Auscultation
Bronchiolitis	Laboured breathing Hyperinflated chest Chest recession	Hyper-resonant	Fine crackles in all zones Wheezes may/may not be present
Pneumonia	Reduced on affected side Rapid, shallow breaths	Dull	Bronchial breathing Crackles
Asthma	Reduced but hyperinflated Use of accessory muscles Chest wall retraction	Hyper-resonant	Wheeze

 Infants with pneumonia may not have any abnormal signs on auscultation.

 Sputum is rarely produced by children, as they swallow it. The main exception is suppurative lung disease from cystic fibrosis.

Palpation

- Chest expansion – this is 3–5 cm in school-aged children. Measure maximal chest expansion with tape measure. Check for symmetry.
- Trachea – checking it is central is seldom helpful and is disliked by children. To be done selectively.
- Location of apex beat to detect mediastinal shift.

Percussion

- needs to be done gently, comparing like with like, using middle fingers
- seldom informative in infants
- localised dullness – collapse, consolidation, fluid.

Auscultation, i.e. ears and stethoscope

- Note quality and symmetry of breath sounds and any added sounds.
- Harsh breath sounds from the upper airways are readily transmitted to the upper chest in infants.
- Hoarse voice – abnormality of the vocal cords.
- Stridor – harsh, low-pitched, mainly inspiratory sound from upper airways obstruction.
- Breath sounds – normal are vesicular; bronchial breathing is higher-pitched and the lengths of inspiration and expiration are equal.
- Wheeze – high-pitched, expiratory sound from distal airway obstruction (Fig. 2.6d).
- Crackles – discontinuous 'moist' sounds from the opening of bronchioles (Fig. 2.6d).

Cardiovascular system

Cyanosis

Observe the tongue for central cyanosis.

Clubbing of fingers or toes

Check if present.

Pulse

Check:
- rate (Fig. 2.7a)
- rhythm – sinus arrhythmia (variation of pulse rate with respiration) is normal
- volume – small in circulatory insufficiency or aortic stenosis; increased in high-output states (stress, anaemia); collapsing in patent ductus arteriosus, aortic regurgitation.

Inspection

Look for:
- respiratory distress
- precordial bulge – caused by cardiac enlargement
- ventricular impulse – visible if thin, hyperdynamic circulation or left ventricular hypertrophy
- operative scars – mostly sternotomy or left lateral thoracotomy.

Palpation

Thrill = palpable murmur.

Apex (4th–5th intercostal space, mid-clavicular line):
- not palpable in some normal infants, plump children or dextrocardia
- heave from left ventricular hypertrophy.

Right ventricular heave at lower left sternal edge – right ventricular hypertrophy.

Percussion

Cardiac border percussion is rarely helpful in children.

CARDIOVASCULAR SYSTEM

Fig. 2.7a Normal resting pulse rate in children.

Age	Beats/min	
<1 year	110–160	Increased with stress, exercise, fever, arrhythmia
2–5 years	95–140	
5–12 years	80–120	
>12 years	60–100	

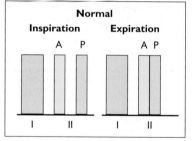

Fig. 2.7b The splitting of the second heart sound is easily heard in children.

Features suggesting a murmur is significant:
- conducted all over the praecordium
- loud
- thrill (equals grade 4–6 murmur)
- any diastolic murmur
- accompanied by other abnormal cardiac signs.

Features of heart failure in infants:
- poor feeding/failure to thrive
- sweating
- tachypnoea
- tachycardia
- gallop rhythm
- cardiomegaly
- hepatomegaly.

Auscultation

Listen for heart sounds and murmurs.

Heart sounds

- Splitting of second sound is usually easily heard and is normal (Fig. 2.7b).
- Fixed splitting of second heart sound in atrial septal defects.
- Third heart sound in mitral area is normal in young children.

Murmurs

- timing – systolic/diastolic/continuous
- duration – mid-systolic (ejection)/pansystolic
- loudness – systolic murmurs graded:
  - 1–2 soft, difficult to hear
  - 3 easily audible, no thrill
  - 4–6 loud with thrill
- site of maximal intensity – mitral/pulmonary/aortic/tricuspid areas
- radiation:
  - — to neck in aortic stenosis
  - — to back in coarctation of the aorta or pulmonary stenosis.

Draw your findings (see Ch. 15 on cardiac disorders).

Hepatomegaly

Important sign of heart failure in infants. An infant's liver is normally palpable 1–2 cm below the costal margin.

Femoral pulses

In coarctation of the aorta:
- decreased volume or may be impalpable in infants
- brachiofemoral delay in older children.

Blood pressure (see p. 19)

 Heart disease is more common in children with other congenital abnormalities or syndromes, e.g. Down's and Turner's syndromes.

Abdomen

Abdominal examination is performed in three major clinical settings:

- routine examination
- an 'acute abdomen' – ?cause (see p. 173)
- abdominal distension/mass – ?cause.

Associated signs

Examine:
- the eyes for signs of jaundice and anaemia
- the tongue for coating and colour
- the fingers for clubbing.

Inspection

The abdomen is protuberant in normal toddlers and young children. The abdominal wall muscles must be relaxed for palpation.

Generalised abdominal distension is most often explained by the five 'F's:

- fat
- fluid (ascites – uncommon in children, most often from nephrotic syndrome)
- faeces (constipation)
- flatus (malabsorption, intestinal obstruction)
- fetus (not to be forgotten after puberty).

Occasionally, it is caused by a grossly enlarged liver and/or spleen or muscle hypotonia.

Causes of localised abdominal distension are:
- upper abdomen – gastric dilatation from pyloric stenosis, hepato/splenomegaly
- lower abdomen – distended bladder, masses.

Other signs:
- dilated veins, abdominal striae
- operative scars (draw a diagram)
- peristalsis – from pyloric stenosis, intestinal obstruction.

Are the buttocks normally rounded, or wasted as in malabsorption, e.g. coeliac disease or malnutrition?

Palpation

- Use warm hands, explain, relax the child and keep the parent close at hand. First ask if it hurts.
- Palpate in a systematic fashion – liver, spleen, kidneys, bladder, through four abdominal quadrants.
- Ask about tenderness. Watch the child's face for grimacing as you palpate. A young child may become more cooperative if you palpate first with his hand or by putting your hand on top of his.

Tenderness

- *Location* – localised in appendicitis, hepatitis, pyelonephritis; generalised in mesenteric adenitis, peritonitis
- *Guarding* – often unimpressive on direct palpation in children. Pain on coughing, on moving about/walking/bumps during car journey suggests peritoneal irritation. Back bent on walking may be from psoas inflammation in appendicitis.

Hepatomegaly (Fig. 2.8a, b)
- palpate from right iliac fossa
- locate edge with tips or side of finger
- edge may be soft or firm
- unable to get above it
- moves with respiration
- measure (in cm) extension below costal margin in mid-clavicular line.

Liver tenderness is likely to be due to inflammation from hepatitis.

Splenomegaly (Fig. 2.8c):
- palpate from right iliac fossa
- edge is usually soft

ABDOMEN

Fig. 2.8a Causes of hepatomegaly

Infection	Congenital, infectious mononucleosis, hepatitis, malaria, parasitic infection
Haematological	Sickle cell anaemia, thalassaemia
Liver disease	Chronic active hepatitis, portal hypertension, polycystic disease
Malignancy	Leukaemia, lymphoma, neuroblastoma, Wilms' tumour, hepatocellular carcinoma
Metabolic	Glycogen and lipid storage disorders, mucopolysaccharidoses
Cardiovascular	Heart failure
Apparent	Chest hyperexpansion from bronchiolitis or asthma

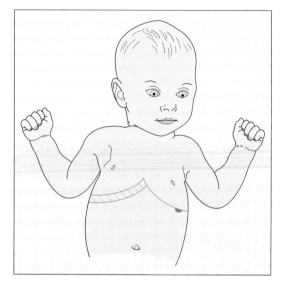

Fig. 2.8b The liver edge is 1–2 cm below the costal margin in infants and young children. The spleen may be 1–2 cm below the costal margin in infants.

Fig. 2.8c Causes of splenomegaly

Infection	Viral, bacterial, protozoal (malaria, leishmaniasis), parasites, infective endocarditis
Haematological	Haemolytic anaemia
Malignancy	Leukaemia, lymphoma
Other	Portal hypertension, Still's disease

On examining the abdomen:
- inspect first, palpate later
- superficial palpation first, deep palpation later
- guarding is unimpressive in children
- silent abdomen – serious!
- immobile abdomen – serious!

- unable to get above it
- notch occasionally palpable if markedly enlarged
- moves on respiration (ask the child to take a deep breath)
- measure size below costal margin (in cm) in mid-clavicular line.

If uncertain whether it is palpable:
- use bimanual approach to spleen
- turn child onto right side.

A palpable spleen is at least twice its normal size!

Kidneys

These are not usually palpable beyond the neonatal period unless enlarged or the abdominal muscles are hypotonic. On examination:

- palpate by balloting bimanually
- they move on respiration
- one can get above them.

Tenderness implies inflammation.

Abnormal masses
- *Wilms' tumour* – renal mass, sometimes visible, does not cross midline
- *neuroblastoma* – irregular firm mass, may cross midline; the child is usually very unwell
- *faecal masses* – mobile, non-tender, indentable
- *intussusception* – acutely unwell, mass may be palpable, most often in right upper quadrant.

Percussion
- *Liver* – dullness delineates upper and lower border. Record span.
- *Spleen* – dullness delineates lower border.
- *Ascites* – shifting dullness. Percuss from most resonant spot to most dull spot.

Auscultation
Not very useful in 'routine' examination, but important in 'acute abdomen':

- increased bowel sounds – intestinal obstruction, acute diarrhoea

- reduced or absent bowel sounds – paralytic ileus, peritonitis.

Genital area is examined routinely in young children, but in older children and teenagers, this is done only if relevant, e.g. vaginal discharge. Is there an inguinal hernia or a perineal rash?

In *males*:
- Is the penis of normal size?
- Is the scrotum well developed?
- Are the testes palpable? With one hand over the inguinal region, palpate with the other hand. Record if the testis is descended, retractile or impalpable.
- Is there any scrotal swelling (hydrocele or hernia)?

In *females*:
- Do the external genitalia look normal?

Does the anus look normal? Any evidence of a fissure?

Rectal examination
- Not part of routine examination.
- Unpleasant and disliked by children.
- Its usefulness in the 'acute abdomen' (e.g. appendicitis) is debatable in children, as they have a thin abdominal wall and so tenderness and masses can be identified on palpation of the abdomen. Some surgeons advocate it to identify a retrocaecal appendix, but interpretation is problematic as most children will complain of pain from the procedure.
- If intussusception is suspected, the mass may be palpable and stools looking like redcurrant jam may be revealed on rectal examination.

 A hyperexpanded chest in bronchiolitis or asthma may displace the liver and spleen downwards, mimicking hepato/splenomegaly.

Neurology/neurodevelopment
Brief neurological screen
A quick neurological and developmental overview should be performed in all children. When doing this:

- use common sense to avoid unnecessary examination
- adapt it to the child's age
- take into account the parent's account of his developmental milestones.

Watch him play, draw or write. Are his manipulative skills normal? Can he walk, run, climb, hop, skip, dance? Are his language skills and speech satisfactory? Are his social interactions appropriate? Does his vision and hearing appear to be normal?

In infants, assess primarily by observation:
- Observe posture and movements of the limbs.
- When picking them up, note their tone. The limbs and body may feel normal, floppy or stiff. Head control may be poor, with abnormal head lag on pulling to sitting.

Most children are neurologically intact and do not require formal neurological examination of reflexes, tone, etc. More detailed neurological assessment is performed only if indicated. Specific problems in development or behaviour require detailed assessment.

More detailed neurological examination
Patterns of movement
Observe walking and running: normal walking is with a heel–toe gait. A toe–heel pattern of walking suggests pyramidal tract (corticospinal) dysfunction (particularly hemiplegia and diplegia), a foot drop (as in a superficial peroneal nerve lesion) or a tight tendo-Achilles (as in a muscle disorder, such as Duchenne's muscular dystrophy), but can be seen intermittently in some normal children. If you are unsure whether a gait is heel–toe or toe–heel, look at the pattern of shoe wear.

A broad-based gait may be due to an immature gait or secondary to a cerebellar disorder.

Observe standing from lying down supine. Children up to 3 years of age will turn prone in order to stand because of poor pelvic muscle fixation; if they continue beyond this age, it suggests neuromuscular weakness (e.g. Duchenne's muscular dystrophy) or low tone due to a central (brain) cause. The need to turn prone to rise or, later, as weakness progresses, to push off the ground with straightened arms and then climb up the legs is known as Gowers' sign.

Coordination
Assess this by:
- asking the child to build one brick upon another or using a peg-board
- asking the child to hold his arms out straight, close his eyes, and observe for drift or tremor
- finger–nose testing (use teddy's nose to reach out and touch if necessary)
- rapid alternating movements of hands and fingers
- touching tip of each finger in turn with thumb
- asking the child to walk heel–toe, jump and hop.

Subtle asymmetries in gait may be revealed by Fog's test – children are asked to walk on their heels, the outside and then the inside of their feet. Watch for the pattern of 'mirrored movement' in the upper limb.

Inspection of limbs
Muscle bulk:
- Wasting may be secondary to cerebral palsy, meningomyelocele or a muscle disorder or from previous poliomyelitis.
- Increased bulk of calf muscles may indicate Duchenne's muscular dystrophy.

Muscle tone
Tone in limbs:
- Best assessed by taking the weight of the whole limb and then bending and extending it around a single joint. Testing is easiest at the knee and ankle

joints. Assess for the range of movement as well as the general feel of it.

- Increased tone in adductors and internal rotators of the hips, clonus at the ankles or increased tone on pronation of the forearms at rest is usually the result of pyramidal dysfunction.
- The posture of the limbs may give a clue as to the underlying tone, e.g. scissoring of the legs, pronated forearms from increased tone.

Truncal tone:
- In pyramidal tract disorders, the trunk and head tend to arch backwards (extensor posturing).
- In muscle disease and some central brain disorders, the trunk may be hypotonic. The child feels floppy to handle and cannot support the trunk in sitting.

Head lag:
- This is best tested by pulling the child up by the arms from the supine position.

Power
Difficult to test in babies. Watch for antigravity movements and note motor function. Both will tell you a lot about power. From 6 months onwards, watch the pattern of mobility and gait. From the age of 4 years, power can be tested formally, first testing proximal muscle and then distal muscle power.

Reflexes
Test with the child in a relaxed position. Brisk reflexes may reflect anxiety in the child or a pyramidal disorder. Absent reflexes may be due to a neuromuscular problem or a lesion within the spinal cord, but may also be due to inexpert examination technique. Children will reinforce reflexes if asked.

Plantar responses
These are an overrated activity as the responses are often equivocal and unpopular with children as it is unpleasant. In any case, they are unreliable under 1 year of age. Upgoing plantar responses provide additional evidence of pyramidal dysfunction.

Sensation
Testing the ability to withdraw to tickle is usually adequate as a screening test. If loss of sensation is likely, e.g. meningomyelocele, more detailed sensory testing is performed.

Cranial nerves
These can usually be tested formally from 4 years of age. Before then ingenuity is required:

I	Need not be tested in routine practice. Can be done by recognising the smell of a hidden mint sweet.
II	Visual acuity – determined according to age. Direct and consensual pupillary response tested to light and accommodation.
III, IV, VI	Full eye movement through horizontal and vertical planes. Is there a squint? Nystagmus – avoid extreme lateral gaze, as it can induce nystagmus in normal children.
V	Clench teeth and waggle jaw from side to side against resistance.
VII	Close eyes tight, smile and show teeth.
VIII	Hearing – ask parents, although unilateral deafness could be missed this way. If in doubt, needs formal assessment in a suitable environment.
IX	Levator palati – saying 'aagh'.
X	Recurrent laryngeal nerve – listen for hoarseness or stridor.
XI	Trapezius and sternomastoid power – shrug shoulders and turn head against resistance.
XII	Put out tongue and waggle it from side to side.

Bones and joints
Presentation of bone and joint disorders include limb pain, unwillingness to use limb, limp, joint or muscle pain, joint swelling and muscle wasting.

- Inspect for – swelling from a joint effusion (loss of joint outline) or synovial thickening, redness, pain on movement, loss of function, muscle wasting above and below any swollen joints.
- Palpate for – heat (comparing joints), tenderness, fluctuation of effusion.
- Movements – active before passive in order not to hurt the child. Explain movements in child-friendly words. If necessary, show on your own joints the movements you wish to test. Record joint movement in degrees.
- Scoliosis – inspect the spine, especially in older children/adolescents. Ask to stand straight (as a soldier!) and then to touch toes.

Neck
Thyroid
- Inspect – swelling uncommon in childhood; occasionally at puberty.
- Palpate from behind and front for swelling, nodule, thrill.
- Auscultate if enlarged.
- Look for signs of hypo/hyperthyroidism.

Lymph nodes
Examine systematically – occipital, cervical, axillary, inguinal. Note size, number, consistency of any glands felt:

- Small, discrete, pea-sized, mobile nodes in the neck, groin and axilla – common in normal children, especially if thin.
- Small, multiple nodes in the neck – common after upper respiratory tract infections (viral/bacterial).
- Multiple lymph nodes of variable size in children with extensive atopic eczema.

- Large, hot, tender, sometimes fluctuant node, usually in neck – infected/abscess.
- Variable size and shape:
  — infections: viral, e.g. infectious mononucleosis, or TB
  — rare causes: malignant disease (usually non-tender), Kawasaki's disease, cat-scratch.

Blood pressure

Indications

Must be closely monitored (Fig. 2.9) if critically ill, if there is renal or cardiac disease or diabetes mellitus, or if receiving drug therapy which may cause hypertension, e.g. corticosteroids. Not measured often enough in children.

Technique

When measured with a sphygmomanometer:

- Show the child that there is a balloon in the cuff and demonstrate how it is blown up.
- Use largest cuff which fits comfortably, covering at least two-thirds of the upper arm.
- The child must be relaxed and not crying.
- Systolic pressure is the easiest to determine in young children and clinically the most useful.
- Diastolic pressure is when the sounds become muffled. May not be possible to discern in young children.

Measurement

Must be interpreted according to a centile chart (see Fig. A.1a,b, Appendix). Blood pressure is increased by tall stature and obesity. Charts relating blood pressure to height are available and preferable; for convenience, charts relating blood pressure to age are often used. An abnormally high reading must be repeated, with the child relaxed, on at least three separate occasions.

Eyes

Examination

Inspect eyes, pupils, iris and sclerae. Are eye movements full and symmetrical? Is nystagmus detectable? If so, may have ocular or cerebellar cause, or testing may be too lateral to the child. Are the pupils equal and central? Is there a squint?

Epicanthic folds are common in Asian ethnic groups.

Ophthalmoscopy

- In infants, the red reflex is seen from a distance of 20–30 cm. Absence of red reflex occurs in corneal clouding, cataract, retinoblastoma.
- Fundoscopy – difficult. Requires experience and cooperation. Mydriatics are needed in young children. Retinopathy of prematurity and retinopathy of congenital infections and choroido-retinal degeneration show characteristic findings. Retinal haemorrhages may be seen in the 'shaken baby syndrome' (non-accidental injury).
- In older children with headaches, diabetes mellitus or hypertension, optic fundi should be examined. Mydriatics are not usually needed.

Ears and throat

Examination is usually left until last, as it can be unpleasant. Explain what you are going to do. Show the parent how to hold and gently restrain a younger child to ensure success and avoid possible injury (Figs 2.10, 2.11).

Throat

Try quickly to get a look at the tonsils, uvula, pharynx and posterior palate. Older children (5 years +) will open their mouths as wide as possible to avoid a spatula. Look for redness, swelling, pus or palatal petechiae. Also check the teeth for dental caries and other gross abnormalities.

Fig. 2.9 Measuring blood pressure in children

Sphygmomanometer
  — stethoscope in older children
  — Doppler ultrasound in infants

Oscillometric (e.g. Dynamapp) – helpful in infants and young children

Invasive – direct measurement from an arterial catheter is mandatory if critically ill

---

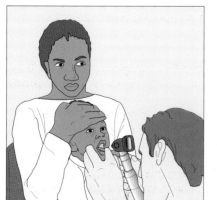

Fig. 2.10 Holding a young child to examine the throat. The mother has one hand on the head and the other across the child's arms.

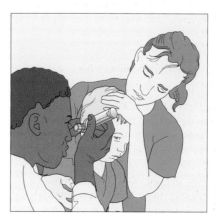

Fig. 2.11 Holding a young child correctly is essential for successful examination of the ear with an auroscope. The mother has one hand on the child's head and the other hand holding the upper arm.

Ears

Examine ear canals and drums gently, trying not to hurt the child. Look for anatomical landmarks on the ear drum and for swelling, redness, perforation, dullness, fluid.

SUMMARY AND MANAGEMENT PLAN

At the end of the history and examination:

- Summarise the key problems (in physical, emotional, social and family terms, if relevant).
- List the diagnoses or differential diagnoses.
- Draw up a management plan to address the problems, both short- and long-term. This could be reassurance, a period of observation, performing investigations or therapeutic intervention.
- Provide explanation to the parents and to the child, if old enough. Provide further information either written or on the internet.
- If relevant, discuss what to tell other members of the family.
- Consider if other professionals should be informed.
- Ensure your notes are dated and signed.

CASE HISTORY

SUMMARY OF AN OUTPATIENT APPOINTMENT

Sean, aged 7 years, has frequent episodic asthma. It is exacerbated by respiratory infections and exercise. There have been significant absences from school and two hospital admissions in the last year. He is on regular, high-dose inhaled steroids and bronchodilator therapy. There are no peak flow measurements, and medical compliance is questionable.

Management plan

- Provided – re-education of family, demonstration of inhaler technique, peak flow meter and diary.
- General practitioner and school nurse informed.
- Review in 2 weeks by general practitioner and 4 weeks at hospital.

FURTHER READING

Gill D, O'Brien N 1998 Paediatric clinical examination, 3rd edn. Churchill Livingstone, Edinburgh

3

Child development, hearing and vision

The main objectives of developmental paediatrics are:

- to help all children achieve their maximum developmental potential
- the early detection and management of delayed development, including specific sensory impairments of hearing and vision; even where there is no specific treatment, the effects of a condition can often be modified
- to act as the entry point for the care and management of the child with special needs.

THE PROCESS OF CHILD DEVELOPMENT

A child's development represents the interaction of heredity and the environment on the developing brain. Heredity determines the potential of the child, while the environment influences the extent to which he achieves that potential. For optimal development, the environment has to meet the child's physical and psychological needs (Fig. 3.1). These vary with age and stage of development:

- an infant is totally physically dependent on his parents and requires a limited number of carers to meet his psychological needs
- a primary school-age child can usually meet some of his physical needs and cope with many social relationships
- teenagers are able to meet most of their physical needs while experiencing increasingly complex emotional needs.

Four areas of development

It is useful to subdivide early childhood development into four functional skill areas (Fig. 3.2):

- gross motor
- fine motor and vision
- speech, language and hearing
- social, emotional, behaviour.

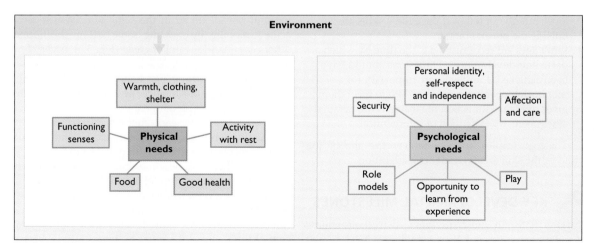

Fig. 3.1 Development can be impaired if the environment is lacking in physical or psychological needs.

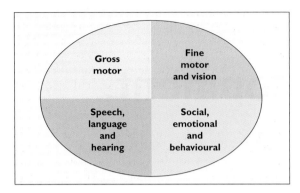

Fig. 3.2 The four functional skill areas of child development.

Gross motor skills are initially the most obvious area of developmental progress. As fine motor skills require good vision, they are grouped together; similarly, normal speech and language development depends on reasonable hearing and so these are also considered together. Social, emotional and behavioural skills are a spectrum of psychological development. A deficiency in any one skill area can have an impact on other areas, e.g. a hearing impairment may affect a child's social skills and behaviour. As the child grows, additional skills become important, such as attention and concentration and how well an individual child's skills are integrated.

Developmental progress in young children is about the acquisition of functional skills. Key principles to this concept are:

- There is a remarkable consistency in the pattern of children's developmental progress, allowing it to be described in terms of developmental milestones comprising crucial sequential skills.
- Always consider developmental progress within each skill area longitudinally over time. Acquisition of sequential skills is like a story.
- There is a wide timescale within the normal range.
- Median ages for skill achievement tell us about when half of a standard population achieve that level, but do not tell us if the child's skills are outside the normal range.
- Limit ages are recognised, i.e. the time by which a particular developmental milestone should have been achieved. Limit ages are important for monitoring development, as failure to meet them gives guidance for action regarding more detailed assessment, investigation or intervention.

These principles apply whatever the age of the child or the skill area(s) under consideration.

🔑 KEY DEVELOPMENTAL MILESTONES

Parents naturally wish to know that their child's development is normal. Young children's development is assessed:

- as part of the child health surveillance programme
- if there is parental concern
- whenever a child is seen by a health professional for another reason, when a brief opportunistic overview is made of the child's development.

Health professionals will need to decide whether the individual child is within the range of normality for his age and stage of development. The range of normal is wide. This adds to the complexity of assessing child development.

Variation in rate of development

This can be demonstrated by considering the age range for the important developmental milestone of walking unsupported. The percentage of children who are walking unsupported is:

- 25% by 11 months
- 50% by 12 months
- 75% by 13 months
- 90% by 15 months
- 97.5% by 18 months.

At 15 months, the majority of the 10% of children not yet walking unsupported will be normal, but in a small proportion there will be an underlying medical problem. At 18 months (two standard deviations from the mean), 97.5% of children will be walking independently. Of those who are not, many will be normal late walkers, but a higher proportion will have an underlying medical problem, such as cerebral palsy, a primary muscle disorder or global developmental delay. Hence, any child who is not walking by 18 months should be carefully examined. Thus 18 months can be set as a 'limit age' for children not walking. Setting the limit age earlier may allow earlier identification of problems, but will also increase the number of children labelled as 'delayed' who are in fact normal.

Variation in pattern of development

The pattern by which children reach key milestones varies, as demonstrated by the variants of locomotor skills. Normal infants progress from immobility to walking, but not all do so in the same way. Whilst most achieve mobility by crawling, some bottom-shuffle and others commando crawl or creep (Fig. 3.3). A very few just stand up and walk. The locomotor pattern (crawling, creeping, shuffling, just standing up and walking) influences the age of walking. The limit age of 18 months for walking applies predominantly to children who have had crawling as their early mobility pattern. Children who bottom-shuffle or commando crawl tend to walk later than crawlers, so that within those not walking at 18 months there will be some children who are simply reflecting variants of normal locomotor patterns.

There is even more variation in the rate of acquisition of social skills and behaviour, e.g. when children can dress themselves or are toilet-trained, but the concept of limit ages still applies to determining whether a child's developmental progress is normal.

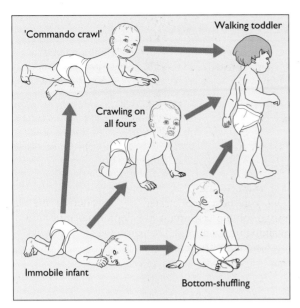

Fig. 3.3 Early locomotor patterns. Most children crawl on all fours *en route* to walking, but some 'bottom-shuffle' and others crawl with their abdomen on the floor, so-called 'commando crawling' or creeping. Bottom-shuffling often runs in families, but the late walking that often goes with this locomotor variant needs to be differentiated from an abnormality such as cerebral palsy.

Eventual level of attainment

This depends on heredity and environment. Lack of stimulation may be associated with developmental delay, particularly in speech and language and social skills.

In addition to the acquisition of skills, their quality is also important. For example, a child may attain a developmental milestone in language, such as putting words and sentences together, but be unskilled and clumsy in trying to converse with other children and adults.

If a child has been born preterm, this should be allowed for when assessing developmental age, by calculating it from the expected date of delivery. This is done up to around 2 years of age, by which time the number of weeks early the child was born is no longer a significant proportion of the child's life and should cease to be counted.

In the following sections, unless stated otherwise, all the ages quoted are median ages.

Gross motor development (Fig. 3.4)

There is rapid progression in gross motor development in the first 18 months of life, from an immobile newborn infant to one who is able to adopt an upright posture and then walk and explore the environment. In order to achieve this, the following sequence of events needs to occur:

1. Acquisition of tone and head control

Muscle tone increases during infancy to enable infants to achieve head control, then sit and stand. In the newborn period, when supine, he will lie with his limbs flexed and kick his arms and legs. Head control is poor, evidenced by marked head lag when pulled up by his arms. When held prone, he can hold his head horizontal. His head control improves so that, when lying prone, by 6 weeks of age he can lift his head and move it from side to side. By 3–4 months of age, he can hold his head upright when held sitting.

2. Primitive reflexes

The newborn infant has a number of primitive spinal or brain stem reflexes (e.g. the Moro on head extension, the grasp reflex when an object is placed across the palm of the hand, the stepping and atonic neck reflexes; see p. 373). These need to disappear to allow motor development to progress, and almost all do so by 4–6 months of age.

3. Sitting

By 6 months of age, the infant will sit without an adult supporting him. To do this, he first needs to have developed protective responses in which he will put out his arm to the side or forwards to protect himself from falling (called sideways or forward propping, or the parachute reflex). He also develops righting responses to bring his head and trunk back to the vertical from tipped positions.

4. Locomotor pattern

He becomes mobile, usually by crawling, but may bottom-shuffle or commando crawl (creep). Initially, he will walk holding onto furniture (10 months) or with his hand held, and if he has been a crawler he is likely to take his first steps unsupported by 12 months.

5. Running, hopping, jumping, pedalling

He subsequently learns to run, kick a ball (20 months), hop on one leg (20 months), go up and down stairs one leg at a time, jump and pedal a bicycle.

Black infants generally achieve their motor milestones at an earlier age than white or Asian infants, but this is not an indicator of later language or cognitive abilities.

Fine motor and vision (Fig. 3.5)

The infant needs to acquire visual attention and a pincer grip to develop the dexterity required to perform complex tasks such as feeding, dressing, writing (and playing computer games!).

1. Fixing, following and visual alertness

The newborn infant will fix and follow a nearby face or light moving across his field of view. By 6 weeks, he will be more visually alert and, when supine, he will turn his head from side to side to follow an object. While some newborn infants have a mild, intermittent squint, any infant with a squint persisting beyond 2 months of age, or a fixed squint at any age, should be referred for a specialist ophthalmological opinion.

2. Hand regard

At 3–4 months, infants show hand regard, spending a lot of time looking at their hands.

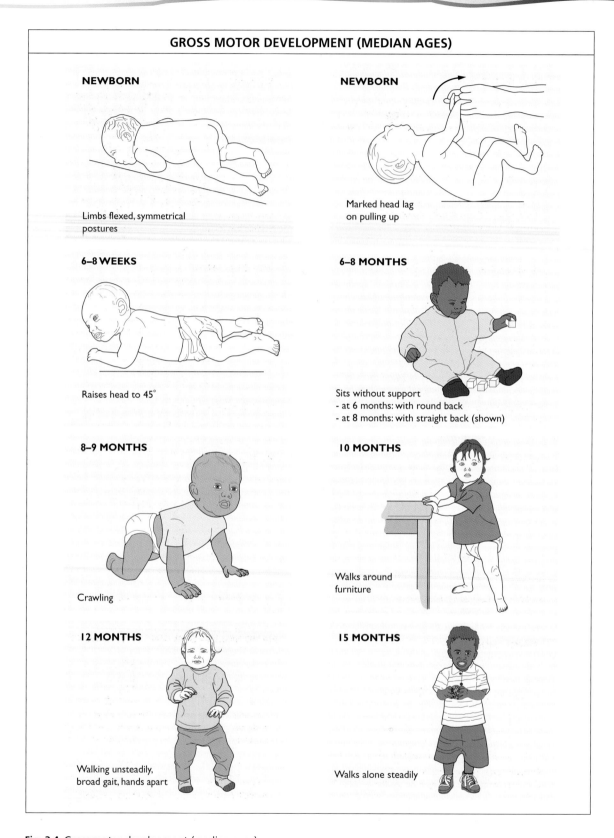

GROSS MOTOR DEVELOPMENT (MEDIAN AGES)

NEWBORN

Limbs flexed, symmetrical postures

NEWBORN

Marked head lag on pulling up

6–8 WEEKS

Raises head to 45°

6–8 MONTHS

Sits without support
- at 6 months: with round back
- at 8 months: with straight back (shown)

8–9 MONTHS

Crawling

10 MONTHS

Walks around furniture

12 MONTHS

Walking unsteadily, broad gait, hands apart

15 MONTHS

Walks alone steadily

Fig. 3.4 Gross motor development (median ages).

FINE MOTOR AND VISION (MEDIAN AGES)

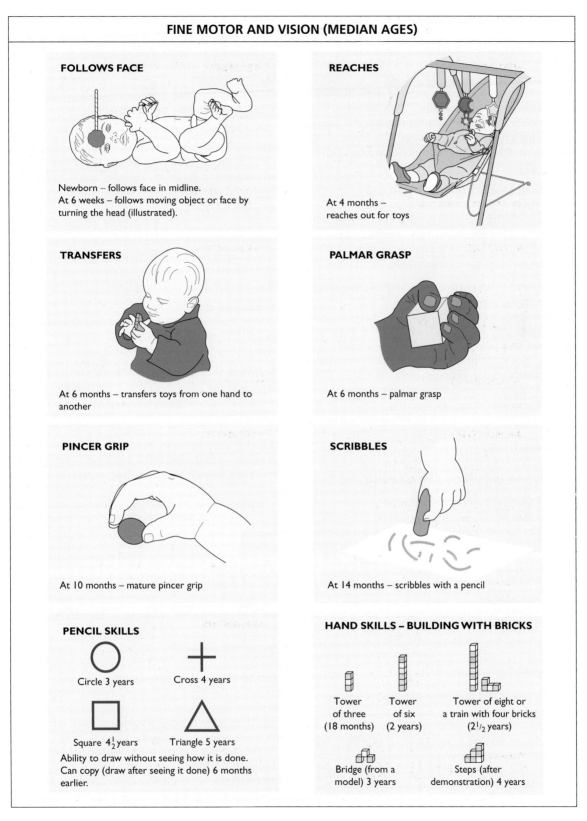

FOLLOWS FACE

Newborn – follows face in midline.
At 6 weeks – follows moving object or face by turning the head (illustrated).

REACHES

At 4 months –
reaches out for toys

TRANSFERS

At 6 months – transfers toys from one hand to another

PALMAR GRASP

At 6 months – palmar grasp

PINCER GRIP

At 10 months – mature pincer grip

SCRIBBLES

At 14 months – scribbles with a pencil

PENCIL SKILLS

Circle 3 years   Cross 4 years

Square $4\frac{1}{2}$ years   Triangle 5 years

Ability to draw without seeing how it is done.
Can copy (draw after seeing it done) 6 months earlier.

HAND SKILLS – BUILDING WITH BRICKS

Tower of three (18 months)   Tower of six (2 years)   Tower of eight or a train with four bricks ($2\frac{1}{2}$ years)

Bridge (from a model) 3 years   Steps (after demonstration) 4 years

Fig. 3.5 Fine motor and vision (median ages).

3. Grasp reflex, voluntary grasping, pincer grasp, pointing

The newborn infant will grasp an object placed across the palm of the hand (the grasp reflex). As this primitive reflex disappears, the infant starts to reach for objects and is able to grasp actively with the whole hand (palmar grasp, 6 months). This becomes more refined, with a good pincer grip (thumb and first or second finger) of a small object at 10 months of age. Soon afterwards, the infant points at objects with the index finger.

4. Handling objects with both hands and transferring

Infants should handle objects with both hands, bang two toys held in either hand by 6 months and transfer objects from one hand to another by 6 months. There should be no hand dominance during the first year.

5. Manipulation of small objects, writing, building bricks, cutting, dressing

The increasing sophistication of infants' hand skills are demonstrated by their pencil skills, their pattern of grip when they hold the pencil, and their ability with building blocks. Pencil skills are initially scribbling (at 14 months), progressing to copying (circle, cross, square or triangle) and subsequently being able to draw these objects or figures. Building with blocks will initially involve making a tower, followed by a bridge or steps. Subsequent skills are dressing, cutting, writing and keyboard skills.

Speech and language and hearing (Fig. 3.6)

1. Sound recognition and vocalisation

The newborn infant stills to voice and startles to loud noises. By 6 weeks of age, he responds to his mother's voice even when she cannot be seen. Vocalisation emerges and by about 4 months the infant is making vowel sounds.

2. Coos and babbles

Babies start to use consonant monosyllables, e.g. 'da' or 'ba', from about 6 months. They turn to a voice at 7–8 months of age (the basis of the distraction test) and acquire two-syllable babble like 'dada' or 'mama' non-specifically.

3. Single words and understanding simple requests

Appropriate use of simple words such as 'dada' or 'mama' and one or two other words usually occurs by 13 months, as well as understanding of simple commands, such as 'no' or 'give me' and responding to their name. By 18 months children can say about ten words and can demonstrate six parts of the body.

4. Joining words, phrases

Combining of two different words usually occurs around 20 months and three words by 24 months.

5. Simple and complex conversation

Conversation becomes increasingly complex, with phrases followed by sentences emerging between 2 and 3 years. At 3 years of age, a child knows his age and a few colours.

Social, emotional, behaviour (Fig. 3.7)

In infancy, social development is mainly gauged by the infant's ability to interact with his family. Subsequently, he will need to acquire self-help skills and imitate adult behaviour patterns. He also needs to learn to enjoy social interaction with other children.

1. Smiling, social responsiveness

Smiling responsively at 6 weeks is an important and remarkably constant milestone. It means that the baby smiles in response to someone smiling directly at him. Infants become increasingly responsive socially. They will wave 'bye-bye' at 10 months when they wish to.

2. Separation anxiety

At about 8 months of age, many infants become anxious and unhappy when separated from their mother or carer. They become wary of strangers.

3. Self-help skills, feeding, toileting, dressing

Infants will put solid food into their mouths at about 6 months of age, drink from a cup by 12 months and hold a spoon and feed themselves safely by 18 months. The age at which bladder and bowel control is reached is very variable. Most achieve it towards the end of the second year, but a significant number only achieve continence at a later age, especially dryness at night.

Children learn to help with dressing and subsequently to dress themselves. They can remove garments at about 24 months and begin to try to dress themselves.

4. Symbolic play

At 18–24 months, children enjoy symbolic play when playing with miniature toys such as a doll, brush, chair and spoon; they play as if they were life-size equivalents.

5. Social behaviour

Once mobile, children start to explore their surroundings and require constant attention and supervision. This raises the issue about parents exercising control and discipline whilst also allowing children to learn from their experiences. Problems may also arise with food refusal, reluctance to go to sleep, waking at night, temper tantrums and antisocial behaviour. Subsequently, they may have difficulty separating from their parents to attend a child-minder, nursery or school and in learning to play and interact with other children. During the second year of life, children play on their own or alongside others (parallel play) and only subsequently learn interactive play (3 years plus).

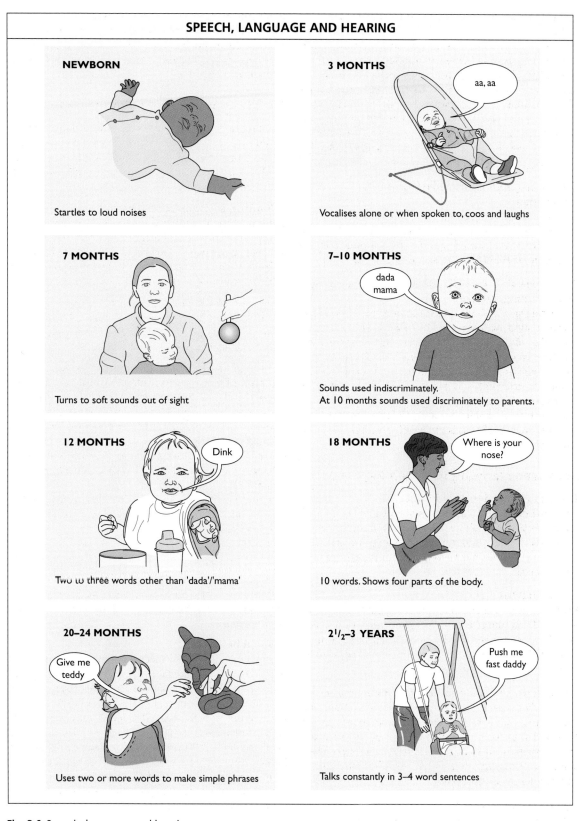

Fig. 3.6 Speech, language and hearing.

SOCIAL, EMOTIONAL AND BEHAVIOUR (MEDIAN AGES)

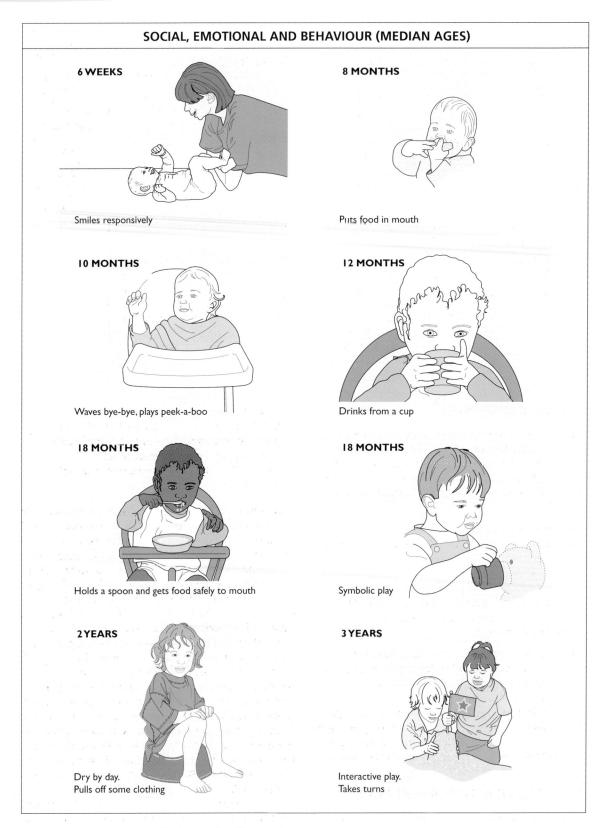

6 WEEKS

Smiles responsively

8 MONTHS

Puts food in mouth

10 MONTHS

Waves bye-bye, plays peek-a-boo

12 MONTHS

Drinks from a cup

18 MONTHS

Holds a spoon and gets food safely to mouth

18 MONTHS

Symbolic play

2 YEARS

Dry by day.
Pulls off some clothing

3 YEARS

Interactive play.
Takes turns

Fig. 3.7 Social, emotional and behaviour (median ages).

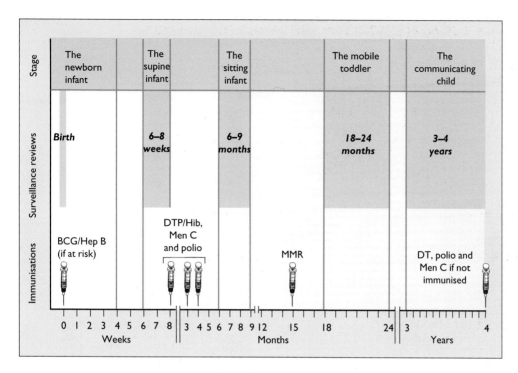

Fig. 3.8 The child health surveillance review and immunisation programme in young children as performed in England and Wales. There is also a surveillance review at age 5–6 years following school entry.

Cognitive development

Cognition refers to higher mental function. This varies markedly with age. In infancy, thought processes are centred around immediate experiences at that time. The thought processes of preschool children, which have been called preoperational thought (by Piaget), tend to be:

- that they are the centre of the world
- that inanimate objects are alive and have feelings and motives
- use of magical thinking
- that everything has a purpose. Toys and other objects are used in imaginative play as aids to thought to help make sense of experience and social relationships.

In middle school children, the dominant mode of thought is practical and orderly, tied to immediate circumstances and specific experiences. This has been called operational thought.

It is only in the mid-teens that an adult style of abstract thought (formal operational thought) begins to develop, with the ability for abstract reasoning, testing hypotheses and manipulating abstract concepts.

CHILD HEALTH SURVEILLANCE

There is a standard child health surveillance and immunisation programme for all young children, comprising a series of checks and reviews. The programme has three main elements:

- immunisation
- health education – to minimise hazards and promote optimum physical and mental health
- screening for the early detection and intervention of physical and developmental problems.

Recently, there has been a shift in emphasis to give greater prominence to health promotion, and the surveillance programme is often now called the child health promotion programme. The programme is a compromise between the desire to detect problems and potentially intervene early whilst avoiding an excessive number of visits. The way it is organised in the UK is shown, with recommended ages, in Figure 3.8. At each review, a check is made for specific physical abnormalities and selected health promotion topics are considered. These are shown in Figure 3.9. At each review, the child's overall development, health and growth are also checked. The emphasis on parental opinion of vision and hearing and speech and language is deliberate, as parents are usually excellent at detecting these problems. Details of each review are entered in the child's 'personal child health record'. These are kept by the parents and they are asked to bring them whenever the child is seen by a health professional.

Surveillance is done in primary care by general practitioners or health visitors. If problems are identified, an action plan is made for the child, which could involve giving advice and monitoring progress or referral to a specialist.

Fig. 3.9 The child health surveillance programme to 5 years old in the UK. (Adapted from Hall D B M, *Health for All Children*, Oxford University Press, Oxford, 1996.)

Age (by whom)	Screening	General examination	Health education
Newborn (usually hospital doctor, may be trained midwife or GP)	Developmental dysplasia of the hips (DDH) Testicular descent in boys Red reflex of fundus	Full physical examination Weight, head circumference and plot centiles Hearing screening if high risk or universal according to local policy	Feeding and nutrition Back to sleep, avoid overheating and parental smoking to reduce SIDS risk Sibling management Crying and sleep problems Car seats
4–7 days (midwife)	Blood test for biochemical screening (phenylketonuria, hypothyroidism for all, haemoglobinopathies if local policy)		
First 2 weeks (GP, good practice, not a review)	Developmental dysplasia of the hips (DDH) Heart murmurs and femoral pulses		Nutrition Immunisation Dangers of shaking baby
6–8 weeks (GP)	Heart murmurs and femoral pulses Developmental dysplasia of the hips (DDH) Testicular descent in boys Red reflex of fundus	Full physical examination Weight, head circumference and plot centiles Vision/hearing – parental concern?	Nutrition Immunisation Recognition of illness Avoid passive smoking
6–9 months (health visitor)	Hearing – distraction test Gait when held standing for hips Testicular descent in boys Eyes for squint	Parental concern – hearing, vision, development	Accident prevention – choking, scalds and burns, safety gates, car seats Nutrition and dental care Developmental needs Avoid sunburn
18–24 months (health visitor)	Walking with normal gait Speech and language appropriate for age Haemoglobin screening in some areas	Parental concern – behaviour, hearing, vision and general development Measure weight and height and plot centiles If special educational needs likely, check that specialist paediatric services have made referral to local education authority	Accident prevention – falls from heights, drowning, poisoning, road safety Need to mix with other children Behaviour problems Toilet training
36–48 months (preschool) (health visitor)		Parental concern – vision, squint, hearing, behaviour, speech and language development Measure height and plot centile	Accidents – roads, fires, drowning Preparation for school Road safety Nutrition and dental care
5–6 years (following school entry) (school nurse)	Vision (Snellen chart) Hearing (sweep test), universal in some areas	Measure height and weight, plot centiles Examination – only selected children where problem identified or parental concern.	

There are, however, a number of problems inherent in developmental screening:

- Much is based on clinical opinion, which is subjective and therefore has its limitations.
- Formal tests (such as 'The Griffiths' or 'The Denver') are time-consuming and have relatively poor predictive value in identifying long-term developmental problems.
- A single observation of development may be affected by the child being tired, hungry, shy or simply not wishing to take part.
- Whilst much of the focus of early development and progress in infants is centred on motor development, this is a poor predictor of problems in cognitive function and later school performance. Development of speech and language is a better predictor of cognitive function.

The reliability of screening tests can be improved by adding a questionnaire completed by parents beforehand. Increasingly, screening is being targeted towards children at high risk or when there are parental concerns.

Although median ages, when half of a standard population of children have achieved a skill, are helpful in thinking about developmental progress, care needs to be taken in their use. For example, when one says that the median age for walking unsupported is 1 year, 50% of parents could feel their child is slow in development and it would be impractical to assess every child doing less well than these median standards.

It is for this reason that limit ages are used. Some important limit ages are shown in Figure 3.10. If the child does not reach any one of these limit ages, further assessment is indicated.

DEVELOPMENTAL DELAY

Features of abnormal development are:

- the child may progress slowly and steadily, but outside the normal range for age, and development may plateau or regress (Fig. 3.11)
- with increasing age, the difference between normal and abnormal development becomes greater and therefore more apparent (Fig. 3.12)
- it can be graded as mild, moderate, severe or profound
- it can involve a specific skill area (specific developmental delay) or affect all skill areas (global developmental delay).

Developmental problems often present at an age when a specific area of development is most rapid and prominent, e.g. motor problems during the first 18 months of age, and speech and language problems at 18 months to 3 years.

Any child whose development is delayed or suboptimal needs assessment to determine the cause and how best to help (Fig. 3.13). Normal developmental progress may be disrupted by a neurological or neurodevelopmental disorder in the child which affects development directly, e.g. cerebral palsy, epilepsy, Down's syndrome or visual impairment; or indirectly through ill-health, e.g. cystic fibrosis, or adverse environmental factors.

Developmental milestone	Age
No responsive smile	8/52
Not achieved good eye contact	3/12
Not reaching for objects	5/12
Not sitting unsupported	9/12
Not walking unaided	18/12
Not saying single words with meaning	18/12
No two or three word sentences	30/12

Further assessment is indicated if these skills have not been acquired by this age

At all ages if there is:
Parental concern
Discordance in different developmental areas
Regression of previously acquired skills

Fig. 3.10 Some important limit ages.

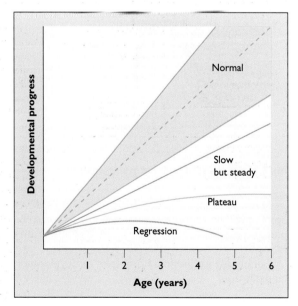

Fig. 3.11 Patterns of abnormal development. These may be slow but steady, plateau or regression.

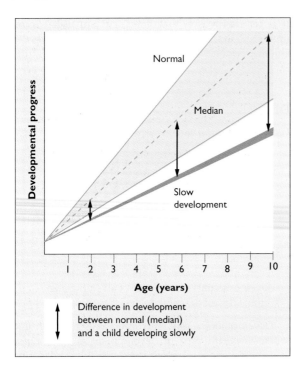

Fig. 3.12 For children with developmental delay, the gap between their abilities and what is normal widens with age.

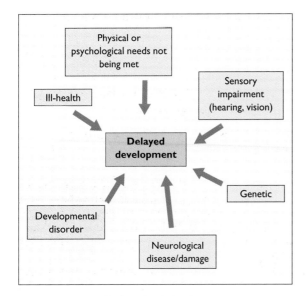

Fig. 3.13 Causes of suboptimal development.

Many parental concerns about their child's development will be variations of normal, in which case the parents need to be reassured or a period of observation set up.

Commonly encountered problems of developmental delay are:

- delayed motor development
- delayed speech and language
- social/communication disorder

Fig. 3.14 Hearing checklist for parents. (Used with permission from Dr Barry McCormick, Children's Hearing Assessment Centre, Nottingham.)

Shortly after birth	Startles and blinks at a sudden noise, e.g. slamming of door
By 1 month	Notices sudden prolonged sounds, e.g. a vacuum cleaner, and pauses and listens when they begin
By 4 months	Quietens or smiles to the sound of your voice even when he cannot see you. He may also turn his head or eyes towards you if you come up from behind and speak to him from the side
By 7 months	Turns immediately to your voice across the room or to very quiet noises made on each side, so long as he is not too occupied with other things
By 9 months	Listens attentively to familiar everyday sounds and searches for very quiet sounds made out of sight. Should also show pleasure in babbling loudly and tunefully
By 12 months	Shows some response to his own name and to other familiar words. May respond when you say 'no' and 'bye-bye' even when he cannot see any accompanying gesture

If you suspect that your baby is not hearing normally, seek advice from your health visitor or doctor.

- global developmental delay
- severe learning difficulties.

The assessment and management of these disorders are considered in Chapter 26 on 'The child with special needs'. Developmental problems of hyperactivity, attention deficit, dyslexia and dyspraxia are considered in Chapter 21 on 'Emotions and behaviour'. Specific sensory deficits can also adversely affect developmental progress.

HEARING

During the later stages of pregnancy, the fetus responds to sound. At birth, a baby reacts to sound, but there is a marked preference for voices. The ability to locate and turn towards sounds comes later in the first year. The early detection of deafness is important (Figs 3.14 and 3.15). If left untreated, the child will have impaired speech, language and learning and behavioural problems stemming from difficulty in communication.

Fig. 3.15 Tests for hearing and auditory function.

Age	Test	Indication
Birth	Otoacoustic emission Brain stem evoked potential Auditory response cradle	Children at high risk, e.g. children of parents with sensorineural hearing loss, preterm or received neonatal intensive care. Universal neonatal screening is being developed nationally
6–9 months	Distraction test (using frequency-specific sounds)	Screening of all children except for a few areas
15 months–4 years	Threshold audiometry (>3 years) Speech discrimination test Impedance audiometry	Children with suspected hearing loss
4 years and upwards	Threshold audiometry	Screening of all children at school entry or if suspected hearing loss

Fig. 3.16 Causes and management of hearing loss.

	Sensorineural	Conductive

Causes	Genetic
	Antenatal and perinatal:
	  Congenital infection
	  Preterm
	  Birth asphyxia
	  Hyperbilirubinaemia
	Postnatal
	  Meningitis/encephalitis
	  Head injury
	  Drugs, e.g. aminoglycosides
	  Neurodegenerative disorders
		Secretory otitis media (glue ear)
		Eustachian tube dysfunction:
		  Down's syndrome
		  Cleft palate
		  Pierre–Robin sequence
		  Mid-facial hypoplasia
		Wax (only rarely a cause of hearing loss)

Hearing loss	May be profound (>90 dB hearing loss)	Maximum of 20–60 dB hearing loss
Natural history	Does not improve or progresses	Intermittent or resolves
Management	Amplification or cochlear implant if necessary	Conservative or medical or surgery

Hearing loss

The causes of hearing loss are listed in Figure 3.16. They can be divided into sensorineural and conductive.

Sensorineural hearing loss

This type of hearing loss is uncommon (1 in 1000 of all births; 1 in 100 in extremely low birthweight infants). It is usually present at birth or develops in the first few months of life. The loss of hearing is usually due to abnormalities of or damage to the cochlea and/or central neural pathways. The hearing loss can be of any severity, including profound.

In newborn infants, hearing impairment can be identified using auditory evoked potentials, which detect brain stem responses to sounds, or the auditory response cradle, which relies on detecting a variety of behavioural responses to sound, such as turning of the head and changes in respiration. More recently, otoacoustic emission testing has been introduced as a screening test and is relatively easy to perform. An earpiece is inserted into the ear canal and produces a sound which evokes an echo or emission from the ear if cochlear function is normal. Audiological tests can be applied if there are risk factors for hearing impairment, although universal neonatal hearing screening is being introduced in the UK.

At 7–9 months of age, the distraction test is used for screening infant hearing in most parts of the UK (Fig. 3.17). This test relies on the baby locating and turning appropriately towards sounds. High- and low-frequency sounds are presented out of the infant's field of vision. Testing is unreliable if not carried out by properly trained staff since it can be difficult to identify hearing-impaired infants as they are particularly adept at using non-auditory cues.

Performance testing using high- and low-frequency stimuli and speech discrimination testing using miniature toys can be used among children with suspected hearing loss at 15 months to 4 years of age (Fig. 3.18). Threshold audiometry can be used to detect and assess

HEARING TESTS

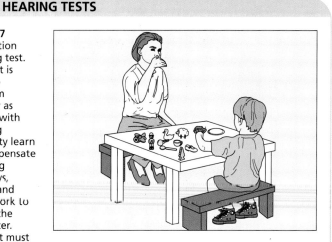

Fig. 3.17 Distraction hearing test. The test is hard to perform reliably as babies with hearing disability learn to compensate by using shadows, smells and guesswork to locate the presenter. The test must be done by well-trained professionals.

Fig. 3.18 Speech discrimination testing using miniature toys to detect hearing loss in children between 15 months and 4 years of age.

the severity of hearing loss in children from 4 years old (Fig. 3.19a–d).

Sensorineural hearing loss is irreversible. The child with severe bilateral hearing impairment will need early amplification with hearing aids for optimal speech and language development. Hearing aid use requires careful supervision, beginning in the home together with the parents and continuing into school. Children often resist wearing hearing aids because background noise can be amplified unpleasantly. Cochlear implants may be required where hearing aids give insufficient amplification. Intensive specialist teaching and support should be provided by peripatetic teachers for children with hearing impairment.

Children with hearing impairment should be placed in the front of the classroom so that they can readily see the teacher. Gesture, visual context and lip movement will also allow children to develop language concepts. Many children with moderate hearing impairment can be educated within the mainstream school system or in partial hearing units attached to mainstream schools. Speech may be delayed, but with appropriate therapy can be of good quality. Modified and simplified signing such as Makaton can be helpful for children who are both hearing-impaired and learning-disabled.

Conductive hearing loss

Conductive hearing loss from middle ear disease is usually mild or moderate, but may be severe. It is much more common than sensorineural hearing loss. In association with upper respiratory tract infections, many children have episodes of hearing loss which are usually self-limiting. In some cases of chronic serous otitis media, the hearing loss may last many months or years. In most affected children there are no identifiable risk factors present, but children with Down's syndrome, cleft palate and atopy are particularly prone to hearing loss from middle ear disease.

Any concern about hearing loss should be taken seriously. Any child with delayed language or speech, learning difficulties or behavioural problems should have his hearing tested, as a mild hearing loss may be the underlying cause without parents or other carers being aware.

Impedance audiometry tests, which measure the air pressure within the middle ear, determine if the middle ear is functioning normally. If the condition does not improve spontaneously, medical treatment (decongestant or a long course of antibiotics or treatment of nasal allergy) can be given. If that fails, then surgery is considered, with insertion of tympanostomy tubes (grommets) with or without the removal of adenoids. The role of surgery remains controversial.

The decision whether to intervene should be based on the degree of functional disability rather than on absolute hearing loss.

 Any child with poor or delayed speech or language must have his hearing checked.

VISION

A newborn infant's vision is limited; the visual acuity is only about 6/200. The retina is well developed but the fovea is immature. Well-focused images on the retina are required for the acquisition of visual acuity and any obstruction to this, e.g. from a cataract, will interfere with the normal development of the optic pathways and visual cortex unless corrected early in life.

Most newborn infants can fix and follow horizontally. There is a preference for patterns such as faces. Initially the eyes may move independently and the

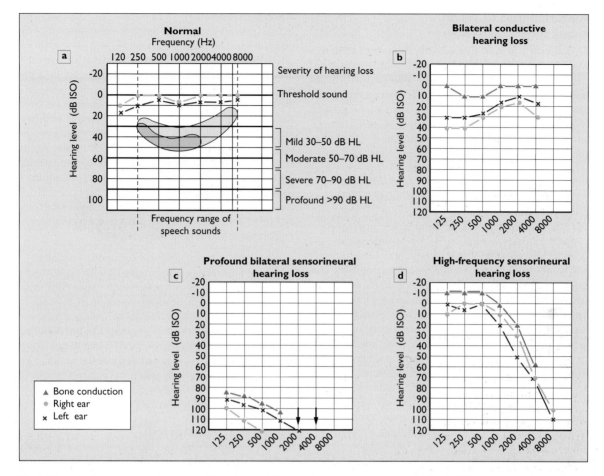

Fig. 3.19 a. Audiogram showing normal hearing and the loudness of normal speech. The light blue area represents the consonants (high-frequency sounds); the green area the vowels (low-frequency sounds). **b.** Audiogram showing bilateral conductive hearing loss. There is a 30–40 dB hearing loss in both the right and left ears. **c.** Audiogram showing bilateral profound sensorineural hearing loss. **d.** Audiogram showing bilateral high-frequency sensorineural hearing loss.

baby may appear to squint; this is particularly noticeable when the baby tries to look at near objects and the eyes over-converge.

By around 6 weeks of age, both eyes should move together when following a light source and no squint should be present. Babies slowly develop the ability to focus at different distances and visual acuity improves from 6/60 at 3 months to adult levels at around 3 years. Testing for abnormalities has to allow for this.

Visual impairment may present in infancy with:

- lack of eye contact with parents
- visual inattention
- random eye movements
- not smiling responsively by 6 weeks post-term
- nystagmus
- squint
- photophobia
- loss of red reflex from a cataract
- a white reflex in the pupil, which may be due to retinoblastoma, cataract or retinopathy of prematurity.

The assessment of vision at different ages is shown in Figure 3.20.

Fig. 3.20 Testing vision at different ages.

Age	Test
Birth	Face fixation and following
	Preferential looking – preference for patterned objects to plain ones
6 weeks	Optokinetic nystagmus demonstrated on looking at a moving, striped target
6 months	Reaches well for toys
2 years	Can identify pictures of reducing size
3 years onwards	Letter matching using single letter charts, e.g. Sheridan Gardiner
5 years onwards	Can identify a line of letters on a Snellen chart by name or matching

Abnormalities of vision

Severe visual impairment

This affects 1 in 1000 births but is important to detect early. A family history of severe visual impairment, developmental delay or extreme prematurity places the infant at an increased risk. In developed countries, about 50% of severe visual impairment is genetic (Fig. 3.21); in developing countries, acquired causes such as infection are more prevalent. The eye examination may be normal, including the pupillary responses when visual impairment is of cortical origin resulting from cerebral damage.

Although few causes of severe visual impairment can be treated, much can be done to help the child and his parents. Parents of a partially sighted or severely visually impaired child need appropriate advice on how to provide non-visual stimulation using speech and touch, on providing a safe home environment and on how to build the child's confidence. In the UK this is usually provided by peripatetic teachers for the visually impaired who provide input at both preschool and school ages. Partially sighted children may be able to attend a mainstream school but require special assistance with low vision aids which include filtered lenses, high-powered magnifiers and small telescopic devices and computers. Severely visually impaired children may need special schooling. Some will need to be taught Braille to enable them to read. While many severely visually impaired children have a visual disability only, at least half have additional neurodevelopmental problems.

Squints (strabismus)

In this common condition there is misalignment of the visual axes. The history may be helpful as squints are often intermittent. The parents are usually correct if they report deviation of the eyes. There may be a history of squint in the family. Newborn babies often give the appearance of having a squint because of overconvergence. In older infants and young children, marked epicanthic folds may cause confusion (pseudosquint). Any infant with a fixed squint or any squint persisting beyond 2 months of age should be referred for a specialist ophthalmological opinion. A squint is usually caused by failure to develop binocular vision due to refractive errors, but cataracts, retinoblastoma and other intraocular causes must be excluded.

Squints are commonly divided into:

- *Concomitant* (non-paralytic, common) – usually due to a refractive error in one or both eyes which is often treated by correction with glasses but may require surgery. Squints are common in children with neurodevelopmental delay. The squinting eye most often turns inwards (convergent), but there can be outward (divergent) or, rarely, vertical deviation.
- *Paralytic* (rare) – due to paralysis of the motor nerves. When rapid in onset, this can be sinister because of the possibility of an underlying space-occupying lesion such as a brain tumour.

Corneal light reflection test

For the non-specialist, the light reflection test is used to detect squints (Fig. 3.22). It is easiest to use a pen

Fig. 3.21 Causes of visual impairment.		
Genetic	**Antenatal and perinatal**	**Postnatal**
Cataract	Congenital infection	Trauma
Albinism	Retinopathy of prematurity	Infection
Retinal dystrophy	Hypoxic-ischaemic encephalopathy	Juvenile idiopathic arthritis
Retinoblastoma	Cerebral abnormality/damage	
	Optic nerve hypoplasia	

SQUINTS

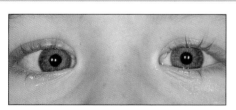

Fig. 3.22 Corneal light reflection test to detect a squint. The reflection is in a different position in the two eyes because of a small convergent squint of the right eye.

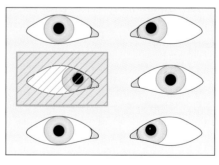

Fig. 3.23 The cover test is used to identify a squint. If the fixing eye is covered, the squinting eye moves to take up fixation. This diagram shows a left convergent squint.

torch held at a distance to produce reflections on both corneas simultaneously. The light reflection should appear in the same position in the two eyes. If it does not, a squint is present. However, a minor squint may be difficult to detect.

Cover test

When a squint is present and the fixing eye is covered, the squinting eye moves to take up fixation (Fig. 3.23). The child's interest can be attracted with a toy or light. The test should be performed with the object near (33 cm) and distant (at least 6 m), as certain squints are present only at one distance. Occlusion should be with a card or plastic occluder. These tests are difficult to perform and reliable results are best obtained by an orthoptist or ophthalmologist.

Refractive errors

All children in the UK are screened for visual acuity and squint at school entry. In some parts of the UK preschool children (at $3^1/_2$–4 years) are screened.

Hypermetropia

This is the most common refractive error in young children and should be corrected early to avoid irreversible damage to vision (amblyopia). This is more likely if accompanied by a squint but may occur without.

Myopia

This is uncommon in young children and is less likely to cause amblyopia unless it is severe or only one eye is affected.

Amblyopia

This is a permanent loss of visual acuity in an eye that has not received a clear image. It affects 2–3% of children. In most cases, it affects one eye; rarely, both are involved. Any interference with visual development may cause amblyopia, such as unilateral or bilateral refractive errors, squint or visual deprivation, e.g. ptosis or cataract. Treatment is by correction of any refractive error with glasses, together with patching of the 'good' eye for specific periods of the day to force the 'lazy' eye to work and therefore develop better vision. It is continued until the vision in the 'lazy eye' no longer improves. The longer treatment is delayed, the less likely it is that normal vision will be obtained. Early treatment is essential, as after 7 years of age improvement is unlikely. Considerable encouragement and support often need to be given to both the child and parents, as young children usually dislike having their eye patched, particularly if vision in the un-patched eye is poor.

FURTHER READING

Hall D M B (ed.) 1996 Health for all children, 3rd edn. Oxford University Press, Oxford. *Describes child health promotion and surveillance, its potential and limitations*

Hall D M B, Hill P, Elliman D 1999 The child surveillance handbook, 2nd edn. Radcliffe Medical Press, Oxford. *A practical guide to child development and surveillance*

Illingworth R S 1988 Basic developmental screening: 0–4. Blackwell Scientific, Oxford. *A short guide to child development*

McCormick B 1994 Hearing screening 0–5 years, 2nd edn. Croom Helm, London. *A practical guide to hearing screening*

4

Care of the sick child

Most sick children are cared for by their parents at home. Medical management is initially given by general practitioners or, in some countries, primary care paediatricians. Most hospital admissions are at secondary care level. A smaller number of children will require tertiary care in a specialist centre, e.g. paediatric intensive care, cardiac or oncology unit. There are a few national centres for very rare and complex treatments, e.g. organ transplantation, craniofacial surgery (Fig. 4.1).

PRIMARY CARE

General practitioner

The majority of acute illness in children is mild and transient (e.g. upper respiratory tract infection, gastroenteritis) or readily treatable (e.g. urinary tract infection). Although serious conditions are uncommon (Fig. 4.2), they must be identified promptly. The condition of sick children, especially infants, may deteriorate rapidly, and parents require rapid access to their general practitioner, who in turn requires ready access to secondary care in a wide range of services for children. Although an individual general practitioner will care for relatively few children with serious chronic illness (e.g. cystic fibrosis, diabetes mellitus) or disability

(e.g. cerebral palsy), each affected child and family are likely to require considerable input from the whole of the primary care team.

HOSPITAL CARE

Accident and emergency

Approximately 1 in 4 children attend an accident and emergency (A&E) department each year in England and Wales. The services which should be provided for children are shown in Figure 4.3. The number of departments able to meet these expectations is increasing, often by creating a dedicated children's A&E department.

Hospital admission

In England and Wales, 1 in 11 children is admitted to hospital each year, representing 16% of all hospital admissions. About 42% of acute admissions are under the care of paediatricians, and the remainder are surgical patients. Most paediatric admissions are of infants and young children and are emergencies, whereas surgical admissions peak at 5 years of age and one-third are elective (Fig. 4.4). The reasons for medical admission are shown in Figure 4.5.

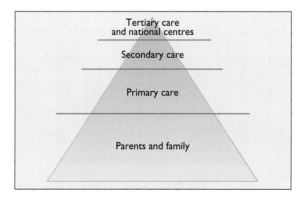

Fig. 4.1 Schematic representation of the 'clinical iceberg' of the provision of care for sick children. (Adapted from Audit Commission, *Children First*, 1993.)

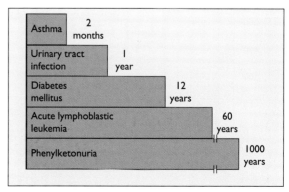

Fig. 4.2 Number of years a general practitioner needs to work before encountering a child newly presenting with these conditions.

Although primary and community health services for children have improved markedly over the last decade, the hospital admission rate has continued to rise (Fig. 4.6). The reasons for this are unclear, but probably include:

- increased hospital admission rate for asthma, one of the commonest causes for in-patient treatment
- lower threshold for admission – there appears to be an increased expectation of hospital

---

Fig. 4.3 Services which should be available for children attending an accident and emergency department. (Adapted from *Welfare of Children in Hospital*, HMSO, London, 1991.)

Environment	Staff	Medical Care
Separate waiting area, play facilities, treatment and recovery areas	Medical and nursing staff trained and experienced in the care and treatment of children	Resuscitation and other equipment for children
Access for parents to examination, X-ray and anaesthetic rooms	Non-paediatric staff trained in communicating with children and families	Priority for prompt treatment
	Effective communication with other health professionals	Rapid transfer if in-patient admission is needed
		Child protection policies
		Procedures and counselling are in place following the sudden death of a child

---

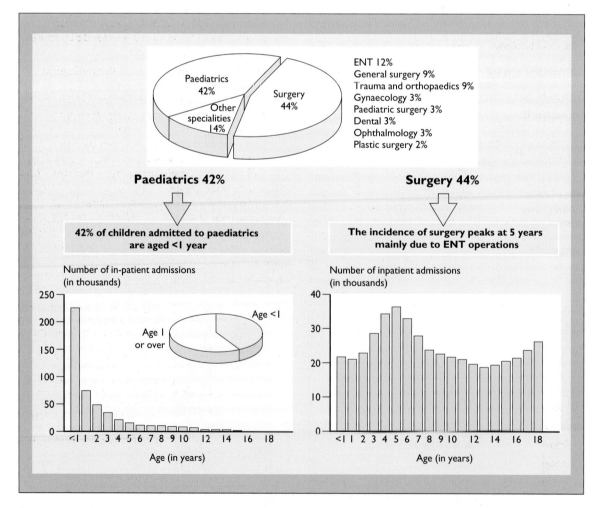

Fig. 4.4 Hospital in-patients of children aged 0–18 years in England and Wales in 1990–91. (Adapted from Audit Commission, *Children First*, 1993.)

admission by parents and medical staff worried that the child's clinical condition may deteriorate

• repeated hospital admission of children with complex conditions who would have died in the past but are now surviving, e.g. very low birthweight infants from neonatal intensive care units, children with cancer or organ failure.

Fig. 4.5 Reason for paediatric medical admissions to a district general hospital.
(Data based on 2160 consecutive admissions to Pinderfields Hospital, Wakefield. Courtesy of Dr Roddy MacFaul.)

Respiratory 31%	Asthma 11% URTI 6% Croup 4% Bronchiolitis 4% Pneumonia 3% Tonsillitis 2.5%
Environment 22%	Head injury 12% Poisoning 8% Child protection 1.5%
Gastroenterology 15%	Gastroenteritis 7% Constipation/soiling 2% Abdominal pain/vomiting 2% Failure to thrive 1%
Infection 10%	Viral infection 6% Septicaemia/meningitis 1.5%
Neurology 8%	Febrile convulsions 3% Epilepsy 3% Apnoea/cyanotic attacks 2%
Kidney and urinary tract 3%	Urinary tract infection 2.5%
Other 11%	

Strenuous efforts are being made to reduce the rate and length of hospitalisation:

• The new speciality of ambulatory paediatrics encompasses specialist, non-in-patient paediatrics and should reduce overnight admission to hospital.

• Dedicated children's short stay beds within or alongside the A&E department are being introduced to allow children to be treated or observed for a number of hours and discharged home directly, avoiding the need for admission to the ward.

• Day-case surgery has been instituted for many operations which used to require overnight stay. Day units are used for complex investigations and procedures.

• Home care teams aim to provide care in the child's home and thereby reduce both the need to attend hospital and the length of stay. Most teams comprise community paediatric nurses, but some include doctors, and they either cover all aspects of paediatric care within a geographical area or are for a specific condition, e.g. cystic fibrosis or malignancy, usually centred around a tertiary referral centre. The problems managed at home by such teams include:

— changing postoperative wound dressings or managing burns
— day-to-day management and support for the family for chronic illnesses, e.g. diabetes mellitus, asthma and eczema
— specialist care, e.g. home oxygen therapy, intravenous infusions via a central venous catheter (e.g. antibiotics or chemotherapy) or peritoneal dialysis
— symptom and pain control and emotional support of terminally ill children (Fig. 4.7).

Some teams provide a 'hospital at home' service for children who are acutely ill, in order to avoid hospitalisation.

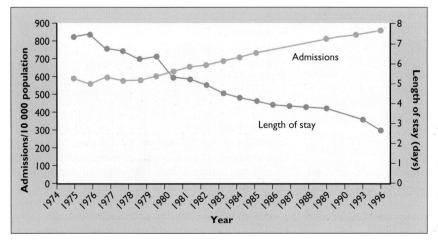

Fig. 4.6 In-patient admission rates for children aged 0–14 years in England. There has been a marked increase in the paediatric admission rate, whereas the surgical admission rate has fallen slightly. In both, there has been a marked reduction in the average length of stay. (Adapted from Audit Commission, *Children First*, 1993.)

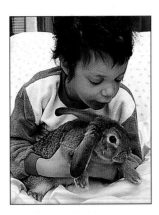

Fig. 4.7 Providing terminal care in a child's home. Although this child required a subcutaneous morphine infusion to control her pain from malignant disease, she was able to remain at home and enjoyed playing with her pet rabbit. (By kind permission of her parents and Dr Ann Goldman.)

Children in hospital

Children should only be admitted to hospital if their care cannot be provided safely at home. Removing young children from their familiar environment to a strange ward is stressful and frightening for the child, parents and family. It also disrupts family routines, not only of the child in hospital, but also of siblings who still need to be looked after at home and transported to and from nursery or school.

Family-centred care
Care in hospital should be child- and family-centred. Parents and siblings should be involved in the child's care, which should be appropriate for the child's physical and emotional maturity and needs. A holistic approach should be adopted towards the child and his family rather than simply focusing on the medical condition. Young children may interpret the pain experienced in hospital and separation from their home or parents as punishment. In general, the distress arising from separating children from their mothers is greatest in young children, and increases the longer the length of stay and the more frequently the child is admitted. Parents should be encouraged to continue to provide the care and support they would give at home. Parents know best about their child's usual behaviour and habits and due attention must be paid to their worries or comments. Many parents rapidly learn some of the nursing skills, e.g. tube feeding, required by their child. Good communication is needed between staff and parents to arrive at a mutually agreed plan of responsibilities for looking after the child. This will avoid parents either feeling pressurised to accept responsibilities they are not confident about or feeling brushed aside and undervalued by staff. Parents should be able to stay overnight with their child.

Child-orientated environment
Children should be cared for within a children's ward. Adolescents should be with others of their own age and not forced to accept ward arrangements designed for babies or adults. Education and facilities for play should be provided.

Information and psychosocial support
Detailed information should be provided, given personally and preferably also written and available in appropriate ethnic languages. Staff should be sensitive to the family's individual needs according to their social, educational, cultural and religious background. Play specialists should be part of the ward team because they can help children understand their illness and its treatment through play. Emotional and psychological support should be given to all. For elective admissions, children and their families should be offered an advance visit and have details of proposed treatment and management explained at an appropriate level.

Skilled staff

Children in hospital should be cared for by specially trained medical, nursing and support staff. Every child admitted to hospital should be supervised by a children's physician or surgeon. Children constitute only a relatively small proportion of the workload in acute surgical specialities, so surgeons and anaesthetists should treat a sufficient number of children to maintain their skills. There should be a 'named nurse' responsible for planning and coordinating care by other nurses to ensure that families receive all the information they need and provide a link with staff involved in discharge planning and post-discharge arrangements.

Multidisciplinary care
Successful management of paediatric conditions often relies on a network of multidisciplinary care, with all the professionals working well together as a coordinated team. If this breaks down, particularly when dealing with complex issues such as child protection, the consequences may be disastrous for the child, family and professionals involved. Child psychiatrists, the community paediatric team and social services are important members of the team.

Pain

It is easy to ignore or underestimate pain in children. Pain should ideally be anticipated and prevented.

Acute pain
This may be caused by:
- tissue damage, e.g. burns or trauma
- disease, e.g. sickle cell crisis
- medical intervention – investigations or procedures
- surgery.

Chronic pain
In children, chronic severe pain sometimes occurs as a result of disease such as malignant disease or juvenile idiopathic arthritis (juvenile chronic arthritis). Intermittent pain of mild or moderate severity, e.g. headache or recurrent abdominal pain, is more common.

Older children can describe the nature and severity of the pain they are experiencing. In younger children,

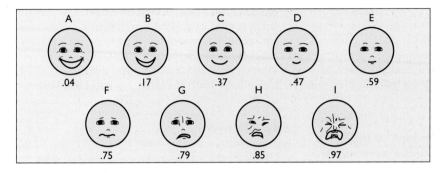

Fig. 4.8 An example of a scoring system for pain assessment in children. (From McGrath P A, DeVeber L L, Hearn M T, Multidimensional pain assessment in children. In: Fields H, Dubner R, Cervero F (eds) *Advances in Pain Research and Therapy*, Raven Press, New York, 1985; p 387–393.)

assessing pain is more difficult. Observation and parental impression are commonly used and a number of self-assessment tools have been designed for children over 3 years old (Fig. 4.8).

Management

The approaches to pain management are listed in Figure 4.9. This should allow pain to be prevented or kept to a minimum. For minor medical procedures, e.g. venepuncture or inserting an intravenous cannula, pain can be alleviated by explanation, the use of a topical anaesthetic to the skin and distraction techniques, such as blowing bubbles, telling stories or computer games. For more invasive procedures, e.g. bronchoscopy, a general anaesthetic should be given.

Postoperative pain can be markedly reduced by local infiltration of the wound, nerve blocks and postoperative analgesics. For severe pain, there was reluctance in the past to use morphine in children for fear of depressing breathing. This should not occur when morphine is given in appropriate dosage under nursing supervision to children with a normal respiratory drive. Intravenous morphine can be given using a patient-controlled delivery system in older children or a nurse-controlled system in young children.

Prescribing drugs

There are marked differences in the absorption, distribution and elimination of drugs between children and adults.

Absorption

In the neonate and infant, oral formulations of drugs can be given as liquids. However, their intake cannot be guaranteed and absorption is unpredictable as it is affected by gastric emptying and acidity, gut motility and the effects of milk in the stomach. Rectal administration can be used for some drugs; absorption is more reliable, but this route is not popular in the UK. In acutely ill neonates and infants, drugs are given intravenously to ensure reliable and adequate blood and tissue concentrations. Intramuscular injections should be avoided if possible as there is little muscle bulk available for injection, absorption is variable and they are painful. Significant systemic absorption can occur across the skin, particularly in preterm infants. Occasionally this can be used therapeutically, but is

---

Fig. 4.9 Approaches to pain management.

Explanation and information

Psychological, by the parent, doctor or nurse
Behavioural
Distraction
Hypnosis

Medical
Local: anaesthetic cream, local infiltration, nerve blocks, warmth or cold, physiotherapy, transcutaneous electrical nerve stimulation (TENS)

Analgesics:
    Mild – paracetamol, NSAIDs
    Moderate – codeine, NSAIDs
    Strong – morphine

Anti-epileptic and anti-depressant drugs for neuropathic pain

---

Consider the route for analgesics – oral if possible, otherwise intravenous, subcutaneous or rectal.

NSAIDs, non-steroidal anti-inflammatory drugs.

---

a potential cause of toxicity, e.g. alcohol and iodine absorption from cleansing solutions applied to the skin for procedures.

Young children find it difficult to take tablets and a liquid formulation is required. Most are glucose-free. Persuading children to take medicines is often a problem. Compliance is improved when medicines are only required once or twice a day.

Distribution

Water comprises a larger percentage of the body in the neonate (80%) than in older children and adults (55%). Drugs which distribute within the extracellular fluid will require a larger dose relative to body weight in infants than in adults. As extracellular fluid correlates with body surface area, this is used when accurate drug dosage is required, e.g. cytotoxic agents. For drugs with a high margin of safety, drug dosages are expressed per kilogram body weight or based on age, with the assumption that the child is of average size. Weight-based dosages should not simply be extrapolated to older children, as the dosage will be excessively large.

In the first few months of life, the plasma protein is low. More of the drug may be unbound and pharmacologically active. In jaundiced babies, bilirubin may compete with some drugs, e.g. sulphonamides, for albumin binding sites.

Elimination

In neonates, drug biotransformation is reduced, as microsomal enzymes in the liver are immature. This leads to a prolonged half-life of drugs metabolised in the liver, e.g. theophylline. Renal excretion is reduced by the low glomerular filtration rate which increases the half-life of some drugs, e.g. gentamicin. Measuring the plasma drug concentration is necessary under these circumstances.

> **Dosages of intravenous drugs are easy to miscalculate as they vary widely in children of different sizes and drugs often need to be diluted. All dosages and dilutions must be checked independently by two trained members of staff.**

Consent

Informed consent of the parent and assent of the older child should be obtained, except in an emergency. In the UK, the legal age of consent to medical treatment is 16 years. In principle, if an older child below 16 years has sufficient understanding, he may accept or refuse to be examined or treated. In practice, problems occur only when the child and parents have strongly opposing views. This is rare and legal advice may then be needed. There is legal precedence in the UK for children with sufficient understanding to agree to treatment against their parents' wishes (Gillick competence). However, when children refuse treatment against the judgement of their parents and doctors, e.g. refusal of a heart–lung transplant by a child with cystic fibrosis, the court has, up until now, overruled the child's wishes. Young children should be provided with as much information as possible in language they can understand, and their wishes should be determined and taken into account as far as possible.

Breaking bad news

Doctors often face the difficult task of imparting bad news to parents and children. In paediatric practice it is often because there is:

- a serious congenital abnormality at birth, e.g. chromosomal disorder

- the diagnosis of a disabling condition, e.g. cerebral palsy, neurodegenerative disorder, gross intracranial abnormality seen at ultrasound in preterm infants
- a serious illness, e.g. meningitis or malignant disease, or an accident, e.g. head injury
- the sudden death of a child, e.g. sudden infant death syndrome (SIDS).

Initial interview

The manner in which the initial interview is conducted is very important. It may have a profound influence on the parents' ability to cope with the problem and their subsequent relationship with health professionals. Parents often continue to recall and recount, for many years, details of the initial interview when they were informed that their child had a serious problem. Parents of children with life-threatening illnesses have said that what they valued most was open, sympathetic, direct and uninterrupted discussion in private that allowed sufficient time for doctors to repeat and clarify information and for them to ask questions (Fig. 4.10).

Discharge from hospital

Children should be discharged from hospital as soon as clinically and socially appropriate. Although there is increasing pressure to reduce the length of hospital stay to a minimum, this must not allow discharge planning to be neglected. Before discharge from hospital, parents and children should be informed of:

- the reason for admission and any implications for the future
- details of medication and other treatment
- any clinical features which should prompt them to seek medical advice, and how this should be obtained
- the existence of any voluntary self-help groups if appropriate
- problems or questions likely to be asked by other family members or in the community. These should be anticipated by the doctor and discussed. What does the nursery or school, baby-sitters or friends need to know? What about sports, etc.?

In addition:

- Suitability of home circumstances needs to be assessed, particularly when the home requires adaptation for special needs.
- Social support may need to be arranged, especially in relation to child protection.
- Medical information should be added to the child's personal health record.
- Consider who else should be informed about the admission and what information it is relevant for them to receive. This must be done before or at the time of discharge. The aim is to provide a seamless service of care, treatment and support, with the family and all the professionals fully

Fig. 4.10 How parents wish to be told the diagnosis of a life-threatening illness.
(Adapted from Woolley H, Stein A, Forrest G C, Baum J D, Imparting the diagnosis of life-threatening illness in children. *British Medical Journal* 298: 1623–1626, 1989.)

Setting
In private
Uninterrupted
Unhurried
Both parents (or friend/relative) present if possible
Senior doctor
Nurse or social worker present

Establish contact
Find out what the family knows or suspects
Respect family's vulnerability
Use the child's name
Do not avoid looking at them
Be direct, open, sympathetic

Provide information
Flexibility is essential
Pace rather than protect from bad news
Name the illness
Describe symptoms relevant to child's condition
Discuss aetiology – parents will usually want to know
Anticipate and answer questions. Don't avoid difficult issues because parents have not thought to ask

Explain long-term prognosis
If child is likely to die, listen to concerns about time, place and nature of death
Outline the support/treatment available

Address feelings
Be prepared to tolerate reactions of shock, especially anger or weeping
Acknowledge uncertainty
How is it likely to affect the family?
What and how to tell other children, relatives and friends?

Concluding the interview
Elicit what parents have understood
Clarify and repeat
Acknowledge that it may be difficult for parents to absorb all the information
Mention sources of support
If available, give parents contact telephone number
Give address of self-help group

Follow-up
Offer early follow-up
Suggest to families that they write down questions in preparation for next appointment
Ensure adequate communication of content of interview to:
other members of staff
general practitioner and health visitor
other professionals, e.g. a referring paediatrician

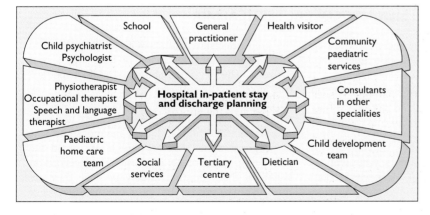

Fig. 4.11 Some of the professionals who may need to be informed on admission or discharge about a child admitted to hospital

informed (Fig. 4.11). This can be facilitated for children with a chronic illness or disability by having a key worker to coordinate their care.

ETHICS

There are many issues in paediatrics that require a good working knowledge of the ethical principles that underpin the practice of medicine. When any decision is made to investigate or to treat, it should be possible to justify that choice in a clear and logical manner. It is the responsibility of the doctor to make this reasoning explicit to patients, families and colleagues. It is helpful to use the language of medical ethics to express this reasoning both verbally and in medical records and correspondence.

Definitions of the principles of medical ethics

These are:

- *non-maleficence* – do no harm
- *beneficence* – do good (these two principles have been part of medical ethics since the Hippocratic Oath)
- *justice*
  — legal justice
  — respect for rights
  — fair distribution of resources, which includes the doctor's time and attention
- *respect for autonomy* – respect for individuals' rights to make informed and thought-out decisions for themselves
- *truth-telling* – an important subset of autonomy that also supports trust, which is so essential in the doctor–patient relationship.

Application of ethical principles to paediatrics

Non-maleficence

Children are more vulnerable to harm. This includes their suffering from fear of procedures, which they may be too young to express verbally. Doctors may do harm from lack of skill or knowledge, especially if they do not treat children frequently.

Beneficence

The child's interest is paramount. In the UK, this is enshrined in the Children Act (1989). This may sometimes conflict with parental autonomy, such as the emergency treatment of a child where the parent is not immediately available or when details are given to social workers in suspected child abuse.

Justice

This involves ensuring a comprehensive child health service, including the prevention of illness and equal access to health care even when poverty, language barriers and parental disability are present.

Autonomy

Children have restricted but developing rights in law. Parents are trusted to make decisions on their child's behalf because they will usually act in the child's best interests.

Truth-telling

It is more difficult to ensure with children than with adults that they understand what is happening to them. For example, it is easy to reassure children falsely that procedures will not hurt; when they find this untrue, trust will be lost for future occasions.

Case histories 4.1 and 4.2 demonstrate some of the ethical problems encountered in paediatrics.

The ethics of research in paediatrics

Where research is part of the child's treatment, e.g. comparing two treatments for a particular cancer, the usual ethical considerations for 'therapeutic' medical research apply. If there is a state of 'equipoise' – i.e. there is no good reason to believe that one of the treatments

---

CASE HISTORY 4.1

MENINGOCOCCAL SEPTICAEMIA

Jack, aged 5 years, has a fever and purpuric rash and you suspect he may have potentially fatal meningococcal septicaemia. Jack hates needles and makes it clear that he rejects any sort of injection. 'No I don't want an injection, go away' is the message, loud and clear, when you try to take blood, do a lumbar puncture, and insert an indwelling intravenous cannula for his antibiotics. Yet with the full and anxious approval of his parents, you go ahead and do these things anyway. But if Jack was 25 years old and made it clear that he refused your interventions, while you'd strongly urge him to give permission and explain that he was in real danger of dying as a result of such refusal, you would not (presumably) treat him against his will, even if his mother and father still urged you to do so.

In contrast to normal adult medical ethics, in paediatrics the autonomy of the patient either is not present at all (as in babies and young infants) or is often not sufficiently developed to be respected if the child's decision conflicts with what appropriate other people consider to be in that child's best interests. The decisions about the child's medical care are generally entrusted to his parents. Why the parents? Not because, as in previous times, the parents, and in particular the father, were regarded as owning the child and thus having some sort of property rights! Rather, parents are given the privilege and responsibility of making decisions on behalf of their children largely because they are most likely to protect and promote the interests of their children. The normal assumption in paediatric practice is that doctors should work closely with parents and give advice that parents may or may not accept. Wherever possible, a mutually trusting and respectful working relationship should be developed and maintained, both because it will be in the best interests of the child and because it will tend to lead to far better experiences of medical care for all involved.

CASE HISTORY 4.2

ACUTE LYMPHATIC LEUKAEMIA, TRUTH-TELLING AND STOPPING TREATMENT

Jane, aged 10 years, has acute lymphoblastic leukaemia which was diagnosed 4 years ago. She has relapsed, with early involvement of the central nervous system. She is well known to the staff of her local children's ward as she has had four relapses of her leukaemia and a previous bone marrow transplant. It is the opinion of her paediatric consultant that no further medical treatment is likely to be curative. Jane asks one of the junior paediatric doctors why her parents had been so upset following a recent discussion with the consultant, at which she had not been present. The parents had made it very clear to all the staff that they did not want their child to be informed of the poor prognosis, nor would they tell her why she was not having further chemotherapy.

The parents have heard of a new drug which is claimed, in some reports on the internet, to help such children. However, it is very expensive, there is evidence that it does not cross the blood–brain barrier and the doctors consider it highly unlikely to be of benefit. The parents insist on a trial of the drug.

Ethical issues to consider are:

- *autonomy* – the parents claim the right to control the information reaching their child on the grounds that it is in her best interests as judged by them
- *truth-telling* – the staff feel that it would be wrong to reassure her falsely

- *non-maleficence* – the parents wish to avoid the shock of the news and the loss of hope in their daughter
- *beneficence* – the staff wish to support the child effectively, which would be difficult is she were to be isolated by ignorance of what is upsetting her family and carers
- *justice* – should scarce resources be used on this new drug? Because her parents are desperate, should Jane be given a drug which, in the specialist's opinion, will not benefit her?

In such situations, further discussion between the parents and staff whom they trust is usually the key to resolving the situation. The parents will need to understand the mutual benfits of adopting as open a pattern of communication as possible. They may be helped by a member of staff being present or helping them talk or listen to the child, who will usually understand more than the parents suspect.

Parents almost always wish to do the best for their child. Detailed explanation is likely to help them see that the child's best interests may not be to seek further cure but to accept a change of focus towards palliative care. A second opinion from an independent specialist may be helpful. If, despite all efforts to reach agreement, the parents reject the doctor's advice, it is fairest to let a court of law decide whether or not to accept the parents' demands.

would be better for the patient – it is justifiable, and many would claim morally desirable, to enrol the child in a trial. Details must be explained to the parent(s), including written information in plain English and other local ethnic languages, and, where applicable, information should be provided for the child in an appropriate form. Parents must have the option to withdraw their child from the research at any stage.

The ethical issues associated with non-therapeutic research in children, e.g. performing a CT scan in a normal child as a control in a trial, and the degree of risk that is justifiable remain controversial. Recently, it has been recognised that the extreme view in which no risk is permissible would exclude children from benefiting fully from medical advances. This position has now been modified to accepting minimal risk provided a number of safeguards are adhered to:

- properly informed consent is obtained from the parent(s)
- the risks are very small, i.e. similar to the risks that are generally encountered and acceptable in

everyday life or, in exceptional circumstances, may be slightly greater than everyday risks if the benefits from the research are sufficiently great
- the research cannot be done on adults.

EVIDENCE-BASED PAEDIATRICS

Clinicians have always sought to base their decisions on the best available evidence. However, such decisions have often been made intuitively, given as clinical opinion, which is difficult to generalise, scrutinise or challenge. Evidence-based practice provides a systematic approach to enable clinicians to efficiently use the best available evidence, usually from research, to help them solve their clinical problems. The difference between this approach and old-style clinical practice is that clinicians need to know how to turn their clinical problems into questions that can be answered by the research literature, to search the literature efficiently, and to analyse the evidence, using epidemiological and biostatistical rules (Figs 4.12 and 4.13).

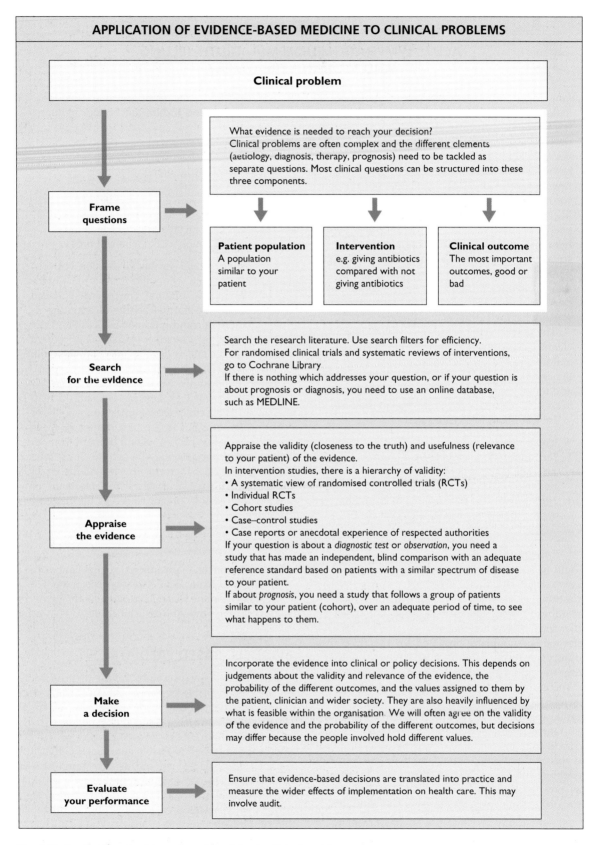

Fig. 4.12 Application of evidence-based medicine to clinical problems.

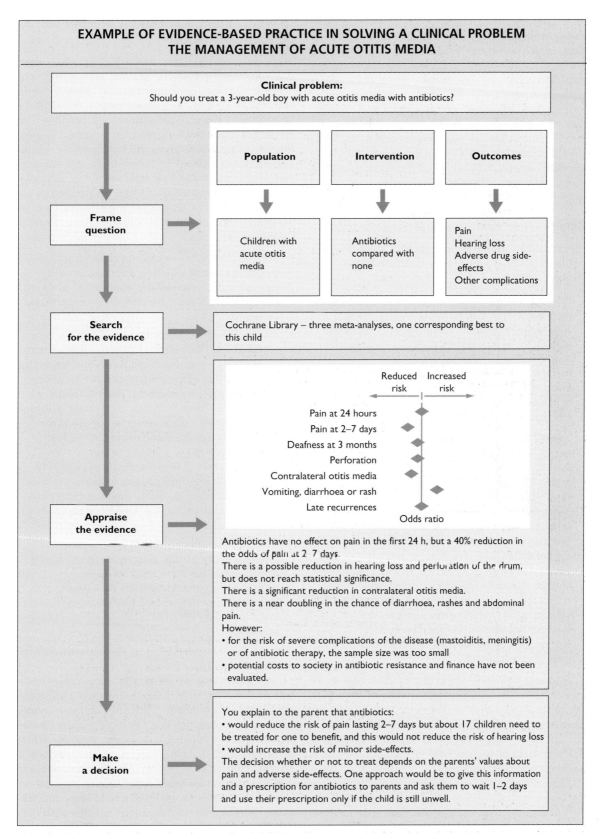

Fig. 4.13 An example of an evidence-based medicine approach to a clinical problem – the treatment of acute otitis media with antibiotics.

Sometimes, the best available evidence will be a high-quality, systematic review of randomised controlled trials, which are directly applicable to a particular patient. For other questions, lack of more valid studies may mean that one has to base one's decision on previous experience with a small number of similar patients. The important factor is that, for any decision, clinicians know the strength of the evidence, and therefore the degree of uncertainty. As this approach requires clinicians to be explicit about the evidence they use, others involved in the decisions (patients, parents, managers and other clinicians) can debate and judge the evidence for themselves.

Why practise evidence-based paediatrics?

There are many examples from the past where, through lack of evidence, clinicians have harmed children, e.g.:

- *Blindness from retinopathy of prematurity*. In the 1950s, following anecdotal reports, many neonatal units started nursing all premature infants in additional ambient oxygen, irrespective of need. Although this reduced mortality, as no properly conducted trials were performed of this new therapy, it took several years for it to be realised that this was also responsible for many thousands of babies needlessly becoming blind from retinopathy of prematurity.

- *Advice that babies should sleep lying on their front (prone), which increases the risk of sudden infant death syndrome (SIDS)*. Medical advice given during the 1970s and 1980s, to put babies to sleep prone, appears to have been based on physiological studies in preterm babies, which showed better oxygenation when nursed prone. Furthermore, autopsies on some infants who died of SIDS showed milk in the trachea, which was assumed to have been aspirated and thought to be more likely if they were lying on their back. However, an accumulation of more valid evidence from cohort and case–control studies showed that nursing term infants prone was associated with an increased risk of SIDS.

Evidence-based medicine allows clinicians to be explicit about the probability (or risk) of important outcomes. For example, in discussing with parents the prognosis of a child who has had a febrile convulsion, one can state that 'the risk of developing epilepsy is 1%' instead of using vague terms, such as 'she is unlikely to develop epilepsy'.

Explicit analysis of evidence has also become more important with the increasing delivery of health care by teams rather than individuals. Each team member needs to understand the rationale for decisions and the probability of different outcomes in order to make their own clinical decisions and to provide consistent information to patients and parents.

To what extent is paediatric practice based on sound evidence?

There are two paediatric specialities in which there is a considerable body of reliable, high-quality evidence underpinning clinical practice, namely paediatric oncology and, to a lesser extent, neonatology. Management protocols of virtually all children with cancer are part of multicentre trials designed to identify which treatment gives the best possible results. The trials are national or, increasingly, international, and include short- and long-term follow up. Examples of the range of evidence available in paediatrics are given in Figure 4.14. In general, the evidence base for paediatrics is poorer than in adult medicine. Reasons for this include:

- The relatively small number of children with significant illness requiring investigation and treatment. To overcome this, multicentre trials are required, which are more difficult to organise and expensive.

- Additional ethical limitations
    — subjecting children to additional investigations or giving a new treatment is severely limited by the inability of the child to give consent. Some parents are concerned that participating in a trial could mean that their child could receive treatment that turns out to be inferior to the standard treatment and could have unknown side-effects.
    — there is concern over the ability of parents to give truly informed consent immediately after the acute onset of serious illness, e.g. the birth of a preterm infant, meningococcal septicaemia or meningitis.

- Limited investment by the pharmaceutical industry in drug trials, as drug use in children is insufficient to justify the cost and ethical difficulties of conducting trials. As a result, approximately 50% of drug treatments in children are unlicensed ('off label').

The consequence is that there is less of a culture of randomised controlled trials in paediatrics compared with adult medicine.

For evidence-based practice to become more widespread, clinicians must recognise the need to ask questions, particularly about procedures or interventions which are common practice. However, evidence-based medicine is not cookbook medicine. Incontrovertible evidence is rare, and clinical decisions complex, which is why clinical care is provided by clinicians and not technicians. Evidence-based health care cannot change this, but is an essential tool to help clinicians make rational, informed decisions together with their patients. In addition, evidence-based paediatrics provides a way for clinicians to articulate their priorities for research and thereby set a research agenda which is relevant to service needs.

Fig. 4.14 Examples of the range of evidence available in paediatrics.

---

1 Clear evidence of benefit

Surfactant therapy in preterm infants

The meta-analysis (see Fig. 9.9, p. 123) from a Cochrane systematic review shows that mortality is halved in preterm infants with respiratory distress syndrome (RDS) treated with surfactant compared with placebo.

This evidence was rapidly produced and introduced into practice as:

- respiratory distress syndrome is the commonest cause of death and disability in a neonatal intensive care unit
- there is a clearly understood disease mechanism for respiratory distress syndrome, i.e. surfactant deficiency
- the effect of surfactant treatment was immediately obvious at the cot-side – ventilator settings often have to be reduced shortly after administration
- potential benefits and side-effects could be clearly defined and identified
- neonatologists are a relatively small group of doctors who meet regularly – national and international studies could be organised and their results quickly disseminated
- there was widespread financial support and involvement from the pharmaceutical industry

2 Clear evidence but need to balance benefits and harms

Antibiotic treatment for children with otitis media

As shown in Figure 4.13, there is a balance of risk and benefits.

3 No clear evidence

Dietary manipulation in the treatment of constipation

It is often recommended that fibre in the diet in children with constipation should be increased. However, this is not based on any clear evidence. One randomised controlled trial of the effect of laxatives plus advice about dietary fibre on chronic constipation showed that this advice increased the intake of dietary fibre, but there was no significant reduction in constipation at 6 months.

Some possible reasons for the lack of evidence on how to treat this common condition are:

- constipation is not a life-threatening disorder
- the causes are multifactorial and the disease mechanism not clearly defined
- there is the belief that there are likely to be few side-effects to increasing fibre and clinicians are willing to prescribe without clear evidence
- there is no support for studies from the pharmaceutical industry
- the research agenda is not driven by such clinical problems

FURTHER READING

Audit Commission 1993 Children first. A study of hospital services. HMSO, London
Welfare of children and young people in hospital. HMSO, London, 1991
Moyer V A, Elliot E J, Davis R L et al 2000 Evidence based paediatrics and child health. BMJ Books, London
Nelson K B, Ellenberg J H 1978 Prognosis in children with febrile seizures. Pediatrics 61: 720–727

Internet

Search filters – http://www.ihs.ox.ac.uk/library/filters.html

5

Paediatric emergencies

There are few situations that provoke greater anxiety than being called to see a child who is seriously ill. This chapter outlines a basic approach to the emergency management of seriously ill children.

THE SERIOUSLY ILL CHILD

The rapid clinical assessment of the seriously ill child will identify if he is in potential respiratory, circulatory or neurological failure (Fig. 5.1). This should take less

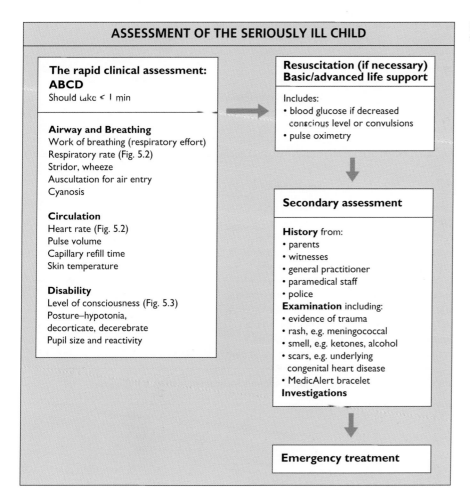

Fig. 5.1 Assessment of the seriously ill child.

ASSESSMENT OF THE SERIOUSLY ILL CHILD

The rapid clinical assessment: ABCD
Should take < 1 min

Airway and Breathing
Work of breathing (respiratory effort)
Respiratory rate (Fig. 5.2)
Stridor, wheeze
Auscultation for air entry
Cyanosis

Circulation
Heart rate (Fig. 5.2)
Pulse volume
Capillary refill time
Skin temperature

Disability
Level of consciousness (Fig. 5.3)
Posture—hypotonia, decorticate, decerebrate
Pupil size and reactivity

Resuscitation (if necessary)
Basic/advanced life support

Includes:
- blood glucose if decreased conscious level or convulsions
- pulse oximetry

Secondary assessment

History from:
- parents
- witnesses
- general practitioner
- paramedical staff
- police

Examination including:
- evidence of trauma
- rash, e.g. meningococcal
- smell, e.g. ketones, alcohol
- scars, e.g. underlying congenital heart disease
- MedicAlert bracelet

Investigations

Emergency treatment

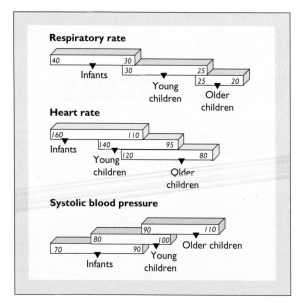

than 1 min. Resuscitation is given immediately if necessary, followed by secondary assessment and emergency treatment.

The four main modes of presentation of serious illness in children are shown in Figure 5.5. In children, the key to a successful outcome is the early recognition and active management of conditions that are potentially life-threatening.

Fig. 5.2 Variation in the normal range for respiratory rate, heart rate and systolic blood pressure with age

Fig. 5.3 Rapid assessment of level of consciousness. A more detailed evaluation is with the Glasgow Coma Scale (Fig. 5.4).	
A	ALERT
V	Responds to VOICE
P	Responds to PAIN
U	UNRESPONSIVE

Fig. 5.4 Glasgow Coma Scale, incorporating the Children's Coma Scale.

	Glasgow Coma Scale (4–15 years)	Children's Coma Scale (<4 years)	
	Response	**Response**	**Score**
Eyes	Open spontaneously	Open spontaneously	4
	Verbal command	React to speech	3
	Pain	React to pain	2
	No response	No response	1
Best motor response			
Verbal command	Obeys	Spontaneous or obeys verbal command	6
Painful stimulus	Localises pain	Localises pain	5
	Withdraws	Withdraws	4
	Abnormal flexion	Abnormal flexion (decorticate posture)	3
	Extension	Abnormal extension (decerebrate posture)	2
	No response	No response	1
Best verbal response	Orientated and converses	Smiles, orientated to sounds, follows objects, interacts	5
	Disorientated and converses	Fewer than usual words, spontaneous irritable cry	4
	Inappropriate words	Cries only to pain	3
	Incomprehensible sounds	Moans to pain	2
	No response	No response to pain	1

A score of < 8 out of 15 means that the airway must be secured and mechanical ventilation is initiated.

Fig. 5.5 The four main modes of clinical presentation of serious illness in children.

Shock		**Surgical emergencies**	
Hypovolaemia	Dehydration – gastroenteritis, diabetic ketoacidosis Blood loss – trauma Plasma loss – burns, nephrotic syndrome	*Acute abdomen*	Appendicitis, peritonitis
		Intestinal obstruction	Intussusception, malrotation
Maldistribution of fluid	Septicaemia Anaphylaxis Bowel obstruction	**The drowsy/unconscious or fitting child** *Post-ictal/status epilepticus*	
		Infection	Meningitis, encephalitis
Cardiogenic	Arrhythmias Heart failure	*Metabolic*	Diabetic ketoacidosis, hypoglycaemia, electrolyte disturbances (calcium, magnesium, sodium), inborn errors of metabolism
Respiratory distress			
Upper airway obstruction (stridor)	Croup (laryngotracheobronchitis), epiglottitis Foreign body Congenital malformations Trauma	*Head injury*	Trauma, non-accidental injury
		Drug/poison ingestion	
Lower airway disorders	Asthma Bronchiolitis Pneumonia Pneumothorax	*Intracranial haemorrhage*	

CARDIOPULMONARY RESUSCITATION

In adults, cardiopulmonary arrest is often cardiac in origin, secondary to ischaemic heart disease. In contrast, children usually have healthy hearts but experience hypoxia from respiratory or neurological failure or shock. If this occurs, irrespective of the cause, basic life support must be started immediately.

 Basic life support (Figs 5.6–5.8)

 Advanced life support (Fig. 5.9)

Children who have been resuscitated successfully should be transferred to a paediatric high-dependency or intensive care unit.

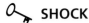 ## THE SERIOUSLY INJURED CHILD

Management of the seriously injured child must allow for potential injury to the cervical spine and other bones and internal injuries (Fig. 5.10)

SHOCK

Shock is present when the circulation is inadequate to meet the demands of the tissues. Critically ill children are often in shock, usually because of hypovolaemia due to fluid loss or maldistribution of fluid, as occurs in sepsis or intestinal obstruction.

The clinical features of shock are due to compensatory physiological mechanisms to maintain the circulation and the direct effects of poor perfusion of tissues and organs. In early compensated shock, the blood pressure is maintained by increased heart and respiratory rates and diversion of blood flow from nonessential tissues such as the skin in the peripheries, which become cold. In late or uncompensated shock, there is failure of compensatory mechanisms, with a fall in blood pressure and increasing acidosis from anaerobic respiration. It is important to recognise early, compensated shock, as this is reversible, in contrast to uncompensated shock, which may be irreversible.

Why are children so susceptible to fluid loss?

Children normally require a much higher fluid intake per kg body weight than adults (Fig. 5.11). This is because they have a higher surface area to volume ratio and a higher basal metabolic rate. Children may therefore become dehydrated if:

- they are unable to take oral fluids
- there are additional fluid losses due to fever, diarrhoea or increased insensible losses (e.g. due to increased sweating or tachypnoea)
- there is loss of the normal fluid-retaining mechanisms, e.g. burns, the permeable skin of premature infants, or increased urinary losses.

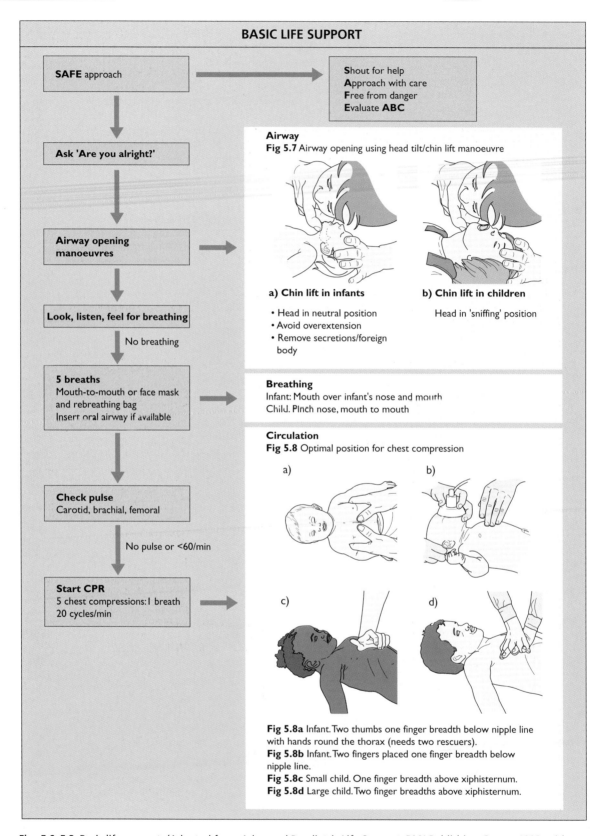

BASIC LIFE SUPPORT

SAFE approach → **S**hout for help / **A**pproach with care / **F**ree from danger / **E**valuate **ABC**

Ask 'Are you alright?'

Airway opening manoeuvres

Look, listen, feel for breathing — No breathing

5 breaths
Mouth-to-mouth or face mask and rebreathing bag
Insert oral airway if available

Check pulse
Carotid, brachial, femoral — No pulse or <60/min

Start CPR
5 chest compressions:1 breath
20 cycles/min

Airway
Fig 5.7 Airway opening using head tilt/chin lift manoeuvre

a) Chin lift in infants
- Head in neutral position
- Avoid overextension
- Remove secretions/foreign body

b) Chin lift in children
Head in 'sniffing' position

Breathing
Infant: Mouth over infant's nose and mouth
Child: Pinch nose, mouth to mouth

Circulation
Fig 5.8 Optimal position for chest compression

a) b) c) d)

Fig 5.8a Infant. Two thumbs one finger breadth below nipple line with hands round the thorax (needs two rescuers).
Fig 5.8b Infant. Two fingers placed one finger breadth below nipple line.
Fig 5.8c Small child. One finger breadth above xiphisternum.
Fig 5.8d Large child. Two finger breadths above xiphisternum.

Figs 5.6–5.8 Basic life support. (Adapted from *Advanced Paediatric Life Support*, BMJ Publishing Group, 1993, with permission.)

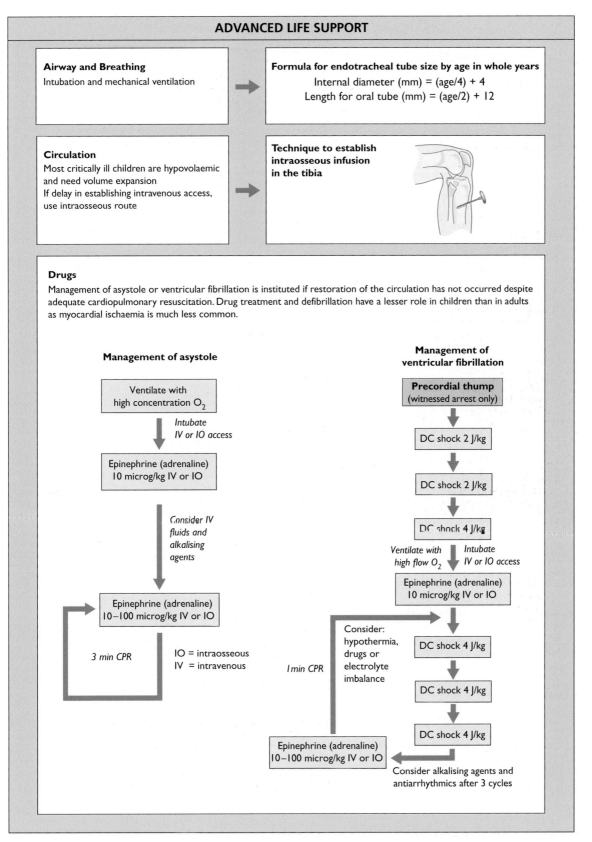

Fig. 5.9 Advanced life support. Management of asystole and ventricular fibrillation. (Adapted from *Advanced Paediatric Life Support*, BMJ Publishing Group, London, 1993, with permission.)

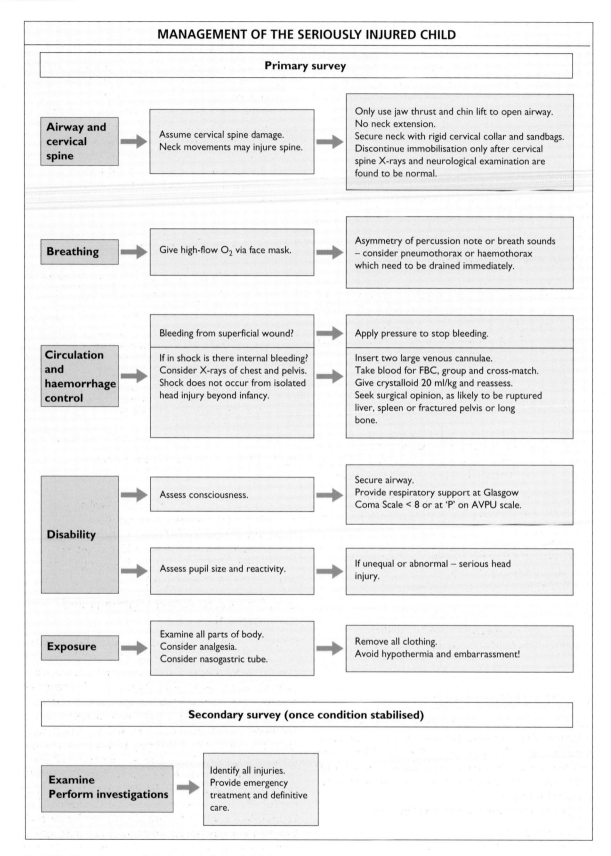

MANAGEMENT OF THE SERIOUSLY INJURED CHILD

Primary survey

Airway and cervical spine
→ Assume cervical spine damage. Neck movements may injure spine.
→ Only use jaw thrust and chin lift to open airway. No neck extension. Secure neck with rigid cervical collar and sandbags. Discontinue immobilisation only after cervical spine X-rays and neurological examination are found to be normal.

Breathing
→ Give high-flow O₂ via face mask.
→ Asymmetry of percussion note or breath sounds – consider pneumothorax or haemothorax which need to be drained immediately.

Circulation and haemorrhage control
→ Bleeding from superficial wound?
→ Apply pressure to stop bleeding.
→ If in shock is there internal bleeding? Consider X-rays of chest and pelvis. Shock does not occur from isolated head injury beyond infancy.
→ Insert two large venous cannulae. Take blood for FBC, group and cross-match. Give crystalloid 20 ml/kg and reassess. Seek surgical opinion, as likely to be ruptured liver, spleen or fractured pelvis or long bone.

Disability
→ Assess consciousness.
→ Secure airway. Provide respiratory support at Glasgow Coma Scale < 8 or at 'P' on AVPU scale.
→ Assess pupil size and reactivity.
→ If unequal or abnormal – serious head injury.

Exposure
→ Examine all parts of body. Consider analgesia. Consider nasogastric tube.
→ Remove all clothing. Avoid hypothermia and embarrassment!

Secondary survey (once condition stabilised)

Examine Perform investigations
→ Identify all injuries. Provide emergency treatment and definitive care.

Fig. 5.10 Management of the seriously injured child.

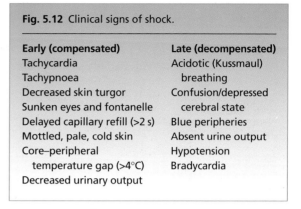

Fig. 5.11 Fluid intake at different ages.

Age	Fluid intake
Infants (> 4 weeks)	100–120 ml/kg per 24 h
Children (1–2 years)	90–120 ml/kg per 24 h
Children (2–15 years)	50–90 ml/kg per 24 h
Adult	20–35 ml/kg per 24 h

Fig. 5.12 Clinical signs of shock.

Early (compensated)	Late (decompensated)
Tachycardia	Acidotic (Kussmaul)
Tachypnoea	breathing
Decreased skin turgor	Confusion/depressed
Sunken eyes and fontanelle	cerebral state
Delayed capillary refill (>2 s)	Blue peripheries
Mottled, pale, cold skin	Absent urine output
Core–peripheral	Hypotension
temperature gap (>4°C)	Bradycardia
Decreased urinary output	

Clinical features (Fig. 5.12)

In shock due to dehydration, there is usually >10% loss of body weight (see Ch. 12). There is a profound metabolic acidosis.

Management priorities

Fluid resuscitation

Rapid restoration of the intravascular circulating volume is the priority (Fig. 5.13). This will usually be with 0.9% saline or blood if following trauma. Colloid solutions, e.g. 4.5% albumin, may be preferable for conditions with increased capillary permeability, e.g. sepsis, but there is controversy regarding the most appropriate fluid to use.

Subsequent management

If there is no improvement following fluid resuscitation, or progression of shock to multi-organ failure, involvement with and then transfer to a paediatric intensive care unit should be arranged as the child will need:

- tracheal intubation and mechanical ventilation
- invasive monitoring including central venous and arterial pressure
- inotropic support
- correction of haematological, biochemical and metabolic derangements
- support for renal or liver failure.

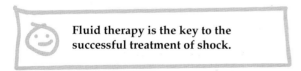

Fluid therapy is the key to the successful treatment of shock.

THE FEBRILE CHILD

Most febrile children have a brief, self-limiting viral infection. Mild localised infections, e.g. otitis media or tonsillitis, may be diagnosed clinically. The clinical problem lies in identifying the relatively few children with a serious invasive bacterial infection which needs prompt treatment.

Factors which need to be considered are:

- past medical history
- illness of other family members
- if a specific illness is prevalent in the community
- immunisation status

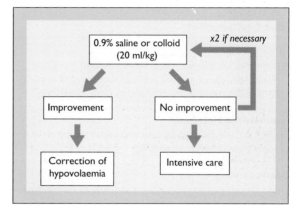

Fig. 5.13 Initial fluid resuscitation in shock.

- recent travel abroad, e.g. malaria, typhoid
- contact with animals, e.g. brucellosis
- predisposition to infection, e.g. nephrotic syndrome, sickle cell disease, HIV infection, chemotherapy for malignant disease or, rarely, a primary immunodeficiency.

Initial assessment, investigations and management

Some diagnostic clues to evaluating the febrile child are shown in Figures 5.14 and 15. Infants and toddlers often present with non-specific signs. If they are suspected of having a severe bacterial infection, urgent investigation called a septic screen (Fig. 5.16) is performed and intravenous antibiotic therapy given immediately to avoid the illness becoming more severe and to prevent rapid spread to other sites of the body. In febrile infants less than 2 months old, identifying serious bacterial infection is unreliable from clinical examination alone, and a septic screen and antibiotic therapy are indicated. Other factors which influence the selection of which children to investigate and treat are shown in Figure 5.17. Children who are not seriously ill can be managed at home with regular review by the parents as long as they are given clear instructions about what clinical features should prompt reassessment by a doctor.

Fig. 5.14 Some diagnostic clues to evaluating the febrile child.

Upper respiratory tract infection
Very common, may be coincidental with another more serious illness

Otitis media
Always examine tympanic membranes in febrile children

Tonsillitis
Erythema or exudate on the tonsils

Stridor
Epiglottitis?
Viral croup?
Bacterial tracheitis?

Pneumonia
In infants, only raised respiratory rate and increased respiratory effort may be present, with no abnormality on auscultation – diagnosis may require chest X-ray

Urinary tract infection
Urine sample needed for any seriouly ill young child or any febrile illness that does not settle

Septicaemia
Can be difficult to recognise in absence of rash before shock develops
Need to start antibiotics on clinical suspicion without waiting for culture results

Meningitis/encephalitis
Lethargy, loss of interest in surroundings, drowsiness/unconscious/seizures?
Neck stiffness, arching of the back, bulging fontanelle, positive Kernig's sign (pain on leg straightening)?
Only non-specific symptoms and signs may be present in young children (<18 months)

Osteomyelitis or septic arthritis
Suspect if painful bone or joint or reluctance to move limb

Periorbital cellulitis
Redness and swelling of the eyelids.
May spread to orbit of the eye

Rash
Viral exanthem?
Purpura from meningococcal infection (Fig. 5.15)?

Abdominal pain
Appendicitis?
Pyelonephritis?
Hepatitis?

Diarrhoea
Gastroenteritis?
Fever with blood and mucus in the stool:
Shigella, *Salmonella*, or *Campylobacter*?

Seizure
Febrile convulsion?
Meningitis?
Encephalitis?

Prolonged fever
Bacterial infection, e.g. UTI, bacterial endocarditis
Other infections – viral, fungal, protozoal
Kawasaki's disease
Drug reaction
Malignant disease
Connective tissue disorder (e.g. Still's disease)

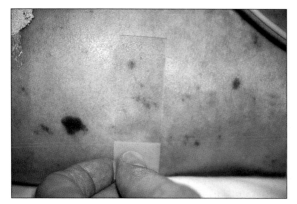

Fig. 5.15 The glass test for meningococcal purpura. Parents are advised to suspect meningococcal disease if their child is febrile and has a rash that does not blanche when pressed under a glass. (Courtesy of Dr Parviz Habibi.)

Fig. 5.16 Septic screen.

Full blood count including differential white cell count
Blood culture
Acute-phase reactant, e.g. C-reactive protein
Urine for microscopy, culture and sensitivity
CSF (unless contraindicated) for microscopy, culture and sensitivity
Chest X-ray

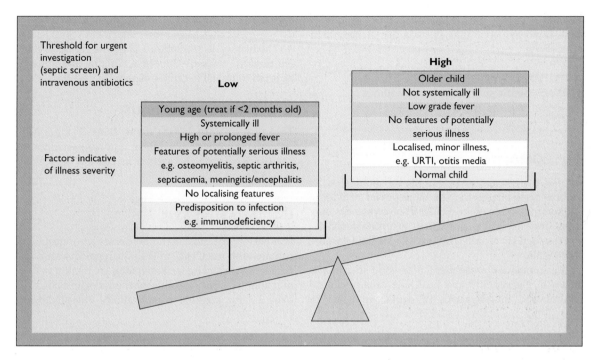

Fig. 5.17 Evaluation of the need for urgent investigation and treatment in the febrile child.

⚷ SEPTICAEMIA

Bacteria may cause a focal infection or proliferate in the bloodstream, leading to septicaemia. In septicaemia, the host response includes the release of inflammatory cytokines and activation of endothelial cells which may lead to septic shock. The commonest cause of septic shock in childhood is meningococcal infection, which may or may not be accompanied by meningitis. *Pneumococcus* is the commonest organism causing bacteraemia, but it is unusual for it to cause septic shock. In neonates, the commonest causes of septicaemia are group B streptococcus or coliforms acquired from the birth canal.

Clinical features

See Figure 5.18.

Management priorities

Children with septic shock will need to be rapidly stabilised and may require transfer to a paediatric intensive care unit.

Antibiotics

Choice depends on the child's age and any predisposition to infection.

Fluids

Significant hypovolaemia is often present, due to fluid maldistribution, which occurs due to the release of vasoactive mediators by host inflammatory and endothelial cells. There is loss of intravascular proteins and fluid which may occur due to the development of a 'capillary leak' caused by endothelial cell dysfunction.

Fig. 5.18 Clinical features of septicaemia.

History	Examination
Fever	Fever
Poor feeding	Purpuric rash
Miserable	(meningococcal
Lethargy	septicaemia)
History of focal infection,	Irritability
e.g. meningitis, osteomyelitis,	Shock
gastroenteritis, cellulitis	Multi-organ
Predisposing conditions,	failure
e.g. sickle cell disease,	
immunodeficiency	

Circulating plasma volume is lost into the interstitial fluid. Central venous pressure monitoring and urinary catheterisation may be required to guide the assessment of fluid balance. Capillary leak into the lungs causes pulmonary oedema, which may lead to respiratory failure, necessitating mechanical ventilation.

Circulatory support

Myocardial dysfunction occurs as inflammatory cytokines and circulating toxins depress myocardial contractility. Inotropic support may be required.

Disseminated intravascular coagulation (DIC)

Abnormal blood clotting causes widespread microvascular thrombosis and consumption of clotting factors. If bleeding occurs, clotting derangement should be corrected with fresh frozen plasma and platelet transfusions.

Steroids

There is no evidence that steroids are of benefit in septic shock.

 Septic shock may occur without meningitis.

COMA

In coma, there is disturbance of the functioning of the cerebral hemispheres and/or the reticular activating system of the brain stem. The level of awareness may range from excessive drowsiness to unconsciousness. It is assessed by rapidly using AVPU or the Glasgow Coma Scale.

The immediate assessment of a child in coma is shown in Figures 5.19 and 5.20. The causes, clinical features and investigations of coma are listed in Figure 5.21. In contrast to adults, most children have a diffuse metabolic insult rather than a structural lesion.

The history, examination and investigation of coma are directed towards the cause. Treatment should be directed to treatable causes, especially infection.

STATUS EPILEPTICUS

This is a seizure lasting more than 30 min. After immediate primary assessment and resuscitation, the priority is to stop the seizure as quickly as possible (Fig. 5.22).

ANAPHYLAXIS

In children, the most common causes are ingestion or contact with nuts, egg, milk and drugs. Urticaria and angioedema causing facial swelling are treated with an oral antihistamine (e.g. chlorphenamine) and observed over 2 h for possible complications. Anaphylaxis is

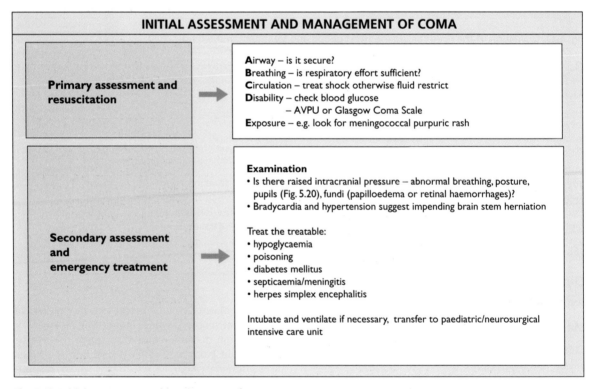

Fig. 5.19 Initial assessment and management of coma.

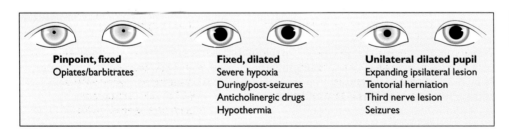

Fig. 5.20 Pupillary signs in coma.

Fig. 5.21 Causes, history and examination, and investigation of coma.

Cause	History and examination	Diagnostic investigations
Infection Meningitis Meningoencephalitis	Fever Irritability, lethargy, drowsiness Poor feeding Rash, e.g. meningococcal purpura Seizures Overseas travel	Full blood count Culture of blood, urine, infected sites, CSF (unless contraindicated) for bacteria and viruses Acute-phase reactant Rapid bacterial antigen/PCR tests for organisms
Metabolic Diabetes mellitus	Previously diagnosed diabetes mellitus Diabetic ketoacidosis	Blood glucose, plasma electrolytes Urine for glucose and ketones Blood gas analysis
Inborn errors of metabolism	Previous history of loss of consciousness Sudden collapse Consanguinity Developmental delay Death or illness of siblings Hepatomegaly	Blood glucose Blood gas analysis Blood ammonia, lactate Urine amino and organic acids Plasma amino acids
Hepatic failure	Jaundice Abnormal bleeding	Abnormal liver function tests Prolonged prothrombin time
Acute renal failure	Oliguria Hypertension	Abnormal creatinine
Hypoglycaemia	Any acutely ill child Known diabetes mellitus Sudden onset of coma	Low blood glucose
Poisoning	Accidental – poison usually identified Deliberate – tablets may be found, also illicit drugs and alcohol	Toxicology screen Plasma level for paracetamol and salicylates
Status epilepticus or post-ictal	Past history of seizures Neurocutaneous lesions on the skin Developmental delay Ongoing seizure activity, e.g. abnormal eye movements Focal neurological signs	Blood glucose Electrolytes – sodium, potassium, calcium, magnesium Drug levels if on anticonvulsants EEG CT scan
Trauma – accidental/ non-accidental	History of road traffic accident, fall, etc. Bruising, haemorrhage Fractures – cervical spine, etc. Focal neurology Retinal haemorrhages	Radiological – plain X-rays or CT/MRI scans
Intracranial tumour or haemorrhage/infarct/ abscess	Raised intracranial pressure: • headache worse on lying down • early morning vomiting • focal neurological signs, e.g. squint, ataxia • personality change • papilloedema/retinal haemorrhage • hypertension	Cranial CT/MRI scan Coagulation screen Screen for procoagulant disorders (protein C and S deficiency) Echocardiogram to exclude infective endocarditis
Hypertension	Symptoms and signs of raised intracranial pressure Fundoscopy – hypertensive changes	High blood pressure Left ventricular hypertrophy on ECG or echocardiography Creatinine and electrolytes

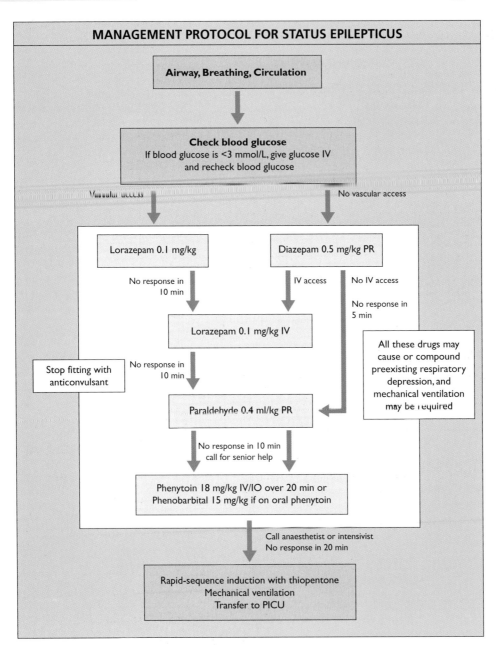

Fig. 5.22 Management protocol for status epilepticus. (Adapted from *Advanced Paediatric Life Support*, BMJ Publishing Group, London, 2001)

life-threatening, from laryngeal oedema, brochoconstriction and shock. Its management is outlined in Figure 5.23.

APPARENT LIFE-THREATENING EVENTS (ALTE)

These occur in infants and are a combination of apnoea, colour change, alteration in muscle tone, choking or gagging, which are frightening to the observer. They may occur on more than one occasion. The relationship of these episodes to sudden infant death syndrome (SIDS) is unclear and the risk of this subsequently occurring is very low. However, ALTEs may be the presentation of a potentially serious disorder, although often no cause is identified.

Management revolves around a detailed history and thorough examination to identify problems with the baby or in care-giving. The infant should be admitted to hospital. Causes and investigations to be considered are listed in Figure 5.24. Multi-channel overnight monitoring is usually indicated.

In most, the episode is brief, with rapid recovery, and the baby is well clinically. Baseline investigations and overnight monitoring of oxygen saturation, respiration and ECG are found to be normal. The parents should be taught resuscitation and will find it helpful to receive follow-up from a specialist paediatric nurse and paediatrician.

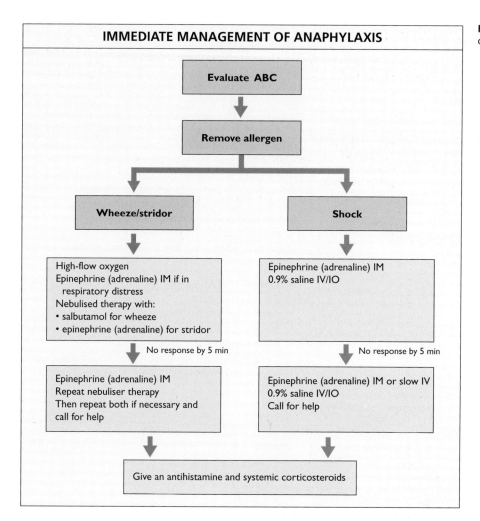

IMMEDIATE MANAGEMENT OF ANAPHYLAXIS

Evaluate ABC

Remove allergen

Wheeze/stridor

Shock

High-flow oxygen
Epinephrine (adrenaline) IM if in
 respiratory distress
Nebulised therapy with:
• salbutamol for wheeze
• epinephrine (adrenaline) for stridor

Epinephrine (adrenaline) IM
0.9% saline IV/IO

No response by 5 min

No response by 5 min

Epinephrine (adrenaline) IM
Repeat nebuliser therapy
Then repeat both if necessary and
call for help

Epinephrine (adrenaline) IM or slow IV
0.9% saline IV/IO
Call for help

Give an antihistamine and systemic corticosteroids

Fig. 5.23 Management
of anaphylaxis.

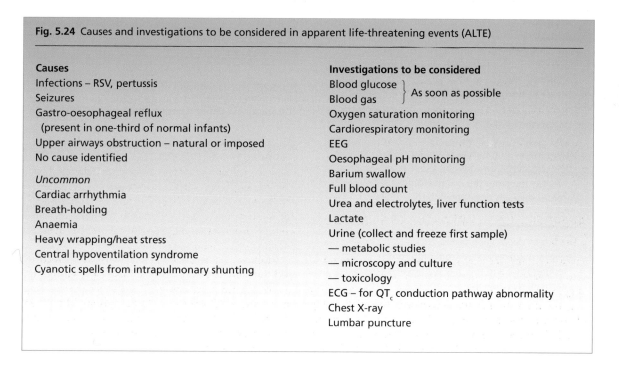

Fig. 5.24 Causes and investigations to be considered in apparent life-threatening events (ALTE)

Causes	Investigations to be considered
Infections – RSV, pertussis	Blood glucose ⎱ As soon as possible
Seizures	Blood gas ⎰
Gastro-oesophageal reflux (present in one-third of normal infants)	Oxygen saturation monitoring
Upper airways obstruction – natural or imposed	Cardiorespiratory monitoring
No cause identified	EEG
	Oesophageal pH monitoring
Uncommon	Barium swallow
Cardiac arrhythmia	Full blood count
Breath-holding	Urea and electrolytes, liver function tests
Anaemia	Lactate
Heavy wrapping/heat stress	Urine (collect and freeze first sample)
Central hypoventilation syndrome	— metabolic studies
Cyanotic spells from intrapulmonary shunting	— microscopy and culture
	— toxicology
	ECG – for QT_c conduction pathway abnormality
	Chest X-ray
	Lumbar puncture

Detailed specialist investigation and assessment will be required if clinical, biochemical or physiological abnormalities are identified.

THE DEATH OF A CHILD

The most common causes of unexpected death in infants are sudden infant death syndrome (SIDS) and undiagnosed congenital abnormalities, such as congenital heart disease. In older children, road traffic or other accidents, malignant disease and acute infections such as meningococcal disease are the main causes.

Sudden infant death syndrome

This is defined as the sudden and unexpected death of an infant or young child for which no adequate cause is found after a thorough postmortem examination. Sudden unexpected death from undiagnosed inherited metabolic disorders (e.g. the fatty acid oxidation defects, medium chain acyl-CoA dehydrogenase deficiency) is rare. Although death by suffocation by parents has received considerable attention in the medical literature and media, it is uncommon.

There is marked variation in the incidence of SIDS in different countries, suggesting that environmental factors are important (Fig. 5.25). SIDS occurs most commonly at 2–4 months of age (Fig. 5.26). The risk for subsequent children is slightly increased.

In the UK, the incidence of SIDS has fallen dramatically during the last few years (Fig. 5.27), coinciding with a national 'Back to Sleep' campaign advocating that infants should be put to sleep on their back (not their front or side), to avoid overheating by heavy wrapping and high room temperature, and that parents should not smoke near their infants.

A recent, large epidemiological study in the UK has suggested additional, less important, possible preventative measures to minimise the risk of SIDS:

- parents to share their bedroom with the baby for the first 6 months
- parents to avoid bringing the baby into their bed when they are tired or have taken alcohol, sedative medicines or illicit drugs
- parents to avoid sleeping with their infant on a sofa, settee or armchair.

Fig. 5.25 Factors associated with SIDS (based on data from Fleming P et al, Sudden unexpected deaths in infancy, The Stationery Office, London, 2000, with permission.)

The infant
Age 1–6 months, peak at 12 weeks
Low birthweight and preterm (but 60% are normal birthweight term infants)
Sex (boys 60%)
Multiple births

The parents
Low income[a]
Poor or overcrowded housing
Maternal age (mother aged <20 years has three times the risk of a mother aged 25–29 years, but 80% of affected mothers are >20 years old)[a]
Single unsupported mother (twice the rate of supported mothers)
High maternal parity[a]
Maternal smoking during pregnancy (1–9 cigarettes/day doubles the risk: >20/day increases the risk fivefold)[a]
Parental smoking after baby's birth

The environment
The infant sleeps lying prone
The infant is overheated from high room temperature and too may clothes and covers, particularly when ill

---

[a]Three of these four factors are present in over 40% of SIDS, but only 8% of control families.

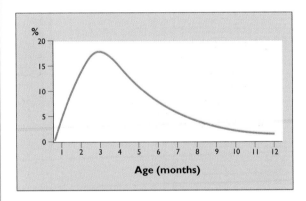

Fig. 5.26 Age distribution of SIDS (based on data from Fleming P et al, Sudden unexpected deaths in infancy, The Stationery Office, London, 2000, with permission.)

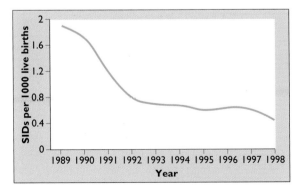

Fig. 5.27 Decline in the number of deaths from SIDS in the UK from 1.9/1000 live births in 1989 to 0.46 in 1998.

Sudden infant death syndrome (SIDS) is the commonest cause of death in children aged 1 month to 1 year.

Following the sudden death of a child

The sudden death of a child is one of the most distressing events that can happen to a family. If close family members are absent, arrangements should be made for them to come, if this is possible. The family should be spoken to sympathetically and in private (see Ch. 3).

Most parents will wish to see and hold their dead child and should be offered the opportunity to do this. This should be encouraged as it helps them accept the reality of their child's death. Even if the child has visible injuries, parents should be supported in seeing their child as their fantasies in the future are usually worse than the reality. They may wish to see the child again within the next few days. The family may wish a minister of religion to be called.

For unexpected deaths in the UK, the coroner has to be notified and will arrange for a postmortem to be performed. The parents should be informed of this, and that details will automatically be forwarded to the police, who will conduct their own inquiry, including interviewing the parents and whoever was looking after the child at the time of death. The parents need to know that this does not imply that they are being blamed or are otherwise responsible for their child's death. The general practitioner, health visitor and other relevant health professionals should be informed and any appointments for the health clinic or hospital cancelled.

Parents should be given written information about the condition from which the child has died, e.g. SIDS, meningococcal disease, and given advice concerning talking about the death to siblings and other family members.

Follow-up should be arranged to provide the family with an opportunity to discuss the results of the postmortem and, when appropriate, consider its implications for future pregnancies. Genetic counselling may be indicated.

The grief following the sudden death of a child will profoundly affect all the members of the family. Bereavement counselling is increasingly available from health professionals in the community or hospital. Parents should be given information about bereavement support from other agencies, e.g. in the UK, the Foundation for the Study of Infant Deaths, Child Death Helpline and CRUSE.

FURTHER READING

Advanced paediatric life support. The practical approach. BMJ Publishing Group, London, 2001. *The core text for the Advanced Paediatric Life Support (UK) course*

Fleming P, Blair P, Bacon C, Berry J 2000 Sudden unexpected deaths in infancy. The Stationery Office, London

Goldman A 1994 Care of the dying child. Oxford Medical Publications, Oxford. *Medical, psychological and practical issues of caring for terminally ill children and their families*

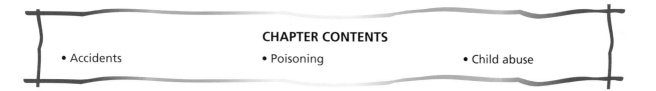

6

Environment

Children need a safe, healthy and nurturing environment to achieve their full potential. Environmental hazards include accidents, poisons and abuse. As far as possible, children should be protected from harm. This is mainly the responsibility of parents and families, but doctors, other professionals and society also play a role. The risk of environmental hazards is increased by:

• poverty
• poor quality, overcrowded homes
• poor parenting skills, which may be due to parental psychiatric illness, violent temperament, poor education or lack of social support.

ACCIDENTS

Accidents (now often called 'unintentional injuries') are extremely common. In the UK, 1 in 4 children attend an accident and emergency (A&E) department each year; about half because of an accident. Most accidents cause only minor injury but some are fatal. Accidents are by far the most common cause of death in children over a year of age (Figs 6.1 and 6.2) and also cause significant disability and suffering, including post-traumatic stress disorders. Head injury with brain damage is the major cause of disability from accidents. Cosmetic damage following burns, scalds and other accidents may cause the child profound psychological harm.

 Accidents are the commonest cause of death in children over a year of age.

Types of accidents affecting children

The type of accident affecting a child depends on the child's age and stage of development. Toddlers constantly explore their immediate environment, usually the home, and are unaware of the consequences of their actions. They are prone to falls, scalds, ingestion of potentially harmful substances and may drown in

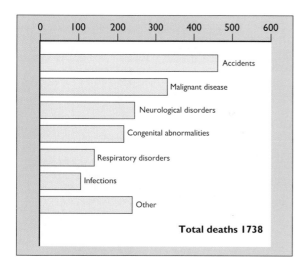

Fig. 6.1 Causes of death in children aged 1–14 years in England and Wales (1997).

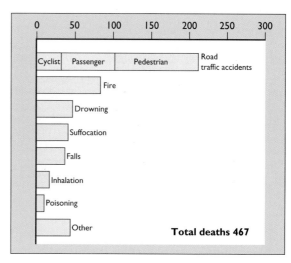

Fig. 6.2 Causes of fatal accidents in children in England and Wales (1997). The most common cause is road traffic accidents.

the bath, ponds or pools. Most serious accidents in babies and toddlers can be anticipated by an observant adult and prevented by vigilant supervision. Older children experience a different range of accidents, mainly as pedestrians or cyclists, while playing sport or from falls while climbing.

 ### Accident prevention

The prevention of childhood accidents is clearly important. Doctors who treat children and see the effects of accidents are particularly well placed to provide the community with advice on appropriate preventive measures (Fig. 6.3). In order to prevent accidents:

- the relationship between an individual type of accident and the child's developmental level must be considered
- specific solutions based on detailed epidemiology (e.g. child-resistant containers for medicines) are more successful than health education
- changes backed by legislation are the most successful.

> **The number of children killed in accidents has declined markedly.**

Road traffic accidents

Road traffic accidents (RTAs) are the most common cause of accidental death in childhood and can be divided into several types.

Pedestrian road traffic accidents

Children's involvement in road traffic accidents is mostly as pedestrians. Boys between the ages of 5 and 9 years are at maximum risk, particularly after school. Children are unable to estimate the speed or dangers of traffic and to foresee dangerous situations. Although it is important to make children aware of the dangers, education about road safety has proved to be of little value in reducing the number of accidents. Primary prevention is required, modifying the environment.

Child passengers in cars

Unrestrained children become missiles inside cars during crashes, even at low speeds. There is good evidence that child restraint systems prevent injury and death.

Bicycle accidents

Bicycle accidents are common during childhood. A boy has a 1 in 80 chance of having a cycling-related head injury severe enough to warrant admission to hospital during childhood.

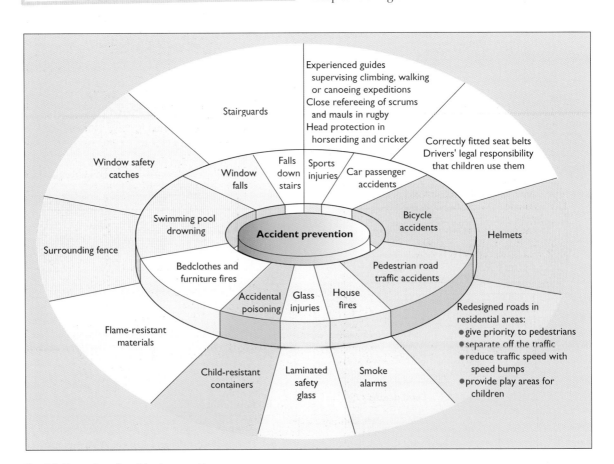

Fig. 6.3 Examples of accident prevention.

Head injuries

Minor head injuries in childhood are common, and the vast majority of children recover without suffering any ill effect. However, about 1 in 800 of these children develop serious problems. The aim of the management of head injuries is to identify those children requiring treatment and to avoid secondary damage to the brain from hypoxia or poor cerebral perfusion

(Fig. 6.4). In infants, as their skull sutures have not fused, their cranial volume may increase from an extradural or subdural bleed before neurological signs or symptoms develop. Their haemoglobin concentration may fall and they may become shocked. In infants and young children, unexplained head injuries may result from child abuse. The presence of retinal haemorrhages is highly suggestive of a shaking injury or severe trauma.

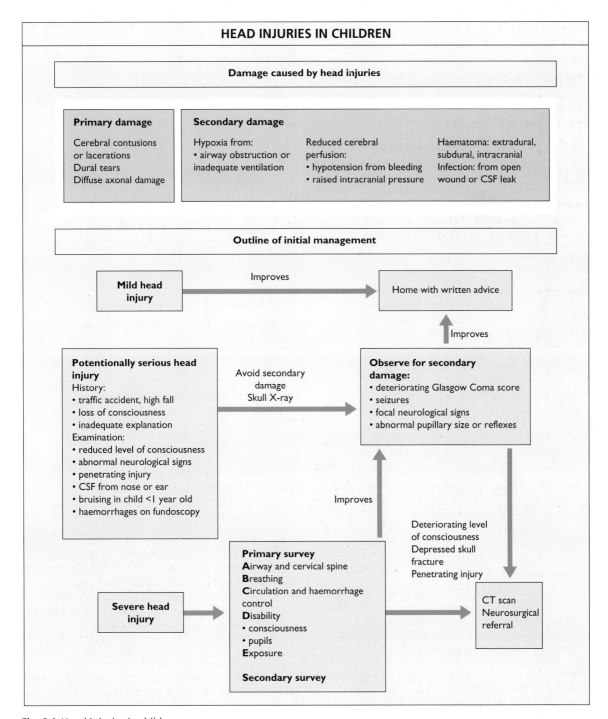

Fig. 6.4 Head injuries in children.

Internal injuries

Children may suffer internal injuries associated with severe trauma. These include:

- Abdominal injuries, including a ruptured spleen, ruptured liver, kidney and bowel. There should be a high index of suspicion for these injuries if there has been abdominal trauma. The child needs close observation. Abdominal ultrasound and X-rays, including CT scan, may be helpful. If there is any doubt, a laparotomy is undertaken.
- Chest injuries, including pneumothorax and haemopericardium, which may require emergency treatment.

These children should be managed in a paediatric intensive care unit.

Burns and scalds

Burns and scalds are the second most common cause of death from accidents. Most of these deaths occur in house fires and are caused by gas and smoke inhalation rather than thermal injury. Scalds in toddlers are common, from knocking over cups of hot liquid or grabbing the handle of a saucepan of boiling water on a cooker, or from bath water which is too hot.

Management

The severity of the injury is assessed:

- *Was there any smoke inhalation?* If this has occurred, there is a danger of subsequent respiratory complications and carbon monoxide poisoning. All affected children should be observed and managed in hospital.
- *Depth of the burn.* In superficial burns, the skin will be epithelialised from surviving cells. In partial-thickness burns, there is some damage to the dermis with blistering, and the skin is pink or mottled. In deep (full-thickness) burns, the skin is destroyed down to and including the dermis and looks white or charred and is painless. Deep burns need assessment and treatment in hospital.
- *Surface area of the burn.* This should be calculated from a surface area chart (Fig. 6.5). The palm and adducted fingers cover about 1% of the body surface. Burns covering more than 10% need assessment and treatment in hospital. Involvement of more than 50% of the body surface carries a poor chance of survival.
- *Involvement of special sites.* Burns to the face may be disfiguring those to the mouth may compromise the airway from oedema, and those to the hand may cause functional loss from scarring. Burns to the perineum are prone to infection.

Treatment

This should be directed at:

- Relieving pain with the use of strong analgesics such as intravenous morphine.

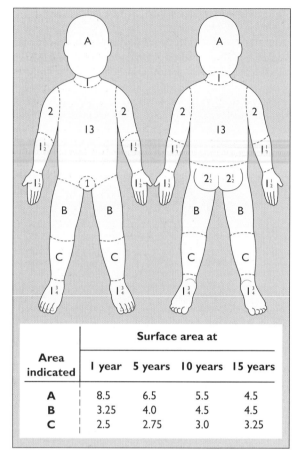

Area indicated	Surface area at			
	1 year	5 years	10 years	15 years
A	8.5	6.5	5.5	4.5
B	3.25	4.0	4.5	4.5
C	2.5	2.75	3.0	3.25

Fig. 6.5 Method of calculating the surface area of a burn (Lund and Browder chart).

- Treating shock with intravenous fluids, preferably plasma expanders, and close monitoring of haematocrit and urinary output. Children with more than 10% burns will require intravenous fluids.
- Providing wound care. Burns should be covered with sterile towels, which reduces pain from contact with cold air and reduces the risk of infection. Blisters should be left alone. Irrigation with cold water should only be used briefly to superficial or partial-thickness burns covering less than 10% of the body as it may rapidly cause excessive cooling.

Severe burns or significant burns to special sites are best dealt with in specialist units. Plastic surgeons will often need to embark on a programme of skin grafts and treatment of contractures. The psychological sequelae of severe burns are often marked and long-lasting, and appropriate psychological support is required.

Drowning and near-drowning

Drowning is the third most common cause of accidental death in children in the UK. Most victims are young children. Drowning is three times more common in boys than in girls. Warmer countries tend to have a

INHALED FOREIGN BODY

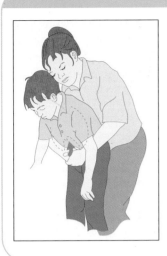

Fig. 6.6 Heimlich manoeuvre in older children to expel an inhaled foreign body. One hand is formed into a fist and placed against the child's abdomen above the umbilicus and below the xiphisternum. The other hand is placed over the fist. Both hands are thrust into the abdomen. This is repeated several times. The child can be standing, kneeling, sitting or supine.

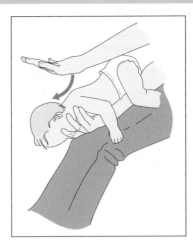

Fig. 6.7 In infants, back blows and chest thrusts are recommended to expel an inhaled foreign body.

higher incidence of drowning than in the UK. Babies may drown in the bath, toddlers may wander into domestic ponds or swimming pools, and older children may get into difficulty in swimming pools, rivers, canals, lakes and in the sea.

Near-drowning

Up to 30% of fatalities can be prevented by skilled on-site resuscitation. Even children who are unconscious with fixed dilated pupils can survive near-drowning episodes, particularly if the water is cold, due to the protective effect of hypothermia. Children who are unconscious with fixed dilated pupils should therefore be fully resuscitated until their temperature is nearly normal. Immediate management at the waterside is with mouth-to-mouth resuscitation and chest compressions. Heat loss should be prevented by covering and warming. Children who may have inhaled water should be admitted to hospital to be observed for signs of respiratory distress and cardiac arrhythmias. Some children who nearly drown aspirate water and develop a pneumonia with secondary infection. Respiratory deterioration can also occur from pulmonary oedema, between 1 and 72 h after the original incident. This is due to surfactant deficiency. It is now thought that there is no difference in outlook for fresh and salt water drowning. Severely ill children require artificial ventilation in a paediatric intensive care unit.

Choking, suffocation and strangulation

Children may choke on vomit, toys or food. Some children may strangle themselves accidentally on curtain cords, bedding and necklaces. Most are accidents but some such injuries are inflicted deliberately as a form of child abuse. Some older boys deliberately hang themselves.

In airway obstruction from an aspirated foreign body, the Heimlich manoeuvre, back blows and chest thrusts, are used in older children to expel the foreign body (Fig. 6.6). Back blows and chest thrusts alone are recommended in infants, as abdominal thrusts may cause intra-abdominal injury (Fig. 6.7).

Dog bites

One in a 100 children present to the A&E department with dog bites. Most dog bites are minor, but severe lacerations, particularly to the face, do occur particularly in the toddler age group. Dog bites usually need only simple wound toilet, but more serious injuries, particularly on the face, may need careful debridement and skilled suturing to avoid unsightly scars. Antibiotics are not usually necessary. Although there has been much publicity about fierce dog breeds such as Rottweilers attacking children in parks or public places, most attacks are by dogs known to the child.

POISONING

Poisoning in children may be:

- accidental – the vast majority
- deliberate self-poisoning in older children
- non-accidental as a form of child abuse
- iatrogenic.

Accidental poisoning

Although many thousands of young children are rushed to doctors' surgeries or hospital for urgent medical attention following accidental ingestion, fortunately most do not develop serious symptoms as they ingest only a small quantity of poison. However, a small percentage of children become seriously ill and a very few children die from poisoning each year.

Most accidental poisoning is in young children, with a peak age of 30 months. Inquisitive toddlers are unaware of the potential danger of taking medicines, household products and eating plants. Most ingestions occur in the child's own home, when supervision is inadequate.

Supervision entails not only reacting to a dangerous situation but prevention through anticipation.

The aim of management of poisoning should be to prevent unnecessary admissions to hospital while maintaining safety. There has been a marked reduction in the hospital admission rate for poisoning. Reasons for this include:

- the introduction of child-resistant containers – in the UK they must be used for paracetamol and salicylate preparations, and certain household products such as white spirit; an alternative container for tablets is opaque blister packs
- a reduction in prescribing potentially harmful medicines, e.g. aspirin and iron.

Education campaigns have not proved successful in preventing accidental child poisoning.

Management
1. Identification of the agent
Parents usually know the identity or can provide containers or tablets.

2. Assessment of the agent's toxicity (Fig. 6.8):
- low – allow home
- intermediate – observe for the recommended time, then discharge home unless symptoms develop
- high – admit to hospital.

Contact the Regional Poisons Information Centre if in doubt about a substance's identity or toxicity.

3. Removal of a poison
There is little evidence that any method is effective if used more than 1 h after ingestion. No method is required if the substance ingested is of low toxicity.

4. Activated charcoal by mouth or nasogastric tube
This is currently seen as the most effective method. It adsorbs some drugs but is ineffective for iron, hydrocarbons and insecticides. It is black, unpalatable and gritty, but may be disguised in flat cola. Aspiration causes pneumonitis.

5. Gastric lavage
This is considered only when a large quantity of a toxic drug has been taken in the previous hour. A cuffed tracheal tube must be used if the patient is drowsy.

6. Induced vomiting with ipecac
This is now rarely used except for young children in whom charcoal cannot be used and who have taken a significantly toxic substance. It is not particularly effective.

7. Specific therapy or antidotes
These are available for only a limited number of poisons (Fig. 6.9). Observation and supportive care is the mainstay of management.

8. Social assessment
This is required in order to prevent further poisoning or accidents. The general practitioner and other health professionals should be contacted.

Fig. 6.8 Potential toxicity in accidental poisoning in infants and young children with some examples.

Toxicity	Medicines	Household products	Plants
Low	Oral contraceptives, most antibiotics	Chalk and crayons, washing powder	Cyclamen, sweet pea
Intermediate	Paracetamol elixir, salbutamol	Bleach, disinfectants, window cleaners	Fuchsia, holly
High	Alcoholic drinks, digoxin, iron, salicylate, tricyclic antidepressants	Acids, alkalis, petroleum distillates, organophosphorus insecticides	Deadly nightshade, laburnum, yew

Fig. 6.9 Potentially harmful poisons.

Poison	Adverse effects	Management
Alcohol (accidental in toddlers, experimenting by older children)	Hypoglycaemia Coma Respiratory failure	Monitor blood glucose. Intravenous glucose if necessary Blood alcohol levels for severity
Acids and alkalis	Inflammation and ulceration of upper gastrointestinal tract leading to stenosis (pylorus – acids; oesophagus – alkalis)	No emesis/gastric lavage No chemical antidotes as they produce heat Early endoscopy. Steroids to suppress inflammation

Fig. 6.9 *(continued)*

Poison	Adverse effects	Management
Bleach (problems seldom arise in children)	Local lesions	No emesis. Milk/antacids orally Endoscopy to identify oesophageal inflammation if indicated Ventilatory support if required
Digoxin	Arrhythmias Hyperkalaemia	ECG monitoring Serum digoxin concentration is a guide to toxicity Purified specific Fab antibody-binding fragments if life-threatening
Disc or button batteries	Mild gastrointestinal symptoms. Oesophageal stricture with large batteries (>20 mm) Corrosion of gut wall and perforation Breaking open with release of mercury – rare	Monitor progress with chest and abdominal X-rays – almost all passed within 2 days, no symptoms Remove batteries if in oesophagus or signs of disintegration. Some authorities recommend removal if not passed within 48 h to avoid danger of disintegration
Iron	*Initial*: vomiting, diarrhoea, haematemesis, melaena, acute gastric ulceration *Latent period of improvement* *Some hours later*: drowsiness, coma, shock, liver failure with hypoglycaemia and convulsions *Long-term complications*: gastric strictures	Serious toxicity if >60 mg/kg elemental iron Abdominal X-ray to count the number of tablets Serum iron levels Gastric lavage considered in severe cases if <1 h after ingestion Intravenous desferrioxamine
Paracetamol – large ingestion uncommon in young children as tablets are difficult to swallow and elixir is too sweet	Gastric irritation Liver failure after 3–5 days	Check plasma concentration after 4 h after ingestion. If >150 mg/kg paracetamol is thought to have been taken, or the plasma concentration is high, start IV acetylcysteine Monitor prothrombin time, liver function tests and plasma creatinine
Petroleum distillates (paraffin/kerosene, white spirit)	Aspiration causing pneumonitis	Emesis contraindicated Usually no treatment required Prophylactic antibiotics and steroids to reduce inflammation – no clear evidence of benefit Aspiration – additional inspired oxygen and intensive care
Salicylates	Tinnitus, deafness, nausea, vomiting, dehydration Hyperventilation causing respiratory alkalosis Later, metabolic acidosis Hypoglycaemia Disorientation	Measure plasma salicylate concentration Gastric lavage if <1 h. Give activated charcoal. Monitor fluid and electrolyte balance. Correct dehydration, electrolyte imbalance and acidosis. Give vitamin K. Forced alkaline diuresis (difficult to achieve without fluid overload). Dialysis
Tricyclic antidepressants	Sinus tachycardia Conduction disorders Dry mouth, blurred vision Agitation, confusion, convulsions, coma Respiratory depression Hypotension	Activated charcoal if within 1 h Cardiac monitoring. Treat arrhythmias conservatively with sodium bicarbonate Correct metabolic acidosis Treat convulsions with diazepam

Deliberate poisoning in older children

These children form one end of the age spectrum of overdose in adults and are more likely to take significant amounts of poison than younger children. Substances that can be regarded as having intermediate toxicity when taken accidentally should be regarded as potentially toxic when taken deliberately. Poisoning in older children should be recognised as a serious symptom and an indication of child and family disturbance, so all children who take poisons deliberately should be assessed by a child or adolescent psychiatrist. Many will also need education or social work assessment.

Chronic poisoning

Children can be poisoned by chronic exposure to chemicals and pollutants. An example from the past is mercury poisoning from teething powders, which used to cause 'pink disease', so called because it resulted in red painful extremities. It also caused anorexia, weight loss and hypotonia. Now the commonest causes are lead ingestion and smoking.

Lead poisoning

In the past, certain paints contained lead. Children are liable to be poisoned from chewing such paintwork or from inhalation when the paint is removed. This is still a problem in parts of the USA. Lead fumes from burning batteries, lead shot for fishing and lead from old water pipes are other potential sources. Children from the Indian subcontinent may be poisoned by surma, the lead-containing eye make-up sometimes used even on young babies. Lead from vehicle exhaust fumes results in higher blood levels in children living in urban compared with rural areas. The change to unleaded petrol has been in response to concern about its potential as an environmental hazard.

Children present with pica (compulsive eating of substances other than food), anorexia, colicky abdominal pain, irritability and failure to thrive and pallor from anaemia. Severe lead poisoning may present with neurological symptoms, including drowsiness, convulsions and coma from lead encephalopathy. Raised intracranial pressure with papilloedema may be present. There is increasing evidence that chronic exposure to relatively low lead levels may be harmful to mental development.

The diagnosis is confirmed by elevated blood lead levels. There may be a hypochromic anaemia and basophil stippling of neutrophils. Radiographs of the knee or wrist may show 'lead lines', which are dense metaphyseal bands. The source of lead should be identified and removed. Chelating agents are used to form non-toxic lead compounds. In mild cases, D-penicillamine is given orally, and in severe cases sodium calcium edetate (EDTA) is indicated.

Smoking

The harmful effects of smoking are well documented, with a greatly increased risk of developing chronic bronchitis, lung cancer and cardiovascular disease. Unfortunately, many children become regular smokers while still at school. Children should be given appropriate health education, although its effectiveness is limited by the poor example set by the widespread smoking of adults. When parents or carers smoke, children have been shown to have a higher incidence of bronchitis, asthma, pneumonia and serous otitis media (glue ear). This particularly applies to babies and young children. Maternal smoking places the infant at increased risk of sudden infant death syndrome (SIDS).

> **Parents' smoking adversely affects their children's health.**

CHILD ABUSE

Children require protection and care. The concept that parents or carers might abuse their children was first recognised as a medical problem only in the 1950s. Although this caused great concern at the time, child abuse is not a new phenomenon. Children have been physically harmed, neglected and subjected to sexual abuse throughout history. What has changed is that society is no longer prepared to accept that parents or care-givers can do whatever they please to their children. Children are now afforded the right to receive recognised and accepted patterns of child care and rearing. Professionals, whether doctors, health visitors, social workers, teachers or others involved in the care of children, now have duties to ensure this. Recognising potential child abuse has to be weighed against the damage of falsely accusing parents of abusing their children. This requires fine judgment.

Types of child abuse

Initially, attention was focused on the 'battered baby', where severe physical injury was inflicted on babies. We now appreciate that in addition to inflicting physical injuries, adults may harm children in a number of different ways. These can be divided into:

- physical abuse (non-accidental injury, NAI) – bruises, burns, lacerations, fractures and internal injuries
- neglect
- emotional abuse
- sexual abuse, including the use of children for pornography
- non-accidental poisoning – where children are deliberately poisoned
- Munchausen's syndrome by proxy – where symptoms or signs of illness in the child are fabricated by the carer.

Although children may present with a single type of abuse, it is more common for children to suffer from a combination of several forms, e.g. physically abused children are often also neglected and emotionally abused. Abuse of all types is very damaging to the emotional development of the child and sexual abuse may also damage the future sexual responses of children. Intervention should aim not only to prevent further injuries but also to provide therapy for any emotional damage inflicted.

Diagnosis

The diagnosis of child abuse is based on assessing the probability that individual injuries or harm have occurred non-accidentally. Serious injuries to children are rarely the initial presentation – they are almost always preceded by minor ones. It is also known that if a particular child in the household has been subjected to abuse, further episodes are more likely to be directed towards the same child. Adults who abuse children do not usually suffer from mental illness, although alcohol, drugs and postnatal depression sometimes contribute. More often, the abuser has a personality disorder, may have experienced poor parenting and abuse as a child and is immature. Factors in the child which may predispose to abuse include disability, low birthweight, the child's age and a demanding personality.

Physical abuse

Most injuries in children follow genuine accidents and must be differentiated from those which are inflicted deliberately. They can usually be differentiated by taking a full history and examining the whole child. It is vital to try to understand exactly how an accident happened and the circumstances surrounding the event. In child abuse there may be:

- a history which is not consistent with the injury
- delay in reporting the injury
- inconsistent histories from care-givers
- inappropriate reaction of parents or care-givers who are vague, elusive, unconcerned or excessively distressed or aggressive
- recurrent injuries
- injuries inconsistent with the child's stage of development.

Presentation of physical abuse
Bruises
These are the commonest mode of presentation (Fig. 6.10a–d). Whereas bruises on the forehead and shins are common in toddlers learning to walk, they are exceptional in non-mobile babies. Bruises on the face, back and buttock are uncommon in genuine accidents.

Some patterns of bruising are suggestive of particular injuries. Bruises from fingertips gripping with excessive force are mostly on the trunk, often on either side of the spine, but may also be seen around the mouth from trying to stop a baby crying, or on the arms from shaking. Slap marks resembling handprints may be seen on the face or buttocks. Bruises may outline a particular object, e.g. a hand, belt or flex used in beating.

Head and abdominal injuries
Head injuries follow whiplash injuries or, less often, from direct blows to the head. Vigorous shaking of babies may rupture the small vessels crossing the subdural space, causing a subdural haemorrhage. There may be a similar injury if the child's head is hit against a soft object such as a bed. There may be no signs of bruising on the surface of the skull. Retinal haemorrhages are often present and are an important sign of non-accidental injury. Clinical features include

CHILD ABUSE – PHYSICAL INJURIES

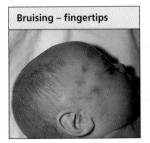

Bruising – fingertips

Fig. 6.10a Bruising from fingertips on a baby's head.

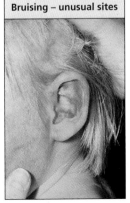

Bruising – unusual sites

Fig. 6.10b Bruising within the pinna is uncommon in accidental injury. Bruising behind the ear may be from blows to the ear.

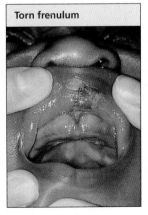

Torn frenulum

Fig. 6.10c A torn frenulum. This may be from forcing a bottle into the mouth or from a blow to the mouth.

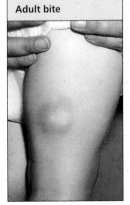

Adult bite

Fig. 6.10d A bite mark on an infant's leg. Adult bite marks may be seen in abuse, but bites from other children are not uncommon.

irritability, poor feeding, increasing head circumference, convulsions, reduced level of consciousness and a full fontanelle.

Direct blows to the head are usually less of a diagnostic problem as there is bruising and there may be an underlying skull fracture. Visceral injuries, particularly to the spleen and liver, may follow blows to the abdomen. They are uncommon and often difficult to diagnose.

Burns or scalds

It is difficult to distinguish burns and scalds inflicted deliberately from those that are accidents. Accidental hot water burns tend to be asymmetrical and spare the flexures and have splash marks. Scalds on the back are uncommon in accidents. The shape of the scald may be suggestive of its aetiology, e.g. a cigarette burn. Burns on the buttocks are unusual but may result from punishment during potty training.

Fig. 6.11 Likelihood of a fracture being due to non-accidental injury.
(Adapted from Kleinman P K, *Current Concepts: a categorical course in paediatric radiology*, SPR, 1994.)

High	Metaphyseal fractures
	Posterior rib fractures
Moderate	Multiple fractures
	Fractures of different ages
	Complex skull fracture
Low	Clavicular fractures
	Long bone shaft fractures
	Linear skull fractures

Fractures

Fractures can be categorised according to their likelihood of being caused by non-accidental injury. The most specific are fractures in infants which require violent handling or shaking (Fig. 6.11). When assessing fractures, it is the history and the child's age, mobility and development that are the crucial features in distinguishing accidental from non-accidental injuries. In infants, relatively little force is required to produce a linear skull fracture, but accidental fractures of the long bones are uncommon. In mobile children, most long-bone fractures are accidental.

Investigation

Fractures in young children may not be detectable clinically. A full radiographic skeletal survey should be performed in all infants with suspected physical abuse. Some lesions may be inconspicuous initially, but can be identified on a radionuclide bone scan or can become evident on a repeat X-ray 1–2 weeks later (Fig. 6.12a,b). In children over 1 year old, a radionuclide bone scan can be substituted for the skeletal survey. Above the age of 5 years, skeletal surveys are of limited value.

Other medical conditions which need to be considered and excluded in suspected child abuse are:

- Coagulation disorders – may result in bruising (Fig. 6.13). Occasionally abuse and a coagulation disorder may coexist.
- Osteogenesis imperfecta – predisposes to fractures. Features that characterise this uncommon condition are generalised osteoporosis, ligamentous laxity, skin fragility, blue sclerae and defective dentition. There may be a family history. Expert assessment of the X-rays is

---

CHILD ABUSE – RIB FRACTURES

Rib fractures – X-ray

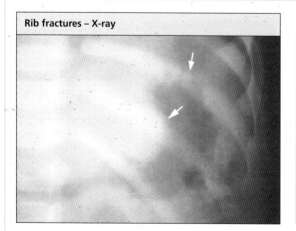

Rib fractures – bone scan

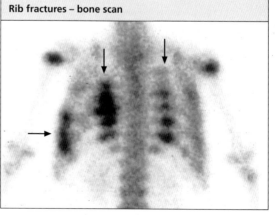

Fig. 6.12a Posterior rib fractures are usually from squeezing rather than direct trauma. They can be seen here in the healing phase with callus formation. Rib fractures are often difficult to identify on an X-ray.

Fig. 6.12b A radionuclide bone scan is more sensitive in detecting fractures in the early stages. This scan clearly shows the multiple rib fractures. (Courtesy of Dr Cathy Owens.)

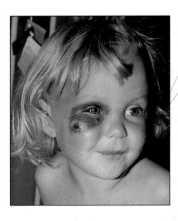

Fig. 6.13 A thorough medical assessment is required in all children when non-accidental injury is suspected. This girl's large bruise followed what was said to be a minor bump. Non-accidental injury was suspected, but examination showed multiple bruises and petechiae. She had immune thrombocytopenic purpura (ITP).

required. Fractures usually affect the shaft of the long bones.

- Copper deficiency – predisposes to fractures. It is rare, but can occur in a preterm or malnourished children.
- Bullous impetigo and scalded skin syndrome – caused by staphylococcal or streptococcal infection; may be mistaken for scalds or cigarette burns.

Neglect

Gross neglect of a child's developmental needs may present clinically as:

- failure to thrive
- inadequate hygiene, including severe nappy rash or infestation
- poor development of emotional attachment to the child's care-giver
- delay in development and speech and language
- poor attendance for immunisations and school.

This will improve if the child's environment is changed to provide adequate food, shelter, affection and stimulation.

Emotional abuse

Emotional abuse includes:

- the withdrawal of love by rejecting the child
- malicious criticism, threats and ridicule
- scapegoating.

Children who have been repeatedly emotionally abused usually present with emotional or behavioural disturbances. There may be excessive compliance or aggressive defiance, poor self-esteem, poor ability to enjoy things or sustain self-occupation, or they may exhibit pseudomature behaviour. Emotional abuse is often associated with physical or sexual abuse.

Non-accidental poisoning

These children are deliberately poisoned by their parents. They present with bizarre symptoms such as:

- hyperventilation after aspirin
- unexplained drowsiness after hypnotics, tranquillisers or alcohol.

The diagnosis is often difficult but can frequently be made by identifying the drug in the blood or urine.

Munchausen's syndrome by proxy

In this uncommon variant of physical abuse, illness in the child is fabricated by a parent, usually the mother. Some of the mothers have connections with health care services. The abuse appears to be a way in which these disturbed parents obtain satisfaction from close association with hospital care. Examples include:

- putting blood in vomit, stool and urine
- placing sugar in the urine so that a diagnosis of diabetes mellitus is made
- contaminating microbiological specimens.

A clue may be that the condition only occurs when the parent is present or following a visit. The condition can be extremely difficult to diagnose, but may be suspected if the child has frequent unexplained illnesses and multiple hospital admissions with symptoms that only occur in the mother's presence and are not substantiated by clinical findings. This disorder can be very damaging to the child, as unnecessary investigations and potentially harmful treatment are likely to be given. The child also learns to live with a pattern of illness rather than health.

Management of suspected child abuse

Abused children may present to doctors in the hospital or to medical or nursing staff in the community. They may also be brought for a medical opinion by social services or the police. In all cases, the procedures of the local area child protection committee should be followed. The medical consultation should be the same as for any medical condition, with a full history and full examination. It is usually most productive when this is conducted in a sensitive and concerned way without being accusatory or condemning. Any injuries or medical findings should be carefully noted, measured, recorded and drawn on a topographical chart. They may need to be photographed with parental consent. The height, weight and head circumference should be recorded and plotted on a centile chart. The interaction between the child and parents should be noted. All notes should be dated, timed and signed. Treatment of specific injuries should be instigated and blood tests and X-rays undertaken.

If abuse is suspected or confirmed, a decision needs to be made as to whether immediate treatment is required and if the child needs immediate protection from further harm. If this is the case, this may be achieved by admission to hospital, which also allows investigations and multidisciplinary assessment. If sympathetically handled, most parents are willing to accept medical advice for hospital admission for

CASE HISTORY 6.1

CHILD ABUSE

A 7-month-old boy was noted by a relative to have a large, unexplained bruise over the side of the head. His mother took him to the nearest A&E department where a skeletal survey showed a normal skull X-ray but a metaphyseal fracture (Fig. 6.14). His mother thought that this must have occurred when he had fallen off his parents' bed the previous day. His mother was training to be a nursery school teacher. Her partner had recently been discharged from prison for burglary. Both parents were interviewed by social services and the police. A child protection conference was held, which the mother attended. The findings were suggestive of non-accidental injury, but definite evidence was lacking.

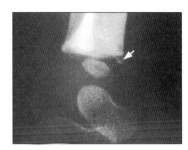

Fig. 6.14
A metaphyseal fracture, usually caused by wrenching, is highly suggestive of non-accidental injury.

The case conference considered the child to be at risk of significant harm and placed him on the Child Protection Register, with close supervision by the health visitor and social services.

---

observation and investigation. Occasionally this is not possible and legal enforcement is required. If medical treatment is not necessary but it is felt to be unsafe for the child to return home, a placement may be found in a foster home.

In addition to a detailed medical assessment, evaluation by social workers and other health professionals will be required. A child protection conference will be convened in accordance with local procedures. In the UK, the conference will be chaired by a senior member of the social services department or of the National Society for the Prevention of Cruelty to Children (NSPCC). Members of the conference may include social workers, health visitors, police, general practitioner, paediatricians, teachers and lawyers. Increasingly, parents attend all or part of the case conference. Details of the incident leading to the conference and the family background will be discussed. Good communication and a trusting working relationship between the professionals are vital as it can be extremely difficult to evaluate the likelihood that injuries were inflicted deliberately and the possible outcome of legal proceedings. The conference will decide:

- whether to place the child's name on the Child Protection Register (see Case history 6.1)
- whether there should be an application to the Court to protect the child
- what follow-up is needed.

If the child is placed on the Child Protection Register, the social services department will produce a child protection care plan which will include medical follow-up in many instances.

 Sexual abuse

A common definition of child sexual abuse is 'involvement of dependent, developmentally immature children

Fig. 6.15 Family risk factors for child sexual abuse.

Poor parental sexual relationship
Maternal depression or physical illness
Mother sexually abused in childhood
Father/abuser either inadequate or aggressive
Family chaotic, disorganised or socially isolated
Parentified daughter who has taken over
    mother's role

and adolescents in sexual activities that they do not fully comprehend, are unable to give informed consent to and that violate social taboos of family roles'. It includes a variety of acts:

- genital exposure
- fondling
- genital, anal or oral sexual activity or intercourse, including rape
- involvement in pornography.

Victims can be of any age and of either sex, but girls outnumber boys, in contrast to other forms of abuse. Risk factors in the family are listed in Figure 6.15. Children may be abused by:

- someone in the family
- a trusted adult, such as a baby-sitter
- someone outside the family, but this is much less common.

Male abusers are more common, but female abusers are being recognised with increasing frequency.

Sexual abuse usually presents as an incidental disclosure by a child, either spontaneously to a trusted adult or as the result of a crisis, such as running away or taking an overdose. It may also present with:

- genital trauma or infection
- sexually transmitted disease
- highly sexualised behaviour towards adults or children
- unexplained pregnancy
- inexplicable change in behaviour or school work.

When child sexual abuse is suspected, the need for and urgency of a medical examination should be assessed. The examination should be conducted by a senior doctor skilled in paediatric examination for child sexual abuse. Assessment of growth, behaviour and development should be made. Examination of the genitalia, which is usually only a detailed inspection and not an internal examination, is done as part of the general clinical examination. Clinical features include:

- bruising around the thighs, genitalia, anus, perineum, buttocks and lower abdomen
- tears and abrasions to the female genitalia – in particular, the hymen may be torn; however, vulval soreness is common in young girls and is rarely due to abuse
- tears and abrasions to the male genitalia
- anal fissures (may be associated with constipation)
- reflex anal dilatation – this is where the buttocks are parted for 30–45 seconds, and in a positive test the anus opens and the rectum can be seen because of incompetence of the internal sphincter. Reflex anal dilatation and anal fissures in isolation are not reliable signs of child sexual abuse as they may have other causes such as constipation.

If appropriate, a forensic physician should also be present to avoid having to repeat the examination.

This allows agreement to be reached about the significance of any minor abnormalities, and allows forensic swabs and samples to be taken. Ideally this should be done within 72 h of the incident.

The examination should be with the knowledge and agreement of the parent, although it may occasionally be performed at the request of the Court. Adolescent girls must give their consent and all children should be accompanied by a trusted adult. In the case of young children, this is usually a parent. It should be performed in privacy, calmly and in a non-threatening environment. The medical examination is rarely diagnostic and significant physical findings are present in less than 30% of sexually abused children. Physical signs must be interpreted in conjunction with the history. There is considerable variation in the normal appearance of the female genitalia. This is partly age-dependent. A normal examination does not exclude abuse.

If sexual abuse is suspected, the procedures of the local area protection committee should be followed. Further information may be obtained from the child during an interview held jointly by a social worker and police officer experienced in child sexual abuse work. Psychological damage secondary to sexual abuse frequently occurs and may need specialist treatment. Post-traumatic stress disorder is a recognised sequel and can persist into adult life.

 At presentation, significant clinical abnormalities are present in less than 30% of sexually abused children.

FURTHER READING

Advanced paediatric life support 2001, 3rd edn. BMJ Publishing, London. *Practical manual*
Hobbs C 1999 Child abuse and neglect: a clinician's handbook, 2nd edn. Churchill Livingstone, London
Hobbs C, Wynne J 2001 Physical signs of child abuse: a colour atlas, 2nd edn. WB Saunders, London
Meadow R (ed) 1997 ABC of child abuse, 3rd edn. BMJ, London. *Collection of review articles*
Morton R, Phillips B 1996 Accidents and emergencies in children, 2nd edn. Oxford University Press, Oxford

7

Genetics

New techniques in molecular biology and cytogenetics and the development of genetic databases have resulted in an explosion of knowledge about the genetic basis of diseases (Fig. 7.1). Clinical application of these advances is now available to families through specialist genetic centres offering diagnosis, investigation, counselling and antenatal diagnosis of an ever-widening range of disorders. Gene therapy trials are underway, bringing hope of improved treatment in the future.

Genetic disorders are:
- common, with 2% of live-born babies having a significant congenital malformation and about 5% a genetic disorder
- burdensome to the affected individual, family and society, as many are associated with severe and permanent disability.

Genetically determined diseases include those resulting from:
- chromosomal abnormalities
- the action of a single gene (Mendelian disorders)
- unusual patterns of inheritance
- interaction of genetic and environmental factors (multifactorial or polygenic disorders).

CHROMOSOMAL ABNORMALITIES

Genes are composed of DNA that is wound around a core of histone proteins and packaged into a succession of supercoils to form the chromosomes. The human chromosome complement was confirmed as recently as 1956. Following the recognition in 1959 of the chromosomal abnormalities in Down's, Klinefelter's and Turner's syndromes, many hundreds of chromosome defects have now been documented. Chromosomal abnormalities are either numerical or structural. They usually, but not always, cause multiple congenital anomalies and learning difficulties.

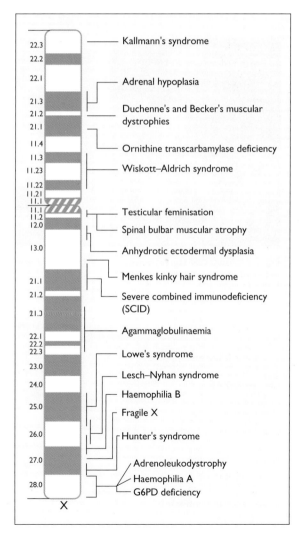

Fig. 7.1 Idiogram of the X chromosome, showing some of the many disorders located on it.

Down's syndrome (Trisomy 21)

This is the most common autosomal trisomy and the most common genetic cause of severe learning difficulties. The incidence in live-born infants is about 1 in 1000.

Clinical features

Down's syndrome is usually suspected at birth because of the baby's facial appearance, but it can be difficult to be certain when relying on clinical characteristics alone. Chromosome analysis takes several days and sufficient certainty about the diagnosis is needed even to take blood for karyotyping. An incorrect suggestion that their baby may have Down's syndrome is potentially damaging for parents, and therefore clinical suspicion about the diagnosis should be confirmed by a senior paediatrician. In addition to the facial appearance, the flat occiput, abnormal dermatoglyphics and hypotonia are helpful diagnostic features (Fig. 7.2a–c and 7.3).

Parents need information about the short- and long-term implications of the diagnosis and of the assistance that is available from both professionals and self-help groups. Parents often find a written explanation of the condition a valuable adjunct to the discussion. They will have a chance to read it with their families and use it as a cue for asking more questions in subsequent discussions. Counselling may also be required to help the family deal with feelings of disappointment, anger or guilt. They will want to understand how and why the condition has arisen, the risk of recurrence and about antenatal diagnosis for future pregnancies.

It is important to note that parents appreciate it when their baby is referred to, not as a diagnostic

DOWN'S SYNDROME

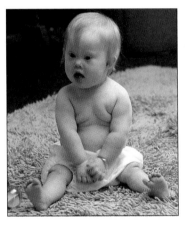

Fig. 7.2a Characteristic facies seen in Down's syndrome. Her posture is due to hypotonia.

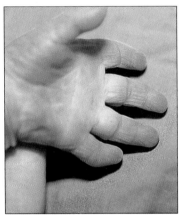

Fig. 7.2b Single palmar crease.

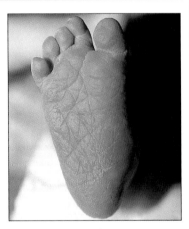

Fig. 7.2c Pronounced 'sandal gap' between the big and first toe.

Fig. 7.3 Characteristic clinical manifestations of Down's syndrome.

Typical facial appearance	Later medical problems include
Round face	Severe learning difficulties
Epicanthic folds	Small stature
Brushfield spots in iris	Recurrent respiratory infections
Protruding tongue	Hearing impairment from secretory otitis media
Small ears	Visual impairment from cataracts, squints
	Increased risk of leukaemia
Other anormalies	Risk of atlantoaxial instability (rare)
Flat occiput	Hypothyroidism
Abnormal creases on palms and soles (dermatoglyphics)	Alzheimer's disease
Hypotonia	
Congenital heart defects (40%)	
Duodenal atresia	

category ('a Down's baby'), but as an individual ('a baby with Down's syndrome').

Cytogenetics

The extra chromosome 21 may result from non-disjunction, translocation or mosaicism.

Non-disjunction (94%)

In non-disjunction:

- most cases result from an error at meiosis
- the pair of chromosomes 21 fails to separate, so that one gamete has two chromosomes 21 and one has none (Fig. 7.4)
- fertilisation of the gamete with two chromosomes 21 gives rise to a zygote with trisomy 21
- the incidence of trisomy 21 due to non-disjunction rises with increasing maternal age (Fig. 7.5), but is independent of paternal age, despite the fact that 5% of non-disjunctions are paternally derived.

Although the incidence of Down's syndrome rises in babies of women over the age of 35 years, a smaller proportion of pregnancies occurs in women over this age and so most affected babies are born to younger mothers. All pregnant women are now offered screening tests measuring biochemical markers in blood samples that may detect an increased risk of Down's syndrome in the fetus. After having one child with trisomy 21 due to non-disjunction, the risk of recurrence of Down's syndrome is 1 in 200 under 35 years and twice the age-specific risk at and above 35 years.

Translocation (5%)

A chromosome 21 is translocated onto a chromosome 14, or more rarely onto a chromosome 15, 22 or 21, and is known as a Robertsonian translocation. In about one-quarter of these, one parent has a balanced translocation, appearing to have only 45 chromosomes, but one chromosome 21 is attached to another chromosome. The affected child has three copies of chromosome 21 (Fig. 7.6).

In translocation Down's syndrome:

- the risk of recurrence is 10–15% if the mother is the translocation carrier and about 2.5% if the father is the carrier
- if a parent carries the rare 21:21 translocation, all the offspring will have Down's syndrome
- if neither parent carries a translocation, the risk of recurrence is <1%.

Fig. 7.5 Risk of Down's syndrome (live births) with maternal age at delivery, prior to screening in pregnancy.

Maternal age (years)	Risk of Down's syndrome
All ages	I in 650
30	I in 900
35	I in 380
37	I in 240
40	I in 110
44	I in 37

INHERITANCE OF DOWN'S SYNDROME

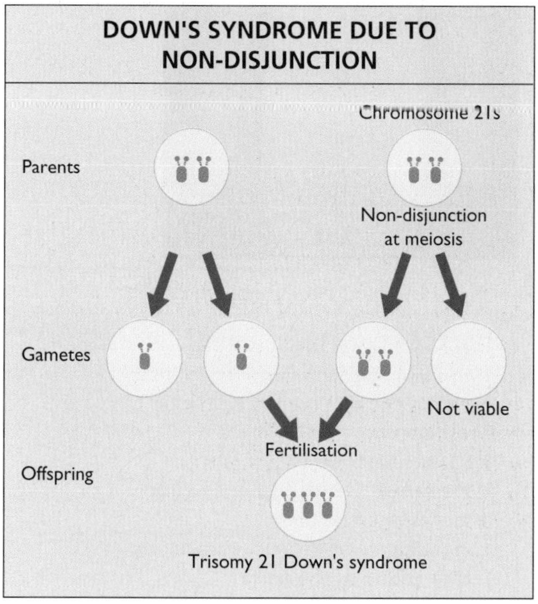

DOWN'S SYNDROME DUE TO NON-DISJUNCTION

Fig. 7.4 Non-disjunction Down's syndrome.

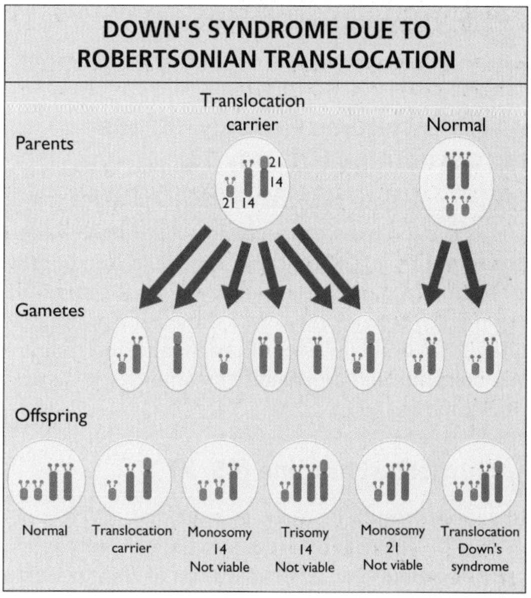

DOWN'S SYNDROME DUE TO ROBERTSONIAN TRANSLOCATION

Fig. 7.6 Translocation Down's syndrome. There is a translocation between chromosomes 21 and 14 inherited from a parent.

EDWARDS' AND PATAU'S SYNDROME

Fig. 7.7a Clinical features of Edwards' syndrome.

Small chin
Low-set ears
Overlapping of fingers
(thumb across palm,
overlapping middle and
ring fingers (Fig. 7.7b))
Rocker-bottom feet
Cardiac and renal
malformations

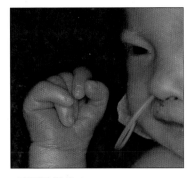

Fig. 7.7b Overlapping of the fingers in Edwards' syndrome.

Fig. 7.8 Clinical features of Patau's syndrome.

Structural defect of brain
Scalp lesions
Small eyes (microphthalmia)
and other eye defects
Polydactyly
Cardiac and renal
malformations

Mosaicism (1%)

In mosaicism some of the cells are normal and some have trisomy 21. This usually arises after the formation of the zygote, by non-disjunction at mitosis. The phenotype may be milder in mosaicism.

The chromosomes of a baby with Down's syndrome must always be examined. If there is free trisomy 21, parental chromosomes need not be examined. If the baby has a translocation, then the parents' chromosomes should be studied, and if one carries a balanced translocation other relatives should also be offered genetic counselling.

   Non-disjunction is the commonest cause of Down's syndrome.

Edwards' syndrome (Trisomy 18) and Patau's syndrome (Trisomy 13)

Although rarer than Down's syndrome (1 in 8000 and 1 in 14 000 live births, respectively), the constellation of severe multiple abnormalities suggests the diagnosis at birth and most die in infancy (Figs 7.7 and 7.8). Many affected fetuses are detected by ultrasound scan during the second trimester of pregnancy and diagnosis can be confirmed antenatally by amniocentesis and chromosome analysis.

Turner's syndrome (45, X)

Most (>95%) result in early miscarriage. Occasional cases may be detected by ultrasound antenatally when a cystic hygroma and other evidence of fetal oedema may be present. In live-born females, the incidence is about 1 in 2500. See Figure 7.9 for the clinical features of Turner's syndrome.

TURNER'S SYNDROME

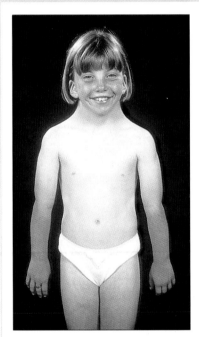

Fig. 7.9a Turner's syndrome, showing neck webbing and widely spaced nipples.

Fig. 7.9b Clinical features of Turner's syndrome.

Lymphoedema of hands and feet in neonate
Short stature
Neck webbing
Wide carrying angle (cubitus valgus)
Widely spaced nipples
Congenital heart defects (particularly coarctation of the aorta)
Ovarian dysgenesis resulting in infertility
Normal intellectual development

Treatment is with:
- growth hormone therapy
- oestrogen replacement for development of secondary sexual characteristics at the time of puberty (but infertility persists).

In about 50% of girls with Turner's syndrome, there are 45 chromosomes, with only one X chromosome. The other cases have a deletion of the short arm of one X chromosome, an isochromosome that has two long arms but no short arm, or a variety of other structural defects of one of the X chromosomes. The incidence does not increase with maternal age and risks of recurrence are very low.

Klinefelter's syndrome (47, XXY)

This disorder occurs in about 1–2 per 1000 live-born males. For clinical features, see Figure 7.10.

Reciprocal translocations

An exchange of material between two different chromosomes is called a reciprocal translocation. When this exchange involves no loss or gain of chromosomal material, the translocation is 'balanced' and has no phenotypic effect. Balanced reciprocal translocations are relatively common, occurring in 1 in 500 of the general population. Unbalanced reciprocal translocations contain an incorrect amount of chromosomal material and cause a combination of dysmorphic features, congenital malformations, developmental delay and learning difficulties. In a newborn baby, the prognosis is difficult to predict, but the effect is usually severe. The parents' chromosomes should be checked to determine whether the abnormality has arisen *de novo*, or as a consequence of a parental rearrangement. Finding a balanced translocation in one parent indicates a recurrence risk for future pregnancies and antenatal diagnosis by chorionic villus biopsy or amniocentesis should be offered as well as testing of relatives.

Deletions

Deletions are another type of structural abnormality. Loss of part of a chromosome usually results in physical abnormalities and learning difficulties. The deletion may involve loss of the terminal or, less commonly, the interstitial part of a chromosome.

An example of a deletion syndrome involves loss of the tip of the short arm of chromosome 5, hence the name 5p- or monosomy 5p. Because affected babies have a high-pitched mewing cry in early infancy, it is also known as *cri du chat* syndrome. Parental chromosomes should be checked to see if one parent carries a balanced chromosomal rearrangement.

An increasing number of syndromes are now known to be due to chromosome deletions too small to be seen by conventional cytogenetic analysis. These submicroscopic deletions can be detected by fluorescent in-situ hybridisation (FISH) studies using DNA probes

Fig. 7.10 Clinical features of Klinefelter's syndrome.

Infertility – most common presentation
Hypogonadism with small testes
Pubertal development apparently normal
   (some males benefit from testosterone therapy)
Gynaecomastia in adolescence
Tall stature
Intelligence – usually in the normal range, but may
   have educational and psychological problems

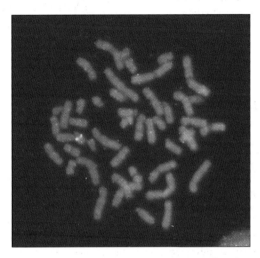

Fig. 7.11 Fluorescent in-situ hybridisation (FISH) demonstrating a microdeletion on chromosome 22 associated with DiGeorge syndrome. Hybridisation signals are seen on one chromosome 22 but not on the other chromosome 22 because of the prescence of a deletion. (Courtesy of L. Gaunt, St Mary's Hospital, Manchester.)

specific to particular chromosome regions. Williams' syndrome is an example of a microdeletion syndrome due to loss of chromosomal material on the long arm of chromosome 7 at band 7q11 (Fig. 7.24a).

MENDELIAN INHERITANCE

Disorders with these patterns of inheritance, described by Mendel in 1865, are rare individually, but collectively numerous, with over 8000 single gene traits or disorders described. For many disorders the Mendelian pattern of inheritance is known. If the diagnosis of a condition is uncertain, its pattern of inheritance may be evident on drawing a family tree (pedigree), which is an essential part of clinical genetics (Fig. 7.12).

Autosomal dominant inheritance

This is the most common mode of Mendelian inheritance (Fig. 7.13a). An affected individual carries the abnormal gene in the heterozygous state on one of

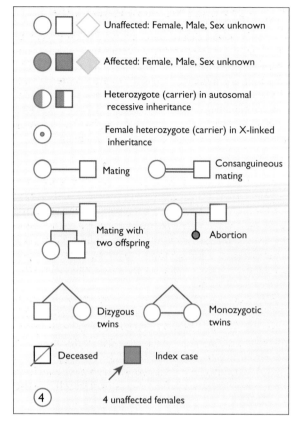

Fig. 7.12 Pedigree symbols

a pair of autosomes (chromosomes 1–22). Male and female offspring each have a 1 in 2 (50%) chance of inheriting the abnormal gene from an affected parent (Fig. 7.13b and c). This is straightforward, but complicating factors include the following.

Variation in expression

Within a family, some affected individuals may manifest the disorder mildly and others more severely. For example, a parent with tuberous sclerosis may have mild skin abnormalities only, but his or her affected child may have, in addition, epilepsy and learning difficulties.

Non-penetrance

Refers to the lack of clinical signs and symptoms in an individual who must have inherited the abnormal gene. An example of this is otosclerosis, in which only about 40% of gene carriers develop deafness (Fig. 7.14).

No family history of the disorder

May be due to:

- A new mutation in one of the gametes leading to the conception of the affected person. This is the most common reason for absence of a family history in dominant disorders, e.g. >80% of individuals with achondroplasia have normal parents.
- Gonadal mosaicism – very occasionally a healthy parent harbours the mutation only in a number of gametes in the gonad. This can account for recurrences of autosomal dominant disorders in

AUTOSOMAL DOMINANT INHERITANCE

Fig. 7.13a Examples of autosomal dominant disorders.

Achondroplasia	Neurofibromatosis
Ehlers–Danlos syndrome	Noonan's syndrome
	Osteogenesis
Familial hyper- cholesterolaemia	imperfecta
	Otosclerosis
Huntington's disease	Polyposis coli
Marfan's syndrome	Tuberous sclerosis
Myotonic dystrophy	

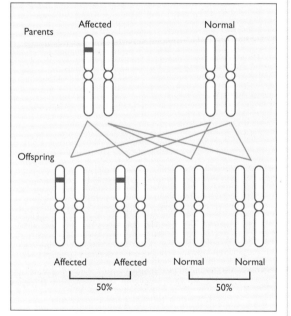

Fig. 7.13b Autosomal dominant inheritance.

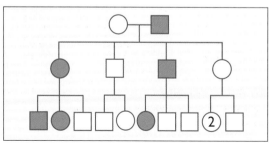

Fig. 7.13c Typical pedigree of an autosomal dominant disorder.

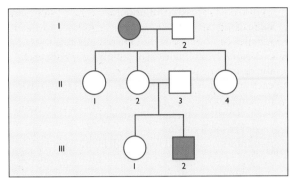

Fig. 7.14 Example of non-penetrance. I1 and III2 have otosclerosis. II2 has normal hearing but must have the gene. The gene is non-penetrant in II2.

siblings born to apparently normal parents. It has been described in congenital lethal osteogenesis imperfecta.

• Non-paternity – if the apparent father is not the biological father.

Homozygosity

In the rare situation where both parents are affected by the same autosomal dominant disorder, there is a 1 in 4 risk that a child will be homozygous for the mutant gene.

Autosomal recessive inheritance

Several hundred disorders resulting from this type of inheritance are known (Fig. 7.15a). An affected individual is homozygous for the abnormal gene, having inherited an abnormal allele from each parent, both of whom are unaffected heterozygous carriers. For two carrier parents, the risk of each child, male or female, being affected is 1 in 4 (25%) (Fig. 7.15b and c). All offspring of affected individuals will be carriers.

Consanguinity

It is thought that we all carry at least one abnormal recessive gene. Fortunately, our spouses usually carry a different one. Marrying a cousin or other relative increases the chance of a couple carrying the same abnormal autosomal recessive gene, inherited from a common ancestor. A couple who are cousins therefore have a small increase in the risk of having a child with a recessive disorder.

Recessive gene frequencies may vary between racial groups. When the gene occurs sufficiently frequently and the gene or its effect can be detected, population-based carrier testing can be performed and antenatal diagnosis offered for high-risk pregnancies. Disorders that can be screened for in this way include cystic fibrosis in north Europeans, sickle cell disease

AUTOSOMAL RECESSIVE INHERITANCE

Fig. 7.15a Examples of autosomal recessive disorders.

Congenital adrenal hyperplasia	Oculocutaneous albinism
Cystic fibrosis	Phenylketonuria
Friedreich's ataxia	Sickle cell disease
Galactosaemia	Tay–Sachs disease
Glycogen storage diseases	Thalassaemia
Hurler's syndrome (MPS I)	Werdnig–Hoffmann disease

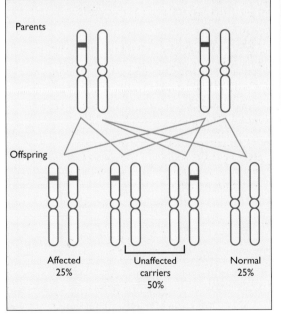

Fig. 7.15b Autosomal recessive inheritance.

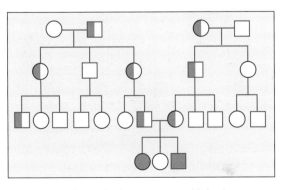

Fig. 7.15c Pedigree to show autosomal inheritance.

in black Africans and Americans, thalassaemias in Mediterranean or Asian ethnicity and Tay–Sachs disease in Ashkenazi Jews.

> **Autosomal recessive disorders often affect metabolic pathways, autosomal dominant disorders usually affect structural proteins.**

X-linked recessive inheritance

Over 250 disorders have been described in which an abnormal recessive gene is carried on the X chromosome (Figs 7.16 and 7.17).

In X-linked recessive inheritance:
- males are affected
- females can be carriers but are usually healthy
- occasionally a female carrier shows mild signs of the disease
- each son of a female carrier has a 1 in 2 (50%) risk of being affected
- each daughter of a female carrier has a 1 in 2 (50%) risk of being a carrier
- daughters of affected males will all be carriers
- sons of affected males will not be affected, since a man passes a Y chromosome to his son.

The family history may be negative, since new mutations and gonadal mosaicism are fairly common. Identification of carrier females in a family requires

X-LINKED RECESSIVE INHERITANCE

Fig. 7.16a Examples of X-linked recessive disorders.

Colour blindness (red–green)
Duchenne's and Becker's muscular dystrophies
Fragile X syndrome
Glucose-6-phosphate dehydrogenase (G6PD) deficiency
Haemophilia A and B
Hunter's syndrome (mucopolysaccharidosis II)

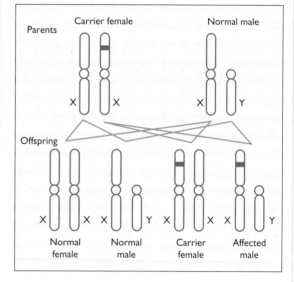

Fig. 7.16b X-linked recessive inheritance.

Fig. 7.17 (below) Typical pedigree for X-linked recessive inheritance, showing Queen Victoria, a carrier for haemophilia A, and her family. It shows affected males in several generations, related through females, and that affected males do not have affected sons (contrast with autosomal dominant inheritance).

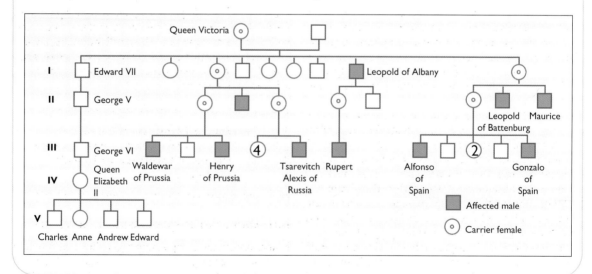

interpretation of the pedigree, looking for mild clinical manifestations and doing specific biochemical or molecular tests. Identifying carriers is important because a female carrier has a high risk of having an affected son regardless of whom she marries, and X-linked recessive disorders are often very severe.

X-linked dominant inheritance

Although dominantly inherited X-linked disorders occur, e.g. a variant of vitamin D-resistant rickets, they are rare. Both males and females are affected.

Y-linked inheritance

No serious genetic defects, apart from some rare forms of intersex and a gene for azoospermia, have been located to the human Y chromosome, which seems reasonable given that half the population live happily without a Y chromosome!

UNUSUAL INHERITANCE PATTERNS

Trinucleotide repeat expansion mutations

A new class of unstable mutations, caused by expansions of trinucleotide repeat sequences inherited in Mendelian fashion, have recently been identified. Fragile X syndrome and myotonic dystrophy were among the first disorders found to be due to such mutations. Other disorders include Huntington's disease, spinocerebellar ataxia and Friedreich's ataxia. These disorders follow different patterns of inheritance but share certain unusual properties due to the nature of the underlying mutation. Clinical anticipation is often seen, with the disorders becoming more severe in successive generations of a family and new mutations being exceedingly rare.

 Fragile X syndrome

The prevalence of severe learning difficulties in males due to fragile X syndrome is about 1 in 4000 (Fig. 7.18a and b). This condition was initially diagnosed on the basis of the appearance of a gap (fragile site) in the distal part of the long arm of the X chromosome. Diagnosis is now achieved by molecular analysis of the CGG trinucleotide repeat expansion in the relevant gene.

Although it is inherited as an X-linked recessive disorder, a high proportion of obligate female carriers have learning difficulties (usually mild to moderate) and around one-fifth of males who inherit the mutation are phenotypically normal but may pass the disorder on to their grandsons through their daughters.

These unusual findings are explained by the nature of the mutation, which occurs in 'pre-mutation' and 'full mutation' forms. The normal copy of the gene contains fewer than 50 copies of the CGG trinucleotide repeat sequence and is stable when transmitted to offspring. Genes with the pre-mutation contain 55–199

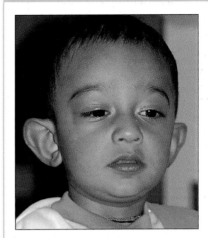

Fig. 7.18a A child with fragile X syndrome. At this age, the main feature is often the prominent ears.

Fig. 7.18b Clinical findings in males in fragile X syndrome.

Moderate learning difficulty (IQ 20–80, mean 50)
Macrocephaly
Macro-orchidism – more common postpubertal than prepubertal
Characteristic appearance – long face, large everted ears, prominent mandible and large forehead, most evident in affected adults. Affected children may not appear to be dysmorphic facially

copies of the repeat sequence. This expansion has no phenotypic effect in male or female carriers, but is unstable and may become larger during transmission through females. Genes with the full mutation contain more than 200 copies of the repeat sequence. This affects gene function, causing the clinical features of fragile X syndrome in virtually all males and around half of the female carriers. These full mutations always arise from expansion of pre-mutations, and never arise directly from normal genes. Hence all mothers of affected males are carriers.

> Fragile X syndrome is the second most common genetic cause of severe learning difficulties after Down's syndrome.

Mitochondrial or cytoplasmic inheritance

Mitochondria are cytoplasmic organelles that function as major energy producers for the cell and contain their own DNA. Mutations in mitochondrial DNA cause several disorders such as Leber hereditary optic neuropathy and various mitochondrial myopathies and encephalopathies. Mitochondrial DNA mutations always show maternal transmission, since only the egg contains cytoplasm and mitochondria. Sperm do not contain mitochondria, so a father with a disorder due to a mitochondrial DNA mutation will not have affected children. On the other hand, all the children of an affected mother will be at risk.

Imprinting and uniparental disomy

In the past, it has been assumed that the activity of a gene is the same regardless of whether it is inherited from the mother or father. Recently, however, it has been shown that some genes are actively expressed only if they have been derived from a parent of a given sex. This phenomenon is called 'imprinting'. An example involves Prader–Willi syndrome (learning difficulties, hypotonia, obesity). The Prader–Willi gene is found in the 15q11–13 region of chromosome 15 (that is, bands 11–13 on the long arm of chromosome 15). Normally, only the paternal copy of the Prader–Willi gene is active. Failure to inherit the active paternal gene will give rise to the syndrome. Failure to inherit the maternal copy of this gene has no effect, since it is inactive. Coincidentally, the gene for the Angelman syndrome (severe learning difficulty, ataxia, happy personality, characteristic facial appearance, epilepsy) is also found in the same chromosome region and is also subject to imprinting. In this case it is the maternal gene that is the active one. Failure to inherit the maternal gene will therefore cause Angelman syndrome.

There are two main ways that a child can fail to inherit the active gene for either syndrome:

- De novo *deletion* (Fig. 7.19). Parental chromosomes are normal, and a deletion occurs as a new mutation in the child. If the deletion occurs on the paternal chromosome 15, the child has Prader–Willi syndrome. If the deletion affects the maternal chromosome 15, the child has Angelman syndrome.
- *Uniparental disomy* (Fig. 7.20). This is when a child inherits two copies of a chromosome from one parent and none from the other parent. In Prader-Willi syndrome the affected child has no paternal (but two maternal) copies of chromosome 15q 11–13. In Angelman syndrome the affected child has no maternal (but two paternal) copies of chromosome 15q11–13. This can be detected with DNA analysis.

 Imprinting is the unusual property of some genes to express only the copy derived from a parent of a given sex.

POLYGENIC OR MULTIFACTORIAL INHERITANCE

There is a spectrum in the aetiology of disease, from environmental factors (e.g. trauma) at one end to purely genetic causes (e.g. Mendelian disorders) at the

---

IMPRINTING

IMPRINTING FROM A DELETION

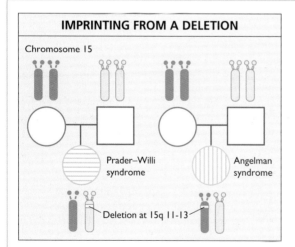

IMPRINTING FROM UNIPARENTAL DISOMY

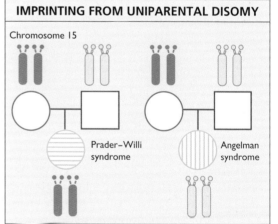

Fig. 7.19 Genetic disorder resulting from deletion of an imprinted gene. If the deletion occurs on chromosome 15 inherited from the father, the child has Prader–Willi syndrome. If the deletion occurs on chromosome 15 from the mother, the child has Angelman syndrome.

Fig. 7.20 Genetic disorder resulting from uniparental disomy affecting imprinted chromosome region. A child who inherits two maternal chromosome 15s will have Prader–Willi syndrome. A child who inherits two paternal chromosome 15s will have Angelman syndrome.

other. Between these two extremes are many disorders which result from the additive effect of several genes (hence the term polygenic) with or without the influence of environmental or other unknown factors (i.e. multifactorial). The two terms are often used interchangeably (Fig. 7.21).

Normal traits such as height and intelligence are also inherited in this way. These parameters show a Gaussian or normal distribution in the population. Similarly, the liability of an individual to develop a disease of multifactorial or polygenic aetiology also has a normal distribution. The condition occurs when a certain threshold level of liability is exceeded. Relatives of an affected person show an increased liability, and so a greater proportion of them than in the general population will fall beyond the threshold and will manifest the disorder (Fig. 7.22).

The risk of recurrence of a multifactorial disorder in a family is usually low and is most significant for first-degree relatives. Empirical recurrence risk data are used for genetic counselling. They are derived from family studies that have reported the frequency at which various family members are affected. Factors that increase the risk to relatives are:

- having a more severe form of the disorder, e.g. the risk of recurrence to siblings is greater in bilateral cleft lip and palate than in unilateral cleft lip alone
- close relationship to the affected person, e.g. overall risk to siblings is greater than to more distant relatives
- multiple affected family members, e.g. the more siblings already affected, the greater the risk of recurrence
- sex difference in prevalence, e.g. in Hirschsprung's; disease the male to female ratio is 3:1; an affected female must have had a greater genetic predisposition, so the risk to siblings is greater than for an affected male.

It is important to note that the phenotype (clinical picture) of a disorder may have a heterogeneous (mixed) basis in different families; for example, hyperlipidaemia leading to atherosclerosis and coronary heart disease can be due to a single gene disorder such as autosomal dominant hypercholesterolaemia, but some forms of hyperlipidaemia are polygenic and result from an interaction of the effect of genes on various lipoproteins.

In many multifactorial disorders, the 'environmental factors' remain obscure. Obvious exceptions include dietary fat intake and smoking in atherosclerosis, and viral infection in insulin-dependent diabetes mellitus. For neural tube defects, the risk of recurrence to siblings is lowered from about 4 to 1% or less in future pregnancies if the mother takes folate before conception and in the early weeks of pregnancy. This is a rare example of the possibility of primary prevention of a genetic disorder.

DNA ANALYSIS

New techniques in DNA testing are continually being developed, making more single gene disorders amenable to molecular analysis. Most molecular testing is performed using polymerase chain reaction (PCR). This involves the amplification of specific DNA sequences, enabling rapid analysis of small samples, which is particularly important in antenatal diagnosis.

The main impact of DNA analysis for genetic counselling is:

- confirmation of a clinical diagnosis
- detection of female carriers in X-linked disorders, e.g. Duchenne's and Becker's muscular dystrophies, haemophilia A and B
- carrier detection in autosomal recessive disorders, e.g. cystic fibrosis

MULTIFACTORIAL INHERITANCE

Fig. 7.21 Conditions with multifactorial inheritance.

Congenital malformations	Adult life
Neural tube defects (anencephaly and spina bifida)	Atherosclerosis and coronary heart disease
Congenital heart disease	Diabetes mellitus
Cleft lip and palate	Asthma
Pyloric stenosis	Epilepsy
Congenital dislocation of the hip	Hypertension
Talipes	
Hypospadias	

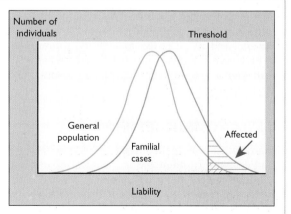

Fig. 7.22 Diagram showing the increased liability to a multifactorial disorder in relatives of an affected person.

- presymptomatic diagnosis in autosomal dominant disorders, e.g. Huntington's disease, myotonic dystrophy
- antenatal diagnosis of an increasing number of Mendelian conditions.

These are accomplished by:

1. Mutation analysis

For an increasing number of disorders, it is possible to directly detect the actual mutation causing the disease. This provides very accurate results for confirmation of diagnosis, and presymptomatic or predictive testing. Identifying the mutation in an affected individual may be very time-consuming, but once this has been done, testing other relatives is usually fairly simple. Examples are:

- Deletions – large deletion mutations are common in a variety of disorders including Duchenne's and Becker's muscular dystrophies, alpha-thalassaemia and 21-hydroxylase deficiency. They can be tested for relatively easily.
- Point mutations and small deletions – these can be readily identified if the same mutation causes all cases of the disorder, as in sickle cell disease. For most disorders, however, there is a very diverse spectrum of mutations. About 78% of cystic fibrosis carriers in the UK possess the ΔF508 mutation, but over 400 other mutations have been identified. Most laboratories test for a certain number of the most common mutations in their given population.
- Trinucleotide repeat expansion mutations – these are readily tested for because the mutation in a given disease is always the same. The only difference is the size of the repeat sequence that can be determined from the size of the DNA fragment containing the repeat.

2. Genetic linkage

If mutation analysis is not available, it may be possible to use DNA sequence variations (markers) located near to, or within, the disease gene to track the inheritance of this gene through a family. This type of analysis requires a suitable family structure and several key members need to be tested to identify appropriate markers before linkage testing can be used predictively. This method is used in some cases of Duchenne's muscular dystrophy.

PRESYMPTOMATIC TESTING

In many autosomal dominant disorders, onset is during adolescence or adult life and clinical expression may not be evident at birth. Relatives of affected individuals may request tests to see if they are likely to develop the disorder in question. Examples include myotonic dystrophy, Huntington's disease, autosomal dominant polycystic kidney disease (adult) and neurofibromatosis.

Assessment may include:

- careful examination of individuals at risk, e.g. evidence of myotonia in myotonic dystrophy; in some disorders in which expression varies and may be mild, it may be impossible to determine clinically whether or not an individual carries the abnormal gene
- investigations, e.g. regular renal scans in individuals at risk of autosomal dominant polycystic kidney disease
- DNA analysis using linked markers or mutation analysis.

It is debatable whether presymptomatic tests (e.g. for myotonic dystrophy) and carrier tests (e.g. for cystic fibrosis) should be performed on children, as these remove the child's future right to choose whether or not to have the information. In Huntington's disease it is generally accepted that children should not be tested.

GENE THERAPY

Gene therapy involves the artificial introduction of genes into disease tissue in order to cure the disease. Success requires:

- Integration of the introduced gene into the chromosomal DNA of recipient cells. The simplest way is to transfer the genes into suitable cells in culture and then insert the transfected cells into the patient
- Delivery to the appropriate tissue. Some tissues, such as blood, are easier to access than others, such as brain or muscle.
- Appropriate expression of the gene.

Gene therapy has been initiated recently in adenosine deaminase deficiency (a rare recessive immune disorder), malignant melanoma and cystic fibrosis, and some clinical benefit has been reported in a few patients. At present, it is generally accepted that gene therapy should be limited to somatic (not germ line) cells, so that the risk of adversely affecting future generations is minimised.

DYSMORPHOLOGY

The term 'dysmorphology' literally means 'the study of abnormal form' and refers to the assessment of birth defects that have their origin during embryogenesis.

Pathogenic mechanisms

Malformation

A primary structural defect occurring during the development of a tissue or organ, e.g. spina bifida and cleft lip and palate.

Deformation

Implies an abnormal intrauterine mechanical force that distorts a normally formed structure, e.g. joint contractures due to fetal compression caused by severe oligohydramnios.

Disruption

Involves destruction of a fetal part which initially formed normally – e.g. amniotic membrane rupture may lead to amniotic bands which may cause limb reduction defects.

Dysplasia

Refers to abnormal cellular organisation or function of specific tissue types, e.g. skeletal dysplasias and dysplastic kidney disease.

Clinical classification of birth defects

Single-system defects

These include single congenital malformations such as spina bifida and are often multifactorial in nature with fairly low recurrence risks.

Sequence

Refers to a pattern of multiple abnormalities occurring after one initiating defect. Potter's syndrome (fetal compression and pulmonary hypoplasia) is an example of a sequence in which all abnormalities may be traced to one original malformation, renal agenesis.

Association

A group of malformations that occur together more often than expected by chance, but in different combinations from case to case, e.g. VATER association (Vertebral anomalies, Anal atresia, Tracheo–oEsophageal fistula, Radial defects) and CHARGE association (Coloboma of the eye, Heart defect, Atresia choanae (choanal atresia), Retardation of growth and development, Genital abnormalities, Ear abnormalities).

Syndrome

When a particular set of multiple anomalies occurs repeatedly in a consistent pattern, this is called a 'syndrome'. Multiple malformation syndromes are often associated with moderate or severe learning difficulties and may be due to:

- chromosomal defects
- a single gene defect (dominant or recessive)
- exposure to teratogens such as alcohol, drugs (valproate, phenytoin) or viral infections during pregnancy
- unknown cause.

Syndrome diagnosis

Although most syndromes are individually rare, recognition of a dysmorphic syndrome may give information regarding:

- risk of recurrence
- prognosis
- likely complications which can be sought and perhaps treated successfully if detected early
- the avoidance of unnecessary investigations
- experience and information which parents can share with other affected families through self-help groups.

Examples of syndromes recognisable by facial appearance are shown in Figures 7.23–7.25.

GENETIC COUNSELLING

The main aim of genetic counselling is to give individuals, couples and families information about hereditary disorders, so that they understand:

- what it means to have the disorder
- their risk of developing or transmitting it to offspring
- measures to treat or prevent the disorder.

A primary goal of genetic counselling is to provide information to allow for greater autonomy and choice in reproductive decisions. Prevention of genetic disease may also result from genetic counselling, but this is not the main aim. The elements of genetic counselling include:

- Establishing the correct diagnosis. This involves detailed history, examination and appropriate investigations that may include chromosome or DNA analysis, biochemical tests, X-rays and clinical photographs.
- Risk estimation. This requires both diagnostic and pedigree information. Drawing a pedigree of three generations is an essential part of genetic counselling. The mode of inheritance may be apparent from the pedigree even when the precise diagnosis is not known.
- Communication. Information must be presented in an understandable and unbiased way. Families often find written information very helpful to refer back to and diagrams are often used to explain patterns of inheritance. The impact of saying 'the recurrence risk is 5%' may be different from saying 'the chance of an unaffected child is 95%', and so both should be presented.
- Discussing options for management and prevention. If there appears to be a risk to offspring, all reproductive options should be discussed. These include not having (more) children or reducing family size, ignoring the risk, artificial insemination by donor or ovum donation if appropriate, preimplantation diagnosis and IVF, or antenatal diagnosis and selective termination of an affected fetus.

Counselling should be non-directive, but should also assist in the decision-making process (Fig. 7.26). This requires:

- time and possibly several sessions for discussion
- a compassionate approach by the professionals
- awareness by the counsellor of psychological issues, such as denial, grief and anger, which are often evoked by genetic illness
- awareness by the counsellor of ethnic, social, religious and educational factors
- follow-up consultations to ensure understanding and to offer support – this is an essential part of genetic counselling, particularly when a family is coming to terms with the diagnosis and the

SYNDROMES RECOGNISED BY 'GESTALT'

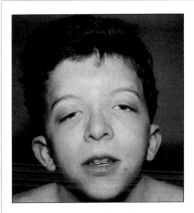

Fig. 7.23a Noonan's syndrome affects males and females. There are some similarities to the phenotype in Turner's syndrome, but it is caused by a faulty autosomal dominant gene and the chromosomes are normal.

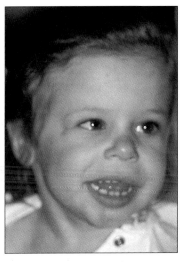

Fig. 7.24a Williams' syndrome is usually sporadic.

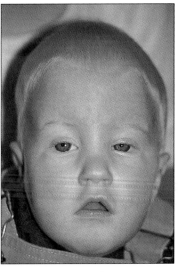

Fig. 7.25a Prader–Willi syndrome.

Fig. 7.23b Clinical features of Noonan's syndrome.

Characteristic facies
Occasional mild learning
  difficulties
Short webbed neck with
  trident hair line
Pectus excavatum
Short stature
Congenital heart disease
  (especially pulmonary
  stenosis, ASD)

Fig. 7.24b Clinical features of Williams' syndrome.

Short stature
Characteristic facies
Transient neonatal
  hypercalcaemia
  (occasionally)
Congenital heart disease
  (supravalvular aortic
  stenosis)
Mild to moderate learning
  difficulties

Fig. 7.25b Clinical features of Prader–Willi syndrome.

Characteristic facies
Hypotonia
Obesity
Hypogonadism
Developmental delay

Fig. 7.26 Influences on decisions regarding options for genetic counselling.

Magnitude of risk
Severity of disorder
Availability of treatment
Person's experience of the disorder
Family size
Availability of a safe and reliable antenatal test
Parental or cultural ethical values

medical staff, specialist health visitors and non-medical counsellors. As more disorders become amenable to genetic diagnosis, it will be important to develop a more coordinated approach in the community which will involve:

- education of the general public and medical profession about genetic issues
- establishment of comprehensive screening programmes (e.g. for cystic fibrosis) in the community, complete with facilities not only for testing but for pre- and post-test counselling
- the non-medical genetic counsellor whose role will become increasingly important.

implications of a genetic disease, after a termination of pregnancy for fetal abnormality or following the death of an affected child.

In the UK, most regional health authorities have a clinical genetics centre where genetic counselling is carried out as a specialist service by consultants, their

Genetic counselling aims to allow parents greater autonomy and choice in reproductive decisions.

CASE HISTORY 7.1

SYNDROME DIAGNOSIS AND GENETIC COUNSELLING

Sean, the second child of healthy parents, was born at term by emergency caesarean section for fetal distress. The pregnancy had been uneventful and no abnormalities were detected on antenatal ultrasound scan. Investigation because of respiratory distress and a cardiac murmur revealed an interrupted aortic arch and ventricular septal defect that required surgical correction in the neonatal period.

The parents asked about recurrence risk for congenital heart disease and were referred to the genetic clinic. At that time, Sean was thriving and early developmental progress appeared normal. On examination there were minor dysmorphic features, including a short philtrum, thin upper lip and prominent ears (Fig. 7.27). There was no family history of congenital heart disease or other significant problems and no abnormalities were detected on examination of the parents.

Because of an association between outflow tract abnormalities of the heart and deletions of chromosome 22, cytogenetic analysis was performed using fluorescent in-situ hybridisation (FISH). A submicroscopic deletion of the long arm of one chromosome 22 (band 22q11) was detected. Other features of DiGeorge's syndrome (hypocalcaemia and T cell deficiency), which occurs at the same chromosome site, were excluded by appropriate tests.

Parental chromosome analysis showed no deletion at chromosome 22q11 in either parent, indicating a low recurrence risk for future pregnancies since gonadal mosaicism for this deletion has not been reported. The older sibling was also normal on testing. Because the parents had normal karyotypes, their own brothers and sisters did not need to be offered tests.

Identification of a 22q11 deletion indicated that other associated problems were likely. Subsequently, Sean required assessment by a multidisciplinary child development team (developmental delay),

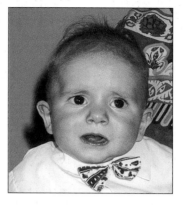

Fig. 7.27 Sean's facial appearance showing the short philtrum, thin upper lip and prominent ears.

educational statementing and recommendation for placement in a school for children with special educational needs (learning difficulty), input from a clinical psychologist when behavioural problems appeared (ritualistic behaviour and obsessional tendencies), input from speech therapist and plastic surgeon (indistinct speech due to velopharyngeal incompetence) and audiology review (conductive hearing loss due to recurrent otitis media).

The impact of the diagnosis and its implications was considerable for the family and the parents needed support from a variety of professionals whilst coming to terms with the various problems as they became apparent. Written information and details of the 22q11 support group were given to the parents. Medical care was coordinated by the paediatrician.

There was the additional worry for the family about a subsequent pregnancy. Fetal echocardiography showed no evidence of congenital heart disease, but invasive tests for cytogenetic analysis were declined because of the low recurrence risk. The baby was born unaffected, with chromosome studies performed on a cord blood sample revealing no abnormality.

FURTHER READING

Aase J M 1990 Diagnostic dysmorphology. Plenum Medical, New York
Baraitser M, Winter R M 1996 Color atlas of congenital malformation syndromes. Mosby-Wolfe, London
Connor J M, Ferguson-Smith M A 1997 Essential medical genetics, 4th edn. Blackwell Scientific Publications, Oxford
Harper P S 1998 Practical genetic counselling, 5th edn. Wright, London. *Book on clinical genetics and counselling*
Jones K L 1997 Smith's recognisable patterns of human malformation, 5th edn. WB Saunders, Philadephia. *Diagnosing syndromes*
Kingston H M 2001 ABC of clinical genetics, 3rd edn. BMJ, London
Mueller R F, Young I D 1998 Emery's elements of medical genetics, 10th edn. Churchill Livingstone, Edinburgh. *General medical genetics*
Strachan T, Read A P 1999 Human molecular genetics, 2nd edn. BIOS Scientific Publishers, Oxford. *Molecular genetics*

Internet

Omim (Online Mendelian Inheritance in Man)
UK: www.hgmp.mrc.ac.uk/omim
US: www.ncbi.nlm.nih.gov/omim

8

Perinatal medicine

The term 'perinatal medicine' acknowledges the continuity of fetal and neonatal life. Using modern technology, such as high-resolution ultrasound and DNA analysis, detailed information about the fetus can now be obtained for a large and increasing number of conditions. There should be close cooperation between the professionals involved in the care of the pregnant mother and fetus and those caring for the newborn infant.

PRE-PREGNANCY CARE

The better a mother's state of health and nutrition, and the higher her socioeconomic living standard and the quality of health care she receives, the greater is the chance of a successful outcome to her pregnancy. This is reflected in the widely varying perinatal mortality rates in different countries. In 1999, the perinatal mortality rate in Costa Rica was 16.5, in the US 8.5, in the UK 8.2 and in Japan 5.3/1000 total births.

Couples planning to have a baby often ask what they should do to optimise their chances of having a healthy child. They can be informed that for the mother:

- *Smoking* reduces birthweight, which may be of critical importance if born preterm. On average, the babies of smokers weigh 170 g less than non-smokers, but the reduction in birthweight is related to the number of cigarettes smoked per day. Smoking is also associated with an increased risk of miscarriage and stillbirth. The infant has a greater risk of sudden infant death syndrome (SIDS).
- *Medication*, either prescribed or proprietary, is best avoided because of potential teratogenic effects.
- *Excess alcohol* ingestion and *drug abuse* may damage the fetus.

- *Congenital rubella* is preventable by maternal immunisation before pregnancy.
- *Exposure to toxoplasmosis* should be minimised by avoiding eating undercooked poultry and wearing gloves when handling cat litter.
- *Listeria infection* can be acquired from eating unpasteurised dairy products, soft ripened cheeses, e.g. brie, camembert and blue veined varieties, patés and ready-to-eat poultry unless thoroughly reheated.
- *Eating liver* during pregnancy is best avoided as it contains a high concentration of vitamin A.
- *Pre-pregnancy folic acid* supplements reduce the risk of neural tube defects in the fetus. Low-dose folic acid supplementation is recommended for all women planning a pregnancy, with a higher dose for women with a previously affected fetus.

Any pre-existing maternal medical condition (e.g. hypertension) or obstetric risk factors for complications of pregnancy or delivery (e.g. recurrent miscarriage or previous preterm delivery) should be identified and treated or monitored. Obesity increases the risk of developing gestational diabetes and pregnancy-induced hypertension.

Couples at risk of inherited disorders should receive genetic counselling before pregnancy. They can then be fully informed, decide whether or not to proceed, and consider antenatal diagnosis if available. Pregnancies at increased risk of fetal abnormality include those in which:

- the mother is over 35 years old, when the risk of Down's syndrome is greater than 1 in 380
- there is a previous abnormal child
- there is a family history of an inherited disorder
- the parents are identified as carriers of an autosomal recessive disorder, e.g. thalassaemia
- a parent carries a chromosomal rearrangement.

Some definitions:
- Stillbirth – fetal death ≥ 24 weeks of pregnancy
- Perinatal mortality rate – stillbirths + deaths within the first 6 days per 1000 live and stillbirths
- Neonatal mortality rate – deaths of live-born infants less than 28 days of age per 1000 live births

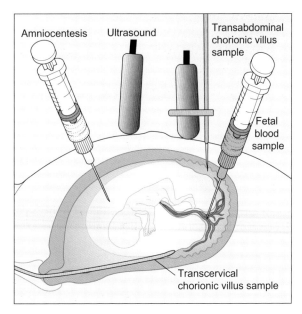

Fig. 8.2 Some of the techniques used for antenatal diagnosis.

ANTENATAL DIAGNOSIS

Antenatal diagnosis has become available for an increasing number of disorders. Screening tests performed on maternal blood and ultrasound of the fetus are listed in Figure 8.1. The main diagnostic techniques for antenatal diagnosis are detailed ultrasound scanning, amniocentesis, chorionic villus sampling and fetal blood sampling (Fig. 8.2). Their indications are listed in Figure 8.3. The structural malformations and some of the other lesions which can be identified on ultrasound are listed in Figure 8.4, with an example in Figure 8.5.

Fig. 8.1 Screening tests for antenatal diagnosis.

Maternal blood	Blood group and antibodies for rhesus and other red cell incompatibilities
	Hepatitis B
	Syphilis
	Rubella
	HIV infection – after counselling and maternal consent
	Testing for neural tube defects – maternal serum alphafetoprotein (MSAFP) is measured in many parts of the UK and other countries. It is raised in about 80% of open neural tube defects and more than 90% of anencephaly. These conditions are increasingly diagnosed or excluded on detailed ultrasound alone
	Testing for Down's syndrome – a risk estimate can be calculated from MSAFP together with human chorionic gonadotrophin (hCG) and unconjugated oestriol (uE_3) measurements (the 'triple' test), adjusted for maternal age. Other hormones can be measured instead, or in addition. If the risk is high, fetal chromosome analysis is offered
Ultrasound screening	Gestational age – can be estimated reliably if performed before 20 weeks
	Multiple pregnancies – can be identified
	Structural malformation – 30–70% of major congenital malformations can be detected. If a significant abnormality is suspected, a more detailed scan by a specialist is advisable
	Fetal growth – can be monitored by serial measurement of abdominal circumference, head circumference and femur length
	Amniotic fluid volume – oligohydramnios may result from reduced fetal urine production (because of dysplastic or absent kidneys or obstructive uropathy), from prolonged rupture of the membranes or associated with severe intrauterine growth retardation. It may cause pulmonary hypoplasia and limb and facial deformities from pressure on the fetus (Potter's syndrome)
	Polyhydramnios is associated with maternal diabetes and gastrointestinal atresia in the fetus

Antenatal diagnosis may allow:

- the option of termination of pregnancy to be offered for severe disorders (see Case history 8.1)
- therapy to be given for a limited number of conditions
- reassurance where disorders are not detected
- optimal obstetric management of the fetus
- neonatal management to be planned in advance.

Parents require accurate medical advice and counselling to help them with these difficult decisions. Many transient or minor disorders are also detected, which may cause considerable anxiety.

Fig. 8.3 Indications for antenatal diagnosis.

Technique	Indication
Detailed ultrasound	Structural malformations and other lesions
Amniocentesis	Chromosomal analysis Alphafetoprotein and acetylcholinesterase for neural tube defects Bilirubin estimation for rhesus disease Enzyme analysis for inborn error of metabolism
Chorionic villus sampling	Chromosomal analysis Enzyme analysis for inborn error of metabolism DNA analysis, e.g. thalassaemia, haemophilia A and B, cystic fibrosis, Duchenne's muscular dystrophy Congenital infection – for virus particles using polymerase chain reaction (PCR)
Fetal blood sampling	Rapid chromosome analysis – if fetal malformations or severe intrauterine growth restriction Severe rhesus and platelet isoimmunisation – assessment Congenital infection serology
Fetal tissue sampling	Skin biopsy for severe congenital skin disorders

Fig. 8.4 Main structural malformations and other lesions detectable by ultrasound.

CNS	Anencephaly – the unexpected birth of an affected infant is now extremely uncommon in the UK Spina bifida – can be difficult to recognise; associated cerebral abnormalities can be helpful Hydrocephalus, microcephaly, encephalocele
Cardiac	A four-chamber view should detect about 60% of severe malformations
Intrathoracic	Diaphragmatic hernia
Facial	Cleft lip and palate
Gastrointestinal	Bowel obstruction – e.g. duodenal atresia, lower bowel obstruction (may be difficult to detect) Exomphalos and gastroschisis
Genitourinary	Dysplastic kidneys Obstructive disorders – readily visualised, but distinguishing mild hydronephrosis from transient, physiological pelvicalyceal dilatation is problematic Oligohydramnios may indicate poor renal function or outflow obstruction
Skeletal	Skeletal dysplasias, e.g. achondroplasia and limb reduction deformities
Hydrops	Oedema of the skin, pleural effusions and ascites
Chromosomal	Down's syndrome – suspected from a thickened fat pad at the back of neck (nuchal thickening), duodenal atresia or an atrioventricular canal defect of the heart Other chromosomal disorders – suspected from identifying multiple abnormalities

ANTENATAL DIAGNOSIS – GASTROSCHISIS

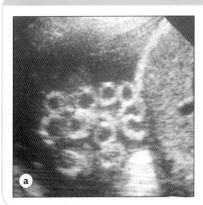
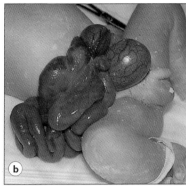

Fig. 8.5 Gastroschisis on antenatal ultrasound showing free loops of small bowel in the amniotic fluid (a) and following delivery (b). Antenatal diagnosis allowed the baby to be delivered at a paediatric surgical unit and the parents to be forewarned about the need for surgery. Satisfactory surgical repair was achieved. (Courtesy of Mr Karl Murphy.)

CASE HISTORY 8.1

ANTENATAL DIAGNOSIS

A routine ultrasound scan at 18 weeks' gestation identified an abnormal 'lemon-shaped' skull (Fig. 8.6). This, together with an abnormal appearance of the cerebellum, is the Arnold–Chiari malformation, which is associated with spina bifida. An extensive spinal defect was confirmed on ultrasound. As the severity of long-term disability varies from mild to severe, advising the parents about the likely outcome is difficult. Dilatation of the cerebral ventricles and talipes already present in this fetus suggested a severe lesion. After counselling, the parents decided to terminate the pregnancy.

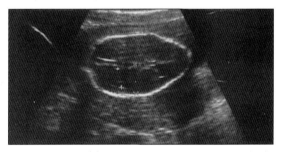

Fig. 8.6 Transverse section showing a 'lemon-shaped' skull on ultrasound instead of the normal oval shape. This is associated with spina bifida. (Courtesy of Mr Guy Thorpe-Beeston.)

> **Congenital malformations which used to be diagnosed at birth or during infancy are increasingly recognised antenatally.**

Fetal medicine

The fetus can sometimes be treated by giving medication to the mother. Examples are as follows:

- Glucocorticoid therapy before preterm delivery accelerates lung maturity and surfactant production, reducing the incidence and severity of respiratory distress syndrome (RDS) and of serious intracranial haemorrhage. For optimal effect, it needs to be given at least 24 h before delivery, but this is often not possible as delivery occurs before this time has elapsed.

- Digoxin or flecainide can be given to the mother to treat fetal supraventricular tachycardia.

There are a few conditions where therapy can be given to the fetus directly:

- *Rhesus isoimmunisation.* The incidence of rhesus incompatibility has fallen markedly since anti-D immunisation of mothers was introduced. Severely affected fetuses become anaemic and may develop *hydrops fetalis*, with oedema and ascites. Infants at risk are identified by maternal antibody screening. Regular ultrasound of the fetus is performed to detect oedema. Mild or moderate disease is monitored by assessing the bilirubin in the amniotic fluid obtained by amniocentesis. Severe disease is best assessed by serially measuring fetal blood haematocrit to detect anaemia. Fetal blood transfusion via the umbilical vein may be required regularly from about 20 weeks' gestation.

- *Perinatal isoimmune thrombocytopenia*. This condition is analogous to rhesus isoimmunisation, but involves maternal anti-platelet antibodies crossing the placenta. It is rare, affecting about 1 in 5000 births. Intracranial haemorrhage secondary to fetal thrombocytopenia occurs in up to 25%, occasionally antenatally. The problem may be anticipated if there was a previously affected infant, and repeated intrauterine platelet transfusions can then be performed.

 Maternal glucocorticoid therapy before preterm delivery markedly reduces morbidity and mortality in the neonate.

Fetal surgery

Fetal surgery is being attempted at a number of centres in the world, but the results have generally been disappointing. Procedures which have been performed include:

- Amnioinfusion of saline for oligohydramnios.
- Surgical correction at hysterotomy. This is when the uterus is opened at 22–24 weeks' gestation to allow surgery on the fetus. It has been performed for diaphragmatic hernia and spina bifida but may precipitate preterm delivery and its efficacy remains highly uncertain.
- Catheter shunts inserted under ultrasound guidance. This is to drain fetal pleural effusions, often from a chylothorax (lymphatic fluid). One end of a looped catheter lies in the chest, the other end in the amniotic cavity.
- Intrauterine shunting for obstruction to urinary outflow. This has yielded disappointing results to date.
- Intrauterine shunting for hydrocephalus. This has largely been abandoned on finding an increased survival rate of severely disabled children.
- Dilatation of stenotic heart valves via a transabdominal catheter inserted under ultrasound guidance into the fetal heart.

Careful case selection and follow-up are required to ensure that these novel forms of treatment are of long-term benefit.

OBSTETRIC CONDITIONS AFFECTING THE FETUS

Preterm delivery

Mothers with pre-eclampsia may require preterm delivery because of the risks of eclampsia and of cerebrovascular accident. The fetus with severe growth restriction may require early delivery to prevent hypoxic damage to the gut and brain, and intrauterine death. Determining the optimal time for preterm delivery requires an evaluation of the risk to the mother and fetus of allowing the pregnancy to continue compared with the neonatal complications associated with preterm birth.

Multiple births

Twins occur naturally in the UK in 1 in 105 deliveries, triplets in 1 in 10 000 and quadruplets in about 1 in every 500 000 deliveries. Over the last decade the number of triplets and higher multiple deliveries has more than doubled, mainly from ovarian stimulation and *in vitro* fertilisation (IVF) programmes.

The main problems associated with multiple births are:
- *Preterm labour*. The median gestation for twins is 36 weeks, for triplets 34 weeks and for quads 32 weeks. Preterm delivery is the most important cause of the greater perinatal mortality of multiple births, especially for triplets and higher order pregnancies.
- *Twin–twin blood transfusions*. These may cause discrepancy in growth, usually of monochorionic (identical) twins.
- *Pre-eclampsia*.
- *Congenital abnormalities*. These occur twice as frequently as in a singleton.
- *Intrauterine growth restriction (IUGR)*. Fetal growth, particularly of the 'second twin', may deteriorate and needs to be monitored regularly.
- *Complicated deliveries*, e.g. due to malpresentation of the second twin at vaginal delivery.

Finding sufficient intensive care cots for preterm multiple births can be problematic.

MATERNAL CONDITIONS AFFECTING THE FETUS

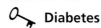 ### Diabetes

Women with insulin-dependent diabetes find it more difficult to maintain good diabetic control during pregnancy and have an increased insulin requirement. Poorly controlled maternal diabetes is associated with polyhydramnios and pre-eclampsia, increased rate of early fetal loss, congenital malformations and late unexplained intrauterine death. Ketoacidosis carries a high fetal mortality. With meticulous attention to diabetic control, the perinatal mortality rate is now only slightly greater than in non-diabetics.

Fetal problems associated with maternal diabetes are:
- *Congenital malformations*. Overall, there is a 6% risk of congenital malformations, a threefold increase compared with the non-diabetic population. The range of anomalies is similar to that for the general population, apart from an increased incidence of cardiac malformations, sacral agenesis (caudal

regression syndrome) and hypoplastic left colon, although the latter two conditions are rare. Studies show that good diabetic control periconceptionally reduces the risk of congenital malformations.

- *Intrauterine growth restriction (IUGR).* There is a threefold increase in growth restriction, probably because of small vessel disease in the mother.

- *Macrosomia* (Fig. 8.7). Maternal hyperglycaemia causes fetal hyperglycaemia as glucose crosses the placenta. As insulin does not cross the placenta, the fetus responds with increased secretion of insulin which promotes growth by increasing both cell number and size. About 25% of such infants have a birthweight greater than 4 kg compared with 8% of non-diabetics. The macrosomia predisposes to cephalopelvic disproportion, shoulder dystocia and birth asphyxia and trauma.

Neonatal problems include:
- *Hypoglycaemia.* Transient hypoglycaemia is common during the first day of life from fetal hyperinsulinism, but can often be prevented by early feeding. The infant's blood glucose should be closely monitored during the first 24 h and hypoglycaemia treated.

- *Respiratory distress syndrome (RDS).* More common as lung maturation is delayed.

- *Hypertrophic cardiomyopathy.* Hypertrophy of the cardiac septum occurs in some infants. It regresses over several weeks but may cause heart failure from reduced left ventricular function.

- *Polycythaemia* (venous haematocrit >0.65). Makes the infant look plethoric. Treatment with partial exchange transfusion to reduce the haemocrit may be required.

Gestational diabetes is when carbohydrate intolerance occurs only during pregnancy. Its definition and method of identification remain controversial. It is more common in women who are obese and in those of Afro-Caribbean and Asian ethnicity. The incidence of macrosomia and its complications is similar to that of the insulin-dependent diabetic mother, but the incidence of congenital malformations is not increased.

 Meticulous control of maternal diabetes during pregnancy markedly reduces fetal and neonatal morbidity and mortality.

Hyperthyroidism

One to two per cent of newborn babies whose mothers have had Graves' disease are hyperthyroid, due to circulating thyroid-stimulating antibody which crosses the placenta and stimulates the fetal thyroid. Hyperthyroidism in the fetus is suggested by fetal tachycardia on a CTG trace, and in the neonate by irritability, weight loss, diarrhoea and exophthalmos lasting several months.

Systemic lupus erythematosus

There is an increased rate of fetal loss in systemic lupus erythematosus (SLE), mostly during the second trimester, in mothers with high titres of antiphospholipid antibodies. Some of the infants born to mothers with antibodies to the Ro (SS-A) or La (SS-B) antigens develop neonatal lupus syndrome, in which there is a self-limiting rash and, rarely, heart block.

Autoimmune thrombocytopenic purpura

In maternal autoimmune thrombocytopenic purpura (AITP), the fetus may become thrombocytopenic because maternal IgG antibodies cross the placenta and damage fetal platelets. Severe fetal thrombocytopenia, which occurs in less than 10% of mothers with proven AITP, places the fetus at risk of intracranial haemorrhage from birth trauma. Infants with severe thrombocytopenia or petechiae at birth should be given intravenous immunoglobulin. Platelet transfusions may be required if there is acute bleeding, but the response to therapy in the neonate is poor. The platelet count continues to fall over the first few days.

MATERNAL DRUGS AFFECTING THE FETUS

Relatively few drugs are known definitely to damage the fetus (Fig. 8.8), but it is clearly advisable for pregnant women to avoid taking medicines unless it is essential. Whilst the teratogenicity of a drug may be recognised if it causes malformations which are severe and distinctive, as with limb shortening following thalidomide ingestion, milder and less distinctive abnormalities may go unrecognised.

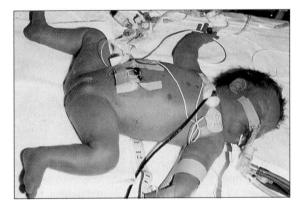

Fig. 8.7 Infant of a diabetic mother showing macrosomia and plethora. Although born at 37 weeks' gestation, she required artificial ventilation for respiratory distress syndrome.

Fig. 8.8 Maternal medication which may adversely affect the fetus.

Cytotoxic agents	Congenital malformations
Diethylstilboestrol (DES)	Clear-cell adenocarcinoma of vagina and cervix
Iodides/propylthiouracil	Goitre, hypothyroidism
Lithium	Congenital heart disease
Phenytoin	Fetal hydantoin syndrome – hypoplastic nails and craniofacial abnormalities
Progestogens (androgenic)	Masculinisation of the female fetus
Tetracycline	Enamel hypoplasia of the teeth
Thalidomide	Limb shortening (phocomelia)
Valproate/carbamazepine	Increased neural tube defects
Vitamin A	Increased spontaneous abortions, abnormal facies
Warfarin	Interferes with cartilage formation (nasal hypoplasia and epiphyseal stippling); cerebral haemorrhages and microcephaly

The problem of establishing a link may be compounded by delay of months or years before any problems present. An example of this is diethylstilboestrol (DES), given in the past for threatened abortion, and its subsequent association with vaginal adenosis and clear-cell carcinoma of the vagina and cervix in female offspring only during adolescence or early adult life.

Alcohol and smoking

Excessive alcohol ingestion during pregnancy is sometimes associated with the 'fetal alcohol syndrome'. Its clinical features are growth restriction, characteristic facies (Fig. 8.9), cardiac defects (up to 70%) and developmental delay. The adverse effects of less severe ingestion and binge drinking remain uncertain. The effects of smoking during pregnancy are described on page 76.

Drug abuse

Maternal drug abuse with narcotics is associated with an increased risk of prematurity and growth restriction. Many narcotic abusers take multiple drugs. Infants of mothers abusing heroin, methadone and other narcotics during pregnancy often show evidence of drug withdrawal, with jitteriness, sneezing, yawning, poor feeding, vomiting, diarrhoea, weight loss and seizures during the first 2 weeks of life. Cocaine abuse rarely causes severe withdrawal in the infant but may result in cerebral infarction and these infants are often restless and difficult to settle. Amphetamine abuse is also associated with gastrointestinal and cerebral infarction. Mothers who abuse drugs and their infants are also at increased risk of hepatitis B and C and HIV infection.

Infants who develop marked features of drug withdrawal will need treatment. Oral morphine, methadone and diazepam are used at different centres. One of the major problems in managing these infants is that the parents' lifestyle and temperament are often not conducive to the needs of babies and young children. Close supervision or alternative care-givers are often required.

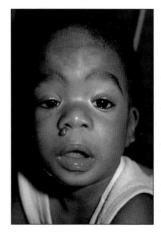

Fig. 8.9 Characteristic facies of fetal alcohol syndrome with a saddle-shaped nose, maxillary hypoplasia, absent philtrum between the nose and upper lip and short thin upper lip. This child also has a strawberry naevus below the right nostril.

Unexplained signs in an infant – consider drug withdrawal.

Drugs given during labour

Potential adverse effects to the fetus of drugs given during labour are:

- *Opioid analgesics/anaesthetic agents.* May suppress respiration at birth and result in delay in establishing normal breathing.
- *Epidural anaesthesia.* May cause maternal pyrexia during labour. It is often difficult to differentiate this from fever caused by an infection. Establishing normal feeding and behaviour during the first few days may also be delayed.
- *Sedatives, e.g. diazepam.* May cause sedation and hypotension in the newborn.
- *Oxytocin.* May cause hyperstimulation of the uterus leading to fetal hypoxia. It is also associated with a small increase in bilirubin levels in the neonate.
- *Intravenous fluids.* May cause neonatal hyponatraemia unless they contain an adequate concentration of sodium.

CONGENITAL INFECTIONS

Intrauterine infection is usually from maternal primary infection. Those that can damage the fetus are:

- rubella
- cytomegalovirus (CMV)
- *Toxoplasma gondii*
- parvovirus
- varicella zoster
- syphilis.

Infants may also become infected in the perinatal period from persistent maternal infection:

- hepatitis B and C
- HIV infection
- herpes simplex virus
- human papilloma virus.

Rubella

The diagnosis of maternal infection must be confirmed serologically as clinical diagnosis is unreliable. The risk and extent of fetal damage are mainly determined by the gestational age at the onset of maternal infection. Infection before 8 weeks' gestation may cause deafness, congenital heart disease, cataracts (Fig. 8.10) and a wide range of defects (Fig. 8.11). About 30% of fetuses of mothers infected at 13–16 weeks' gestation have impaired hearing; beyond 18 weeks' gestation the risk to the fetus is minimal. Viraemia after birth continues to damage the infant. Tests used to confirm the diagnosis are shown in Figure 8.12.

Congenital rubella is preventable. In the UK, it has become rare since the measles/mumps/rubella (MMR) vaccine was introduced into the childhood immunisation programme, but this is dependent on the maintenance of a high vaccine uptake rate.

Cytomegalovirus

CMV is the most common congenital infection, affecting 3–4/1000 live births in the UK, with higher rates reported in parts of the USA. In Europe, 50% of pregnant women are susceptible to CMV. About 1% of susceptible women will have a primary infection during pregnancy, and in about 40% of them the infant becomes infected. The infant may also become infected following recurrent infection in a pregnant woman who is immune, but this is much less likely to damage the fetus.

When an infant is infected:
- 90% are normal at birth and develop normally
- 5% have clinical features of infection at birth (see Fig. 8.11), most of whom will have neurodevelopmental disabilities such as sensorineural hearing loss, cerebral palsy, epilepsy and developmental delay

CONGENITAL INFECTIONS

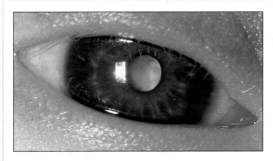

Fig. 8.10 Cataract from congenital rubella. Congenital heart disease and deafness are the other common defects.

Fig. 8.12 Diagnosis of congenital rubella, cytomegalovirus (CMV) and *Toxoplasma* infection.

Urine	Rubella, CMV culture
Blood	Rubella-specific IgM
	CMV-specific IgM
	Toxoplasma-specific IgM and persistently raised *Toxoplasma* IgG

Fig. 8.11 Clinical features of congenital rubella, cytomegalovirus (CMV) and *Toxoplasma* infection.

Clinical features	Rubella	CMV	Toxoplasma
Growth restriction	+++	+++	+
Anaemia	+	++	++
Petechiae, purpura	++	+++	+
Jaundice	+	+++	++
Hepatosplenomegaly	+++	+++	++
Congenital heart disease	+++	–	–
Pneumonitis	+	++	+
Eye			
Glaucoma	++	–	–
Retinopathy	+	+	+++
Cataract	++	–	+
CNS			
Encephalitis	+	++	+
Microcephaly	–	++	+
Intracranial calcification	–	++	++
Hydrocephalus	–	–	++
Bone lesions	++	–	–
Sensorineural deafness	+++	++	–

- 5% develop problems later in life, mainly sensorineural hearing loss.

Infection in the pregnant woman is usually asymptomatic or causes a mild non-specific illness. Identification of infection in all pregnant women would require regular serological testing during pregnancy and might miss fetal infection following recurrence of CMV. As most infected infants develop normally, screening in pregnancy is not considered justified at present in the UK.

Toxoplasmosis

Acute infection with *Toxoplasma gondii*, a protozoan parasite, may result from the consumption of raw or undercooked meat and from contact with the faeces of recently infected cats. In the UK, fewer than 20% of pregnant women have had past infection, in contrast to 80% in France and Austria.

Transplacental carriage may occur during the parasitaemia of a primary infection, and about 40% of fetuses become infected. In the UK, the incidence of congenital infection is only about 0.1 per 1000 live births. Most infected infants are asymptomatic. About 10% have clinical manifestations, of which the most common are:

- hydrocephalus
- cerebral calcification
- retinopathy, an acute fundal chorioretinitis which sometimes interferes with vision
- other features as shown in Figure 8.11. These infants usually have long-term neurological disabilities. Asymptomatic infants remain at risk of developing chorioretinitis into adulthood.

As the specific IgM antibody test has a low sensitivity, serial IgG antibody tests are needed to differentiate passively acquired maternal antibody from fetal infection. In some countries, e.g. France and Austria, pregnant women are screened serologically for *Toxoplasma* infection during pregnancy. During early pregnancy, confirmation of fetal infection is obtained from cordocentesis and, if positive, termination of pregnancy or treatment with the antibiotic spiramycin can be offered. The severely affected fetus may also have evidence on ultrasound of a fetal anomaly, e.g. hydrocephalus. Infected newborn infants are given treatment. In the UK, in view of the low incidence and the lack of data on the efficacy of treatment, pregnant women are not routinely screened.

Varicella zoster

Fifteen per cent of pregnant women are susceptible to varicella (chickenpox). Usually, the fetus is unaffected, but is at risk if the mother develops chickenpox:

- in the first half of pregnancy (<20 weeks), when there is a <2% risk of the fetus developing severe scarring of the skin and possibly ocular and neurological damage

- within 5 days before or 2 days after delivery, when the fetus is unprotected by maternal antibodies and the viral dose is high. About 25% develop a vesicular rash. The illness has a mortality as high as 5%. Exposed susceptible women can be protected with varicella zoster immune globulin and treated with aciclovir. Infants born in the high-risk period should also receive zoster immune globulin and are often also given aciclovir prophylactically.

Susceptible pregnant women should be given passive immunisation (VZIG, varicella zoster immune globulin) if in contact with chickenpox.

 If there is maternal chickenpox shortly before or after delivery – the infant needs protection from infection.

Syphilis

Congenital syphilis is now rare in the UK, but in the 1980s there was a marked, but transient, increase in the number of cases reported in the USA, mainly among HIV-infected mothers. If mothers with syphilis identified on antenatal screening are fully treated a month or more before delivery, the infant does not require treatment and has an excellent prognosis. If there is any doubt about the adequacy of maternal treatment, the infant should be treated with penicillin.

ADAPTATION TO EXTRAUTERINE LIFE

Fetal lungs are filled with fluid. Fetal catecholamines released during labour reduce the secretion of this lung fluid. During delivery, the thorax is squeezed and lung fluid drained. Once the infant gasps, the remaining lung fluid is absorbed via the lymphatic and pulmonary circulation. The combination of delivery and umbilical cord occlusion results in a gasp, on average, 6 s after delivery. Lung expansion is generated by marked intrathoracic negative pressure and a functional residual capacity is established. The mean time to establish regular breathing is 30 s. After an elective caesarean section, when the mother has not been in labour and the infant's chest has not been squeezed through the birth canal, it may take several hours for the lung fluid to be completely absorbed.

In the fetus, oxygenated blood bypasses the lungs (Fig. 8.13). Pulmonary expansion at birth is associated with a falling pulmonary vascular resistance and subsequent increase in pulmonary blood flow. Increased left atrial filling results in a rise in the left atrial pressure which further contributes to the closure of the foramen ovale. The flow of oxygenated blood through the ductus arteriosus causes physiological, and eventual anatomical, ductal closure.

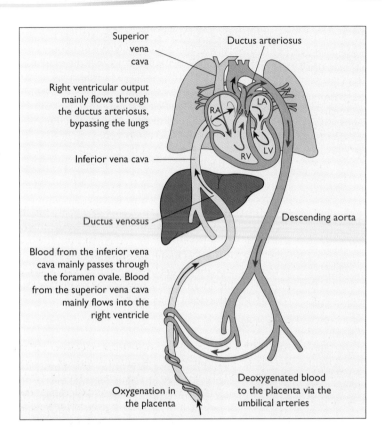

Fig. 8.13 The fetal circulation.

Superior vena cava

Ductus arteriosus

Right ventricular output mainly flows through the ductus arteriosus, bypassing the lungs

RA   LA

RV   LV

Inferior vena cava

Ductus venosus

Descending aorta

Blood from the inferior vena cava mainly passes through the foramen ovale. Blood from the superior vena cava mainly flows into the right ventricle

Oxygenation in the placenta

Deoxygenated blood to the placenta via the umbilical arteries

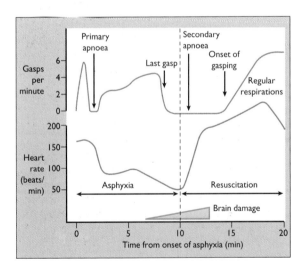

Fig. 8.14 The changes in respiration and heart rate following continuous total asphyxia in a newborn animal. Once the infant has stopped gasping and has a marked bradycardia, resuscitation with lung expansion is required to establish regular respirations and restore the circulation. (Adapted from Dawes G S, *Foetal and Neonatal Physiology*, Year-Book Publishers, Chicago, 1968.)

Under experimental conditions, it is known that if a newborn animal is continuously asphyxiated and deprived of oxygen at birth, it will initially gasp before becoming apnoeic (primary apnoea), during which time the heart rate is maintained. This is followed by irregular gasping and then a second period of apnoea (secondary apnoea), when the heart rate and blood pressure fall. At this stage, the infant will only recover if help with lung expansion is provided, e.g. by tracheal intubation and positive pressure ventilation (Fig. 8.14).

The human fetus rarely experiences a continuous asphyxial insult, except after severe antepartum haemorrhage or complete occlusion of umbilical blood flow in a cord prolapse. More commonly, asphyxia which occurs during labour and delivery is intermittent; only when it is severe and prolonged is an infant born whose clinical condition resembles 'secondary apnoea'. Although birth asphyxia is an important cause of failure to establish breathing which requires resuscitation at birth, there are other causes, including birth trauma, maternal analgesic or anaesthetic agents, retained lung fluid or the infant is preterm or has a congenital malformation which interferes with breathing.

The Apgar score is used to describe a baby's condition at 1 and 5 min after delivery (Fig. 8.15). It is also measured at 5-min intervals thereafter if the infant's condition remains poor. The most important components are the heart rate and respiration.

NEONATAL RESUSCITATION

Most infants do not require any resuscitation. Shortly after birth, the baby will gasp or cry, establish normal breathing and become pink. The baby can be handed

Fig. 8.15 The Apgar score.

	Score		
	0	1	2
Heart rate	Absent	<100 beats/min	>100 beats/min
Respiratory effort	Absent	Gasping or irregular	Regular, strong cry
Muscle tone	Flaccid	Some flexion of limbs	Well flexed, active
Reflex irritability	None	Grimace	Cry, cough
Colour	Pale/blue	Body pink, extremities blue	Pink

directly to his mother, covering him with a warm towel to ensure he does not become cold.

A newborn infant who does not establish normal respiration quickly will need to be transferred to a resuscitation table for further assessment (Fig. 8.16). There should be an overhead radiant heater and the infant should be dried and partially covered and kept warm. The mouth and nose are gently suctioned to remove any fluid or blood. Vigorous suction of the back of the throat may provoke bradycardia from vagal stimulation and should be avoided. If the infant's breathing in the first minute of life is irregular or shallow, but the heart rate is satisfactory (>100 beats/min), additional oxygen is given and breathing encouraged with gentle tactile stimulation.

If the infant does not start to breathe, or if the heart rate drops below 100 beats/min airway positioning and breathing by mask ventilation are started (Fig. 8.16b, c and d). If the baby's condition does not improve promptly with basic resuscitation, or if the infant is clearly in very poor condition at birth, tracheal intubation and artificial ventilation should be performed immediately (Fig. 8.16e). If at any time the heart rate drops below 60 beats/min, external cardiac compression should be given (Fig. 8.16f and g). If the response to ventilation and external cardiac compression remains inadequate, drugs are given (Fig. 8.16h). Evidence for their efficacy is poor.

> **Providing optimal ventilation is the key to successful neonatal resuscitation.**

Meconium aspiration

The passage of meconium becomes increasingly common the greater the infant's gestational age. Infants who inhale thick meconium may develop meconium aspiration syndrome, so any thick meconium present at delivery should be removed from the upper airway by suction immediately after the head is delivered to try to prevent aspiration. If the infant cries at birth and establishes regular respiration, he should be treated as normal and no attempt made to intubate. If respiration is not established, the cords should be inspected under direct vision and any meconium present should be aspirated by suctioning a large-bore suction catheter passed below the cords, or intubated and the tracheal tube aspirated. As much meconium as possible is removed, but if the infant becomes bradycardic, positive pressure ventilation will need to be initiated despite the presence of meconium.

Naloxone

Infants born to mothers who have received opiate analgesia within a few hours of delivery may occasionally develop respiratory depression which can be reversed by naloxone. It is only given if respiration continues to be depressed following initial resuscitation. As the half-life of naloxone is shorter than that of the maternal opiate, the infant's breathing must be monitored, as further doses of naloxone may be required. With modern obstetric practice, naloxone is rarely needed.

Failure to respond to resuscitation

Poor response to tracheal intubation is usually because the tracheal tube is misplaced or has become blocked with secretions or meconium. Chest wall movement is the best guide to air entry to the lungs. If there is any uncertainty about the adequacy of ventilation and resuscitation continues to be unsuccessful, it is essential to remove the tracheal tube, give mask ventilation and then re-intubate. The decision to stop resuscitation is always difficult and should be made by a senior paediatrician. The longer it takes a baby to respond to resuscitation, the less likely he is to survive. If there is no respiratory effort or cardiac output after 20 min of effective resuscitation, further efforts are likely to be fruitless. If prolonged resuscitation is required, the infant should be transferred to the neonatal unit for assessment and monitoring.

Resuscitation of the preterm infant

Preterm infants are particularly liable to hypothermia, and every effort must be made to keep them warm during resuscitation. Very premature infants often develop respiratory distress syndrome, and early administration of surfactant has been shown to reduce mortality. Resuscitation of infants at the threshold of viability, at 22–24 weeks' gestation, raises particularly

---

NEONATAL RESUSCITATION

Preparation
• All health professionals dealing with newborn infants should be proficient in basic resuscitation, i.e. **A**irway, **B**reathing with mask ventilation, **C**irculation with cardiac compressions.
• Additional skilled assistance is needed if the baby does not respond rapidly and should be called without delay.
• A person proficient in advanced resuscitation (**A**irway, **B**reathing via tracheal ventilation, **C**irculation, **D**rugs) should be available at short notice in a maternity unit at all times.
• The need for resuscitation can usually be anticipated and a person proficient in advanced resuscitation should be in attendance at all high-risk deliveries.
• A clock should be started at birth for accurate timing of changes in the infant's condition and for determining the Apgar scores.
• Babies should be prevented from becoming cold.

(a)

The inverted pyramid showing the relative frequency of procedures in neonatal resuscitation. (Adapted from *Pediatric Advanced Life Support*, American Heart Association, 1997)

Airway and breathing
Airway – opened by placing the infant's head in the neutral position (Fig. 8.16b)

Breathing – mask ventilation
• Mask over mouth and nose (Fig. 8.16c)
• Head slightly extended
• Connect to breathing bag or ventilator circuit (Fig. 8.16d)
• Rate – 30–40 breaths/min
• Pressure – to achieve chest wall movement (15–25 cmH$_2$O, 0.5s inflation time). The first few breaths may require higher pressures, (30 cmH$_2$O or more)
• Reassess every 30s. If not responding, check mask position, head position and circuit

Intubation
If effective mask ventilation not established, intubate and start artificial ventilation (Fig. 8.16e). If adequate ventilation still not achieved, consider:
• **D**isplaced tube (often in oesophagus or right main bronchus)
• **O**bstructed tube (especially meconium)
• **P**neumothorax or other patient problems
  — lung immaturity/respiratory distress syndrome, diaphragmatic hernia, pleural effusion
  — shock from blood loss
  — upper airway obstruction e.g. choanal atresia
• **E**quipment failure, e.g. exhausted gas supply

(b)   (c)

Infant's head is placed slightly extended, avoiding over extension or flexion which cause upper airway obstruction

The face mask must cover the nose

(d)

The oxygen is given via a pressure regulator. Pressure is delivered when the T-piece is occluded. Alternatively, the mask may be attached to a rebreathing bag

(e)

Tracheal intubation of a newborn infant. The laryngoscope blade is advanced to lift the epiglottis, as shown, and the laryngoscope is then lifted upwards. Gentle pressure on the trachea with the little finger or by an assistant helps bring the vocal cords into view

Fig. 8.16 Resuscitation of the newborn.

difficult ethical and management issues. They should be taken by experienced paediatricians, with as much involvement with the parents as possible.

⟋ SIZE AT BIRTH

An infant's gestation and birthweight influence the nature of the medical problems likely to be encountered in the neonatal period. In the UK, 7% of babies are of low birthweight (<2.5 kg). However, they account for about 70% of neonatal deaths.

Babies with a birthweight below the 10th centile for their gestational age are called small for gestational age or small-for-dates (Fig. 8.17). The majority of these infants are normal, but small. The incidence of congenital abnormalities and neonatal problems is higher in those whose birthweight falls below the second or third centile (approximately two standard deviations below the mean), and some authorities restrict the term to this group of babies. An infant's birthweight may also be low because of preterm birth, or because the infant is both preterm and small for gestational age.

NEONATAL RESUSCITATION (CONT.)

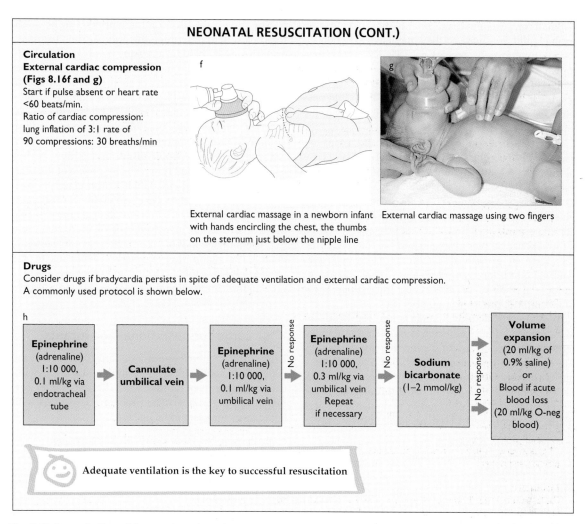

Circulation
External cardiac compression (Figs 8.16f and g)
Start if pulse absent or heart rate <60 beats/min.
Ratio of cardiac compression:
lung inflation of 3:1 rate of
90 compressions: 30 breaths/min

External cardiac massage in a newborn infant with hands encircling the chest, the thumbs on the sternum just below the nipple line

External cardiac massage using two fingers

Drugs
Consider drugs if bradycardia persists in spite of adequate ventilation and external cardiac compression. A commonly used protocol is shown below.

Epinephrine (adrenaline) 1:10 000, 0.1 ml/kg via endotracheal tube → Cannulate umbilical vein → Epinephrine (adrenaline) 1:10 000, 0.1 ml/kg via umbilical vein → *No response* → Epinephrine (adrenaline) 1:10 000, 0.3 ml/kg via umbilical vein Repeat if necessary → *No response* → Sodium bicarbonate (1–2 mmol/kg) → *No response* → Volume expansion (20 ml/kg of 0.9% saline) or Blood if acute blood loss (20 ml/kg O-neg blood)

Adequate ventilation is the key to successful resuscitation

Fig. 8.16 Resuscitation of the newborn (cont.).

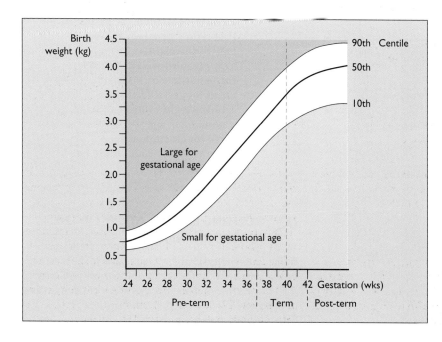

Fig. 8.17 The birthweight of small-for-gestational-age infants is below the 10th centile for their gestation. Small-for-gestational-age infants may be preterm, term or post-term.

Small-for-gestational-age infants may have grown normally but are small, or they may have experienced intrauterine growth restriction (IUGR), when they appear thin and malnourished. Babies with a birthweight above the 10th centile may also be malnourished, e.g. a fetus growing along the 80th centile who develops growth failure and whose weight falls to the 20th centile.

Growth restriction in both the fetus and infant has traditionally been classified as symmetrical or asymmetrical. In the more common asymmetrical growth restriction, the weight or abdominal circumference lies on a lower centile than that of the head. This occurs when the placenta fails to provide adequate nutrition late in pregnancy but brain growth is relatively spared at the expense of liver glycogen and skin fat (Fig. 8.18). This form of growth restriction is associated with maternal pre-eclampsia, cardiac or renal disease or multiple gestation, or it may be idiopathic. These infants rapidly put on weight after birth.

In symmetrical growth retardation, the head circumference is equally reduced. It suggests a prolonged period of poor intrauterine growth. This is usually due to a small but normal fetus, but may be due a fetal chromosomal disorder or syndrome, a congenital infection, maternal smoking, drug and alcohol abuse or a chronic medical condition or malnutrition. These infants are more likely to remain small permanently.

The fetus with IUGR is at risk from:
- intrauterine hypoxia and death
- birth asphyxia.

After birth, these infants are liable to:
- hypothermia because of their relatively large surface area
- hypoglycaemia from poor fat and glycogen stores
- hypocalcaemia
- polycythaemia (venous haematocrit >0.65).

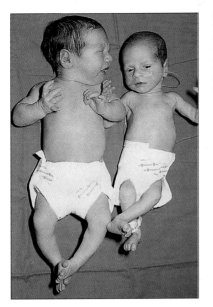

Fig. 8.18
Twins, one of whom suffered from severe intrauterine growth restriction.

The growth-restricted fetus will need to be monitored closely to determine the optimal time for delivery. This will include assessing fetal size clinically (symphysis to fundal height measurement) and serial ultrasound measurements of fetal growth. Antenatal cardiotocography (CTG) to detect evidence of fetal hypoxia may be combined with an ultrasound assessment of fetal activity, breathing and amniotic fluid volume to form a biophysical profile to identify high-risk pregnancies. Doppler ultrasound is now widely used to obtain a blood flow velocity profile of the uterine artery (maternal circulation to the placental bed) and the umbilical artery (fetal circulation). Absence or reversal of flow velocity in the umbilical artery during diastole carries an increased risk of morbidity from hypoxic damage to the gut or brain, or of intrauterine death. The blood flow velocity waveforms in the fetal descending aorta, cerebral and other arteries may give an indication of fetal circulatory redistribution in response to hypoxia.

Large-for-gestational-age infants

Large-for-gestational-age infants are those above the 90th weight centile for their gestation. Macrosomia is a feature of infants of mothers with diabetes, either permanent or gestational. The problems associated with being large for gestational age are:

- birth asphyxia from a difficult delivery
- birth trauma especially from shoulder dystocia at delivery
- hypoglycaemia due to hyperinsulinism
- polycythaemia.

> **Some definitions:**
>
> **Neonate** – infant ≤28 days old
> **Preterm** – gestation <37 weeks
> **Post-term** – gestation ≥42 weeks
> **Low birthweight** – <2500 g
> **Very low birthweight** – <1500 g
> **Extremely low birthweight** – <1000 g
> **Small for gestational age** – birthweight <10th centile for gestational age
> **Large for gestational age** – birthweight >90th centile for gestational age

ROUTINE EXAMINATION OF THE NEWBORN INFANT

Immediately after a baby is born, parents are naturally anxious to know if their baby is all right. To answer this, the midwife (or the paediatrician or obstetrician, if present) will briefly but carefully check that the baby is pink, breathing normally and has no major abnormalities. If the mother has had hydramnios, a feeding tube needs to be passed into the stomach to exclude oesophageal atresia. If a significant problem is identified, an experienced paediatrician needs to explain the situation to the parents. If the baby is markedly preterm, small or ill, admission to a neonatal unit will be required. Should there be any uncertainty about the child's sex, it is best not guess but to explain to the parents that further tests are necessary. In most hospitals, babies are given vitamin K at birth to prevent haemorrhagic disease of the newborn.

Within 24 h of birth every baby should have a full and thorough medical examination, the 'routine examination of the newborn infant'. Its purpose is to:

- detect congenital abnormalities not already identified at birth, e.g. congenital heart disease, developmental dysplasia of the hip
- check for potential problems arising from maternal disease or familial disorders
- provide an opportunity for the parents to discuss any questions about their baby.

Before approaching the mother and baby, the obstetric and neonatal notes must be checked to identify relevant information. The examination (Fig. 8.19) should be performed with the mother or ideally both parents present. Many lesions in the newborn resolve spontaneously (Fig. 8.20). Some of the abnormalities detectable at birth are noted in Figure 8.21. A serious congenital anomaly is present at birth in about 10–15/1000 live births (Fig. 8.22). In addition, many congenital anomalies, especially of the heart, present clinically at a later age.

Procedures in newborn infants

Testing for developmental dysplasia of the hip (DDH), also called congenital dislocation of the hip (CDH)

The infant needs to be relaxed, as kicking or crying results in tightening of the muscles around the hip and prevents satisfactory examination. The pelvis is stabilised with one hand. With the other hand, the examiner's middle finger is placed over the greater trochanter and the thumb around the distal medial femur. The hip is held flexed and adducted. The femoral head is gently pushed downwards. If the hip is dislocatable, the femoral head will be pushed posteriorly out of the acetabulum (Fig. 8.23a).

The next part of the examination is to see if the hip can be returned from its dislocated position back into the acetabulum. With the hip abducted, upward leverage is applied (Fig. 8.23b). A dislocated hip will return with a 'clunk' into the acetabulum. Ligamentous clicks without any movement of the head of femur are of no significance. It should be possible to abduct the hips fully, but this may be restricted if the hip is dislocated. Clinical examination does not identify some infants who have hip dysplasia from lack of development of the acetabular shelf. DDH is more common in girls (sixfold increase), if there is a positive family history (20% of affected infants), if the birth is a breech presentation (30% of affected infants) or if the infant has a neuromuscular disorder.

Early recognition of DDH is important as it reduces long-term morbidity. A specialist orthopaedic opinion should be sought in the management of this condition. Ultrasound examination of the hip joint is performed increasingly in many hospitals, either following an abnormal examination or to screen babies at increased risk (breech presentation or positive family history). Ultrasound examination can be performed to screen all babies, but this requires considerable resources and there are false positives. It will, however, identify some babies missed on clinical examination. Studies are in progress to ascertain the desirability of universal ultrasound screening.

Vitamin K therapy

Vitamin K deficiency may result in haemorrhagic disease of the newborn. This disorder can occur early, during the first week of life, or late, from 1 to 8 weeks of age. In most affected infants, the haemorrhage is mild, such as bruising, haematemesis and melaena, or prolonged bleeding of the umbilical stump or after a circumcision. However, some suffer from intracranial haemorrhage, half of whom are permanently disabled or die.

Breast milk is a poor source of vitamin K, whereas infant formula milk has a much higher vitamin K content. Haemorrhagic disease of the newborn may occur in infants who are wholly breast-fed but not if fed with an infant formula. Infants of mothers taking anticonvulsants, which impair the synthesis of vitamin K-dependent clotting factors, are at increased risk of haemorrhagic disease, both during delivery and soon after birth. Infants with liver disease are also at increased risk.

The disease can be prevented if vitamin K is given by intramuscular injection, and in the UK was widely given to all newborn infants immediately after birth. A few years ago, a study suggested a possible association between vitamin K given intramuscularly and the development of cancer in childhood, but this has not been found in other, much larger studies. The initial study has led to the recommendation that vitamin K should be given orally rather than by intramuscular injection. As absorption via the oral route is variable, several doses are needed over the first few weeks of life to achieve adequate liver storage. Mothers on anticonvulsant therapy should receive oral prophylaxis from 36 weeks' gestation and the baby given intramuscular vitamin K.

 Vitamin K should be given to all newborn infants to prevent haemorrhagic disease of the newborn.

ROUTINE EXAMINATION OF THE NEWBORN INFANT

Fig. 8.19a The routine examination of the newborn infant

Birthweight, gestational age and birthweight centile are noted.

General observation of the baby's appearance, posture and movements provides valuable information about any abnormalities. The baby must be fully undressed during the examination.

The head circumference is measured with a paper tape measure and its centile noted. This is a surrogate measure of brain size.

The fontanelle and sutures are palpated. The fontanelle size is very variable. The sagittal suture is often separated and the coronal sutures may be overriding. A tense fontanelle when the baby is not crying may be due to raised intracranial pressure and cranial ultrasound should be performed to check for hydrocephalus. A tense fontanelle is also a late sign of meningitis.

The facies is observed. If abnormal, this may represent a syndrome, particularly if other anomalies are present. Down's syndrome is the most common, but there are hundreds of syndromes. When the diagnosis is uncertain, a book or a computer database may be consulted and advice should be sought from a senior paediatrician or geneticist.

If plethoric or pale, the haematocrit should be checked to identify polycythaemia or anaemia. Central cyanosis, which always needs urgent assessment, is best seen on the tongue.

Jaundice within 24 h of birth requires further evaluation.

The eyes are checked for cataracts (red reflex checked with an ophthalmoscope) and other abnormalities.

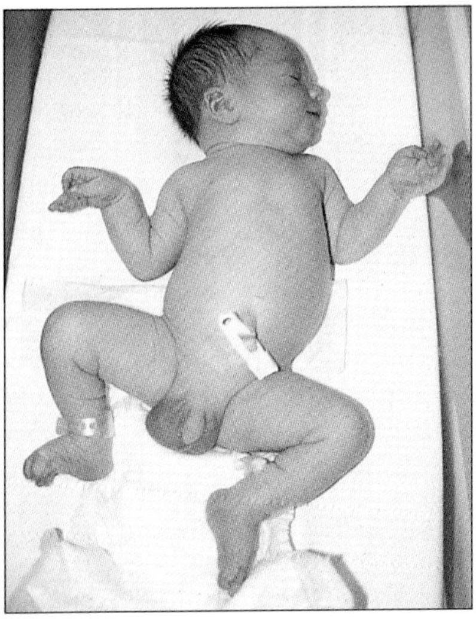

The palate needs to be inspected, including posteriorly to exclude a posterior cleft palate, and palpated to detect an indentation of the posterior palate from a submucous cleft.

Breathing and chest wall movement are observed for signs of respiratory distress.

On auscultating the heart, the normal rate is 110–150 beats/min in term babies, but may drop to 85 beats/min during sleep.

On palpating the abdomen the liver normally extends 1–2 cm below the costal margin, the spleen tip may be palpable as may the kidney on the left side. Any intrabdominal masses, which are usually renal in origin, need further investigation.

The genitalia and anus are inspected on removing the nappy. In boys the presence of testes in the scrotum is confirmed.

The femoral pulses are palpated. Their pulse pressure is:

- reduced in coarctation of the aorta. This can be confirmed by measuring the blood pressure in the arms and legs
- increased if there is a patent ductus arteriosus.

Fig. 8.19b Term newborn.
Median measurements:
Birth weight 3.5 kg
Head circumference 35 cm
Length 50 cm

Muscle tone is assessed by observing limb movements and on picking up the baby while supporting the head. Most babies will support their weight with their feet. On turning the baby prone, the head is lifted to the horizontal and the back straightened.

The whole of the back and spine is observed, looking for any midline defects of the skin.

The hips are checked for developmental dysplasia of the hips (DDH). This is left until last as the procedure is uncomfortable.

LESIONS IN THE NEWBORN

Fig. 8.20a Lesions in newborn infants which resolve spontaneously.

Peripheral cyanosis of the hands and feet – common in the first day.

Traumatic cyanosis from a cord round the baby's neck or from a face or brow presentation – causes blue discoloration of the skin, petechiae over the head and neck or affected part but not the tongue.

Swollen eyelids and distortion of shape of the head from the delivery.

Subconjunctival haemorrhages – occur during delivery.

Small white pearls along the midline of the palate (Epstein's pearls).

Cysts of the gums (epulis) or floor of the mouth (ranula).

Breast enlargement – may occur in newborn babies of either sex (Fig. 8.20b). A small amount of milk may be discharged.

White vaginal discharge or small withdrawal bleed in girls. There may be a prolapse of a ring of vaginal mucosa.

Capillary haemangioma or 'stork bites' – pink macules on the upper eyelids, mid-forehead and nape of the neck are common and arise from distension of the dermal capillaries. Those on the eyelids gradually fade over the first year; those on the neck become covered with hair.

Neonatal urticaria (erythema toxicum) – a common rash appearing at 2–3 days of age, consisting of white pinpoint papules at the centre of an erythematous base. Microscopy of the fluid contents reveals eosinophils. The lesions are concentrated on the trunk; they come and go at different sites.

Milia – white pimples on the nose and cheeks, from retention of keratin and sebaceous material in the pilaceous follicles.

Mongolian blue spots – blue/black macular discoloration at the base of the spine and on the buttocks (Fig. 8.20c) occasionally occur on the legs and other parts of the body. Usually but not invariably in Afro-Caribbean or Asian infants. They fade slowly over the first few years. They are of no significance unless misdiagnosed as bruises.

Umbilical hernia – common, particularly in Afro-Caribbean infants. No treatment is indicated, as it usually resolves within the first 2–3 years.

Positional talipes – the feet often remain in their *in-utero* position. Unlike true talipes equinovarus, the foot can be fully dorsiflexed to touch the front of the lower leg.

Harlequin colour change – when lying sideways, there is reddening down one half of the body with sharply demarcated blanching down the other side, lasting for a few minutes (Fig. 8.20d). It is thought to be due to vasomotor instability.

Caput succedaneum (see page 121)

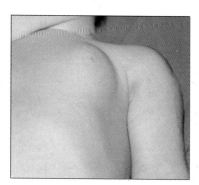

Fig. 8.20b Breast enlargement in a newborn infant.

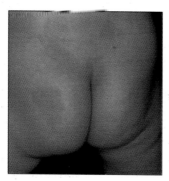

Fig. 8.20c A Mongolian blue spot.

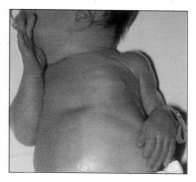

Fig. 8.20d Harlequin colour change.

SIGNIFICANT ABNORMALITIES DETECTED ON ROUTINE EXAMINATION

Fig. 8.21a Some abnormalities detected on routine examination.

Port wine stain (naevus flammeus). Present from birth and usually grows with the infant (Fig. 8.21b). It is due to a vascular malformation of the capillaries in the dermis. Rarely, if along the distribution of the trigeminal nerve, it may be associated with intracranial vascular anomalies (Sturge–Weber syndrome), or severe lesions on the limbs with bone hypertrophy (Klippel–Trenaunay syndrome). Disfiguring lesions can now be improved with laser therapy.

Strawberry naevus (cavernous haemangioma). Not usually present at birth, but appears in the first month of life (Fig. 8.21c). It is more common in preterm infants. It increases in size until 3–9 months old, then gradually regresses. No treatment is indicated unless the lesion interferes with vision or the airway. Ulceration or haemorrhage may occur. Thrombocytopenia may occur with large lesions, when therapy with systemic steroids or interferon-α may be required.

Natal teeth consisting of the front lower incisors – may be present at birth. If loose they should be removed to avoid the risk of aspiration.

Extra digits – are usually connected by a thin skin tag but may be completely attached containing bone and should be removed by a plastic surgeon. Skin tags anterior to the ear and accessory auricles should be removed by a plastic surgeon.

Heart murmur – poses a difficult problem, as most murmurs audible in the first few days of life resolve shortly afterwards. However, some are caused by congenital heart disease. If there are any features of a significant murmur (see Ch. 15), an echocardiogram is indicated. Otherwise, a follow-up examination is arranged and the parents warned to seek medical assistance if their baby feeds poorly, develops laboured breathing or becomes cyanosed.

Midline abnormality over the spine or skull, such as a tuft of hair, swelling or naevus – requires further evaluation as it may indicate an underlying abnormality of the vertebrae, spinal cord or brain.

Palpable and large bladder – if there is urinary outflow obstruction, particularly in boys with a posterior urethral valve.

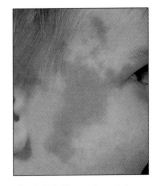

Fig. 8.21b Port wine stain in an infant.

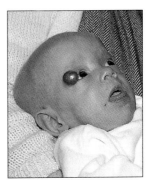

Fig. 8.21c Strawberry naevus.

Fig. 8.22 Prevalence of serious congenital anomalies per 1000 live births (England and Wales).

Anomaly	Prevalence
Congenital heart disease	6–8 (0.8 on the first day of life)
Developmental dysplasia of the hip	1.5 (but about 6/1000 have an abnormal initial clinical examination)
Talipes	1.0
Down's syndrome	1.0
Cleft lip and palate	0.8
Urogenital (hypospadias, undescended testes)	1.2
Spina bifida/anencephaly	0.1

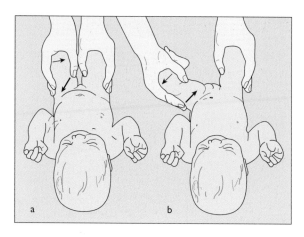

Fig. 8.23 (a) The hip is dislocated posteriorly out of the acetabulum (Barlow manoeuvre). **(b)** The dislocated hip is relocated back into the acetabulum (Ortolani manoeuvre).

Biochemical screening (Guthrie test)

Biochemical screening is performed on every baby. A blood sample, usually a heel prick, is taken when feeding has been established on day 5–9 of life. It was introduced to screen for phenylketonuria, which is rare, but is now also used to screen for hypothyroidism, which is more common. Screening for galactosaemia, maple syrup urine disease and homocystinuria can also be performed. The blood spot can also be used to screen for haemoglobinopathies (mainly sickle cell and thalassaemia), and this is done where the disease is prevalent. It is also possible to screen for cystic fibrosis, but this is not performed routinely throughout the UK.

 In the UK all babies are screened for congenital hypothyroidism and phenylketonuria.

FURTHER READING

James D K, Steer P J, Weiner C P, Gonik B 1999 High risk pregnancy. Management options. WB Saunders, London.
A comprehensive textbook on perinatal medicine
Rennie J M, Roberton N R C 1999 Textbook of neonatology. Churchill Livingstone, Edinburgh
Resuscitation at birth. The newborn life support provider course manual. Resuscitation Council, UK. 2001

9

Neonatal medicine

The dramatic reduction in neonatal mortality throughout the developed world has resulted from advances in the management of newborn infants together with improvements in maternal health and obstetric care. Neonatal intensive care became increasingly available in the UK from 1975, and it is since that time that the mortality of very low birthweight infants has fallen (Fig. 9.1).

About 10% of babies born in the UK require special medical and nursing care. This can be provided in special care baby units or in transitional care units on postnatal wards, which have the advantage that they avoid separating mothers from their babies. About 1–3% of babies require intensive care, which is undertaken in neonatal intensive care units, many of which are situated in tertiary referral centres serving a number of maternity departments. Modern technology allows even tiny preterm infants to benefit from the full range of intensive care, anaesthesia and surgery. If it is anticipated during pregnancy that the infant is likely to require long-term intensive care or surgery, it is preferable for the transfer to the tertiary centre to be made *in utero*. When a baby requires transfer postnatally, transport should be by an experienced team of doctors and nurses. Arrangements should also be made for parents to be close to their infant during this stressful time.

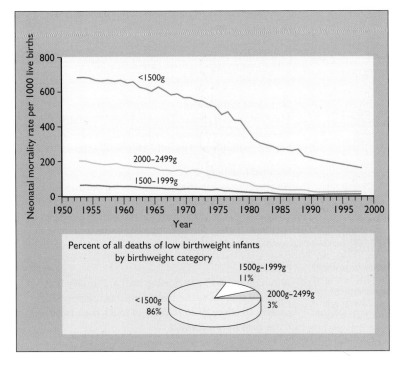

Fig. 9.1 The dramatic fall in neonatal mortality rate in England and Wales, according to birthweight. In very low birthweight infants, the marked fall in the mortality rate has been relatively recent. (Adapted from the Audit Commission. Data from OPCS.)

STABILISING THE PRETERM OR SICK INFANT

Preterm infants of less than 34 weeks' gestation and newborn infants who become seriously ill require monitoring. Many of them will need respiratory and circulatory support (Fig. 9.2). If the preterm infant is allowed to develop respiratory failure, a vicious cycle of lung collapse, secondary surfactant deficiency and later circulatory failure may follow.

BIRTH ASPHYXIA

The incidence of this serious condition has fallen markedly in recent years in the UK to about 1.5/1000 live births. It remains an important cause of brain damage in children and its prevention is one of the key aims of modern obstetric care.

Asphyxia, meaning suffocation, is characterised by reduced oxygen delivery to the tissues. It has a number of different manifestations in the fetus and newborn infant. The fetal cardiotocograph (CTG) may be abnormal, but is poor at assessing the severity of asphyxia unless it is profound. However, when normal, the CTG is highly predictive of the absence of asphyxial problems in the neonate. Fetal blood sampling or cord blood analysis may identify a metabolic acidosis, but is also poor at predicting neonatal outcome unless the acidosis is very severe. Low Apgar

STABILISING THE PRETERM OR SICK INFANT

Additional oxygen and artificial ventilation
Many infants with respiratory distress require additional inspiratory oxygen and ventilatory support. In preterm infants this is often for respiratory distress syndrome (surfactant deficiency), but even in the absence of this disorder, many infants <30 weeks' gestation require artificial ventilation because of lung immaturity or to avoid recurrent apnoea.

Circulatory support
Circulatory support is often given with blood transfusion, saline infusion or inotropic drugs. Echocardiography can provide information on ventricular function.

Monitoring
The heart rate, respiratory rate and temperature are monitored continuously. Oxygenation is measured indirectly by pulse oximetry for oxygen saturation. The arterial O_2 and CO_2 tensions can also be measured transcutaneously. Blood gas analysis is performed on arterial samples from a peripheral or umbilical artery catheter. The arterial oxygen tension is maintained at 8–12 kPa (60–90 mmHg) and the CO_2 tension at 4.5–6.5 kPa (35–50 mmHg).

Chest X-ray
A chest X-ray is required to help diagnose respiratory disorders and confirm the position of the tracheal tube and umbilical artery catheter.

Avoiding hypothermia
Hypothermia increases mortality and should be prevented by placing the baby under a radiant warmer or in an incubator.

Antibiotics
Infants requiring intensive care are usually given broad-spectrum antibiotics.

Metabolic disturbance
Blood glucose is checked regularly and IV dextrose given to prevent hypoglycaemia. Fluid requirements are very variable and must be closely monitored.

Minimal handling
All procedures, especially painful ones, adversely affect oxygenation and the circulation. Sedation and analgesia, e.g. an IV infusion of morphine, are given as required. Handling is kept to a minimum and done as rapidly and efficiently as possible.

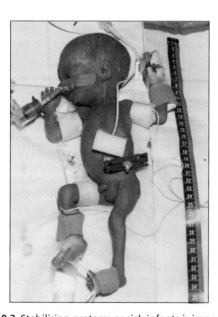

Fig. 9.2 Stabilising preterm or sick infants is important to prevent complications. This preterm infant has leads on his limbs for monitoring heart rate and respiratory rate, temperature and oxygen saturation. There are arterial and intravenous cannulae and a nasotracheal tube for artificial ventilation.

Parents
Although medical and nursing staff are usually fully occupied stabilising the baby, time must be found for parents to allow them to see and touch their baby and to be kept fully informed.

scores at 1 and 5 min, reflecting delayed onset of respiration and circulatory failure at birth, are also poor at predicting outcome, but if the score remains low at 15–20 min of age, the risk of long-term disability or mortality is greatly increased. Hypoxic-ischaemic encephalopathy is the term used to describe the clinical manifestation of brain injury immediately or up to 48 h after asphyxia, whether antenatal, intrapartum or postnatal. Hypoxic-ischaemic encephalopathy can be graded as:

- mild – the infant is irritable, responds excessively to stimulation, may have staring of the eyes and hyperventilation and has impaired feeding
- moderate – the infant is lethargic, with reduced spontaneous movements of the limbs and seizures
- severe – there are no spontaneous movements or response to pain; tone in the limbs may fluctuate between hypotonia and hypertonia; seizures are prolonged and often refractory to treatment; multi-organ failure is present.

Management

Skilled resuscitation and stabilisation of sick infants will minimise asphyxial damage. Infants with hypoxic-ischaemic encephalopathy may need:

- respiratory support
- treatment of seizures with anticonvulsants
- fluid restriction because of transient renal impairment to avoid exacerbating cerebral oedema
- treatment of hypotension by volume and inotrope support
- monitoring and treatment of hypoglycaemia and electrolyte imbalance.

Prognosis

When hypoxic-ischaemic encephalopathy is mild, complete recovery can be expected. The prognosis is usually good if the condition is moderate, but more variable if severe. Several weeks after the insult, cystic lesions or ventricular dilation from cerebral atrophy may be identified on cranial ultrasound, CT or magnetic resonance imaging (MRI) scans. Information about cerebral metabolism suggests that there is a delay in cell damage which may in the future offer therapeutic intervention shortly after the hypoxic insult. The potential benefit of reducing cerebral metabolism by active cooling of the whole baby or the baby's head is being evaluated. Those infants who have recovered fully on clinical neurological examination and are feeding normally by 10 days of age have an excellent long-term prognosis. Severe hypoxic-ischaemic encephalopathy has a mortality approaching 12%, and, of the survivors, 20% have neurodevelopmental disabilities, particularly cerebral palsy (Fig. 9.3).

In view of the potential medicolegal implications, it has been suggested that infants who fail to breathe at birth or develop seizures or other abnormal neurological

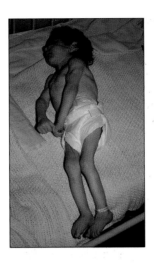

Fig. 9.3 Brain damage from severe birth asphyxia following a sudden, severe antepartum haemorrhage caused this child to become microcephalic, blind and deaf and to have spastic quadriplegia. However, less than 15% of cerebral palsy has an identifiable perinatal cause.

signs should be diagnosed as having 'neonatal encephalopathy', as this does not imply that birth asphyxia was the cause. The diagnosis of birth asphyxia would then only be made if there is:

- evidence of severe antenatal or intrapartum hypoxia
- resuscitation needed at birth
- features of encephalopathy
- evidence of hypoxic damage to other organs
- no other prenatal or postnatal cause identified.

🔑 BIRTH INJURIES

Infants may be injured at birth, particularly if they are malpositioned or too large for the pelvic outlet. Injuries may also occur during manual manoeuvres, from forceps blades or at Ventouse deliveries. Fortunately, now that caesarean section is available in every maternity unit, heroic attempts to achieve a vaginal delivery with resultant severe injuries to the infant have become extremely rare.

Soft tissue injuries

These include:
- Caput succedaneum (Fig. 9.4) – bruising and oedema of the presenting part extending beyond the margins of the skull bones, resolves in a few days.
- Cephalhaematoma (Figs 9.4 and 9.5) – bleeding below the periosteum, confined within the margins of the skull sutures. It usually involves the parietal bone. The centre of the haematoma feels soft. It resolves over several weeks. It is occasionally accompanied by a linear skull fracture.
- Chignon – bruising oedema from a Ventouse delivery.
- Bruising to the face after a face presentation and to the genitalia and buttocks after breech delivery. Preterm infants bruise readily from even mild trauma.

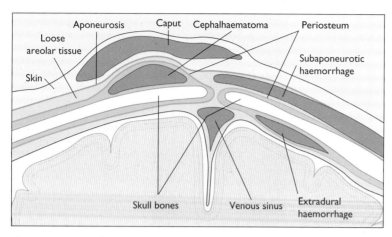

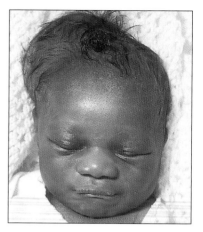

Fig. 9.4 Location of extracranial and extradural haemorrhages.

Fig. 9.5 A large cephalhaematoma.

- Abrasions to the skin from scalp electrodes applied during labour or from accidental scalpel incision at caesarean section.
- Subaponeurotic haemorrhage (very uncommon) – may be accompanied by serious blood loss.
- Severe or fatal injury (very rare) from a tear of the *tentorium cerebelli* or *falx cerebri*.

Nerve palsies

These result from traction to the cervical nerve roots. They may occur at breech deliveries or with shoulder dystocia. Upper nerve root (C5 and C6) injury results in an Erb's palsy (Fig. 9.6). Less often, the lower roots are injured, resulting in weakness of the wrist extensors and intrinsic muscles of the hand (Klumpke's palsy). Most palsies resolve completely over a few weeks. Occasionally, following severe injury, paralysis is permanent. Surgical reconstruction of the nerves is increasingly attempted. Rarely, nerve palsies may be from damage to the cervical spine. A facial nerve palsy may result from compression of the facial nerve by forceps blades or against the mother's pelvis. It is usually transient.

Fractures

Clavicle

Usually from shoulder dystocia. A snap may be heard at delivery or the infant may have reduced arm movement on the affected side, or a lump from callus formation may be noticed over the clavicle at several days of age. The prognosis is excellent.

Humerus/femur

Usually mid-shaft, occurring at breech deliveries. They heal rapidly with immobilisation.

THE PRETERM INFANT

The appearance, the likely clinical course, chances of survival and long-term prognosis depend on the gestational age at birth. Very preterm infants have

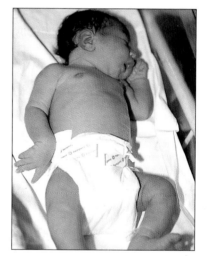

Fig. 9.6 Erb's palsy. The affected arm lies straight, limp and with the hand pronated and the fingers flexed (waiter's tip position).

very thin, dark red, transparent skin, no palpable breast tissue and shapeless, soft ears. The testes of males have not yet descended into the scrotum and females have widely separated labia majora and protruding labia minora. They lie with their arms and legs extended and have poor muscle tone. The external appearance and neurological findings can be scored to provide an estimate of an infant's gestational age (see Appendix).

The rate and severity of problems associated with prematurity decline markedly with increasing gestation. Infants born at 23–26 weeks' gestation encounter many problems (Fig. 9.7), require many weeks of intensive (Fig. 9.8) and special care in hospital and have a high overall mortality. With modern intensive care, the prognosis is excellent after 32 weeks' gestational age. The severity of an infant's respiratory disease largely determines the neonatal course and outcome.

Respiratory distress syndrome

In respiratory distress syndrome (RDS), also called hyaline membrane disease, there is a deficiency of surfactant, the mixture of lipoproteins excreted by the

Fig. 9.7 Medical problems of preterm infants.

Need for resuscitation at birth
Respiratory
 Respiratory distress syndrome (RDS)
 Pneumothorax
 Apnoea and bradycardia
Hypotension
Patent ductus arteriosus
Temperature control
Metabolic
 Hypoglycaemia
 Hypocalcaemia
 Electrolyte imbalance
 Osteopenia of prematurity
Nutrition
Infection
Jaundice
Intracranial haemorrhage/periventricular leucomalacia
Necrotising enterocolitis
Retinopathy of prematurity
Anaemia of prematurity
Iatrogenic
Bronchopulmonary dysplasia (chronic lung disease)
Inguinal hernias

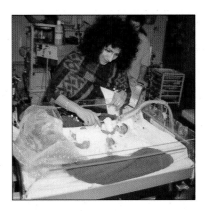

Fig. 9.8
A preterm infant receiving intensive care. Even during this period, parents need to be given the opportunity to get to know their baby.

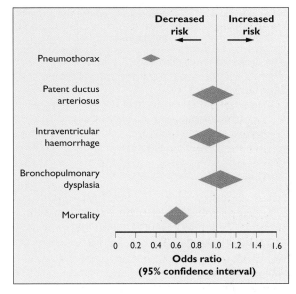

Fig. 9.9 Meta-analysis of treatment of preterm infants with natural surfactant, showing a dramatic reduction in pneumothoraces and mortality.

type II pneumocytes of the alveolar epithelium, which lowers surface tension. There is alveolar collapse and inadequate gas exchange. The more preterm the infant, the higher the incidence of RDS. The majority of infants born before 28 weeks' gestation have RDS, which tends to be more severe in boys than girls. Surfactant deficiency is rare at full term but may occur secondary to hypoxia, acidosis or hypothermia, particularly in the infant of a diabetic mother. The term hyaline membrane disease derives from a proteinaceous exudate seen in the airways of postmortem specimens. Glucocorticoids, given antenatally to the mother, stimulate fetal surfactant production and are used if preterm delivery is anticipated. A 24 h period is ideal to allow the drug to act.

The recent development of exogenous surfactant therapy has been a major advance. The preparations are derived from extracts of calf or pig lung or are synthetic. They are instilled directly into the lung via the tracheal tube. Multinational placebo-controlled trials show that exogenous surfactant treatment reduces mortality from RDS by about 40%, without increasing the morbidity rate (Fig. 9.9).

At delivery or within 4 h of birth, babies with RDS develop clinical signs of:

- tachypnoea
- chest recession with retraction of the subcostal and intercostal muscles and diaphragm, causing in-drawing of the ribs

- expiratory grunting in order to try to create positive airway pressure during expiration and maintain functional residual capacity
- tachycardia
- cyanosis.

The characteristic chest X-ray appearance is shown in Figure 9.10. Treatment with raised ambient oxygen is required, which may need to be supplemented with continuous positive airway pressure (delivered via nasal cannulae or face mask) or artificial ventilation via a tracheal tube. Considerable expertise is required to manage preterm babies with severe RDS. The ventilatory requirements need to be adjusted according to the infant's oxygenation (which is measured continuously), chest wall movements and blood gas analyses. Artificial ventilation may be synchronised as far as possible with the infant's respiration, or the infant's breathing may be partially or completely suppressed with sedatives and muscle relaxants. Whereas ventilators used in adults tend to be volume-cycled, pressure-limited ventilators are usually used in neonates as there

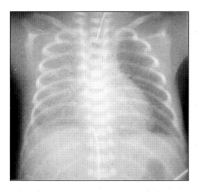

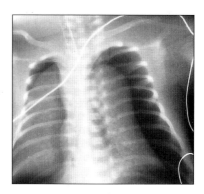

Fig. 9.11 Chest X-ray showing right-sided pulmonary interstitial emphysema and bilateral pneumothoraces in a preterm infant with respiratory distress syndrome.

Fig. 9.10 Chest X-ray in respiratory distress syndrome showing a diffuse granular or 'ground glass' appearance of the lungs and an air bronchogram, where the larger airways are outlined. The heart border becomes indistinct or obscured completely. The diagnosis of respiratory distress syndrome is made on the basis of a characteristic chest X-ray and the clinical course.

is an air leak around uncuffed tracheal tubes. New modes of ventilation, such as high-frequency oscillation, provide an alternative to intermittent positive pressure ventilation and their role is under evaluation.

> **Surfactant therapy markedly reduces the mortality of preterm infants with respiratory distress syndrome.**

Pneumothorax

In respiratory distress syndrome (RDS), air from the overdistended alveoli may track into the interstitium, resulting in pulmonary interstitial emphysema (PIE) (Fig. 9.11). In up to 20% of infants ventilated for RDS, air leaks into the pleural cavity and causes a pneumothorax. When this occurs, the infant's oxygen requirement usually increases, the tidal volume decreases and the breath sounds and chest movement on the affected side are reduced, although this can be difficult to detect clinically. A pneumothorax may be readily demonstrated by transillumination with a bright fibre-optic light source applied to the chest wall. A tension pneumothorax is treated by inserting a chest drain. In order to try and prevent pneumothoraces, infants are ventilated with the lowest pressures that provide adequate chest movement and satisfactory blood gases, and ventilation is adjusted to avoid the infant breathing against the ventilator.

Apnoea and bradycardia

Episodes of apnoea and bradycardia are common in very low birthweight infants until they reach about 32 weeks' gestational age. An episode of bradycardia may occur either when an infant stops breathing for sufficiently long or when the infant continues to breathe

but against a closed glottis. An underlying cause (hypoxia, infection, anaemia, electrolyte disturbance, hypoglycaemia, convulsions, heart failure or aspiration due to gastro-oesophageal reflux) needs to be excluded, but in many no cause is identified. Treatment with a respiratory stimulant such as theophylline or caffeine often helps. Breathing will usually start again after gentle physical stimulation. Occasionally, respiratory support with continuous positive airways pressure (CPAP) or artificial ventilation is required.

Patent ductus arteriosus

The ductus arteriosus remains patent in many preterm infants. Shunting of blood across the ductus, from the left to the right side of the circulation, is most common in infants with RDS. It may produce no symptoms or it may cause apnoea and bradycardia, increased oxygen requirement and difficulty in weaning the infant from artificial ventilation. The pulses are 'bounding' from an increased pulse pressure, the precordial impulse becomes prominent and a systolic murmur may be audible. With increasing circulatory overload, signs of heart failure may develop. More accurate assessment of the infant's circulation can be obtained on echocardiography. Treatment, if necessary, is with fluid restriction and indomethacin. Indomethacin is a prostaglandin synthetase inhibitor which has widespread effects on the circulation, including reduced renal function. If these measures fail to close a symptomatic duct, surgical ligation will be required.

Temperature control

Newborn infants have a larger surface area relative to their body weight than older children. The skin of preterm infants is thin and poorly keratinised and in the first week of life it is an important source of water and heat loss. Preterm infants are unable to shiver, cannot curl up and are usually nursed naked. This adds to their difficulty in maintaining body temperature. Oxygen consumption is increased if the environment is too cold or too hot. There is a neutral temperature range in which an infant's oxygen consumption is lowest. In the very immature baby, the

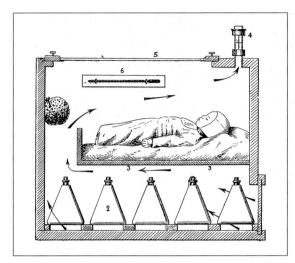

Fig. 9.12 The importance of avoiding hypothermia in newborn infants has long been recognised. This incubator was used in the late 19th century to keep newborn infants warm. The sponge is to increase ambient humidity.

neutral temperature is highest during the first few days of life. The temperature of these small babies is maintained using incubators (Fig. 9.12) or overhead radiant heaters.

Radiant heaters allow better access to the baby, but evaporative heat loss through the skin is greater and this makes fluid balance more difficult to control. Heat loss is reduced by covering the baby with a thermal blanket or plastic shield, providing humidity and clothing the baby whenever practical. Closed incubators provide a more constant environment where ambient humidity can be readily provided, reducing evaporative heat loss.

Fluid balance

A preterm infant's fluid requirements will vary with gestational age, clinical condition and whether he is nursed in a closed or open incubator. On the first day of life, about 60 ml/kg are usually required, increasing by 30 ml/kg per day to 150–180 ml/kg per day. This is adjusted according to the infant's clinical condition, plasma electrolytes, urine output and weight change.

Nutrition

Preterm infants have a high nutritional requirement because of their rapid growth. A preterm infant at 28 weeks' gestation doubles his birthweight in 6 weeks and trebles it in 12, whereas a term baby doubles his weight in 4.5 months and trebles it in a year.

Infants of 35–36 weeks' gestational age are mature enough to suck and swallow milk. Less mature infants will need to be fed via an oro- or nasogastric tube. Even in very preterm infants, enteral feeds, preferably breast milk, are introduced as soon as possible. The

breast milk may need to be supplemented with protein, calories and minerals. There are also special infant formulas designed to meet the increased requirements of preterm infants. In the very immature or sick infant, parenteral nutrition is often required. This is usually given through a central venous catheter, paying strict attention to aseptic technique both during insertion and when fluids are changed.

Poor bone mineralisation (osteopenia of prematurity) was previously common but is prevented by provision of adequate phosphate, calcium and vitamin D. Because iron is mostly transferred to the fetus during the last trimester, preterm babies have low iron stores and are at a risk of iron deficiency. This is in addition to loss of blood from sampling and an inadequate erythropoietin response. Recombinant human erythropoietin may reduce transfusion requirements; its indications and safety are currently being determined. Iron and folic acid supplements are started at about 4 weeks of age.

Infection

Preterm infants are at increased risk of infection, either during or shortly after birth from organisms acquired from the maternal birth canal. Infections later on are nosocomial (hospital-derived) and often associated with indwelling catheters or artificial ventilation.

Intracranial lesions

Periventricular haemorrhages occur in 25% of very low birthweight infants and are easily recognised on intracranial ultrasound scans (Fig. 9.13). Typically, they occur in the germinal matrix above the caudate nucleus, which supports a fragile network of blood vessels. Fortunately, the majority of haemorrhages are small and harmless, but larger haemorrhages may extend into the lateral ventricles or even involve the brain parenchyma. Most haemorrhages occur within the first 72 h of life. They are more common following birth asphyxia and in infants with severe RDS. Pneumothorax is a significant risk factor.

Dilatation of the ventricles which may follow an intraventricular bleed is also readily detected on ultrasound. This dilatation may resolve spontaneously or progress to hydrocephalus, which may cause the sutures to separate, the head circumference to increase rapidly and the anterior fontanelle to become tense. Convulsions or other symptoms may develop at this stage. Removal of CSF by lumbar puncture or ventricular tap may provide symptomatic relief until a ventriculoperitoneal shunt is inserted.

Ischaemic lesions are more difficult to detect by ultrasound. There may initially be an echodense area or 'flare' within the brain parenchyma. This may resolve, or cystic lesions may be noted some weeks later. Multiple widespread cysts, also called periventricular leucomalacia (PVL), are associated with a poor developmental outcome.

INTRACRANIAL ULTRASOUND IN PRETERM INFANTS

Coronal section   **Parasagittal section**

a) Normal anatomy

Sylvian fissure · Choroid plexus · Lateral ventricle · Third ventricle

b) Intra- and periventricular haemorrhage with dilatation of both lateral and third ventricles

Germinal layer haemorrhage · Intraparenchymal haemorrhage · Germinal layer haemorrhage · Dilated lateral ventricles · Intraventricular haemorrhage

c) Severe periventricular leucomalacia

Periventricular cysts and increased echodensity of white matter

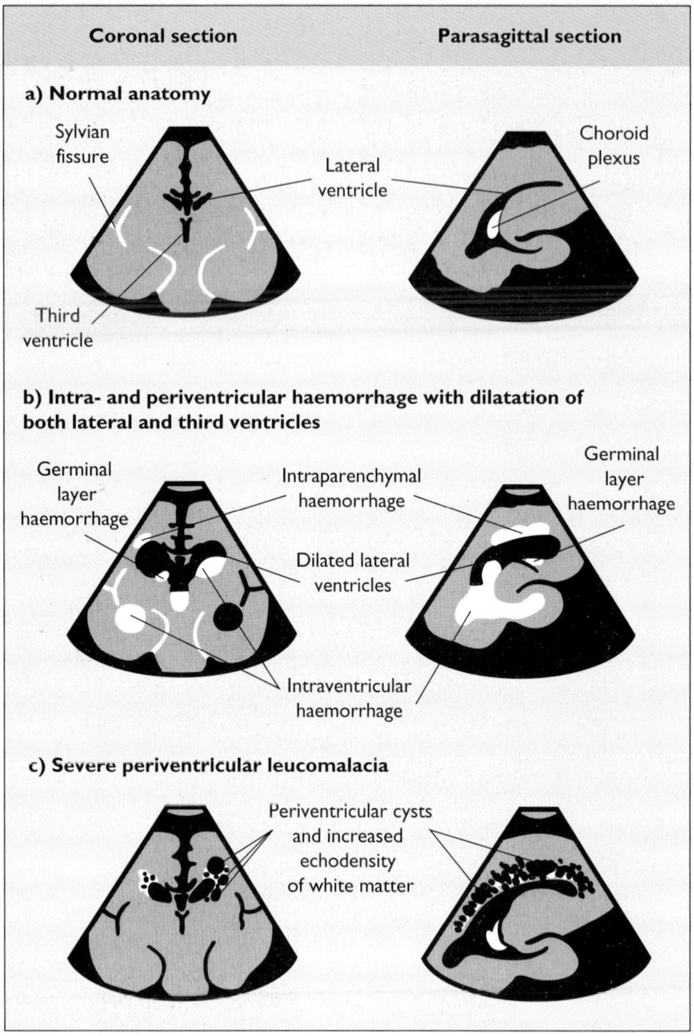

Fig. 9.13a Intracranial ultrasound in preterm infants.

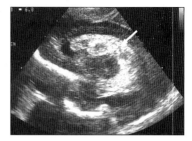

Fig. 9.13b Large intraventricular haemorrhage.

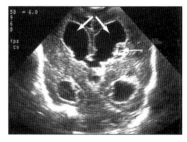

Fig. 9.13c Marked ventricular dilatation (↑). Haemorrhage is visible within the ventricles (↑).

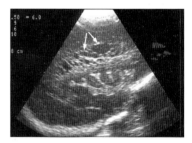

Fig. 9.13d Periventricular leucomalacia, following ischaemic damage (↑).

Necrotising enterocolitis

Necrotising enterocolitis is a serious illness mainly affecting preterm infants in the first few weeks of life. It is caused by ischaemia of the bowel wall and infection from organisms colonising the bowel and may be accelerated by feeding with milk. The infant stops tolerating feeds, milk is aspirated from the stomach and there may be vomiting, which may be bile-stained. The abdomen becomes distended (Fig. 9.14a) and the stool sometimes contains fresh blood. The infant may rapidly become shocked and require ventilatory support because of apnoeic attacks or respiratory failure. The characteristic X-ray features are distended loops of bowel, thickening of the bowel wall with intramural air and air in the portal tract (Fig. 9.14b). The disease may progress to bowel perforation which can be detected by X-ray or by transillumination of the abdomen (Fig. 9.14c).

Treatment is to stop oral feeding and give broad-spectrum antibiotics to cover both aerobic and anaerobic organisms. Parenteral nutrition is always needed and artificial ventilation and circulatory support are often needed. Surgery is performed for bowel perforation. The disease has significant morbidity and a mortality of about 20%. Long-term sequelae include the development of strictures and malabsorption if extensive bowel resection has been necessary.

Retinopathy of prematurity

Retinopathy of prematurity (ROP) affects developing blood vessels at the junction of the vascular and non-vascularised retina. There is vascular proliferation

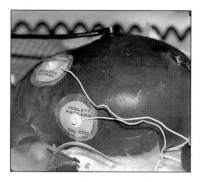

Fig. 9.14a Necrotising enterocolitis showing gross abdominal distension and tense and shiny skin over the abdomen.

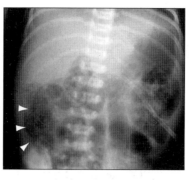

Fig. 9.14b Abdominal X-ray showing the characteristic features of distended loops of bowel and thickening of the bowel wall with intramural air (arrow).

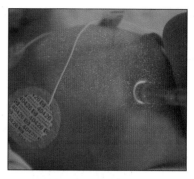

Fig. 9.14c Bowel perforation may be identified on X-ray or by transillumination.

which may progress to retinal detachment, fibrosis and blindness. It was initially recognised that the condition can be caused by giving additional oxygen given in an uncontrolled way. Now, even with careful monitoring of the infant's oxygenation, evidence of retinopathy of prematurity is still found in about 20% of all very low birthweight infants, with a higher percentage in the very immature. It is first detected at the equivalent of 32–38 weeks' gestational age. All very low birthweight infants should have their eyes screened 6–7 weeks after birth by indirect ophthalmoscopy. The early stages of the disease are more frequent and usually resolve completely. Cryosurgery or laser therapy may be indicated for severe disease. Severe visual impairment occurs in about 1% of very low birthweight infants.

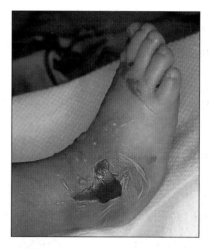

Fig. 9.15 Iatrogenic disease. Extravasation of a peripheral infusion containing calcium.

Iatrogenic disease

Preterm infants, particularly those of very low birthweight or with severe lung disease, need intensive care for many days or weeks. Adverse events are inevitable when such complex techniques are used. Iatrogenic disease may result in significant morbidity and mortality unless all staff are highly skilled and pay meticulous attention to detail (Fig. 9.15).

Bronchopulmonary dysplasia

Infants who have a prolonged oxygen requirement are described as having bronchopulmonary dysplasia (BPD) or chronic lung disease of prematurity. It was initially defined as an additional oxygen requirement beyond 28 days of life, but, more recently, the gestational age of 36 weeks is increasingly used. The lung damage comes from pressure and volume trauma from artificial ventilation, oxygen toxicity, infection and the accumulation of lung secretions. The chest X-ray characteristically shows widespread areas of opacification, often with cystic changes (Fig. 9.16). Some infants need prolonged artificial ventilation, but most are weaned onto continuous positive airways

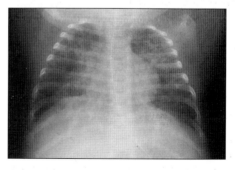

Fig. 9.16 Chest X-ray of bronchopulmonary dysplasia (BPD) showing fibrosis and lung collapse, cystic changes and overdistension of the lungs.

pressure (CPAP) followed by additional ambient oxygen, sometimes over several months. Corticosteroid therapy may facilitate earlier weaning from the ventilator and often reduces the infant's oxygen requirements, but concern about side-effects limits its use. Some babies go home while still receiving additional oxygen. Infants with very severe disease may die of intercurrent infection or cor pulmonale.

Problems following discharge

In general, the children born premature are shorter and thinner than infants born at full term, although neonatal unit graduates are much better nourished than previously. Readmission to hospital during the first year of life is increased approximately fourfold in very low birthweight infants. Those with broncho-pulmonary dysplasia (chronic lung disease of prematurity) are more susceptible to recurrent wheezing, bronchiolitis and chest infections. A monoclonal antibody to RSV, the commonest cause of bronchiolitis, is now available (palivizumab, given monthly by intramuscular injection); its use reduces the hospital admission rate of preterm infants, but its high cost limits its use. Inguinal hernias, usually in boys, may appear in the first few months of life.

Very low birthweight infants are at increased risk of a wide range of neurodevelopmental problems. These include visual impairment, hearing loss, cerebral palsy and learning difficulties (Fig. 9.17). Although only 5–10% have a serious disability, they are more prone to specific learning difficulties, particularly delayed language development, poor attention span, difficulty with fine motor skills and have more behavioural problems than siblings born at term. The risk of developing these problems increases markedly if born at very early gestational age. Gross abnormalities on intracranial ultrasound and abnormal neurological examination at term indicate an increased risk of long-term disability. All very low birthweight infants should have their developmental progress monitored to allow early detection and treatment of any problems.

✎ JAUNDICE

Over 60% of all newborn infants become visibly jaundiced. This is because:

- the haemoglobin concentration falls rapidly in the first few days after birth from haemolysis

Fig. 9.17 Follow-up at 3 years of age of survivors (54%) of extremely preterm infants born at <28 weeks' gestation admitted to a neonatal intensive care unit between 1980 and 1989.
(Adapted from Cooke RWI, Factors affecting survival and outcome at 3 years in extremely preterm infants. *Archives of Diseases in Childhood* 71: F28–31, 1994.)

Normal	72%
Lesser disabilities	9%
Moderate or severe disabilities	19%
Cerebral palsy	13%
Cognitive delay	10%
Deafness	2%
Visual impairment	6%
Seizures	2%
Multiple disabilities	8%

(1 g of haemoglobin yields 640 μmol [35 mg] of bilirubin) (Fig. 9.18)
- the red cell life span of newborn infants (70 days) is markedly shorter than that of adults (120 days)
- hepatic bilirubin metabolism is less efficient in the first few days of life.

Jaundice is important as:

- it may be a sign of another disorder, e.g. infection
- unconjugated bilirubin can be deposited in the brain, particularly in the basal ganglia, causing kernicterus.

Kernicterus

This is bilirubin neurotoxicity, which may occur when the level of unconjugated bilirubin exceeds the albumin-binding capacity of the blood. As this free bilirubin is fat-soluble, it can cross the blood–brain barrier. The neurotoxic effects vary in severity from transient

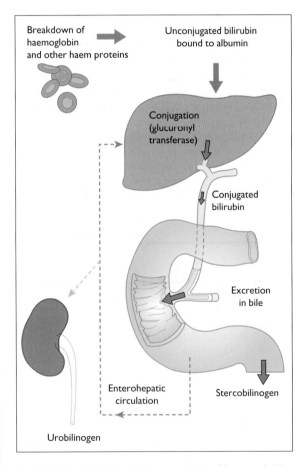

Fig. 9.18 The initial breakdown product of haemoglobin is unconjugated bilirubin (indirect bilirubin) which is insoluble in water but soluble in lipids. It is carried in the blood bound to albumin. It is taken up by the liver and conjugated by the enzyme glucuronyl transferase to conjugated bilirubin (direct bilirubin), which is water-soluble and excreted in bile into the gut and is detectable in urine when blood levels rise. Reabsorption of bilirubin from the gut (enterohepatic circulation) is increased when milk intake is low.

disturbance to catastrophic damage and death. Early manifestations are lethargy and poor feeding. In severe cases, there is irritability and increased muscle tone and the baby may lie with an arched back (opisthotonus). Infants who survive may develop choreoathetoid cerebral palsy (due to damage to the basal ganglia), learning difficulties and sensorineural deafness. Kernicterus used to be an important cause of brain damage in infants with severe haemolytic disease, but has become rare since the introduction of prophylactic anti-D immunoglobulin for rhesus-negative mothers.

Clinical evaluation

Babies become clinically jaundiced when the bilirubin level reaches 80–120 µmol/L. Management varies according to the infant's gestational age, age at onset, bilirubin level and rate of rise and the overall clinical condition.

1. Age at onset

The age of onset is a useful guide to the likely cause of the jaundice (Fig. 9.19).

Jaundice <24 hours of age

Jaundice starting within 24 h of birth usually results from haemolysis. This is particularly important to

Fig. 9.19 Causes of neonatal jaundice.

Jaundice starting at <24 h of age	Haemolytic disorders: Rhesus incompatibility, ABO incompatibility, G6PD deficiency, Spherocytosis, pyruvate kinase deficiency, Congenital infection
Jaundice at 24 h to 2 weeks of age	Physiological jaundice, Breast milk jaundice, Infection, e.g. urinary tract infection, Haemolysis, e.g. G6PD deficiency, ABO incompatability, Bruising, Polycythaemia, Crigler–Najjar syndrome
Jaundice at >2 weeks of age	*Unconjugated:* Physiological or breast milk jaundice, Infection (particularly urinary tract), Hypothyroidism, Haemolytic anaemia, e.g. G6PD deficiency, High gastrointestinal obstruction; *Conjugated (>15% of total bilirubin):* Bile duct obstruction, Neonatal hepatitis

identify as the bilirubin is unconjugated and can rise very rapidly reaching extremely high levels.

Haemolytic disorders
Rhesus haemolytic disease. Affected infants are usually identified antenatally and given fetal therapy if necessary (see Ch. 8). The birth of a severely anaemic infant with hydrops and hepatosplenomegaly who rapidly develops severe jaundice has become rare. Antibodies may develop to rhesus antigens other than D and to the Kell and Duffy blood groups, but haemolysis is usually much less severe.

ABO incompatibility. This is now more common than rhesus haemolytic disease. Most ABO antibodies are IgM and do not cross the placenta, but some group O women have an IgG anti-A-haemolysin in the blood which can cross the placenta and may haemolyse the red cells of a group A infant. Occasionally group B infants are affected by anti-B haemolysins. Haemolysis is usually less severe than in rhesus disease. The infant's haemoglobin level is usually normal or only slightly reduced and, in contrast to rhesus disease, hepatosplenomegaly is absent. The direct antibody test (Coombs' test) is usually weakly positive and haemolysins are usually detectable in the blood. The jaundice usually peaks in the first 12–72 h.

G6PD deficiency. The Mediterranean and Middle- and Far-Eastern variants may cause neonatal jaundice (see Ch. 20). Parents of affected infants should be given a list of drugs to be avoided as they may precipitate haemolysis.

Spherocytosis is considerably less common than G6PD deficiency (see Ch. 20). There is often, but not always, a family history. The disorder can be identified by recognising spherocytes on the blood film.

Congenital infection
Jaundice at birth can also be from congenital infection. In this case the bilirubin is conjugated and the infants have other abnormal clinical signs.

Jaundice at 2 days–2 weeks of age
Physiological jaundice
This accounts for most babies who become jaundiced during this period. Other conditions need to be considered before it can be assumed that the baby's jaundice is physiological.

Breast milk jaundice
Breast milk may exacerbate jaundice in healthy infants. The hyperbilirubinaemia is unconjugated and may be prolonged. The cause is unknown. In some infants the jaundice appears to be exacerbated if milk intake is poor from delay in establishing breast-feeding and the infant becomes dehydrated. Breast-feeding should be continued, although the bilirubin level will fall if it is interrupted.

Infection
An infected baby may develop an unconjugated hyperbilirubinaemia from poor fluid intake, haemolysis,

reduced hepatic function and an increase in the entero-hepatic circulation. If infection is suspected, appropriate investigations and treatment should be instigated. In particular, urinary tract infections may present in this way.

Other causes
Although jaundice from haemolysis usually presents in the first day of life, it may occur during the first week. Bruising and polycythaemia (venous haematocrit is >0.65) will exacerbate the infant's jaundice. The very rare Crigler–Najjar syndrome, when the enzyme glucuronyl transferase is deficient or absent, may result in extremely high levels of unconjugated bilirubin.

Jaundice at >2 weeks of age (persistent neonatal jaundice)
Jaundice in babies more than 2 weeks old is called persistent or prolonged neonatal jaundice. In most infants the hyperbilirubinaemia will still be unconjugated, but this needs to be confirmed on laboratory testing.

In prolonged unconjugated hyperbilirubinaemia:

- 'breast milk jaundice' is the most common cause, affecting about 15% of healthy breast-fed infants; the jaundice gradually fades and disappears by 3–4 weeks of age
- infection, particularly of the urinary tract, needs to be considered
- congenital hypothyroidism needs to be excluded as it may present with prolonged jaundice before the clinical features of coarse facies, dry skin, hypotonia and constipation become evident. Affected infants should be identified on neonatal biochemical screening (Guthrie test).

Conjugated hyperbilirubinaemia is suggested by the baby passing dark urine and unpigmented pale stools. Its causes include neonatal hepatitis syndrome and biliary atresia. It is important to diagnose biliary atresia promptly, as delay in surgical treatment adversely affects outcome (see Ch. 18 for further details).

2. Severity of jaundice
Jaundice can be observed most easily by blanching the skin with the finger. The jaundice tends to start on the head and face and then spreads down the trunk and limbs. A transcutaneous jaundice meter is used in some centres, but if the jaundice appears clinically significant or there is any doubt about its severity, a bilirubin level should be checked on a blood sample. It is easy to underestimate jaundice in Afro-Caribbean, Asian and preterm babies, and a low threshold should be adopted for measuring the bilirubin of these infants.

3. Rate of change
The rate of rise tends to be linear until a plateau is reached, so serial measurements can be plotted on a chart and used to anticipate the need for treatment before it rises to a dangerous level.

4. Gestation
Preterm infants are more susceptible to damage from raised bilirubin so the intervention threshold is lower.

5. Clinical condition
Jaundice may make infants drowsy. Infants who experience severe hypoxia, hypothermia or any serious illness may be more susceptible to damage from severe jaundice. Drugs which may displace bilirubin from albumin, e.g. sulphonamides and diazepam, are rarely used in newborn infants.

Management
Poor milk intake and dehydration will exacerbate jaundice, but studies have failed to show that supplementing breast-feeding with water or dextrose solution will reduce it. Phototherapy is the most widely used therapy, with exchange transfusion for severe cases.

Phototherapy
Light (wavelength 450 nm) from the blue band of the visible spectrum converts unconjugated bilirubin by photodegradation into a harmless water-soluble pigment. Although no long-term sequelae of phototherapy from overhead light have been reported, it is disruptive to normal nursing of the infant and should not be used indiscriminately. The infant's eyes are covered, as a bright light is uncomfortable and has been shown to cause retinal damage in animals. Phototherapy can result in hypo- or hyperthermia, dehydration, a macular rash and diarrhoea.

More recently a fibreoptic blanket has been developed which can be applied directly to the skin. Both an overhead light and blanket can be used simultaneously (intensive (double) phototherapy).

Exchange transfusion
Exchange transfusion is required if the bilirubin rises to levels which are considered dangerous, particularly if there is associated anaemia. Exchange transfusions have been performed traditionally via an umbilical venous catheter by alternately withdrawing 10–20 ml aliquots of the baby's blood and replacing them with donor blood. The procedure can be performed more efficiently, and avoiding the complications associated with umbilical vein cannulation, by infusing the blood via a peripheral vein while extracting blood from an arterial line. Twice the infant's blood volume (80 ml/kg) is exchanged. Donor blood should be as fresh as possible and screened to exclude CMV, hepatitis B and C and HIV infection. The procedure has a low complication rate but does carry some risk of morbidity and mortality.

There are no bilirubin levels which are known to be safe or which will definitely cause kernicterus. In rhesus haemolytic disease, it was found that kernicterus could be prevented if the bilirubin was kept below 340 µmol/L (20 mg/dl). As there is no consensus among paediatricians in the UK on the bilirubin levels at which phototherapy and exchange transfusion should be performed, each department should have clear guidelines for the management of jaundice.

RESPIRATORY DISTRESS IN TERM INFANTS

Newborn infants with respiratory problems develop the following signs of respiratory distress:

- tachypnoea
- laboured breathing, with chest wall recession and nasal flaring
- expiratory grunting
- tachycardia
- cyanosis.

The causes in term infants are listed in Figure 9.20.

Affected infants should be admitted to the neonatal unit for monitoring of heart and respiratory rates, oxygenation and circulation. A chest X-ray will be required to help identify the cause, especially those which may need immediate treatment, e.g. pneumothorax or diaphragmatic hernia. Additional ambient oxygen, mechanical ventilation and circulatory support are given as required.

Transient tachypnoea of the newborn

By far the commonest cause of respiratory distress in term infants is transient tachypnoea of the newborn, caused by delay in the resorption of lung liquid. It is more common after birth by caesarean section. The

Fig. 9.20 Causes of respiratory distress in term infants.

Pulmonary

Common	Transient tachypnoea of the newborn
Less common	Meconium aspiration Pneumonia Pneumothorax Persistent pulmonary hypertension of the newborn Milk aspiration
Rare	Diaphragmatic hernia Tracheo-oesophageal fistula (TOF) Respiratory distress syndrome (RDS) Pulmonary hypoplasia Airways obstruction, e.g. choanal atresia Pulmonary haemorrhage

Non-pulmonary

	Congenital heart disease Intracranial birth trauma/asphyxia Severe anaemia Metabolic acidosis

chest X-ray may show fluid in the horizontal fissure. Additional ambient oxygen may be required. The condition usually settles within the first day of life but can take several days to resolve completely.

Meconium aspiration

Meconium is passed before birth by 8–20% of babies. It is rarely passed by preterm infants, and occurs increasingly the greater the gestational age, affecting 20–25% of deliveries by 42 weeks. It may be passed in response to fetal hypoxia. At birth these infants may inhale thick meconium, which should be aspirated from the airway immediately after the head has been delivered. However, asphyxiated infants may already start gasping and aspirate meconium before delivery. Meconium is a lung irritant and results in both mechanical obstruction and a chemical pneumonitis, as well as predisposing to infection. In meconium aspiration the lungs are over-inflated, accompanied by patches of collapse and consolidation. There is a high incidence of air leak, leading to pneumothorax and pneumomediastinum. Artificial ventilation is often required. Infants with meconium aspiration may develop persistent pulmonary hypertension of the newborn which may make it difficult to achieve adequate oxygenation despite high pressure ventilation. Severe meconium aspiration has a high morbidity and mortality.

Pneumonia

Prolonged rupture of the membranes, chorioamnionitis and low birthweight predispose to pneumonia. Infants with respiratory distress will usually require investigation to identify any infection. Broad-spectrum antibiotics are started early until the results are available.

Pneumothorax

A pneumothorax may occur spontaneously in up to 2% of deliveries. It is usually asymptomatic. Pneumothoraces also occur secondary to meconium aspiration, RDS or as a complication of ventilation. Management is described on page 124.

Milk aspiration

This occurs more frequently in preterm infants and those with respiratory distress or neurological damage. Babies with bronchopulmonary dysplasia often have gastro-oesophageal reflux which predisposes to aspiration. Infants with a cleft palate are prone to aspirate respiratory secretions or milk.

Persistent pulmonary hypertension of the newborn

This life-threatening condition is usually associated with birth asphyxia, meconium aspiration, septicaemia or RDS. It sometimes occurs as a primary disorder. As a result of the high pulmonary vascular resistance, there is right-to-left shunting within the lungs and at

131

atrial and ductal levels. Cyanosis occurs soon after birth. Heart murmurs and signs of heart failure are often absent. A chest X-ray shows that the heart is of normal size and there may be pulmonary oligaemia. An urgent echocardiogram is required to establish that the child does not have congenital heart disease.

Most infants require mechanical ventilation and circulatory support in order to achieve adequate oxygenation. Inhaled nitric oxide, a potent vasodilator, may be beneficial. New modes of artificial ventilation, such as high-frequency or oscillatory ventilation, may be tried. Extracorporeal membrane oxygenation (ECMO), where the infant is placed on heart and lung bypass for several days, is indicated for severe cases.

Diaphragmatic hernia

This occurs in about 1 in 4000 births. Many are now diagnosed on antenatal ultrasound screening. In the newborn period, it usually presents with failure to respond to resuscitation or respiratory distress. In most cases there is a left-sided herniation of abdominal contents through the posterolateral foramen of the diaphragm. The apex beat and heart sounds will then be displaced to the right side of the chest, with poor air entry in the left chest. Vigorous resuscitation may cause a pneumothorax in the normal lung, thereby aggravating the situation. The diagnosis is confirmed by X-ray of the chest and abdomen (Fig. 9.21). Once the diagnosis is suspected, a large nasogastric tube is passed and suction is applied to prevent distension of the intrathoracic bowel. After stabilisation, the diaphragmatic hernia is repaired surgically, but in most infants with this condition the main problem is pulmonary hypoplasia – where compression by the herniated viscera throughout pregnancy has prevented development of the lung in the fetus. This lung hypoplasia is the main cause of the high mortality (30–60%). ECMO has been used pre- and postoperatively to provide respiratory support.

Other causes

Other causes of respiratory distress are listed in Figure 9.20. When due to heart failure, abnormal heart sounds and/or heart murmurs may be present on auscultation. An enlarged liver from venous congestion is a helpful sign. The femoral arteries must be palpated, as coarctation of the aorta and interrupted aortic arch are important causes of heart failure in newborn infants.

INFECTION

Infants are exposed to a wide range of potential pathogens from the birth canal. The risk of infection is increased if there has been prolonged rupture of the membranes, especially if chorioamnionitis has developed, if the mother develops a fever and if the infant is preterm.

Presentation is usually non-specific (see Fig. 9.22). If systemic infection is suspected, investigation and treatment must be started promptly. A chest X-ray is performed if there is respiratory distress, together with a septic screen comprising a full blood count to detect neutropenia, blood cultures and urine and CSF for microscopy and culture. An acute-phase reactant (C-reactive protein) is also measured in many centres. Antibiotics are started immediately without waiting for culture results. Intravenous antibiotics are given to cover group B streptococci, *Listeria monocytogenes* and other Gram-positive organisms (usually penicillin or amoxicillin), combined with cover of Gram-negative organisms (an aminoglycoside or third-generation cephalosporin). The initial choice of antibiotics and length of treatment will depend on the site of infection and the pattern of pathogens in the unit. If cultures are negative and the infant has recovered clinically, antibiotics can be stopped after 48 h.

Neonatal meningitis, although uncommon, has a mortality of 20–50%, with one-third of survivors having serious sequelae. Presentation is the same as for

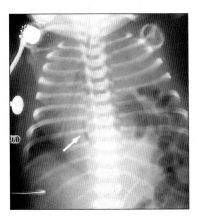

Fig. 9.21 Chest X-ray in diaphragmatic hernia showing loops of bowel in the chest and displacement of the mediastinum. There is a tracheal tube and a nasogastric tube (↑) which lies within the chest.

Fig. 9.22 Clinical features of neonatal sepsis.

Fever or temperature instability or hypothermia
Poor feeding
Vomiting
Apnoea and bradycardia
Respiratory distress
Abdominal distension
Jaundice
Neutropenia
Hypo-/hyperglycaemia
Shock
Irritability
Seizures
Lethargy, drowsiness
In meningitis:
    Tense or bulging fontanelle
    Head retraction (opisthotonus)

other forms of neonatal sepsis. A bulging fontanelle and lying with the back hyperextended (opisthotonus) are late signs. If meningitis is thought likely, ampicillin or penicillin and a third-generation cephalosporin (e.g. cefotaxime) are given. Serial measurements of an acute-phase reactant are useful to monitor response to therapy. Complications include cerebral abscess, ventriculitis, hydrocephalus, hearing loss and neurodevelopmental impairment.

Nosocomially acquired infections are an inherent risk in a neonatal unit or postnatal ward. All staff must adhere strictly to effective handwashing to prevent cross-infection. In intensive care, the other main sources of infection are indwelling catheters for parenteral nutrition or arterial blood gas sampling, tracheal tubes and invasive procedures which break the protective barrier of the skin. Infection of indwelling catheters usually develops after the first week of life. Coagulase-negative *Staphylococcus* (*Staph. epidermidis*) is the most common pathogen in this situation, but the range of organisms is very broad, and includes *Candida* and other fungal infections. Broad-spectrum antibiotics are used but should include flucloxacillin or vancomycin to cover coagulase-negative staphylococcal infection.

Some specific infections

 ### Group B streptococcal infection

Up to 30% of pregnant women have faecal or vaginal carriage of group B streptococci. Up to half of the infants born to these mothers carry the organism on their skin, but only 1% of them become ill. The incidence of disease varies widely between countries, from 1 to 5 per 1000 live births. Early-onset disease typically presents on day 1–3 with pneumonia, septicaemia and, occasionally, meningitis. Mortality is up to 10%. Transmission from mother to infant occurs during delivery or by ascending infection shortly before birth. Late-onset disease, from 1 week to 3 months of age, is less common. It usually causes meningitis but may present with focal infections such as osteomyelitis or septic arthritis.

Antibiotics can be given during labour to mothers whose infants are at increased risk of infection. They can be identified from maternal colonisation of group B *Streptococcus* on universal screening at 35–38 weeks' gestation, as is practised widely in the USA. Alternatively, at-risk infants can be identified if risk factors are present such as preterm delivery, intrapartum maternal fever ≥38°C, prolonged rupture of the membranes, chorioamnionitis or a previously affected infant.

> **Group B streptococcal infection may mimic respiratory distress syndrome.**

Listeria monocytogenes infection

Perinatal and neonatal *Listeria* infection is uncommon but serious. It is transmitted to the mother in food, such as unpasteurised milk, soft cheeses and undercooked poultry. It can cause a mild, influenza-like illness in the mother, or there may be asymptomatic faecal and vaginal carriage. Infection in pregnancy may cause spontaneous abortion, preterm delivery or fetal infection. The fetus usually acquires infection transplacentally, but also by ascending infection from the genital tract or at delivery. A characteristic feature of *Listeria* infection, even in preterm infants, is meconium staining of the liquor, which is otherwise unusual at an early gestation. There may be placental abscesses from which the organism can be cultured.

In early-onset disease, presentation is at delivery or within the first few hours of life with septicaemia and pneumonia, a widespread rash and meningitis. The mortality is 30%. In late-onset disease, presentation is at 1–8 weeks of age, most often with meningitis, and has a better prognosis.

Gram-negative infections

Escherichia coli and other Gram-negative organisms, which are present in faeces and carried vaginally, used to be the most common cause of early-onset sepsis in the newborn. In the UK and the USA, group B streptococcal infection is now more common.

Conjunctivitis

Sticky eyes are common in the neonatal period, starting on the third or fourth day of life. Cleaning with saline or water is all that is required and the condition resolves spontaneously. A more troublesome discharge may be due to staphylococcal or streptococcal infection and can be treated with a topical antibiotic eye ointment, e.g. neomycin.

Purulent discharge with swelling of the eyelids within the first 48 h of life is most likely to be due to gonococcal infection. The discharge should be Gram-stained urgently as well as cultured and treatment started immediately. In countries such as the UK and the USA where penicillin resistance is a problem, a third-generation cephalosporin is given intravenously. The eye needs to be cleansed frequently.

Chlamydia trachomatis eye infection usually presents with a purulent discharge and swelling of the eyelids (Fig. 9.23) towards the end of the first week of life, but may also present shortly after birth. The organism can be identified with a monoclonal antibody test on the pus. Treatment is with topical tetracycline eye ointment and oral erythromycin, both for 2 weeks. Both gonococcal and chlamydial eye infections need to be treated vigorously to avoid damage to the eye. The mother and partner also need to be checked and treated.

Umbilical infection

The umbilicus dries and separates during the first few days of life. If the skin surrounding the umbilicus

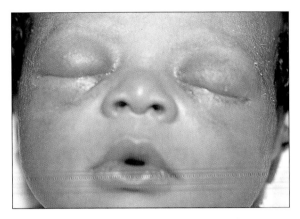

Fig. 9.23 Purulent discharge and swollen eyelids in an 8-day-old infant. This is the characteristic presentation of conjunctivitis from *Chlamydia trachomatis*. *Neisseria gonorrhoea* was absent.

becomes inflamed, systemic antibiotics are indicated. Sometimes the umbilicus continues to be sticky, as it is prevented from involuting by an umbilical granuloma. This can be removed by applying silver nitrate while protecting the surrounding skin.

Herpes simplex virus (HSV) infections
Neonatal HSV infection is uncommon, occurring in 1 in 3000 to 1 in 20 000 live births. HSV infection is usually transmitted during passage through an infected birth canal or by ascending infection. Most infections are caused by HSV-2. The risk to an infant born to a mother with a primary genital infection is high, about 40%, while the risk from recurrent maternal infection is less than 3%. In most infants who develop HSV infection, the condition is unexpected as the mother's primary infection is asymptomatic or causes a non-specific illness.

The infection is more common in preterm infants. Presentation is at any time up to 4 weeks of age, with localised herpetic lesions on the skin or eye, or with encephalitis or disseminated disease. Mortality due to localised disease is low, but disseminated disease has a high mortality with considerable morbidity in survivors. If the mother is recognised as having primary disease or develops genital herpetic lesions at the time of delivery, elective caesarean section is indicated. Women with a history of recurrent genital infection can be delivered vaginally as the risk of neonatal infection is very low. Aciclovir can be given prophylactically to the baby during the at-risk period, but its efficacy is unproven.

Hepatitis B
Infants of mothers who are hepatitis B surface antigen (HBsAg)-positive should receive hepatitis B vaccination shortly after birth to prevent vertical transmission. The vaccination course needs to be completed during infancy and antibody response checked. Babies are at highest risk of becoming chronic carriers when their mothers are 'e' antigen-positive but have no

'e' antibodies. Infants of 'e' antigen-positive mothers should also be given passive immunisation with hepatitis B immunoglobulin within 24 h of birth.

 Infants of HBsAg-positive mothers should be vaccinated against hepatitis B.

NEONATAL SEIZURES

Many babies startle or are slightly jittery, which must be differentiated from seizures. Seizure activity has very variable features and may be tonic, clonic or more subtle, e.g. cycling movements of the limbs or apnoea and bradycardia. About 90% of cases have a detectable cause. An EEG may be helpful in identifying seizures. The causes of seizures are listed in Figure 9.24.

Whenever seizures are suspected, a low blood glucose, calcium, magnesium and sodium need to be excluded immediately. A cerebral ultrasound is performed to identify haemorrhage or cerebral malformations. A septic screen, including a lumbar puncture, will be needed to exclude meningitis or a subarachnoid haemorrhage unless a cause has been identified. Treatment is directed at the cause whenever possible. Ongoing or repeated seizures are treated with an anticonvulsant, although their efficacy in suppressing seizures is much poorer than in older children. The prognosis depends on the underlying cause.

HYPOGLYCAEMIA

Hypoglycaemia is particularly likely to occur in the first 24 h of life in babies who had intrauterine growth restriction, who are preterm, born to mothers with diabetes mellitus, are large-for-dates, hypothermic, polycythaemic or ill for any reason. Growth-restricted

Fig. 9.24 Causes of neonatal seizures.

Hypoxic-ischaemic encephalopathy
Birth trauma
Septicaemia/meningitis
Metabolic
   Hypoglycaemia
   Hypo-/hypernatraemia
   Hypocalcaemia
   Hypomagnesaemia
   Inborn errors of metabolism
   Pyridoxine dependency
Intracranial haemorrhage
Cerebral malformations
Drug withdrawal, e.g. maternal opiates
Congenital infection
Kernicterus

and preterm infants have poor glycogen stores, whereas the infants of a diabetic mother have sufficient glycogen stores, but hyperplasia of the islet cells in the pancreas causes high insulin levels. Symptoms are jitteriness, irritability, apnoea, lethargy, drowsiness and seizures.

There is no agreed definition of hypoglycaemia in the newborn. Many babies tolerate low blood glucose levels in the first few days of life, as they are able to utilise lactate and ketones as energy stores. Recent evidence suggests that blood glucose levels above 2.6 mmol are desirable for optimal neurodevelopmental outcome, although during the first 24 h after birth many asymptomatic infants transiently have blood glucose levels below this level. There is good evidence that prolonged, symptomatic hypoglycaemia can cause permanent neurological disability.

Hypoglycaemia can usually be prevented by early and frequent milk feeding. In infants at increased risk of hypoglycaemia, blood glucose is regularly monitored at the bedside using a reagent strip. If this suggests that the blood glucose is low, a blood sample should be checked in the laboratory for confirmation, while treatment is initiated without delay. If the infant cannot be fed or the hypoglycaemia persists or becomes symptomatic, glucose is given by intravenous infusion. The concentration of the intravenous dextrose may need to be increased from 10 to 15% or even 20%, but the latter concentration is given only via a central venous catheter. Resolution of the hypoglycaemia should be confirmed on repeat laboratory blood glucose measurement. Intravenous infusions with a high concentration of glucose need to be monitored carefully; if there is extravasation into the tissues, there is a risk of reactive hypoglycaemia as well as skin necrosis. If there is difficulty or delay in starting the infusion, or a satisfactory response is not achieved, glucagon can be given.

CRANIOFACIAL DISORDERS

Cleft lip and palate

A cleft lip (Fig. 9.25a) may be unilateral or bilateral. It results from failure of fusion of the frontonasal and maxillary processes. In bilateral cases the premaxilla is anteverted. Cleft palate results from failure of fusion of the palatine processes and the nasal septum. Cleft lip and palate affect about 0.8 per 1000 babies. Most are inherited polygenically, but they may be part of a syndrome of multiple abnormalities, e.g. chromosomal defects. Some are associated with maternal anticonvulsant therapy. They may be detected on antenatal ultrasound scanning.

Surgical repair of the lip (Fig. 9.25b) may be performed within the first week of life for cosmetic reasons, although some surgeons feel that better results are obtained if surgery is delayed. The palate is usually repaired at several months of age. A cleft palate may make feeding more difficult, but some affected infants can still be breast-fed successfully. In bottle-fed babies, if milk enters the nose and causes choking, special teats and feeding devices may be helpful. Orthodontic advice and a dental prosthesis may help with feeding. Secretory otitis media is relatively common and should be sought on follow-up. Infants are also prone to acute otitis media. Adenoidectomy is best avoided, as the resultant gap between the abnormal palate and nasopharynx will exacerbate feeding problems and the nasal quality of speech. A multidisciplinary team approach is required, involving plastic and ENT surgeons, paediatrician, orthodontist, audiologist and speech therapist. Parent support groups can provide valuable support and advice for families (Cleft Lip and Palate Association, CLAPA).

Pierre–Robin sequence

The Pierre–Robin sequence is an association of micrognathia (Fig. 9.26), posterior displacement of the tongue (glossoptosis) and midline cleft of the soft palate. There may be difficulty feeding and, as the tongue falls

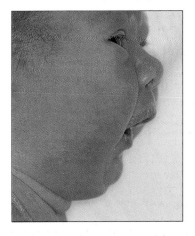

Fig. 9.26 Micrognathia in Pierre–Robin sequence.

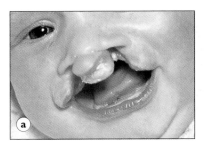

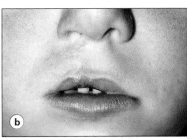

Fig. 9.25 Before (a) and after (b) operation for cleft lip. Photographs showing the impressive results of surgery help many parents cope with the initial distress at having an affected infant. (Courtesy of Mr N. Waterhouse.)

back, there is obstruction to the upper airways which may result in cyanotic episodes. The infant is at risk of failure to thrive during the first few months. If there is upper airways obstruction, the infant may need to lie prone, allowing the tongue and small mandible to fall forward. Persistent obstruction can be treated using a nasopharyngeal airway. Eventually the mandible grows and these problems resolve. The cleft palate can then be repaired.

GASTROINTESTINAL DISORDERS

Oesophageal atresia

Oesophageal atresia is usually associated with a tracheo-oesophageal fistula (Fig. 9.27). It occurs in 1 in 3500 live births and is associated with polyhydramnios during pregnancy. If suspected, a wide-calibre feeding tube is passed and checked to see if it reaches the stomach. If not diagnosed at birth, clinical presentation is with persistent salivation and drooling from the mouth after birth, associated with choking and cyanotic episodes. If the diagnosis is not made at this stage, the infant will cough and choke when fed. There may be aspiration into the lungs of saliva (or milk) from the upper airways and acid secretions from the stomach. Almost half of the babies have other congenital malformation, e.g. as part of the VACTERL association (Vertebral, Anorectal, Cardiac, Tracheo-oEsophageal, Renal and Radial Limb anomalies). In oesophageal atresia, a chest X-ray will confirm that a wide-calibre feeding tube has failed to reach the stomach. Continuous suction is applied to the tube to reduce aspiration of saliva and secretions pending transfer to a neonatal surgical unit.

Small bowel obstruction

This may be recognised antenatally on ultrasound scanning. Otherwise, small bowel obstruction presents with persistent vomiting, which is bile-stained unless the obstruction is above the ampulla of Vater. Meconium may initially be passed, but subsequently its passage is usually delayed or absent. Abdominal distension becomes increasingly prominent the more distal the bowel obstruction. High lesions will present soon after birth, but lower obstruction may not present for some days.

Small bowel obstruction may be caused by:

- atresia or stenosis of the duodenum (Fig. 9.28) – a third of such babies have Down's syndrome and it is also associated with other congenital malformations
- atresia or stenosis of the jejunum or ileum – there may be multiple atretic segments of bowel
- malrotation with volvulus – a dangerous condition as it may lead to infarction of the entire midgut
- meconium ileus – thick inspissated meconium, of putty-like consistency, becomes packed into the lower ileum; almost all affected neonates have cystic fibrosis
- meconium plug – a plug of inspissated meconium causes lower intestinal obstruction.

The diagnosis is made on clinical features and abdominal X-ray showing intestinal obstruction. Atresia or stenosis of the bowel and malrotation are treated surgically, after correction of fluid and electrolyte depletion. A meconium plug will usually pass spontaneously. Meconium ileus may be dislodged using gastrograffin contrast medium.

Large bowel obstruction

This may be caused by:

- *Hirschsprung's disease*. Absence of the myenteric nerve plexus in the rectum which may extend along the colon. The baby often does not pass meconium within 48 h of birth and subsequently the abdomen distends. About 15% present as an acute enterocolitis (see Ch. 12).

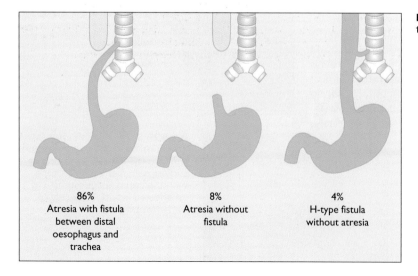

Fig. 9.27 Oesophageal atresia and tracheo-oesophageal fistula.

86%
Atresia with fistula between distal oesophagus and trachea

8%
Atresia without fistula

4%
H-type fistula without atresia

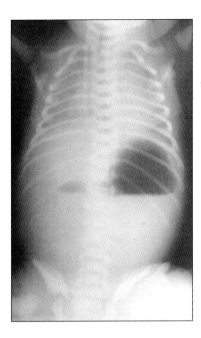

Fig. 9.28 Abdominal X-ray in duodenal atresia slowing a 'double bubble' from distension of the stomach and duodenal cap. There is absence of air distally.

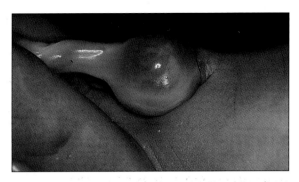

Fig. 9.29 Small exomphalos, with loops of bowel confined to the umbilicus. Care needs to be taken not to put a cord clamp across these lesions.

Exomphalos/gastroschisis

These lesions are often diagnosed antenatally (see Ch. 8). In exomphalos, the abdominal contents protrude through the umbilical ring, covered with a transparent sac formed by the amniotic membrane and peritoneum (Fig. 9.29). It is often associated with other major congenital abnormalities. In gastroschisis the bowel protrudes through a defect in the anterior abdominal wall, adjacent to the umbilicus, and there is no covering sac. It is not associated with other congenital abnormalities.

Gastroschisis carries a much greater risk of dehydration and protein loss, so the abdomen of affected infants should be wrapped in several layers of clingfilm to minimise fluid and heat loss. A nasogastric tube is passed and aspirated frequently and an intravenous infusion of dextrose established. Colloid support is often required to replace protein loss. Many lesions can be repaired by primary closure of the abdomen. With large lesions, the intestine is enclosed in a silastic sac sutured to the edges of the abdominal wall and the contents gradually returned into the peritoneal cavity.

- *Rectal atresia*. Absence of the anus at the normal site. Lesions are high or low, depending whether the bowel ends above or below the *levator ani* muscle. In high lesions there is a fistula to the bladder or urethra in boys, or the vagina or bladder in girls. Treatment is surgical.

 Bile-stained vomiting is from intestinal obstruction until proved otherwise.

FURTHER READING

Fanaroff A A, Martin R J 2001 Neonatal perinatal medicine. Diseases of the fetus and infant, 7th edn. Mosby, St Louis

Klaus M H, Fanaroff A A 2001 Care of the high-risk neonate, 5th edn. Saunders, Philadelphia

Rennie J M, Roberton N R C 1999 Textbook of neonatology, 3rd edn. Churchill Livingstone, Edinburgh. *Comprehensive textbook*

Speidel B D, Fleming P J, Henderson J et al 1998 A neonatal vade-mecum, 3rd edn. Edward Arnold, London

Stephenson T, Marlow N, Watkin S, Grant J 2000 Pocket neonatology, 1st edn. Churchill Livingstone, Edinburgh

10

Growth and puberty

There are four phases of human growth (Fig. 10.1).

Fetal

This is the fastest period of growth, accounting for about 30% of eventual height. Size at birth is determined by the size of the mother and by placental nutrient supply, which in turn modulates fetal growth factors (IGF-2, human placental lactogen and insulin). Severe intrauterine growth restriction and extreme prematurity can result in permanent short stature.

The infantile phase

Growth during infancy to around 18 months of age is also largely dependent on adequate nutrition. Good health and normal thyroid function are also necessary. This phase is characterised by a rapid but decelerating growth rate, and accounts for about 15% of eventual height. An inadequate rate of weight gain during this period is called 'failure to thrive'.

Childhood phase

This is a slow, steady but prolonged period of growth which contributes 40% of final height. Pituitary growth hormone (GH) secretion acting to produce insulin-like growth factor 1 (IGF-1) at the epiphyses is the main determinant of a child's rate of growth, provided there is adequate nutrition and good health. Thyroid hormone, vitamin D and steroids also affect cartilage cell division and bone formation. Profound chronic unhappiness can decrease GH secretion and accounts for psychosocial short stature.

Pubertal growth spurt

Sex hormones, mainly testosterone and oestradiol, cause the back to lengthen and boost GH secretion. This adds 15% to final height. The same sex steroids cause fusion of the epiphyseal growth plates and a cessation of growth. If puberty is early, which is not

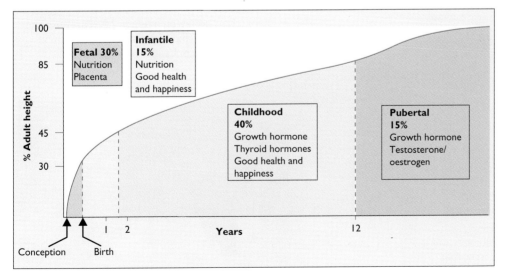

Fig. 10.1 Diagrammatic representation of the phases of growth in childhood. The fetal and infantile phases are mainly dependent on adequate nutrition, whereas the childhood and pubertal phases are dependent on growth hormone and other hormones.

uncommon in girls, the final height is reduced because of early fusion of the epiphyses.

🔑 MEASUREMENT

Growth must be measured accurately with attention to correct technique and accurate plotting of the data:

- Weight – readily and accurately determined with electronic scales but must be performed on a naked infant or a child dressed only in underclothing as an entire month's or year's weight gain can be represented by a wet nappy or heavy jeans, respectively.

- Height – the equipment must be regularly calibrated and maintained. In children over 2 years of age, the standing height is measured as illustrated (Fig. 10.2). In children under 2, length is measured lying horizontally (Fig. 10.3), using the mother to assist. Accurate length measurement in infants can be difficult to obtain, as the legs need to be held straight and infants often dislike being held still. For this reason, routine measurement of length in infancy is often omitted from child surveillance, but it should always be performed whenever there is doubt about an infant's growth.

- Head circumference – the occipitofrontal circumference is a measure of head and brain growth. The mean of three measurements is used. It is of particular importance in developmental delay or suspected hydrocephalus.

These measurements should be plotted as a simple dot on an appropriate growth centile chart. Standards for a population should be constructed and updated every generation to allow for the trend towards earlier puberty and taller adult stature from improved childhood nutrition. Height in a population is normally distributed and the deviation from the mean can be measured as a centile or standard deviation (Fig. 10.4). The bands on the current UK 1990 growth reference charts have been chosen to be two-thirds of a standard deviation apart and correspond approximately to the 25th, 9th, 2nd and 0.4th centiles below the mean, and the 75th, 91st, 98th and 99.6th centiles above the mean. The further these centiles lie from the mean, the more likely it is that a child has a pathological cause for his short or tall stature. For instance, values below the 0.4th or above the 99.6th centile will occur by chance in only 4 per 1000 children and can be used as a criterion for referral from primary to specialist care. A single growth parameter should not be assessed in isolation of the other growth parameters, e.g. a child's low weight may be in proportion to his height if he is short, but abnormal if he is tall. Serial measurements are used to show the pattern and determine the rate of growth. This is helpful in diagnosing or monitoring many paediatric conditions.

🔑 PUBERTY

Puberty follows a well-defined sequence of changes that may be assigned stages as shown in Figure 10.5.

In *females* the features of puberty are:
- breast development – the first sign, usually starting between 8.5 and 12.5 years
- pubic hair growth and a rapid height spurt – occur almost immediately after breast development
- menarche – occurs on average 2.5 years after the start of puberty and signals the end of growth (only around 5 cm height gain remaining).

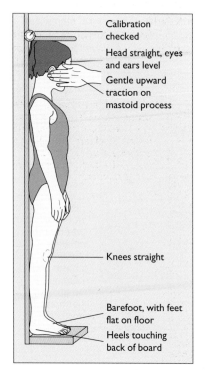

Fig. 10.2 Measuring height accurately in children.

Calibration checked

Head straight, eyes and ears level

Gentle upward traction on mastoid process

Knees straight

Barefoot, with feet flat on floor

Heels touching back of board

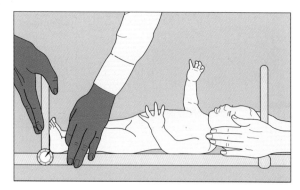

Fig. 10.3 Measuring length in infants and young children. An assistant is required to hold the legs straight.

In *males:*

- testicular enlargement to greater than 4 ml volume measured using an orchidometer (Fig. 10.6) – the first sign of puberty
- pubic hair growth – follows testicular enlargement, usually between 10 and 14 years of age
- height spurt – when the testicular volume is 12–15 ml, after a delay of around 18 months.

The height spurt in males occurs later and is of greater magnitude than in females, accounting for the greater final average height of males than females.

In *both sexes* there will be development of acne, axillary hair, body odour and mood changes.

If puberty is abnormally early or late, it can be further assessed:

- bone age measurement from a hand and wrist X-ray to determine skeletal maturation (Fig. 10.7)
- in females – pelvic ultrasound to assess uterine size and endometrial thickness.

SHORT STATURE

Short stature is usually defined as a height below the second (i.e. two standard deviations below the mean) or 0.4th centile (–2.6SD). Only 1 in 50 children will be shorter than the second centile and 1 in 250 shorter than the 0.4th centile. Most such children will be normal, though short, but the further the child is below these centiles, the more likely it is that there will be a pathological cause. However, the rate of growth may be pathological long before a child's height falls below these values. This growth failure can be identified from the child's height falling across centile lines plotted on a growth chart. This allows growth failure to be identified even though the child's height is still above the second centile.

Measuring height velocity is a sensitive indicator of growth failure. Two **accurate** measurements at least 6 months but preferably a year apart allow calculation of height velocity in cm/year (Fig. 10.8). This is plotted at the midpoint in time on a height/velocity chart. A height velocity persistently below the 25th centile is abnormal and that child will eventually become short. (A tall child with a height on the 98th centile will grow at approximately the 75th velocity centile; a short child with a height on the second centile will grow at approximately the 25th velocity centile – hence the boundaries of normal growth approximate to the 25th–75th centile.) A disadvantage of using height velocity calculations is that they are highly dependent on the accuracy of the height measurements and so tend not to be used outside specialist growth units.

The height centile of a child must be compared with the weight centile and an estimate of their genetic target centile and range calculated from the height of their parents (Fig. 10.9).

Most short children are psychologically well adjusted to their size. However, there may be problems from being teased or bullied at school, poor self-esteem and they are at a considerable disadvantage in competitive sport. They are also assumed by adults to be younger than their true age and may be treated inappropriately.

Causes (Fig. 10.9)

Familial

Most short children have short parents and fall within the centile target range allowing for mid-parental height. Care needs to be taken, though, that both the child and a parent do not have an inherited growth disorder.

Intrauterine growth restriction (IUGR) and extreme prematurity

About one-third of children born with severe intrauterine growth restriction or who were extremely premature remain short.

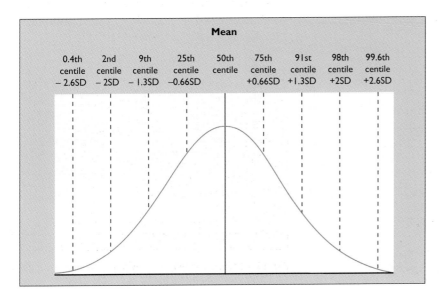

Fig. 10.4 Interpretation of the UK growth reference charts. The lines show the mean and bands which are two-thirds of a standard deviation (SD) apart. The centiles are shown in the diagram.

0.4th centile – 2.6SD	2nd centile – 2SD	9th centile – 1.3SD	25th centile –0.66SD	50th centile	75th centile +0.66SD	91st centile +1.3SD	98th centile +2SD	99.6th centile +2.6SD

Mean

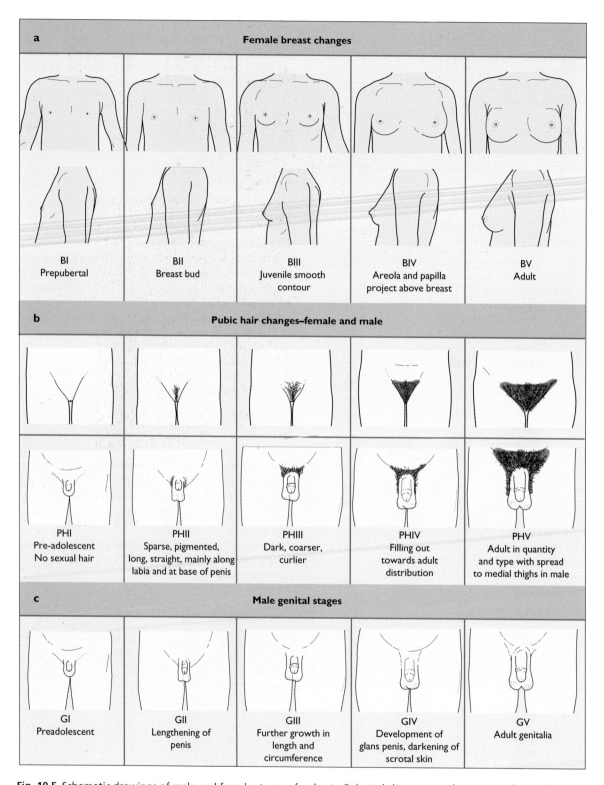

Fig. 10.5 Schematic drawings of male and female stages of puberty. Pubertal changes are shown according to the Tanner stages of puberty.

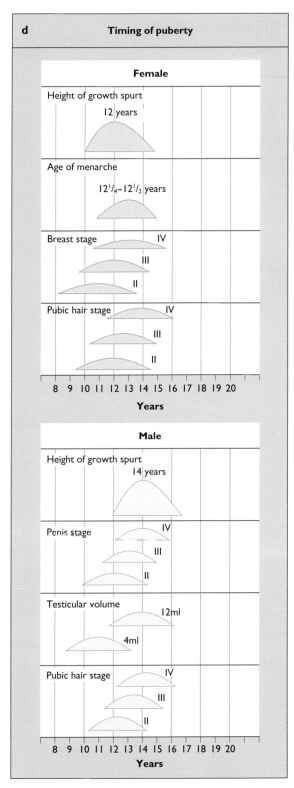

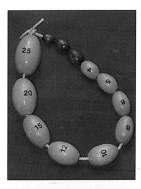

Fig. 10.6 Orchidometer to assess testicular volume (in ml). (From Wales J K H, Rogol A D, Wit J M, *Pediatric Endocrinology and Growth*, Mosby-Wolfe, London, 1996, with permission.)

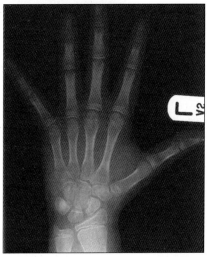

Fig. 10.7 An X-ray of the left wrist and hand to determine bone age. It allows assessment of skeletal maturation from the time of appearance or maturity of the epiphyseal centres, using a standardised rating system. The child's height can be compared with skeletal maturation and an adult height prediction made.

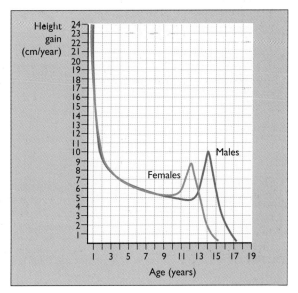

Fig. 10.8 Male and female height velocity charts (50th centile) showing that adult males are taller than females as they have a longer childhood growth phase, their peak height velocity is higher and their growth ceases later.

Fig. 10.5d Timing of puberty. Pubertal changes are shown according to the Tanner stages of puberty. (Diagrams based on Zitelli B J, Davis H W *Atlas of Pediatric Physical Diagnosis*, 2nd edn, Lippincott, Philadelphia, 1992 and Johnson T R, Moore W M, Jeffries J E *Children are Different*, 2nd edn, Ross Laboratories, Division of Abbot Laboratories, Columbus, OH, 1978.)

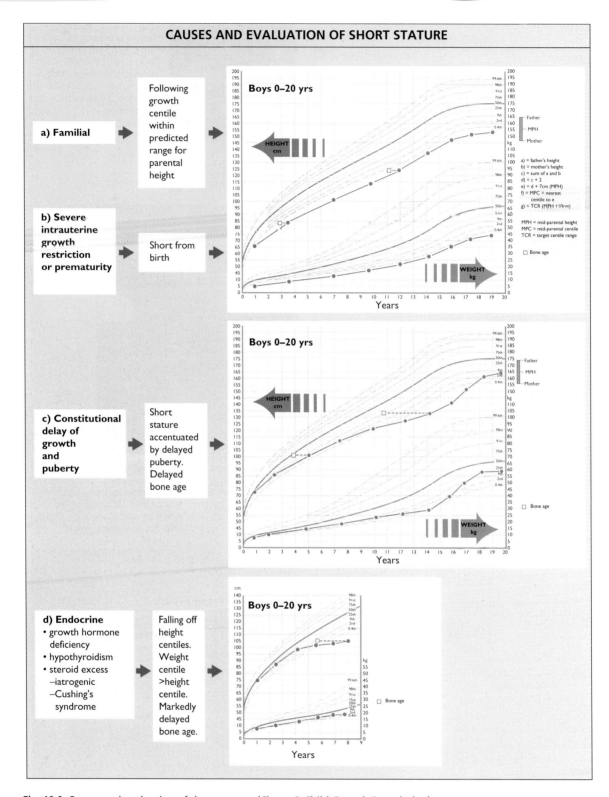

Fig. 10.9 Causes and evaluation of short stature. (Charts © Child Growth Foundation)

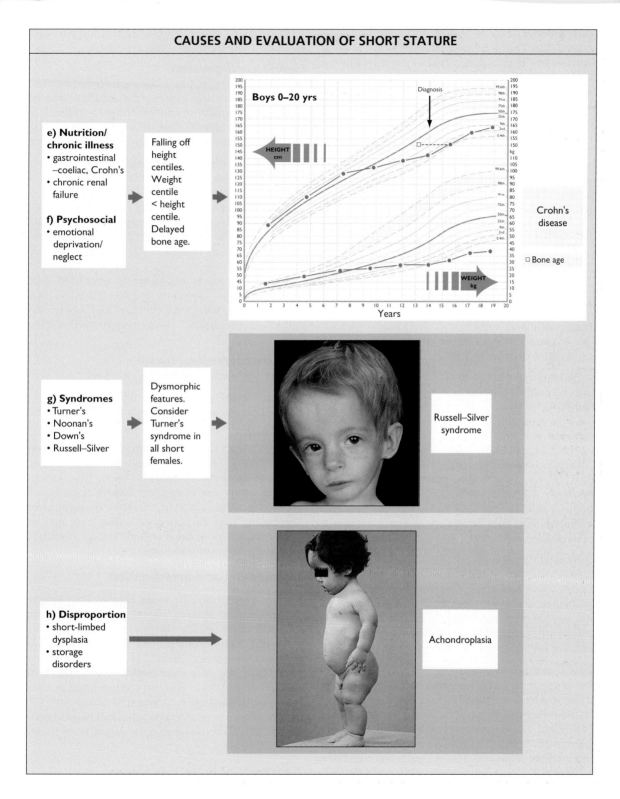

CAUSES AND EVALUATION OF SHORT STATURE

e) Nutrition/chronic illness
• gastrointestinal —coeliac, Crohn's
• chronic renal failure

f) Psychosocial
• emotional deprivation/neglect

Falling off height centiles. Weight centile < height centile. Delayed bone age.

Boys 0–20 yrs

Diagnosis

HEIGHT cm

Crohn's disease

□ Bone age

WEIGHT kg

Years

g) Syndromes
• Turner's
• Noonan's
• Down's
• Russell–Silver

Dysmorphic features. Consider Turner's syndrome in all short females.

Russell–Silver syndrome

h) Disproportion
• short-limbed dysplasia
• storage disorders

Achondroplasia

Fig. 10.9 Causes and evaluation of short stature *(cont.)*.

Constitutional delay of growth and puberty

These children have delayed puberty, which is often familial, usually having occurred in the parent of the same sex. It is commoner in males. It is a variation of the normal timing of puberty rather than an abnormal condition. It may also be induced by dieting or excessive physical training. An affected child will not show the same sexual changes as his peers, and bone age would show moderate delay. The legs will be long in comparison to the back. Eventually the target height will be reached. The condition may cause psychological upset The onset of puberty can be induced with androgens or oestrogens.

Endocrine

Hypothyroidism, growth hormone (GH) deficiency and steroid excess are uncommon causes of short stature. They are associated with children being relatively overweight, i.e. their weight on a higher centile than their height.

Hypothyroidism

This is usually congenital in infancy or caused by autoimmune thyroiditis during childhood.

Growth hormone deficiency

This may be an isolated defect or secondary to panhypopituitarism. Pituitary function may be abnormal in congenital mid-facial defects or as a result of a craniopharyngioma (a tumour affecting the pituitary region), a hypothalamic tumour or cranial irradiation. Craniopharyngioma usually presents in late childhood and may result in abnormal visual fields (characteristically a bitemporal hemianopia as it impinges on the optic chiasma), optic atrophy or papilloedema on fundoscopy. In GH deficiency, the bone age is markedly delayed.

Corticosteroid excess

This is usually iatrogenic, as corticosteroid therapy is a potent growth suppressor. This effect is greatly reduced by alternate day therapy, but some growth suppression may be seen even with relatively low doses of inhaled steroids in susceptible individuals. Non-iatrogenic Cushing's syndrome is very unusual in childhood.

Nutritional/chronic illness

This is a relatively common cause of abnormal growth. These children are usually short and underweight, i.e. their weight is on the same or a lower centile than their height. Inadequate nutrition may be due to insufficient food, restricted diets or poor appetite associated with a chronic illness, or from the increased nutritional requirement from a raised metabolic rate. Chronic illnesses which may present with short stature include:

- coeliac disease, which usually presents in the first 2 years of life
- Crohn's disease
- chronic renal failure – may be present in the absence of a history of renal disease
- cystic fibrosis.

Both Crohn's and coeliac disease may result in short stature without gastrointestinal symptoms.

Psychosocial deprivation

Children subjected to physical and emotional deprivation may be short and underweight and show delayed puberty. This condition may be extremely difficult or impossible to identify, but affected children show catch-up growth if placed in a nurturing environment.

Chromosomal disorder/syndromes

Many chromosomal disorders and syndromes are associated with short stature. Down's syndrome is usually diagnosed at birth, but Turner's, Noonan's and Russell–Silver syndromes may present with short stature. Turner's syndrome may be particularly difficult to diagnose clinically and *should be considered in all short females*.

Whereas Turner's syndrome is associated with 45XO karyotype, Noonan's and Russell–Silver syndromes have no recognised chromosomal abnormality and diagnosis requires recognition of their clinical features.

Disproportionate short stature

This is confirmed by measuring:

- sitting height – base of spine to top of head
- subischial leg length – subtraction of sitting height from total height.

Charts exist to assess the normality of body proportions. These conditions are rare and may be caused by disorders of the formation of bone. They include achondroplasia and other short-limbed dysplasias. If the legs are extremely short, treatment by surgical leg lengthening may be appropriate. The back may be short from severe scoliosis or some storage disorders, such as the mucopolysaccharidoses.

Examination and investigation

Plotting present and previous heights and weights on appropriate growth charts together with the clinical features usually allows the cause to be identified without any investigations. Previous height and weight measurements should be available from the parent-held personal child health record. The bone age may be helpful as it is markedly delayed in some endocrine disorders, e.g. hypothyroidism and GH deficiency, and is used to estimate adult height potential. Investigations which may be indicated are shown in Figure 10.10.

Treatment of endocrine causes

Growth hormone deficiency is treated with biosynthetic GH, which is given by subcutaneous injection, usually daily. GH is expensive and the management of GH deficiency is undertaken at specialist centres. The best response is seen in children with the most severe hormone deficiency. There is no longer a risk of transmission of prion diseases, e.g. Creutzfeldt–Jakob

Fig. 10.10 Investigation of short stature.

Investigation	Significance
X-ray of wrist and hand for bone age	Some delay in constitutional delay of growth and puberty. Marked delay for hypothyroidism or growth hormone deficiency or other endocrine causes
Full blood count	Anaemia in coeliac or Crohn's disease
Creatine and electrolytes	Creatinine raised in chronic renal failure
Thyroid-stimulating hormone (TSH)	Raised in hypothyroidism
Karyotype in females	Turner's syndrome shows 45XO
Endomysial and gliadin antibodies	Usually present in coeliac disease
CRP (acute-phase reactant)	Raised in Crohn's disease
Growth hormone provocation tests (using insulin, glucagon or arginine in specialist centres)	Growth hormone deficiency
MRI scan if neurological symptoms/signs	Craniopharyngioma or intracranial tumour

disease, which unfortunately occurred in a number of instances before 1985 when cadaveric GH was used. Other applications of GH therapy under study include Turner's syndrome, chronic renal failure and intrauterine growth restriction (IUGR).

Hypothyroidism is treated with thyroxine replacement therapy.

TALL STATURE

This is a less common presenting complaint than short stature, as many parents are proud that their child is tall. However, some adolescents (mainly females) become concerned about excessive height during their pubertal growth spurt. The causes are shown in Figure 10.11. Most tall stature is inherited from tall parents. Overeating in childhood leading to obesity 'fuels' early growth and may result in tall stature; however, because puberty is often somewhat earlier than average, final height is usually not excessive.

Secondary endocrine causes are rare. Both congenital adrenal hyperplasia and precocious puberty lead to early epiphyseal fusion so that eventual height is reduced after an early excessive growth rate.

Marfan's (a disorder of loose connective tissue) and Klinefelter's (XXY) syndromes both cause long-legged tall stature, and in XXY there is also infertility and learning difficulties.

Tall children may be disadvantaged by being treated as older than their chronological age. Excessive height in prepubertal or early pubertal adolescent females can be treated with oestrogen therapy to induce premature fusion of the epiphyses, but as it produces variable results and has potentially serious side-effects it is seldom undertaken. Surgical destruction of the epiphyses in the legs may also be considered in extreme cases.

Fig. 10.11 Causes of excessive growth or tall stature.

Familial	Most common cause
Obesity	Puberty is advanced so final height centile is less than in childhood
Secondary	Hyperthyroidism
	Excess sex steroids – precocious puberty from whatever cause
	Excess adrenal androgen steroids – congenital adrenal hyperplasia
	True gigantism (excess GH secretion)
Syndromes	Long-legged tall stature:
	Marfan's syndrome
	Homocystinuria
	Klinefelter's syndrome
	(47 XXY and XXY karyotype)
	Proportionate tall stature at birth:
	Maternal diabetes
	Primary hyperinsulinism
	Beckwith's syndrome
	Sotos syndrome – associated with large head, characteristic facial features and learning difficulties

ABNORMAL HEAD GROWTH

Most head growth occurs in the first 2 years of life and 80% of adult head size is achieved before the age of 5 years. This largely reflects brain growth, but small or large heads may be familial and the mid-parental head percentile may need to be calculated. At birth, the sutures and fontanelles are open. During the first few months of life, the head circumference may increase across centiles, especially if small for gestational age.

The posterior fontanelle closes by 8 weeks, and the anterior fontanelle by 12–18 months. If there is a rapid increase in head circumference, raised intracranial pressure should be excluded.

Microcephaly

Microcephaly, a head circumference below the second centile, may be:

- familial – when it is present from birth and development is often normal
- an autosomal recessive condition – when it is associated with developmental delay

CASE HISTORY 10.1

MICROCEPHALY

Figure 10.12 shows the head circumference chart of Tim, who was healthy and was developing normally. At 18 months of age, he was rushed to hospital as he was unrousable from profound hyoglycaemia secondary to the deliberate administration of insulin by his mother, who had diabetes. Although Tim was taken into care and had no further hypoglycaemic episodes, his head circumference shows cessation of growth. He has developed moderate learning difficulties and mild cerebral palsy.

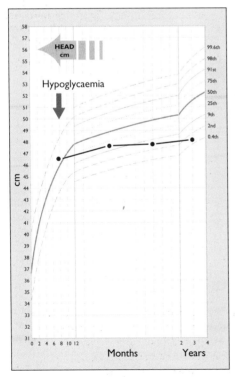

Fig. 10.12 Tim's head circumference chart. (Chart © Child Growth Foundation)

- caused by a congenital infection
- acquired after an insult to the developing brain, e.g. perinatal hypoxia, hypoglycaemia or meningitis; there is often accompanying cerebral palsy and seizures. (See Case history 10.1.)

Macrocephaly

Macrocephaly is a head circumference above the 98th centile. The causes of a large head are listed in Figure 10.13. Most are normal children and often the parents have large heads. A rapidly increasing head circumference, even if the head circumference is still below the 98th centile, suggests raised intracranial pressure and may be due to hydrocephalus, subdural haematoma or brain tumour. It must be investigated promptly by intracranial ultrasound if the anterior fontanelle is still open, otherwise by CT or MRI scan.

Asymmetric heads

Skull asymmetry may result from an imbalance of the growth rate at the coronal, sagittal or lambdoid sutures, although the head circumference increases normally. Occipital plagiocephaly, a parallelogram-shaped head, is seen with increased frequency since the advice that babies should sleep lying on their back. It improves with time as the infant becomes more mobile. Plagiocephaly is also seen in infants with hypotonia, e.g. preterm infants may develop long, flat heads from lying on their sides for long periods on the hard surface of incubators (Fig. 10.14). Under these circumstances, it is not associated with abnormal development.

Craniosynostosis

The sutures of the skull bones do not finally fuse until about 12 years of age. Premature fusion of a suture (craniosynostosis) may lead to distortion of the head shape (Fig. 10.15). The craniosynostosis may be a feature of a syndrome or may be an isolated finding. The fused suture may be felt or seen as a palpable ridge and confirmed on skull X-ray or cranial CT scan. If necessary, the condition can be treated surgically because of raised intracranial pressure or for

---

Fig. 10.13 Causes of a large head.

Tall stature
Familial macrocephaly
Raised intracranial pressure
    Hydrocephalus – progressive or arrested
    Chronic subdural haematoma
    Cerebral tumour
Neurofibromatosis
Cerebral gigantism (Sotos syndrome)
CNS storage disorders, e.g. mucopolysaccharidosis
    (Hurler's syndrome)

cosmetic reasons. Such operations are performed in specialist centres for craniofacial reconstructive surgery (Fig. 10.16).

PREMATURE SEXUAL DEVELOPMENT

The development of secondary sexual characteristics before 8 years old in females and 9 years old in males is outside the normal range. It may be due to:

- precocious puberty when it is accompanied by a growth spurt
- premature breast development (thelarche)
- premature pubic hair development (adrenarche).

Precocious puberty (PP) may be categorised according to the levels of the pituitary-derived gonadotrophins, follicle-stimulating hormone (FSH) and luteinising hormone (LH), as:

- gonadotrophin-dependent (central, 'true' PP) from premature activation of the hypothalamic–pituitary–gonadal axis
- gonadotrophin-independent (pseudo, 'false' PP) from excess sex steroids.

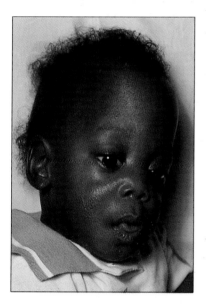

Fig. 10.14 Long flat head of a preterm infant. This can be avoided by lying preterm infants on a soft surface and regularly changing their head position.

Precocious puberty

Females

This is usually idiopathic or familial and follows the normal sequence of puberty. Organic causes (Fig. 10.17) are rare and are associated with:

- dissonance when the sequence of pubertal changes is abnormal, e.g. isolated pubic hair with virilisation of the genitalia, suggesting excess androgens from either congenital adrenal hyperplasia or an androgen-secreting tumour
- rapid onset
- neurological symptoms and signs, e.g. neurofibromatosis.

Ultrasound examination of the ovaries and uterus is helpful in establishing the cause of precocious puberty. In the premature onset of normal puberty, multicystic ovaries and an enlarging uterus will be identified.

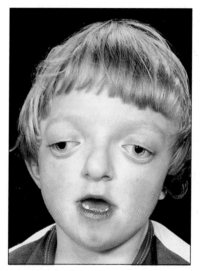

Fig. 10.16 Crouzon's syndrome showing the typical shallow orbits and exophthalmos. Craniofacial reconstructive surgery is required to prevent visual loss and cerebral damage from raised intracranial pressure.

Fig. 10.15 Forms of craniosynostosis.

Localised
Coronal suture only – asymmetrical skull
Sagittal suture only – a long narrow skull

Generalised
Multiple sutures resulting in microcephaly and developmental delay
Genetic syndromes, e.g. with syndactyly in Apert's syndrome, with exophthalmos in Crouzon's syndrome.

Fig. 10.17 Causes of precocious puberty.

Gonadotrophin-dependent (↑LH > FSH↑)
Idiopathic/familial
CNS abnormalities
   Congenital anomalies, e.g. hydrocephalus
   Acquired, e.g. post-irradiation, infection, surgery
   Tumours, e.g. microscopic hamartomas
Hypothyroidism

Gonadotrophin-independent (↓FSH, ↓LH, rare)
Adrenal disorders – tumours, congenital, adrenal hyperplasia
Ovarian – tumour (granulosa cell)
Testicular – tumour (Leydig cell)
Exogenous sex steroids

Precocious puberty in females is usually due to the premature onset of normal puberty.

Males (see Case history 10.2)
This is uncommon and usually has an organic cause, particularly intracranial tumours. Examination of the testes may be helpful:

- bilateral enlargement suggests gonadotrophin release, usually from an intracranial lesion
- small testes suggest an adrenal cause (e.g. a tumour or adrenal hyperplasia)
- a unilateral enlarged testis suggests a gonadal tumour.

Tumours in the hypothalamic region are best investigated by cranial MRI scan.

Central precocious puberty in males usually has an organic cause.

Management
The management of precocious puberty is directed towards:

- Detection and treatment of any underlying pathology, e.g. intracranial tumour in males,

reducing the rate of skeletal maturation if necessary. Skeletal maturation is assessed by bone age. An early growth spurt may result in early cessation of growth and a reduction in adult height.
- Addressing psychological/behavioural difficulties associated with early progression through puberty.

Deciding whether to treat a girl who is simply going through puberty early needs consideration of all these factors. If treatment is required for gonadotrophin-dependent disease, GnRH analogues are the treatment of choice. In gonadotrophin-independent cases, the source of excess sex steroids needs to be identified. Inhibitors of androgen or oestrogen production or action (e.g. medroxyprogesterone acetate, cyproterone acetate, testolactone, ketoconazole) may be used.

Premature breast development (thelarche)

This usually affects females between 6-months and 2 years of age. The breast enlargement may be asymmetrical. It is differentiated from precocious puberty by the absence of axillary and pubic hair and of a growth spurt. It is self-limiting. Investigations are not usually required (see Case history 10.3).

Premature adrenarche

This occurs when pubic hair develops before 8 years of age in females and before 9 years in males but with no other signs of sexual development. It is more common in Asian and Afro-Caribbean children. There may be a slight increase in growth rate. It is usually

---

CASE HISTORY 10.2

PRECOCIOUS PUBERTY IN A BOY

This 6-year-old boy presented with precocious puberty (Fig. 10.18a and b). He was noted to have multiple *café au lait* spots consistent with a diagnosis of neurofibromatosis type 1. An MRI scan showed a mass in the hypothalamus which proved to be an optic glioma. He was treated with radiotherapy, although full remission was not possible to achieve. The site of injection of gonadotrophin superagonist treatment to suppress his sexual development is covered by the plaster.

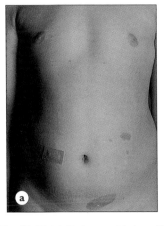 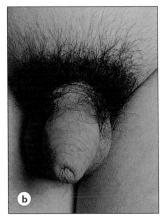

Fig. 10.18 (a) He has multiple *café au lait* spots. Neurofibromatosis type 1 was diagnosed. (b) Genitalia showing stage 3 genitalia and pubic hair with 12 ml testicles bilaterally. He also had adult body odour. (From Wales J K H, Rogol A D, Wit J M, *Pediatric Endocrinology and Growth*, Mosby-Wolfe, London, 1996, with permission.)

CASE HISTORY 10.3

PREMATURE THELARCHE

This 18-month-old female developed enlargement of both breasts (Fig. 10.19). There was no pubic hair growth, sweatiness or body odour and her height was in the mid-parental range. Her bone age was only mildly advanced (21 months) and a pelvic ultrasound showed a pre-pubertal uterus, small volume ovaries with two cysts in the left ovary. Her subsequent growth rate was normal. A diagnosis of premature thelarche was made.

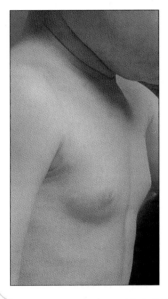

Fig. 10.19 Premature breast development in a 18-month-old girl. The absence of a growth spurt and axillary and pubic hair differentiates it from precocious puberty. It is self-limiting and often resolves. (From Wales J K H, Rogol A D, Wit J M, *Pediatric Endocrinology and Growth*, Mosby-Wolfe, London, 1996, with permission.)

Fig. 10.20 Causes of delayed puberty.

Constitutional delay of growth and puberty/familial
By far the commonest

Low gonadotrophin secretion
Systemic disease
Cystic fibrosis, severe asthma, Crohn's disease, organ failure, anorexia nervosa, starvation, excess physical training
Hypothalamopituitary disorders
Panhypopituitarism
Isolated gonadotrophin or growth hormone deficiency
Intracranial tumours (including craniopharyngioma)
Kallmann's syndrome (LHRH deficiency and inability to smell)
Aquired hypothyroidism

High gonadotrophin secretion
Chromosomal abnormalities
Klinefelter's syndrome (47 XXY)
Turner's syndrome (45 XO)
Steroid hormone enzyme deficiencies
Acquired gonadal damage
Post-surgery, chemotherapy, radiotherapy, trauma, torsion of the testis, autoimmune disorder

self limiting. An ultrasound scan of the ovaries and uterus and a bone age should be obtained to exclude central precocious puberty.

DELAYED PUBERTY

Delayed puberty is often defined as the absence of pubertal development by 14 years of age in females and 15 years in males. The causes of delayed puberty are listed in Figure 10.20. In contrast to precocious puberty, the problem is common in males, in whom it is mostly due to constitutional delay. Affected males are short during childhood and have delayed skeletal maturity on bone age. There is often a family history of delayed puberty in the boy's father. Eventually puberty will occur and a near predicted height attained, as growth will continue for longer than his peers. The boys may suffer from teasing, poor self-esteem and do badly in competitive sports. Assessment in boys includes:

- pubertal staging, especially testicular volume
- identification of chronic systemic disorders.

In girls, karyotype should be performed to identify Turner's syndrome and thyroid and sex steroid hormones measured.

The aims of management are to:
- identify and treat any underlying pathology
- ensure normal psychological adaptation to puberty and adulthood
- accelerate growth and promote entry into puberty if necessary.

Following reassurance that puberty will occur, treatment is often not required. Should treatment be wanted, oral oxandrolone can be used in young males. This weakly androgenic anabolic steroid will induce some catch-up growth but not secondary sexual characteristics. In older boys, low-dose testosterone will accelerate growth as well as inducing secondary sexual characteristics. Females may be treated with oestradiol.

DISORDERS OF SEXUAL DIFFERENTIATION

The fetal gonad is initially bipotential (Fig. 10.21) In the male, a testis-determining gene on the Y chromosome (SRY) is responsible for the differentiation of the gonad into a testis. The production of testosterone

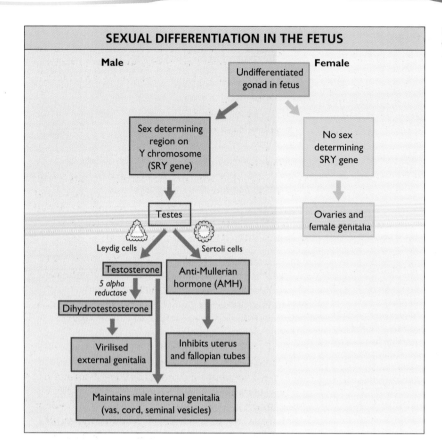

Fig. 10.21 Sexual differentiation in the fetus.

and its metabolite, dihydrotestosterone, results in the development of male genitalia. In the absence of SRY, the gonads become ovaries and the genitalia female.

Rarely, newborn infants may be born with ambiguous genitalia and there may be uncertainty about the infant's sex. Ambiguous external genitalia may be secondary to:

- excessive androgens producing virilisation in a female – the commonest cause of this is congenital adrenal hyperplasia
- inadequate androgen action, producing undervirilisation in a male – this can result from inability to convert testosterone to dihydrotestosterone (5-α-reductase deficiency) or abnormalities of the androgen receptor (androgen insensitivity syndrome)
- gonadotrophin insufficiency, which is also seen in several syndromes, e.g. Prader–Willi syndrome and congenital hypopituitarism, which result in a small penis and cryptorchidism
- true hermaphroditism, caused by chromosomal rearrangement leading to both testicular and ovarian tissue being present and a complex external phenotype; this is rare.

All parents and their relatives are desperate to know the sex of their newborn baby. However, if the genitalia are ambiguous, the infant's sex must not be assigned until detailed assessment by medical, surgical and psychological specialists has been performed. Birth registration must be delayed until this has been completed. Incorrect assignment of sex may have lifelong medical and legal consequences.

Sexuality is complex and depends on more than the phenotype, chromosomes and hormone levels. Before the most appropriate sex of rearing is decided upon, the karyotype needs to be determined, adrenal and sex hormone levels measured, and ultrasound of the internal structures and gonads performed. Sometimes laparoscopic imaging and biopsy of internal structures are necessary. In many intersex conditions, it is usual to raise the child as a female, as it is easier to fashion female external genitalia, whereas it is not possible surgically to create an adequately functioning penis. However, it may be impossible to predict the sexual identity of the child in eventual adult life and further support or gender reassignment may be required. This is a controversial area and is best managed by experienced multi-disciplinary teams.

 The most common cause of ambiguous genitalia in newborn infants is congenital adrenal hyperplasia leading to female virilisation.

Congenital adrenal hyperplasia

A number of autosomal recessive disorders of adrenal steroid biosynthesis result in congenital adrenal hyperplasia. Its incidence is about 1 in 5000 births, and it is commoner in the offspring of consanguineous marriages. Over 90% have a deficiency of the enzyme 21-hydroxylase which is needed for cortisol biosynthesis; 80% of cases are also unable to produce aldosterone (Fig. 10.22). In the fetus, the resulting cortisol deficiency stimulates the pituitary to produce ACTH, which drives overproduction of adrenal androgens.

Presentation is with:
- virilisation of the external genitalia in females, with clitoral hypertrophy and variable fusion of the labia (see Case history 10.4)
- in the male, the penis may be enlarged and the scrotum pigmented, but these changes are seldom identified
- a salt-losing adrenal crisis in the 80% of males who are salt losers; this occurs at 1–3 weeks of age, presenting with vomiting and weight loss, floppiness and circulatory collapse.
- tall stature in the 20% of male non-salt losers; they also develop a muscular build, adult body odour, pubic hair and acne from excess androgen production, leading to precocious puberty.

There may be a family history of neonatal death if a salt-losing crisis had not been recognised and treated.

Diagnosis

This is made by finding markedly raised levels of the metabolic precursor 17α-hydroxyprogesterone in the blood. In salt losers, the biochemical abnormalities are:
- low plasma sodium
- high plasma potassium
- metabolic acidosis
- hypoglycaemia in a salt-losing crisis.

Management

Affected females will require corrective surgery to their external genitalia, but as they have a uterus and ovaries, they should be reared as girls and are able to have children. Males in a salt-losing crisis require saline, dextrose and hydrocortisone intravenously.

The long-term management of both sexes is with:
- lifelong glucocorticoids to suppress ACTH levels to allow normal growth and maturation
- mineralocorticoids (fludrocortisone) if there is salt loss; before weaning, infants may need added sodium chloride
- monitoring of growth, skeletal maturity and, in many centres, plasma androgens and 17α-hydroxyprogesterone – insufficient hormone replacement results in increased ACTH secretion and androgen excess, which will cause rapid initial growth and skeletal maturation at the expense of final height; excessive hormonal replacement will result in skeletal delay and slow growth

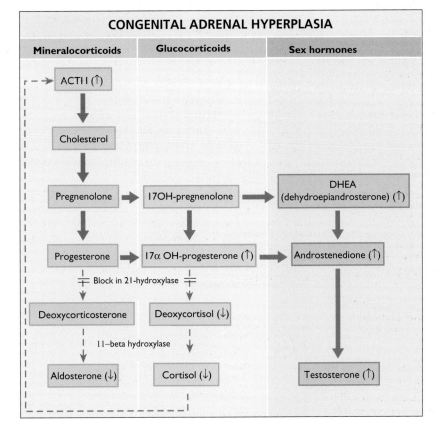

Fig. 10.22 Abnormal adrenal steroid biosynthesis in the commonest form of congenital adrenal hyperplasia.

CONGENITAL ADRENAL HYPERPLASIA

Mineralocorticoids	Glucocorticoids	Sex hormones

ACTH (↑)

Cholesterol

Pregnenolone → 17OH-pregnenolone → DHEA (dehydroepiandrosterone) (↑)

Progesterone → 17α OH-progesterone (↑) → Androstenedione (↑)

╪ Block in 21-hydroxylase ╪

Deoxycorticosterone   Deoxycortisol (↓)

11–beta hydroxylase

Aldosterone (↓)   Cortisol (↓)   Testosterone (↑)

CASE HISTORY 10.4

AMBIGUOUS GENITALIA AT BIRTH

The appearance of this newborn infant's genitalia is shown in Figure 10.23. Investigation revealed:

- a normal female karyotype, 46XX
- the presence of a uterus on ultrasound examination
- a markedly raised plasma 17α-hydroxyprogesterone concentration, confirming congenital adrenal hyperplasia.

Plasma electrolytes were checked every few days for the first 4 weeks to check for salt loss, which was absent. After detailed explanation with her parents, she was started on oral hydrocortisone replacement therapy. Surgery was performed at 9 months of age to reduce clitoral size and separate

 Severe hypospadias and bilateral undescended testes – a male or virilised female? The karyotype is required.

the labia. Her growth, biochemistry and bone age were monitored frequently at follow-up and she attained normal adult height. Psychological counselling and support were offered around puberty and further genital surgery was needed before she became sexually active.

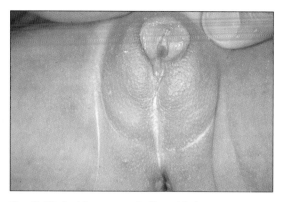

Fig. 10.23 Ambiguous genitalia at birth. Investigation established that this was a female infant with congenital adrenal hyperplasia causing clitoral hypertrophy with fusion of the labia.

- additional hormone replacement to cover illness or surgery, as they are unable to mount a cortisol response.

Death can occur from adrenal crisis at the time of illness or injury. Females require surgery to reduce cliteromegaly and a vaginoplasty before sexual intercourse is attempted. Females often experience psychosexual problems, which may relate to the high androgen levels experienced *in utero* and prior to diagnosis.

Prenatal diagnosis and treatment are possible when a couple have had a previously affected child.

Dexamethasone may be given to the mother around the time of conception, and continued if the fetus is found to be female, in order to reduce fetal ACTH drive and hence the virilisation.

 Salt-losing adrenal crisis needs urgent treatment with hydrocortisone, saline and glucose given intravenously.

FURTHER READING

Brook C G D 1993 A guide to the practice of paediatric endocrinology. Cambridge University Press, Cambridge
Brook C G D 1995 Clinical paediatric endocrinology. Blackwell Science, Oxford
Kappy M S, Blizzard R M, Migeon C J 1994 The diagnosis and treatment of endocrine disorders in childhood and adolescence. Charles C. Thomas, Springfield, IL
Wales J K H, Rogol A D, Wit J M 1996 A color atlas of pediatric endocrinology and growth. Mosby-Wolfe, London

11

Nutrition

Children need food of appropriate quantity and quality for optimal growth and development. If their nutritional intake is inadequate they will fail to gain or lose weight and will subsequently fail to grow in height. Prolonged or severe nutritional deficiency will result in malnutrition.

THE NUTRITIONAL VULNERABILITY OF INFANTS AND CHILDREN

Infants and children are more vulnerable to poor nutrition than are adults. There are a number of reasons for this.

Low nutritional stores
Newborn infants, particularly those born before term, have poor stores of fat and protein (Fig. 11.1). The smaller the child, the less is his calorie reserve and the shorter the period he will be able to withstand starvation.

High nutritional demands for growth
The nourishment children require, per unit body size, is greatest in infancy (Fig. 11.2), because of their rapid growth during this period. At 4 months of age, 30% of an infant's energy intake is used for growth, but by 1 year of age this falls to 5%, and by 3 years to 2%. The risk of growth failure from restricted energy intake is therefore greater in the first 6 months of life than in later childhood. Even regular small deficits in early childhood will lead to a cumulative deficit in weight and height.

Rapid neuronal development
The brain grows rapidly during the last trimester of pregnancy and throughout the first 2 years of life. The complexity of interneuronal connections also increases substantially during this time. This process appears to be sensitive to undernutrition. Even modest energy

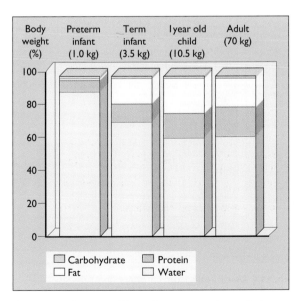

Fig. 11.1 Body composition of preterm and term infants, children and adults. Newborn infants, particularly the preterm, have poor stores of fat and protein.

Fig. 11.2 Reference values for energy and protein requirements.		
Age	**Energy** (kcal/kg per 24 h)	**Protein** (g/kg per 24 h)
0–6 months	115	2.2
6–12 months	95	2.0
1–3 years	95	1.8
4–6 years	90	1.5
7–10 years	75	1.2
Adolescence		
11–14 years (male/females)	65/55	1.0
15–18 years	60/40	0.8

deprivation during periods of rapid brain growth and differentiation are thought to lead to an increased risk of adverse neurodevelopmental outcome. This is not surprising when one considers that at birth the brain accounts for approximately two-thirds of basal metabolic rate, and at 1 year for about 50% (Fig. 11.3). Many studies have drawn attention to the delayed development seen in children suffering from protein energy malnutrition due to inadequate food intake, although inadequate psychosocial stimulation may also contribute.

A child's nutrition may be compromised following an acute illness or surgery. After a brief anabolic phase, when catecholamine secretion is increased, the metabolic rate and energy requirement are increased. Urinary nitrogen losses may become so great that it is impossible to achieve a positive nitrogen balance and weight is lost. After uncomplicated surgery this phase may last for a week, but it can last several weeks after extensive burns, complicated surgery or severe sepsis. Thereafter, previously lost tissue is replaced and a positive energy and nitrogen balance can be achieved. However, infants may not show catch-up growth unless their energy intake is as high as 150–200 kcal/kg per day.

The weight of a term infant doubles by 4 months and trebles by 1 year.

Long-term outcome of early nutritional deficiency

Linear growth of populations

Growth and nutrition are closely related, such that the mean height of a population reflects its nutritional status. Thus, in the developed world, people have got taller. Height is adversely affected by lower socio-economic status and increasing number of children in families. Children's size increases amongst populations emigrating from poor to more affluent countries.

Disease in adult life

Evidence suggests that undernutrition *in utero* resulting in growth restriction is associated with an increased incidence of coronary heart disease, stroke, non-insulin-dependent diabetes, hypertension and chronic airway obstruction in later life (Fig. 11.4). There is also a similar but weaker association with low weight at 1 year of age. For example, there is a twofold reduction in death rates from coronary heart disease and stroke between the lower and upper ends of birthweight distribution, and coronary heart disease doubles in men who weighed less than 8 kg at 1 year compared with those over 12.2 kg. The mechanism is unclear, but it is recognised that fetal undernutrition leads to redistribution of blood flow and changes in fetal hormones, such as insulin-like growth factors and cortisol. These observations lend weight to the importance of protecting the nutrition of child-bearing women and their babies.

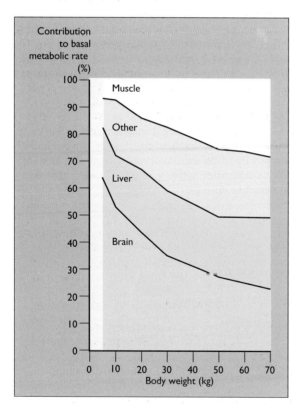

Fig. 11.3 The relative contribution to basal metabolic rate derived from brain, liver and muscle changes with growth. Whereas the brain accounts for two-thirds of the basal metabolic rate at birth, this falls to 25% in adults. (Adapted from Halliday M A 1971 Pediatrics 47(1) Suppl 2: 169.)

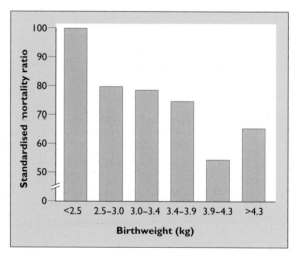

Fig. 11.4 Death rates from coronary heart disease according to birthweight. (After Barker D J, *Fetal Origins of Adult Disease*. In: *Growing up in Britain: Ensuring the Healthy Future for our Children. A Study of 4–5 year olds*, BMJ Books, London, 1999.)

INFANT FEEDING

Breast-feeding

There can be no doubt that breast milk is the best diet for babies, although the popularity of breast-feeding has frequently reflected the whim of fashion.

Advantages (Fig. 11.5)

In developing countries, where the environment is often highly contaminated, breast-feeding dramatically improves survival during infancy as a result of reduced gastrointestinal infection. Consequently, breast-feeding is one of the four most important World Health Organization strategies for improving infant and child survival. The superiority of breast milk over modern adapted cow's milk formulae is less easy to prove in developed countries. This is partly because it is impossible to conduct randomised studies and partly because of confounders such as social class, education and smoking.

There is now convincing evidence that gastrointestinal infection is less common in breast-fed infants even in developed countries. There is also evidence that human milk feeds reduce the incidence of necrotising enterocolitis in preterm infants.

Many mothers who breast-feed find that it helps them establish an intimate, loving relationship with their baby. However, establishing breast-feeding is not always straightforward, and many mothers need help and encouragement.

Breast-feeding may confer an advantage in long-term neurological development in preterm infants, although there are many confounding variables in this relationship. The most likely nutrients in breast milk for conferring this advantage are probably long-chain polyunsaturated fatty acids. These are now added to some formula feeds.

Breast-feeding is associated with a reduced incidence of inflammatory bowel disease and diabetes mellitus in children when they grow up, and a reduction in breast cancer in mothers who breast-feed. Claims that breast-feeding reduces the incidence of allergic disorders and sudden infant death syndrome (SIDS) have not been substantiated.

Disadvantages (Fig. 11.6)

As one cannot readily tell how much milk a baby is taking from the breast, the baby's weight should be checked regularly, every few days in the first couple of weeks, then weekly until feeding is well established. Successful breast-feeding of twins can be achieved, but is more difficult (Fig. 11.7). It is rarely possible to totally breast-feed triplets and higher-order births. Preterm infants can be breast-fed, but the milk will need to be expressed from the breast until the infant can suck. Maintaining the supply of milk can be a problem for mothers of preterm babies.

Whilst two-thirds of mothers in the UK initially breast-feed, this proportion rapidly declines during the first few months (Fig. 11.8). Nearly 90% of social class I mothers start breast-feeding, compared with less than half of mothers from social class V. Breast-feeding is restrictive for the mother as others cannot take charge of her baby for any length of time. This is particularly important if she goes to work. Facilities for breast-feeding in public places are still limited. Although breast-feeding avoids the preparation needed for infant formulae, it is not necessarily cheaper for the family if it delays a mother returning to work.

> **Exclusive breast-feeding in early infancy is life-saving in developing countries.**

Establishing breast-feeding

Colostrum, rather than milk, is produced for the first few days. Colostrum differs from mature milk in that the content of protein and immunoglobulin is much higher. Volumes are low but water or formula supplements are not required whilst the supply of breast milk is becoming established.

The first breast-feed should take place as soon as possible after birth. Subsequently, frequent suckling is beneficial as it enhances the secretion of the hormones initiating and promoting lactation.

Primates probably do not breast-feed instinctively. Monkeys bred in captivity in zoos have to be taught how to breast-feed by their keepers. It is therefore important that breast-feeding should have as high a public profile as possible. Women who have never seen an infant being breast-fed are less likely to want to breast-feed themselves. Education in schools and during pregnancy about the advantages of breast-feeding is important. Advice and support from other women who have breast-fed may be important in dealing with early problems such as engorgement or cracked nipples.

'Bonding', a critical period shortly after birth in establishing a mother–infant relationship, is seen in many animals. In humans, there is no evidence for a similar critical period and there is considerable flexibility in the timing and manner in which this close relationship develops.

Formula feeding

Infants who are not breast-fed require a formula feed based on cow's milk. Unmodified cow's milk is unsuitable for feeding in infancy as it contains too much protein and electrolyte and inadequate iron and vitamins. Even after considerable modification, differences remain between formula feeds and breast milk (Fig. 11.9).

Most modern cow's milk-based formulae may be divided into two types, depending upon whether or not the casein to non-casein ratio has been modified by the addition of demineralised whey (soluble protein).

BREAST FEEDING

Fig. 11.5 Why breast is best – the advantages of breast milk.

Anti-infective properties			
Humoral		Breast milk lipase	Enhanced lipolysis
Secretory IgA	Comprises 90% of immunoglobulin in human milk. Provides mucosal protection, but of uncertain benefit	Calcium: phosphorus ratio of 2:1	Prevents hypocalcaemic tetany and improves calcium absorption
Bifidus factor	Promotes growth of *Lactobacillus bifidus*, which metabolises lactose to lactic and acetic acids. The resulting low pH may inhibit growth of gastrointestinal pathogens	Low renal solute load	
		Iron content	Bioavailable (40–50% absorption)
		Long-chain polyunsaturated fatty acids	Structural lipids, important in retinal development
Lysozyme	Bacteriolytic enzyme		
Lactoferrin	Iron binding protein. Inhibits growth of *E. coli*	**Other advantages**	
Interferon	Antiviral agent	Emotional	If successful, promotes close attachment between mother and baby
Cellular			
Macrophages	Phagocytic. Synthesise lysozyme, lactoferrin, C3, C4	Contraceptive effects	Not a reliable contraceptive, but, overall, increases the time interval between children. Important in reducing birth rate in developing countries
Lymphocytes	T-cells may transfer delayed hypersensitivity responses to infant. B-cells synthesise IgA		
Nutritional properties		Reduction in disease occurrence in later life	Insulin-dependent diabetes mellitus, inflammatory bowel disease, sudden infant death syndrome (unproven)
Protein quality	More easily digested curd (60:40 whey : casein ratio)		
Hypoallergenic	May reduce subsequent atopic disease. Conflicting evidence	Maternal health	Possible reduction in premenopausal breast cancer
Lipid quality	Rich in oleic acid (with palmitate in C-2 position). Improved digestibility and fat absorption		

Fig. 11.6 Disadvantages of breast-feeding.

Unknown intake	Volume of milk intake not known	Vitamin K deficiency	There is insufficient vitamin K in breast milk to prevent haemorrhagic disease of the newborn
Transmission of infection	CMV, hepatitis and HIV in an infected mother can be identified in breast milk and increases the risk of transmission to the baby		
		Potential transmission of environmental contaminants	Nicotine, alcohol, caffeine, etc.
Breast milk jaundice	Mild, self-limiting, unconjugated hyperbilirubinaemia and not a contraindication	Less flexible	Other family members cannot help or take part. More difficult in public places
Transmission of drugs	Antithyroid drugs, cathartics, antimetabolites	Emotional upset if unsuccessful	Breast-feeding can be problematic to establish. Difficulties or lack of success can be upsetting if mother is determined to breast-feed
Nutrient inadequacies	Prolonged breast-feeding without timely introduction of appropriate solids may lead to poor weight gain and rickets		

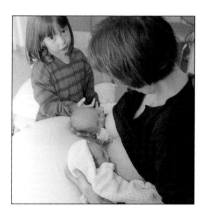

Fig. 11.7
Successful
breast-feeding
of preterm
twins.

Fig. 11.9 A comparison of human milk, cow's milk and infant formula (per 100 ml).

	Breast milk at term	Cow's milk	Infant formula (modified cow's milk)
Energy (kcal)	70	67	60–65
Protein (g)	1.3	3.5	1.5–1.9
Carbohydrate (g)	7.0	4.9	7.0–8.6
Casein : whey	40:60	63:37	40:60–63:37
Fat (g)	4.2	3.6	2.6–3.8
Sodium (mmol)	0.65	2.3	0.65–1.1
Calcium (mmol)	0.88	3.0	0.88–2.1
Phosphorus (mmol)	0.46	3.2	0.9–1.8
Iron (μmol)	1.36	0.9	8–12.5

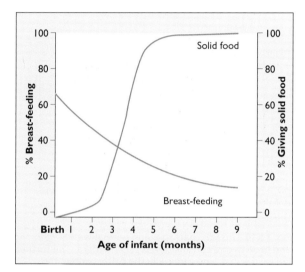

Fig. 11.8 Prevalence of breast-feeding and proportion of infants given solid feeds during the first 9 months of life in the UK (1995).

A casein : whey ratio of 40:60 forms a smaller curd and provides an amino acid profile more like breast milk than a higher casein milk.

All milks currently available in the UK have been modified to make their mineral content and renal solute load comparable with that of mature human milk. Since these changes were introduced in the UK (in the 1970s), there has been an impressive reduction in the incidence of hypernatraemic dehydration in infants with gastroenteritis. There is no evidence that any one of the many brands is superior to any other.

Introduction of whole, pasteurised cow's milk

Breast or formula feeding is recommended until the age of 12 months, and there are advantages in continuing to 18 months of age. Pasteurised cow's milk is deficient in vitamins A, C and D and in iron, and if introduced in the first year will require supplements unless the infant is having a good diet of mixed solids. Alternatively, 'follow-on' formulae can be used from

6 months of age. They contain more protein and sodium than infant formulae and, in contrast to cow's milk, are fortified with iron and vitamins.

Soya formulae

Soya formulae have been widely used instead of cow's milk formulae in the belief that they may help to prevent atopic manifestations such as eczema or asthma. However, there is no compelling evidence that their use leads to a reduced risk of these disorders. Although modern soya protein formulae are nutritionally adequate and support normal growth, there are a number of disadvantages associated with their use and they cannot be regarded as a satisfactory, routine alternative to cow's milk formulae. Approximately 10–30% of infants with cow's milk protein intolerance who are fed on a soya milk will subsequently develop clinical soya intolerance. Soya formulae contain a higher aluminium content, and the infants have lower serum immunoglobulin levels and a poorer response to vaccinations than those fed cow's milk formula.

Weaning

Solid foods are usually introduced between the ages of 3 and 6 months (see Fig. 11.8). Although human milk may be nutritionally adequate until 6 months of age, many babies will exhibit behavioural changes from 3 to 4 months, such as increased crying and poor sleeping, which may represent hunger and a need for solid food. After 6 months of age, breast milk becomes increasingly nutritionally inadequate as a sole feed, leading to deficiencies in energy, vitamins and iron. Early weaning foods such as puréed non-wheat cereals, fruit and vegetables tend to be high in energy, vitamins and minerals. Once babies can chew (at about 6 months), more lumpy foods and a variety of tastes and textures should be introduced. Added sugar and salt are best avoided in weaning foods because early exposure may produce unhealthy dietary preferences in later childhood and adult life.

Breast- or formula-fed infants obtain about half their energy from fat. After 1 year of age, whole cow's milk still provides a major contribution to the diet of most children. Some nutritionists have suggested that dietary fat intake should be reduced to supply less than 35% of energy requirements and fibre intake increased. The later introduction of solids, more breast-feeding and the fact that many weaning foods are gluten-free may be responsible for the reduction in the incidence of coeliac disease in infancy. A lower incidence of gastroenteritis may also be a factor.

FAILURE TO THRIVE

The term 'failure to thrive' is used to describe sub-optimal weight gain or growth in infants and toddlers. Recognition of the entity depends upon demonstration of inadequate weight gain when plotted on a centile chart, with mild failure to thrive being a fall across two centile lines and severe a fall across three centile lines. Between 6 weeks and 1 year of age, only 5% of children will cross two lines, and only 1% will cross three. The weight of a child with 'failure to thrive' may fall within the normal range, but most are below the 2nd centile when identified. Repeated observations are therefore essential and are usually available in the child's personal child health record. A single observation of weight is difficult to interpret unless markedly discrepant from the head circumference or length, although the further the weight is below the 2nd centile, the more likely it is that the child is 'failing to thrive'. Weighing infants is of relatively little value unless the weights are accurate and plotted on a centile chart.

Differentiating the infant who is failing to thrive from a normal but small or thin baby is often a problem (Fig. 11.10). Normal but short infants have no symptoms, are alert, responsive and happy, and their development is satisfactory. The parents may be short (low mid-parental height) or the infant may have been extremely preterm or growth-restricted at birth. Any intercurrent illness will be accompanied by a temporary failure to gain weight.

An additional diagnostic problem is 'catch-down' (as opposed to 'catch-up') weight. This is when an infant's weight falls from the birth centile, which is affected by the intrauterine environment, to a lower, genetically determined growth centile. These infants need only close monitoring of their growth over a few months.

Causes

It has been traditional to divide the causes of failure to thrive into organic and non-organic categories (Fig. 11.11). *Non-organic* failure to thrive is associated with a broad spectrum of psychosocial and environmental deprivation and is often accompanied by a delay in those aspects of development which rely on

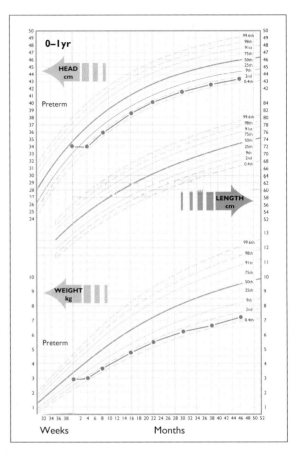

Fig. 11.10 Growth chart showing normal weight gain and growth in a constitutionally small infant. The further below the 2nd, and especially the 0.4th, centile, the more likely it is that there will be an organic cause. (Chart © Child Growth Foundation)

environmental stimulation, e.g. speech. Undernutrition is the final common pathway for poor weight gain in non-organic failure to thrive, usually from a combination of inadequate or inappropriate feeding as well as psychosocial factors. The mother may be depressed, have an eating disorder herself or have poor understanding of her baby's needs. It is estimated that 5–10% of children with failure to thrive will be on a child protection register or be subjected to abuse or neglect, while a somewhat larger proportion will have socioeconomic deprivation as an important factor. This may be poor housing, poverty, inadequate social support and lack of an extended family, which make good child care even more difficult. However, some studies suggest that failure to thrive is not necessarily more common in deprived than in non-deprived communities, and that identification of deprivations leads inappropriately to the application of that diagnostic label.

The commonest *organic* causes of failure to thrive are gastro-oesophageal reflux, coeliac disease (see Fig. 12.16), cystic fibrosis (see Figs 14.26–28), cardiac disease and renal failure. Less than 5% of children with 'failure to thrive' will be found to have an organic cause.

Fig. 11.11 The main causes of failure to thrive.

Non-organic causes
Feeding problems – insufficient breast milk or poor technique
Maternal stress
   Inadequate food consumed
   Lack of awareness of how much consumed
   Tense, poorly feeding child
   Intolerance of normal feeding behaviours leading to early cessation of meals
   Social exclusion and financial difficulties
Lack of stimulation and undernutrition – infant or toddler not demanding food
Munchausen's syndrome by proxy – deliberate underfeeding to generate failure to thrive

Organic
Inability to feed
   Mechanical problem, e.g. cleft palate
   Lack of coordination, e.g. cerebral palsy
Poor retention of food
   Vomiting
   Gastro-oesophageal reflux
Illness-induced anorexia – any chronic disorder, e.g. cystic fibrosis, renal failure, congenital heart disease, renal tubular disorders
Impaired nutrient absorption, e.g. coeliac disease, cystic fibrosis, cow's milk protein intolerance
Increased energy requirements, e.g. cystic fibrosis, malignancy
Metabolic – hypothyroidism, congenital adrenal hyperplasia, amino acid and organic acid disorders
Miscellaneous – chromosomal disorders, syndromes, congenital infection

Fig. 11.12 Investigations to be considered in failure to thrive.

Investigation	Significance of an abnormality
Full blood count and differential	Anaemia, infection, inflammation, immune deficiency
Plasma creatinine and electrolytes	Renal failure, renal tubular acidosis, metabolic disorders
Liver function tests	Liver disease, malabsorption, metabolic, disorders
Thyroid function tests	Hypothyroidism
Acute-phase reactant	Inflammation, e.g. Crohn's disease
Ferritin	Iron deficiency anaemia
Immunoglobulins	Immune deficiency
Anti-endomysial and anti-gliadin antibodies	Coeliac disease
Urine microscopy and culture and dipsticks	Urinary tract infection, renal disease
Stool microscopy and culture	Intestinal infection, parasites
Chromosomal analysis in girls	Turner's syndrome
Chest X-ray and sweat test	Cystic fibrosis

Clinical features and investigation

Studying the growth chart in combination with the history and examination of the child is the key to its evaluation. A detailed dietary history is required. Further information about the child and family from the health visitor, general practitioner or other professionals involved with the family can be particularly helpful. Organic causes are almost invariably suggested by the presence of abnormal symptoms or signs. Investigations to be considered are listed in Figure 11.12.

Failure to thrive is a description, not a diagnosis.

Management

The management of most non-organic failure to thrive is multidisciplinary and can be carried out in primary care. The health visitor is well placed to make home visits to assess eating behaviours and provide support. A paediatric dietician may be helpful in assessing the quantity and composition of food intake and recommending strategies for increasing energy intake. Input from social services may also be appropriate.

Hospital admission may occasionally be necessary for a period of assessment and observation of the child and family, or when detailed investigations are required.

Outcome

Follow-up studies suggest that children with non-organic failure to thrive continue to under-eat (see Case history 11.1). Although there is usually a gradual

CASE HISTORY 11.1

NON-ORGANIC FAILURE TO THRIVE

Jamie, aged 11 months, was causing concern to his health visitor as he was not putting on any weight (Fig. 11.13). She arranged for him to be assessed by his general practitioner, who found that he was otherwise well. His mother was a single parent who left school at 16 years and had Jamie at the age of 18. They lived in a high rise flat and Jamie's mother received income support. Her own mother lived on the other side of the city.

On visiting the home, the health visitor found Jamie's mother to be tense and anxious. In particular, she was worried about making ends meet. She fed Jamie the same food as she ate herself, together with pasteurised milk which she had started at 6 months of age. The meals were chaotic. After a few mouthfuls, Jamie stopped eating and his mother did not coax him but became frustrated and angry.

Jamie's health visitor suggested strategies for increasing Jamie's food intake (Fig. 11.14). She continued to provide support and encouragement to his mother and arranged a nursery placement for Jamie. By 2 years of age he had caught up by one centile line, but still ate erratically.

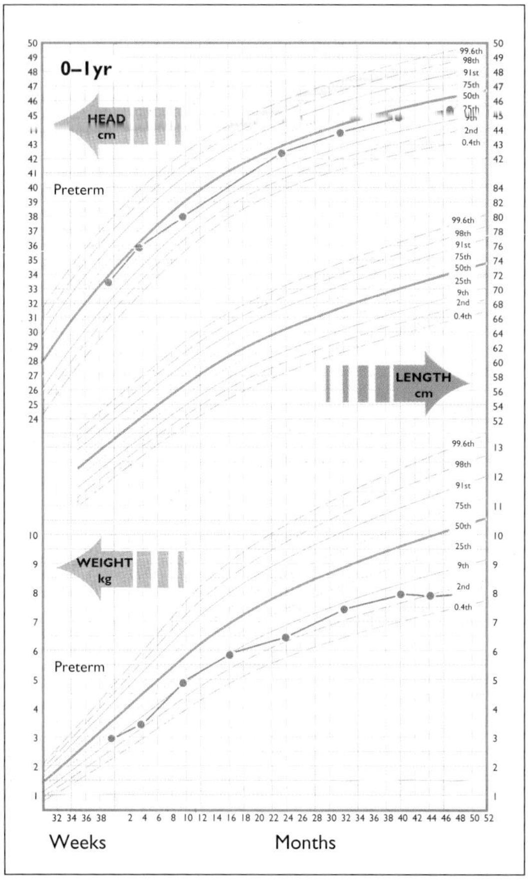

Fig. 11.13 Jamie's growth chart. (Chart © Child Growth Foundation)

Fig. 11.14 Strategies for increasing energy intake. (After Wright C M, Identification and management of failure to thrive: a community perspective. *Archives of Disease in Childhood* 82: 5–9, 2000.)

Dietary
Three meals and two snacks each day
Increase number and variety of foods offered
Increase energy density of usual foods
   (e.g. add cheese, margarine and cream)
Decrease fluid intake, particularly squash

Behavioural
Have meals at regular times, eaten with other
   family members
Praise when food is eaten
Gently encourage child to eat, but avoid conflict
Never force-feed

---

improvement in the preschool years, a lasting deficit is common and these children tend to remain underweight. In contrast, impairment of development is only short term.

MALNUTRITION

Worldwide, malnutrition is common and is responsible directly or indirectly for about half of all deaths of children under 5 years of age. Primary malnutrition also continues to occur in developed countries as a result of poverty, parental neglect or poor education. Specific nutritional deficiencies, particularly of iron, remain common in developed countries. Restrictive diets may be iatrogenic as a result of exclusion diets or parental food fads, or may be self-inflicted.

Malnutrition is far from rare in hospital, affecting 20–40% of patients in a children's hospital. The chronically ill are at particular risk, especially preterm infants and those children with congenital heart disease or chronic gut or respiratory disorders. In these children, malnutrition may result from a combination of anorexia, malabsorption and increased requirements because of infection or inflammation. Anorexia nervosa and other feeding disorders cause malnutrition in older children and adolescents. The diencephalic syndrome, which is extremely rare, comprises severe protein-energy malnutrition in association with a cerebral tumour, usually of the hypothalamus. Food intake is often high, suggesting a possible defect in energy metabolism.

Assessment of nutritional status

Malnutrition must be recognised and accurately defined for rational decisions to be made about refeeding. Evaluation is divided into assessment of past and present dietary intake, anthropometry and laboratory assessments (Fig. 11.15).

Dietary assessment

Parents are asked to record as best they can all food the child eats during several days. This gives a reasonably accurate assessment of habitual food intake. Children under 12 years are likely to give unreliable information if questioned directly.

Anthropometry

Regular growth measurements are valuable as a fall-off of a growth parameter is one of the earliest indicators of incipient malnutrition. Height, weight, triceps skinfold thickness and mid-arm circumference are basic measures which permit a reasonably accurate assessment of nutritional status. The World Health Organization recommends that nutritional status is expressed as:

- height for age – a measure of stunting and an index of chronic malnutrition
- weight for height – a measure of wasting and an index of acute malnutrition (Fig. 11.16).

Subcutaneous fat stores can be assessed by measuring skinfold thickness, whilst upper arm circumference in conjunction with triceps skinfold thickness is an indication of skeletal muscle mass. However, it is difficult to measure skinfold thickness accurately in young children, so this reduces its use in reflecting short-term changes in body composition.

Laboratory investigations

These are useful in the detection of early physiological adaptation to malnutrition, but clinical history, examination and anthropometry are of greater value than any single biochemical or immunological measurement.

Consequences of malnutrition

Malnutrition is a multisystem disorder. When severe, immunity is impaired, wound healing is delayed and operative morbidity and mortality increased. Malnutrition worsens the outcome of illness, e.g. respiratory muscle dysfunction may delay a child being weaned from mechanical ventilation. Malnourished children are less active, less exploratory and more apathetic. These behavioural abnormalities are rapidly reversed with proper feeding, but prolonged and profound malnutrition probably does cause some permanent delay in intellectual development.

The role of intensive nutritional support

Malnutrition from many childhood disorders is due to inadequate nutrient intake and responds to tube

NUTRITIONAL ASSESSMENT

Fig. 11.15

Anthropometry
- Weight
- Height
- Mid-arm circumference
- Skinfold thickness

Laboratory
- Low plasma albumin
- Low concentration of specific minerals and vitamins

Food intake
- Dietary recall
- Dietary diary

Immunodeficiency
- Low lymphocyte count
- Impaired cell-mediated immunity

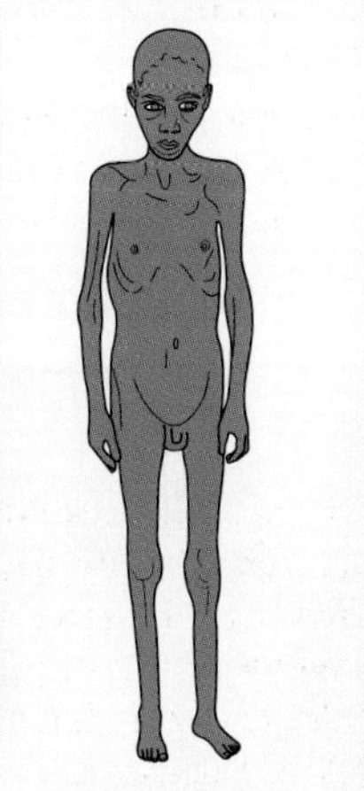

Fig. 11.16

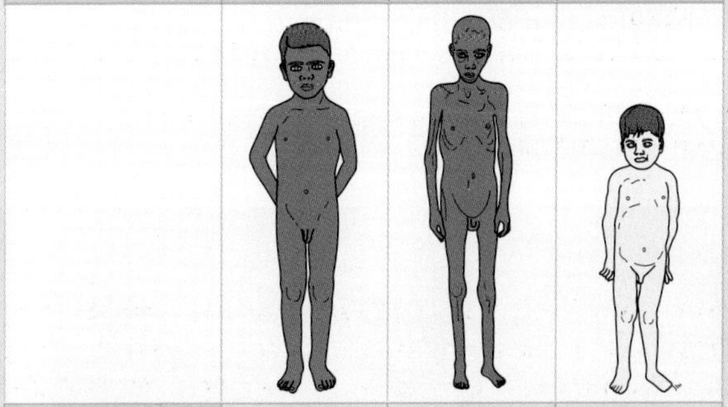

	Normal	Wasted	Stunted
Weight/age %	100	70	70
Weight/height%	100	70	100
Height/age %	100	100	84

Fig. 11.15 Assessment of nutritional status. This cannot be determined by a single measurement, but is a composite of a number of variables.

Fig. 11.16 Comparison of a normal, wasted and stunted child at 1 year. Low weight for height reveals a child of normal height, but who is thin and wasted, whereas low height for age reveals a short, non-wasted child.

feeding nasogastrically or by gastrostomy. Thus malnourished children with cystic fibrosis, malignancy, inflammatory bowel disease, advanced liver disease, congenital heart disease, cerebral palsy and chronic renal failure will all grow if given supplementary enteral feeds. Other than for Crohn's disease, whether such nutritional support alters prognosis or quality of life remains uncertain.

Marasmus and kwashiorkor

Severe protein-energy malnutrition in children usually leads to marasmus, with a weight less than 60% of the mean for age, and a wasted, wizened appearance (Fig. 11.17). Oedema is not present. Skinfold thickness and mid-arm circumference are markedly reduced, and affected children are often withdrawn and apathetic.

Kwashiorkor is another manifestation of severe protein malnutrition (Fig. 11.18), in which body weight is 60–80% of expected and oedema is present. In addition, there may be:

- a 'flaky-paint' skin rash with hyperkeratosis and desquamation
- a distended abdomen and enlarged liver
- angular stomatitis
- hair which is sparse and depigmented
- diarrhoea, hypothermia, bradycardia and hypotension
- low plasma albumin, potassium, glucose and magnesium.

It is unclear why some children with protein-energy malnutrition develop kwashiorkor and others develop marasmus. Kwashiorkor is a feature of children reared in traditional, polygamous societies, where infants are not weaned from the breast until about 12 months of age. The subsequent diet tends to be relatively high in starch. Kwashiorkor often develops after an acute intercurrent infection, such as measles or gastroenteritis. There is some evidence that kwashiorkor is a manifestation of primary protein deficiency with energy intake relatively well maintained or, alternatively, that it results from excess generation of free radicals.

Management

Urgent treatment for severe malnutrition involves correcting dehydration, acid–base disturbance and hypocalcaemia and treating infection. Hypothermia is common and children require careful wrapping, particularly at night. Children with severe malnutrition are deficient in potassium and magnesium and these should be supplemented. Diarrhoea is a frequent complication of refeeding, but parenteral nutrition is not usually required. Overzealous treatment with fluids may lead to cardiac failure. In kwashiorkor, severe hypoglycaemia is frequently associated with coma, hypothermia and infection and carries a high mortality. Feeding 2- to 4-hourly, including during the night, has reduced the frequency of hypoglycaemia and the mortality. The overall mortality of severe malnutrition among children treated in hospital is about 30%.

Rickets

Rickets, derived from the old English word 'wrickken', meaning to twist, is used to describe the clinical syndrome arising from an excess of undermineralised bone matrix in growing bone (Fig. 11.19). It usually results from deficient intake or defective metabolism of vitamin D (Fig. 11.20). It can also occur from a nutritional deficiency of calcium, particularly in developing countries, or, in preterm infants, from a deficiency of phosphate in breast milk or unsupplemented cow's milk formulae.

Mineralisation of osteoid is impaired, and the epiphyseal growth area becomes disorganised and hypertrophic. The clinical features are listed in Figure 11.21. Bones are soft and the long bones easily deformed. Skull bones can be indented easily by finger pressure (craniotabes), and expansion of the costochondral junctions produces a 'rickety rosary'. In-drawing of

---

MALNUTRITION

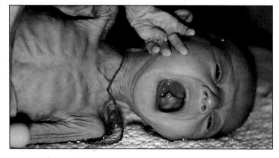

Fig. 11.17 Marasmus in a 3-month-old baby who was unable to establish breast-feeding because of a cleft palate.

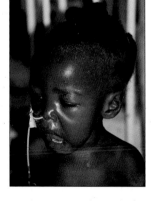

Fig. 11.18 Kwashiorkor, a particular manifestation of severe protein-energy malnutrition in some developing countries where infants are weaned late from the breast and the young child's diet is high in starch. There is hyperkeratosis and depigmentation of the skin and redness of the hair. (Courtesy of Dr Sharon Taylor.)

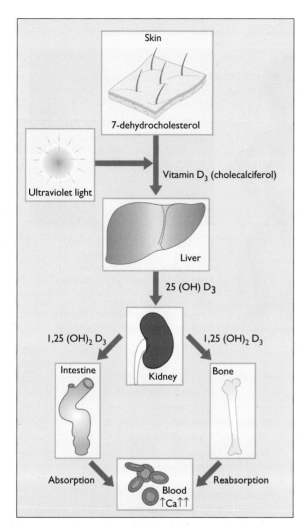

Fig. 11.19 *Vitamin D metabolism*. In most countries, sunlight is the most important source of vitamin D. Vitamin D is not abundant naturally in food except in fish liver oil, fatty fish and egg yolk. Vitamin D_2 (ergocalciferol) is the form used to fortify food such as margarine. Vitamin D_3 is hydroxylated in the liver and again in the kidney to produce 1–25 dihydroxyvitamin D $(1,25(OH)_2D_3)$, the most active form of the vitamin. It is produced following parathormone secretion in response to a low plasma calcium.

Fig. 11.20 Causes of rickets.

Nutritional (primary) rickets
Risk factors
  Living in northern latitudes
  Decreased exposure to sunlight, e.g. in some Asian children living in the UK
  Diets low in calcium, phosphorus and vitamin D, e.g. exclusive breastfeeding into late infancy or, rarely, toddlers on unsupervised 'dairy-free' diets
  Prolonged parenteral nutrition in infancy with an inadequate supply of parenteral calcium and phosphate

Intestinal malabsorption
Defective production of 25(OH)D_3 – liver disease
Increased metabolism of 25(OH)D_3 – enzyme induction by anticonvulsants

Defective production of 1,25(OH)$_2$D$_3$
  Hereditary type I vitamin D- resistant (or dependent) rickets (mutation which abolishes activity of renal hydroxylase)
  Familial (X-linked) hypophosphataemic rickets (renal tubular defect in phosphate transport)
  Chronic renal disease
  Fanconi's syndrome (renal loss of phosphate)

Target organ resistance to 1,25(OH)$_2$D$_3$
  Hereditary vitamin D-dependent rickets type II (due to mutations in vitamin D receptor gene)

radiographically. The disorder can be prevented by health education about a balanced diet, exposure to sunlight and vitamin D supplementation when indicated, e.g. in preterm infants.

Vitamin A (retinol)

In developed countries, biochemical vitamin A deficiency is seen as a complication of fat malabsorption when supplementation has been inadequate. Clinical manifestations under these circumstances are rare, except for impaired dark adaptation. Vitamin A deficiency is common in many developing countries, where it causes eye damage from corneal scarring and acceleration of malnutrition from impairment of mucosal function and immunity. A number of community-based trials of supplementation have shown a marked reduction in mortality by reducing the incidence of infection.

OBESITY

About 1 in 5 children in the UK and the USA is now overweight, reflecting the epidemic in obesity which is present in adults in many affluent countries. In children, the prevalence doubled in the 1980s and continues to increase. Obesity in children is important,

the softened ribs along the attachment of the diaphragm produces a hollowing called Harrison's sulcus (Fig. 11.22).

Diagnosis
Serum calcium is low or normal, phosphorus is low, and plasma alkaline phosphatase activity is greatly increased. X-ray of the wrist joints shows cupping and fraying of the metaphyses and a widened epiphyseal plate (Fig. 11.23).

Treatment
Nutritional rickets is treated with oral supplements of vitamin D and correction of the predisposing risk factors. Response is monitored biochemically and

RICKETS

Fig. 11.21 Clinical features of rickets.

Misery
Failure to thrive/short stature
Frontal bossing
Craniotabes
Delayed closure of anterior fontanelle
Delayed dentition
Rickety rosary
Harrison's sulcus
Expansion of metaphyses
  (especially wrist)
Bowing of weight-bearing bones
Hypotonia
Seizures (late)

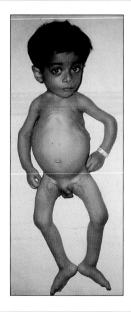

Fig. 11.22 Rickets in a 3-year-old boy secondary to coeliac disease. He has frontal bossing, a Harrison's sulcus and bow legs.

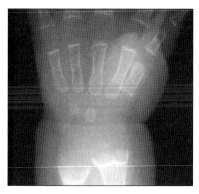

Fig. 11.23 An X-ray of the wrist showing rickets. The ends of the radius and ulna are expanded, rarefied and cup-shaped and the bones are poorly mineralised. This infant was exclusively breast-fed until 12 months of age, when he presented with a hypocalcaemic seizure.

as it predicts not only obesity in adult life, but also an increased risk of complications (Fig. 11.24), and reduces life expectancy.

Body mass index (BMI=weight [kg]/height^2[m^2]) is the best single index of obesity. It is easy to measure, centile charts are available, and a BMI above the 95th centile predicts both an increased risk of persistence of obesity into adult life and abnormalities in blood lipids and blood pressure.

Exogenous causes of obesity are rare. As over-nutrition accelerates growth and the onset of puberty, most obese children are also above the 50th centile for height. This makes the differentiation from hypo-thyroidism or Cushing's syndrome easier, as these conditions are associated with short stature from a decline in growth velocity. There are a number of uncommon syndromes associated with obesity, such as Prader–Willi syndrome (poor linear growth, developmental delay, dysmorphic facial features, hypotonia and undescended testicles in males).

Emotional disturbance is seen in some affected children and unhappiness may lead to further excessive eating. The child or teenager may be teased and develop a poor self-image, adversely affecting self-confidence, particularly in establishing relationships with the opposite sex. Psychological support may be required.

Management

There is disagreement about how best to manage childhood obesity. Population-based interventions may be more effective than approaches targeted at fat children. Moreover, there is concern about the palatability of lower fat diets, which may also compromise

Fig. 11.24 Complications of obesity.

Orthopaedic
  Slipped femoral epiphysis
  Tibia vara (bow legs)
Benign intracranial hypertension
  Headaches
  Blurred optic disc margins
Hypoventilation syndrome
  Daytime somnolence
  Sleep apnoea
  Snoring
  Hypercapnia
  Heart failure
Gall bladder disease
Polycystic ovary disease
Non-insulin-dependent diabetes mellitus
Hypertension
Abnormal blood lipids
Psychological sequelae
  Low self-esteem
  Teasing

intake of iron and calcium. In particular, low-energy diets may impair growth and nutritious food choices should not be completely eliminated on the basis of their fat content.

Targeted treatment of fat children should therefore be considered for those children with a BMI above the 85th centile, particularly if associated with hypertension, or a sudden increase in weight without linear growth. Those children with a BMI above the 95th centile require evaluation, as this is associated with an increased risk of obesity-related disease and later mortality. Achieving weight reduction is a difficult challenge for the child, his family and health professionals. Even when some weight reduction is achieved, this is often temporary. A general approach to management is to:

- begin early, in preschool children
- consider deferring treatment until the family is ready to make changes
- educate about the medical complications of obesity
- involve all family members in the programme
- institute permanent changes, not short-term fixes aimed at rapid weight loss
- reduce inactivity
  — limit TV and computer games
  — walk to school if possible
  — play with friends
  — encourage the family to take 30 min of activity a day
- reduce calorie intake
  — calorie counting is difficult and inaccurate
  — initially only one or two energy-dense foods per day, with emphasis on increasing the intake of low calorie foods
- have clearly defined but realistic goals:
  — weight goals: maintenance of baseline weight to allow a gradual decline in BMI as linear growth occurs
  — behaviour goals: development of awareness and motivation of current eating habits, parents and problem behaviours
  — medical goals: resolution of complications, such as abnormal lipid profiles or blood pressure
- monitor eating and exercise activities – joining a group of others with the same problem may be helpful; the more frequent the follow-up, the more likely that weight loss is achieved and maintained
- give encouragement and avoid criticism.

DENTAL CARIES

Dental destruction occurs as a result of exposure to organic acids produced by bacterial fermentation of carbohydrate, particularly sucrose (Fig. 11.25). Prevalence is now rising in young children. It is strongly related to socioeconomic deprivation.

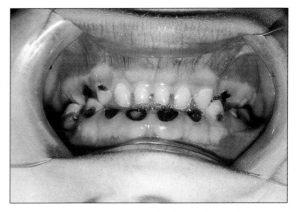

Fig. 11.25 Dental caries. Prop feeding infants when put to sleep with a bottle containing milk or other fermentable liquids places them at high risk of severe dental caries and should be discouraged.

Prevention involves:
- a reduction in plaque bacteria (brushing and flossing)
- less frequent ingestion of carbohydrates
- regular inspection by a dentist
- an optimal intake of fluoride up to puberty to improve the resistance of the tooth to damage; water fluoridation is one of the most effective ways of achieving this.

Incorporation of fluoride in enamel by ionic substitution leads to replacement of calcium hydroxyapatite with calcium fluorapatite, which is less soluble in organic acids. In areas where drinking water contains a low concentration of fluoride, supplementation with fluoride drops or tablets is needed. Additionally, topical fluoride in toothpaste or mouthwashes is also advisable. Excess fluoride administration, before enamel has formed, may lead to mottled enamel (dental fluorosis).

Infants and children who are put to bed with a bottle containing fermentable liquid (milk or a sucrose-containing fruit juice) are at particular risk of developing severe dental caries. Characteristically, fluid collects around the upper anterior and posterior teeth, which become extensively damaged. Because of reduced salivation and swallowing during sleep, clearance and neutralisation of organic acids are also reduced. So called 'prop feeding' should therefore be energetically discouraged.

FURTHER READING

Barker D J 1999 Fetal origins of adult disease. In: Growing up in Britain: ensuring the healthy future for our children. A study of 4–5 year olds. BMJ Books, London

British Paediatric Association (Standing Commission on Nutrition) 1994 Is breast-feeding beneficial in the UK? (Statement). Archives of Disease in Childhood 71: 276–280

Department of Health 1991 Dietary reference values for food energy and nutrients in the United Kingdom. HMSO, London

Foster K, Lader D, Cheesbrough S 1997 Infant feeding 1995. The Stationery Office, London

Wright C M 2000 Identification and management of failure to thrive: a community perspective. Archives of Disease in Childhood 82: 5–9

Internet

www.who.dk/tech/nutemg.htm – How to breastfeed, World Health Organization.

12

Gastroenterology

Few children reach adulthood without experiencing gastrointestinal disorders such as vomiting, gastro-enteritis, episodes of abdominal pain or constipation. In most instances, the symptoms are mild and transient, but serious causes need to be excluded. Chronic gastrointestinal disorders are a potent cause of weight loss and poor growth in spite of the enormous reserve capacity of the gut.

VOMITING

Posseting and *regurgitation* are terms used to describe the non-forceful return of milk, but differ in degree. Posseting describes the small amounts of milk which often accompany the return of swallowed air ('wind'), whereas regurgitation describes larger, more frequent losses. Posseting occurs in nearly all babies from time to time, whereas regurgitation usually indicates the presence of gastro-oesophageal reflux.

Vomiting is the forceful ejection of gastric contents. It is a common problem in infancy and childhood (Figs 12.1 and 12.2). It is usually benign and is often caused by feeding disorders or mild gastro-oesophageal reflux or gastroenteritis. Potentially serious disorders need to be excluded if the vomiting is bilious or prolonged, or if the child is systemically unwell. In infants, vomiting may be associated with infection outside the gastro-intestinal tract, especially in the urinary tract and central nervous system. In intestinal obstruction, the more proximal the obstruction, the more prominent the vomiting and the sooner it becomes bile-stained (unless the obstruction is proximal to the ampulla of Vater). When intestinal contents have been stagnant for a long time, the vomitus may become faeculant.

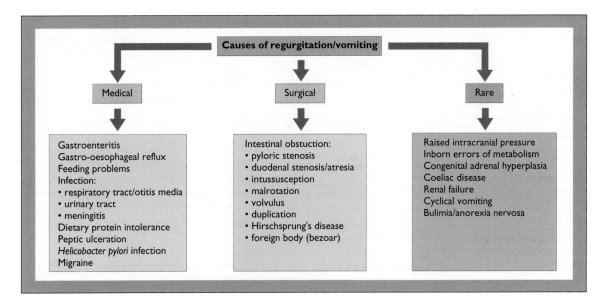

Causes of regurgitation/vomiting

Medical	Surgical	Rare
Gastroenteritis Gastro-oesophageal reflux Feeding problems Infection: • respiratory tract/otitis media • urinary tract • meningitis Dietary protein intolerance Peptic ulceration *Helicobacter pylori* infection Migraine	Intestinal obstuction: • pyloric stenosis • duodenal stenosis/atresia • intussusception • malrotation • volvulus • duplication • Hirschsprung's disease • foreign body (bezoar)	Raised intracranial pressure Inborn errors of metabolism Congenital adrenal hyperplasia Coeliac disease Renal failure Cyclical vomiting Bulimia/anorexia nervosa

Fig. 12.1 Causes of regurgitation/vomiting.

Gastro-oesophageal reflux

Physiological, asymptomatic reflux may occur in any child or adult but it is infrequent. Measurement of lower oesophageal pH shows that in normal individuals there is acidity from reflux of stomach contents for less than 4% of a 24-h period. Reflux occurring more frequently than this results from functional immaturity of the lower oesophageal sphincter leading to episodes of inappropriate relaxation. A short intra-abdominal length of oesophagus probably also contributes. It is common in the first year of life. By 12 months of age, nearly all symptomatic reflux will have resolved spontaneously, presumably due to a combination of maturation of the lower oesophageal sphincter, assumption of an upright posture and more solids in the diet. A sliding hiatus hernia is present in some symptomatic infants, but many children with a hiatus hernia are symptom-free.

Severe reflux is uncommon, but may be associated with potentially serious complications (Fig. 12.3). Reflux is common:

- in children with cerebral palsy, when energetic management, surgically if necessary, may transform the child's quality of life
- in newborn infants with bronchopulmonary dysplasia (chronic lung disease of prematurity)
- following surgery for oesophageal atresia or diaphragmatic hernia.

Management

Patients with mild, uncomplicated reflux can be diagnosed clinically and treated without further investigation. However, when the history is atypical or when complications are present, further investigation is indicated (Case history 12.1). The best diagnostic test is 24-h oesophageal pH monitoring. Contrast studies of the upper gastrointestinal tract are performed to exclude underlying anatomical abnormalities in the oesophagus, stomach and duodenum, such as malrotation.

Endoscopy and oesophageal biopsy are performed in some centres if oesophagitis is suspected.

It is worthwhile treating all infants with symptomatic reflux; repeated regurgitation is smelly and unpopular with the family. Mild reflux responds well to the addition of inert thickening agents to feeds (e.g. Nestargel, Carobel), and positioning in a 30° head-up prone position after feeds. Drugs which enhance gastric emptying (e.g. domperidone) are useful in more severe forms of reflux, as are H$_2$-antagonists (e.g. ranitidine) to reduce oesophagitis. Surgery, called fundoplication, in which the fundus of the stomach is wrapped around the intra-abdominal oesophagus, is reserved for those patients with complications failing to respond to intensive medical treatment, oesophageal stricture or recurrent respiratory symptoms, especially aspiration.

Pyloric stenosis

In pyloric stenosis, there is hypertrophy of the pylorus causing gastric outlet obstruction. It presents at between 2 and 7 weeks of age, irrespective of gestational age. It is more common in boys (4:1), particularly first-borns, and there may be a family history, especially on the maternal side. Clinical features are:

- projectile vomiting (not bile-stained), which increases in frequency and severity with time
- constant hunger even after vomiting; only when markedly dehydrated do they refuse to feed
- a hypochloraemic alkalosis with a low plasma potassium from vomiting acid stomach contents
- weight loss or poor weight gain if presentation is delayed.

Diagnosis

Unless immediate fluid resuscitation is required, a test feed is performed. The baby is given a milk feed, which will calm the hungry infant, allowing examination. Gastric peristalsis may be seen as a wave moving from

CASE HISTORY 12.1

SEVERE GASTRO-OESOPHAGEAL REFLUX

This infant (Fig. 12.4a) had a history of frequent regurgitation from the first few days of life. He developed two chest infections. Some of the vomits contained altered blood. A 24-h oesophageal pH study showed severe gastro-oesophageal reflux (Figs 12.4b and c). Endoscopy showed oesophagitis. He had probably had episodes of aspiration pneumonia. Symptoms resolved on treatment with feed thickeners and ranitidine. His parents also commented on how much better he slept at night. Treatment was reduced from 14 months of age and symptoms did not recur.

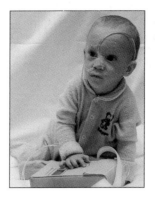

Fig. 12.4a The pH study in progress.

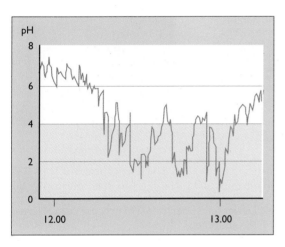

Fig. 12.4b Part of the 24-h oesophageal pH study showing severe reflux, with frequent drops in pH below 4.

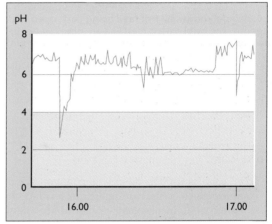

Fig. 12.4c Part of a normal oesophageal pH study. The lower oesophageal pH is above 4 for most of the time.

left to right across the abdomen (Fig. 12.5a). The pyloric mass or 'olive' is usually palpable in the right upper quadrant (Fig. 12.5b). If the stomach is overdistended with air, it will need to be emptied by a nasogastric tube to allow palpation. Ultrasound examination is increasingly used to confirm the diagnosis (Fig. 12.5c). A barium meal is only performed when the diagnosis remains in doubt.

Management

Initial management is to correct any fluid and electrolyte disturbance with intravenous fluids. The chloride and potassium deficits should be replaced. Treatment is by pyloromyotomy, when the muscle but not the mucosa of the pylorus is cut (Fig. 12.5d). The operation can be performed through a variety of incisions, including through the umbilicus or laparoscopically. Postoperatively the child can be fed the next day and is usually discharged within 2–3 days of surgery.

CRYING

Excessive crying in infants is distressing for all concerned. Advice on appropriate feeding, wrapping and reassurance will usually suffice. The emotional climate within a home is readily transmitted to a baby, and tense, anxious or irritable care-givers are likely to have similar babies. Organic causes should not be overlooked. Crying of sudden onset may be due to a urinary tract, meningeal or middle ear infection, to pain from an unrecognised fracture, oesophagitis or torsion of the testis. Severe nappy rash, constipation or coeliac disease may produce a miserable, crying infant. The complaint that a baby is 'always crying' may be a pointer to potential or actual non-accidental injury. On the basis of countless reports of parents, there seems little doubt that the eruption of teeth is painful in some infants. However, teething does not cause vomiting, diarrhoea, high fever or convulsions.

PYLORIC STENOSIS

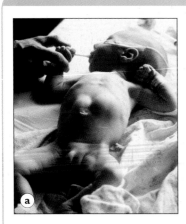
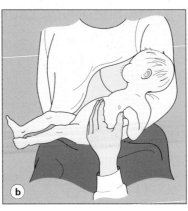
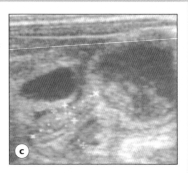
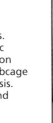

Fig. 12.5 (a) Visible gastric peristalsis in an infant with pyloric stenosis. (b) Diagram showing a test feed being performed to diagnose pyloric stenosis. The pyloric mass feels like an 'olive' on gentle, deep palpation halfway between the midpoint of the anterior margin of the right ribcage and the umbilicus. (c) Ultrasound examination showing pyloric stenosis. (d) Pyloric stenosis at operation showing pale, thick pyloric muscle and pyloromyotomy incision.

Infant 'colic'

The term 'colic' is used to describe a common symptom complex which occurs during the first few months of life. Paroxysmal, inconsolable crying or screaming accompanied by drawing up of the knees takes place several times a day, particularly in the evening. There is no firm evidence that the cause is intestinal, but this is often suspected. The condition usually resolves by 4 months of age. Occasionally, cow's milk protein intolerance or gastro-oesophageal reflux may be responsible. Sympathetic advice is helpful. The condition is essentially benign, although it may precipitate non-accidental injury in infants already at risk. Therapies such as gripe water are of unproven benefit. In severe, persistent cases an empirical 2-week trial of a cow's milk-free diet followed by a trial of anti-reflux treatment may be worthwhile.

ACUTE ABDOMINAL PAIN

Managing acute abdominal pain in children requires considerable skill. In nearly half the children admitted to hospital, the pain resolves undiagnosed. In young children it is essential not to delay the diagnosis and treatment of acute appendicitis, as progression to perforation can be rapid. It is easy to belittle the clinical signs of abdominal tenderness in young children. Of the surgical causes, appendicitis is by far the commonest. It needs to be differentiated from mesenteric adenitis and the other surgical and medical conditions listed in Figure 12.6. The testes, hernial orifices and hip joints must always be checked. It is noteworthy that:

- Lower lobe pneumonia may cause pain referred to the abdomen.
- Primary peritonitis is seen in patients with ascites from nephrotic syndrome or liver disease.
- Diabetic ketoacidosis may cause severe abdominal pain.
- Urinary tract infection, including acute pyelonephritis, is a relatively uncommon cause of acute abdominal pain, but must not be missed. It is important to test a urine sample in order to identify not only diabetes mellitus but also conditions affecting the liver and urinary tract.

Acute appendicitis

Acute appendicitis is the commonest cause of abdominal pain in childhood requiring surgical intervention (Fig. 12.7). Although it may occur at any age, it is very uncommon in children less than 3 years old. The clinical features of acute uncomplicated appendicitis are:

- *Symptoms*
  - anorexia
  - vomiting (usually only a few times)
  - abdominal pain, initially central and colicky (appendicular midgut colic) but then localising to the right iliac fossa (from localised peritoneal inflammation)

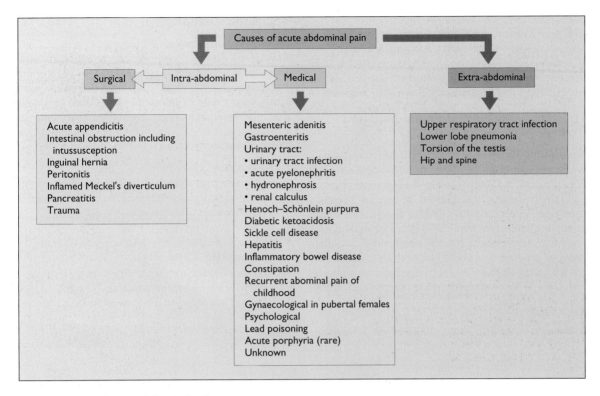

Fig. 12.6 Causes of acute abdominal pain.

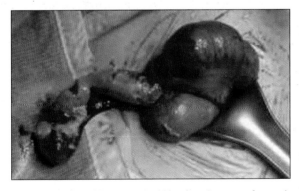

Fig. 12.7 Appendicitis at operation showing a perforated acutely inflamed appendix covered in fibrin.

- *Signs*
  — flushed face with oral foetor
  — low-grade fever 37.2–38°C
  — abdominal pain aggravated by movement
  — persistent tenderness with guarding in the right iliac fossa (McBurney's point).

In preschool children:
- the diagnosis is more difficult, particularly early in the disease
- faecoliths are more common and can be seen on a plain abdominal X-ray
- perforation is more common, as the omentum is less well developed and fails to surround the appendix.

 In young children with appendicitis, it is easy to underestimate abdominal signs and progression to perforation may be rapid.

With a retrocaecal appendix, localised guarding may be absent, and in a pelvic appendix there may be few abdominal signs.

Appendicitis is a progressive condition and so repeated observation and clinical review every few hours are key to making the correct diagnosis, avoiding delay on the one hand and unnecessary laparotomy on the other.

No laboratory investigation or imaging is consistently helpful in making the diagnosis. A neutrophilia is not always present on a full blood count. White blood cells or organisms in the urine are not uncommon in appendicitis as the inflamed appendix may be adjacent to the ureter or bladder. In some centres, laparoscopy is available to see whether or not the appendix is inflamed. Appendicectomy is straightforward in uncomplicated appendicitis.

Complicated appendicitis includes the presence of an appendix mass, an abscess or perforation. If there is generalised guarding consistent with perforation, fluid resuscitation and intravenous antibiotics are given prior to laparotomy. If there is a palpable mass in the right iliac fossa and there are no signs of generalised peritonitis, it may be reasonable to elect for conservative management with intravenous antibiotics, with appendicectomy being performed after several weeks. If symptoms progress, laparotomy is indicated. If an abscess is confirmed on abdominal ultrasound, operative drainage and appendicectomy will be required.

Non-specific abdominal pain and mesenteric adenitis

Non-specific abdominal pain (NSAP) is abdominal pain which resolves in 24–48 h. The pain is less severe than in appendicitis, and tenderness in the right iliac fossa is variable. It is often accompanied by an upper respiratory tract infection with cervical lymphadenopathy. In some of these children, the abdominal signs do not resolve and an appendicectomy is performed. The diagnosis of mesenteric adenitis can only be made definitively in those children in whom large mesenteric nodes are seen at laparotomy or laparoscopy and whose appendix is normal.

Intussusception

Intussusception describes the invagination of proximal bowel into a distal segment. It most commonly involves ileum passing into the caecum and colon through the ileocaecal valve (Fig. 12.8a). Intussusception is the commonest cause of intestinal obstruction in infants after the neonatal period. It usually occurs between 2 months and 2 years of age and resuscitation and reduction are urgent.

Presentation is with:
- paroxysmal, severe colicky pain and pallor – during episodes of pain, the child becomes pale, especially around the mouth, and draws up his legs
- a sausage-shaped mass – often palpable in the abdomen (Fig. 12.8b)
- passage of a characteristic redcurrant jelly stool comprising blood-stained mucus – this is a characteristic sign but tends to occur later

INTUSSUSCEPTION

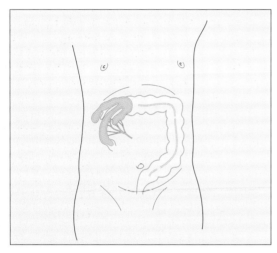

Fig. 12.8a Intussusception, showing why the blood supply to the gut rapidly becomes compromised, making relief of this form of obstruction urgent.

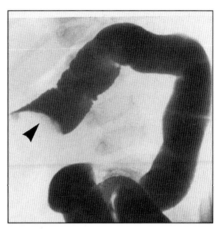

Fig. 12.8c An abdominal X-ray demonstrating an intussusception (see arrow), taken during reduction by air insufflated per rectum.

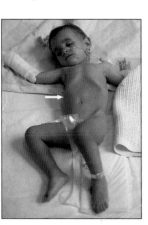

Fig. 12.8b A child with an intussusception. The mass can be seen in the upper abdomen. The child has become shocked.

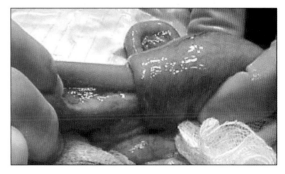

Fig. 12.8d Intussusception at operation showing the ileum entering the caecum. The surgeon is squeezing the colon to reduce the intussusception.

in the illness and may be first seen after a rectal examination

- abdominal distension and shock.

Usually, no underlying intestinal cause for the intussusception is found, although there is some evidence that viral infection leading to enlargement of Peyer's patches may form the lead point of the intussusception. An identifiable lead point such as a Meckel's diverticulum or polyp is more likely to be present in children over 2 years old. Intravenous volume expansion is likely to be required immediately as there is often pooling of fluid in the gut, which may lead to hypovolaemic shock.

An X-ray of the abdomen may show distended small bowel and absence of gas in the distal colon or rectum. Sometimes the outline of the intussusception itself can be visualised. Unless there are signs of peritonitis, reduction of the intussusception by rectal air insufflation is usually attempted (Fig. 12.8c). The success rate of this procedure is about 75%. The remaining 25% require operative reduction (Fig. 12.8d). Recurrence of the intussusception occurs in less than 5% but is more frequent after hydrostatic reduction.

> **Shock is an important complication of intussusception.**

Meckel's diverticulum

Two per cent of individuals have an ileal remnant of the vitellointestinal duct, in the form of a Meckel's diverticulum, which contains ectopic gastric mucosa or pancreatic tissue. Most are asymptomatic but they may present with severe rectal bleeding which is neither bright red nor true melaena. Other forms of presentation include intussusception, volvulus around a band, or diverticulitis which mimics appendicits. A technetium scan will demonstrate increased uptake by ectopic gastric mucosa in 70% of cases (Fig. 12.9). Treatment is by surgical resection.

Malrotation

If the small bowel mesentery is not fixed at the duodenojejunal flexure or in the ileocaecal region, its base is shorter than normal, predisposing to volvulus. It may arise in the fetus from the duodenojejunal flexure failing to rotate adequately to the left around the superior mesenteric vessels or the caecum failing to rotate and descend on the right. Ladd's bands may cross the duodenum, contributing to an obstruction (Fig. 12.10). There are two presentations:

- obstruction
- obstruction with a compromised blood supply.

If there is infarction of the bowel, blood may be seen in the gastric aspirates or in the stool. Obstruction with bilious vomiting usually presents in the first few days of life but can be seen at a later age. Any child with dark green vomiting needs an upper gastrointestinal contrast study to assess intestinal rotation, unless signs of vascular compromise are present, when an urgent laparotomy is needed.

MECKEL'S DIVERTICULUM

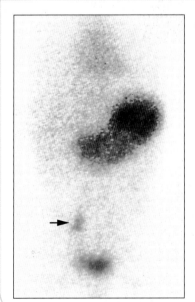

Fig. 12.9 A technetium scan showing uptake by ectopic gastric mucosa in a Meckel's diverticulum in the right iliac fossa.

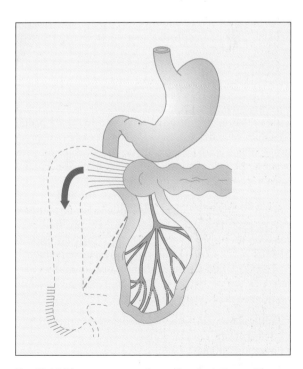

Fig. 12.10 The commonest form of malrotation, with the caecum remaining high and fixed to the posterior abdominal wall. There are Ladd's bands obstructing the duodenum.

At operation, the volvulus is untwisted, the duodenum mobilised and the bowel placed in the non-rotated position with the duodenojejunal flexure on the right and the caecum and appendix on the left. The malrotation is not 'corrected', but the mesentry broadened. The appendix may be removed to avoid later diagnostic confusion in the event of appendicitis.

RECURRENT ABDOMINAL PAIN

Recurrent pain, sufficient to interrupt normal activities and lasting for at least 3 months, occurs in 10% of school-age children. Less than 10% of these children will have a definable organic cause. The widely held belief that the remainder have psychogenic pain is without foundation. A number of studies have failed to show a difference between such children and their families and controls. However, in some children, it may be a manifestation of stress (see p. 321) or it may become part of a vicious cycle of anxiety and escalating pain leading to family distress and demands for increasingly invasive investigations. There is evidence that anxiety may lead to altered motility, which may be perceived by the child as pain.

Over 90% of children with recurrent abdominal pain have no structural or mucosal abnormality in the gastrointestinal tract. Their pain is characteristically central, around the umbilicus, and the children are otherwise entirely well. It is increasingly recognised, however, that some have one of three recognisable symptom constellations resulting from functional abnormalities of gut motility or enteral neurones – irritable bowel syndrome, non-ulcer dyspepsia or abdominal migraine.

Irritable bowel syndrome

This disorder, also common in adults, is associated with altered gastrointestinal motility and an abnormal sensation of intra-abdominal events. Studies of pressure changes within the small intestine of children with irritable bowel syndrome suggest that abnormally forceful contractions occur. It has also been shown that affected adults experience pain from the inflation of balloons in the intestine at substantially lower volumes than do controls. There is therefore an interplay between these two factors, both of which are modulated by psychosocial factors such as stress and anxiety.

There is often a positive family history and a characteristic set of symptoms, although not all patients experience every symptom:

- abdominal pain, often worse before or relieved by defaecation
- mucousy stools
- bloating
- feeling of incomplete defaecation
- constipation, often alternating with normal or loose stools.

Non-ulcer dyspepsia

Some children with abdominal pain have symptoms suggesting an upper gastrointestinal disorder:

- epigastric pain
- postprandial vomiting
- belching
- bloating
- early satiety
- heartburn.

If endoscopy is performed, it fails to reveal an ulcer or other mucosal disease in the stomach or duodenum, but gastric motility is abnormal.

Abdominal migraine

Classical cranial migraine is often associated with abdominal pain in addition to headaches, and in some children the abdominal pain predominates. The attacks of pain are midline, paroxysmal, stereotypic and associated with facial pallor. There is usually a personal or family history of migraine. Pizotifen, a serotonin receptor antagonist, is a helpful prophylactic agent in those children with frequent, severe symptoms.

Management of recurrent abdominal pain

It is important that a full history and examination are not only done, but seen to be done, otherwise reassurance will be unconvincing. It will also establish that the child is growing normally and that there are no abnormalities on examination. In children with irritable bowel syndrome and non-ulcer dyspepsia, it can be helpful to explain to both the child and parents that 'sometimes the insides of the intestine become so sensitive that some children can feel the food going round the bends'. It is also necessary to make a distinction between 'serious' and 'dangerous'. These disorders can be serious, if, for example, they lead to substantial loss of schooling, but they are not dangerous.

Investigations should be guided by the clinical features. Although there are many potential organic causes, most are rare and investigations are only performed if indicated. A urine microscopy and culture is mandatory as urinary tract infections may cause pain in the absence of other symptoms or signs.

The long term prognosis is:
- about half of affected children rapidly become free of symptoms
- in one-quarter, the symptoms take some months to resolve
- in one-quarter, symptoms continue or return in adulthood as irritable bowel syndrome, non-ulcer dyspepsia or cranial migraine.

Gastritis and peptic ulceration

The greater use of endoscopy in children and the identification of the Gram-negative organism, *Helicobacter pylori*, in association with antral gastritis have focused attention on it as a potential cause of abdominal pain in children. In adults, there is substantial evidence that *H. pylori* is a strong predisposing factor to duodenal ulcers. This association in children is much less clear. Duodenal ulcers are uncommon in children but should be sought in those with night pain, particularly if it wakes them, or when there is a history of peptic ulceration in a first-degree relative.

H. pylori causes a nodular antral gastritis which may be associated with abdominal pain and nausea. It is usually identified in gastric antral biopsies, but may also be present on microaerophilic culture. The organism produces urease, which forms the basis for a laboratory test on biopsies and the ^{13}C breath test following the administration of ^{13}C-labelled urea by mouth. Serological tests are generally unreliable in children. Treatment comprises various therapy regimens (e.g. a proton pump inhibitor, clarithromycin, and either amoxicillin or metronidazole).

GASTROENTERITIS

Infective diarrhoea and vomiting remain an important cause of morbidity in developed countries, although mortality is very low. In developing countries, gastroenteritis still claims the lives of 5 million children under the age of 5 each year.

The commonest cause of gastroenteritis in developed countries is rotavirus infection, which accounts for up to 60% of cases in children less than 2 years of age, particularly during the winter months. Other viruses, particularly adenovirus, calicivirus, corona and astroviruses, have been implicated in outbreaks but are much less common and their role as pathogens is less clear.

Bacterial causes are less common in developed countries, and are suggested by the presence of blood in the stools. *Campylobacter jejuni* infection, usually the commonest of the bacterial infections in developed

countries, is often also associated with severe abdominal pain. *Shigella* and some salmonellae produce a dysenteric type of infection, with blood and pus in the stool, pain and tenesmus. *Shigella* may be accompanied by high fever causing a febrile convulsion. Cholera and enterotoxigenic *E. coli* infection are associated with profuse, rapidly dehydrating diarrhoea. However, clinical features act as a poor guide to the pathogen.

A number of disorders may masquerade as gastroenteritis (Fig. 12.11) and, when in doubt, hospital referral is essential. Dehydration and its complications are the usual cause of death in gastroenteritis, and its correction is the fundamental aim of treatment. Accurate clinical assessment of dehydration is important but difficult (Figs 12.12 and 12.13).

Fig. 12.11 Conditions which can mimic gastroenteritis.

Systemic infection	Septicaemia, meningitis
Local infections	Respiratory tract infection, otitis media, hepatitis A, urinary tract infection
Surgical disorders	Pyloric stenosis, intussusception, acute appendicitis, necrotising enterocolitis, Hirschsprung's disease
Metabolic disorder	Diabetic ketoacidosis
Renal disorder	Haemolytic uraemic syndrome
Other	Coeliac disease, cow's milk protein intolerance, adrenal insufficiency

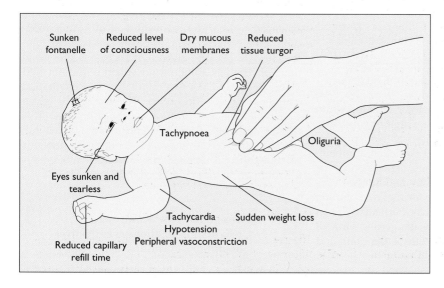

Fig. 12.12 Clinical features of dehydration in an infant.

Sunken fontanelle · Reduced level of consciousness · Dry mucous membranes · Reduced tissue turgor · Tachypnoea · Oliguria · Eyes sunken and tearless · Tachycardia Hypotension Peripheral vasoconstriction · Sudden weight loss · Reduced capillary refill time

Fig. 12.13 Clinical assessment of dehydration.

	Moderate dehydration	Severe dehydration
Body weight loss	5–10%	>10%
General appearance	Thirsty, restless or lethargic	Drowsy, cold, sweating
Tears	Reduced/absent	Absent
Tissue elasticity	Reduced/absent	Absent
Mucous membranes	Dry	Very dry
Capillary refill time	Normal/prolonged	Prolonged (>2 s)
Blood pressure	Normal or low	Low or unrecordable
Urine output	Reduced	Marked oliguria
Pulse	Rapid	Rapid, weak, may be impalpable
Eyes	Sunken	Grossly sunken
Anterior fontanelle	Sunken	Very sunken

Infants are at particular risk of dehydration because of their:

- greater surface area to weight ratio, leading to greater insensible water losses (300 ml/m² per day, equivalent in infants to 15–17 ml/kg per day)
- inability to gain access to fluids when thirsty
- higher basal fluid requirements (100–120 ml/kg per day, i.e. 10–12% of body weight)
- immature renal tubular reabsorption processes.

Isonatraemic and hyponatraemic dehydration

In dehydration, there is a total body deficit of sodium and water. In most instances, the losses of sodium and water are proportional and plasma sodium remains within the normal range (isonatraemic dehydration). When sodium losses exceed those of water, plasma sodium falls (hyponatraemic dehydration) and this is associated with a shift of water from extra- to intracellular compartments. The increase in intracellular volume leads to an increase in brain volume, sometimes resulting in convulsions, whereas the marked extracellular depletion leads to a greater degree of shock per unit of water loss. This form of dehydration is more common in poorly nourished infants in developing countries.

Hypernatraemic dehydration

Infrequently, water loss exceeds the relative sodium loss and plasma sodium concentration increases (hypernatraemic dehydration). This usually results from high insensible water losses (high fever or hot, dry environment) or from profuse, low-sodium diarrhoea. The extracellular fluid becomes hypertonic with respect to the intracellular fluid and there is a shift of water into the extracellular space from the intracellular compartment. Signs of extracellular fluid depletion are therefore less per unit of fluid loss, and depression of the fontanelle, reduced tissue elasticity and sunken eyes are less obvious. This makes this form of dehydration more difficult to recognise clinically, particularly in an obese infant. It is a particularly dangerous form of dehydration as water is drawn out of the brain and cerebral shrinkage within a rigid skull may lead to multiple, small cerebral haemorrhages and convulsions.

Fig. 12.14 Composition (mmol/L) of oral rehydration solutions.

	Standard solution	WHO/UNICEF
Sodium	60	90
Potassium	20	20
Chloride	50	80
Citrate	10	10
Glucose	75–110	110

The WHO/UNICEF solution is designed principally for use in developing countries in children with moderate to severe dehydration. The sodium concentration is too high for routine use in developed countries.

Transient hyperglycaemia occurs in some patients with hypernatraemic dehydration; it is self-correcting and does not require insulin.

Management

Mild dehydration (<5% body weight loss)

In most cases of gastroenteritis in infants and toddlers in developed countries, dehydration is mild, with less than 5% loss of body weight, and there are few, if any, clinical signs of dehydration. It can usually be managed by short-term substitution of normal feeds with a maintenance type of glucose–electrolyte solution (Fig. 12.14). The glucose or sucrose is present in oral rehydration solutions to enhance sodium and water absorption, not as a calorie source. Rehydration solutions may be rice-based. The solution is given until vomiting and profuse diarrhoea subside. This usually lasts less than 24 h and a normal diet can then be introduced immediately. Contrary to previous teaching, there is no need to re-introduce milk gradually or to avoid milk or milk-containing foods.

 Throughout the world, oral rehydration solution saves the lives of millions of children each year.

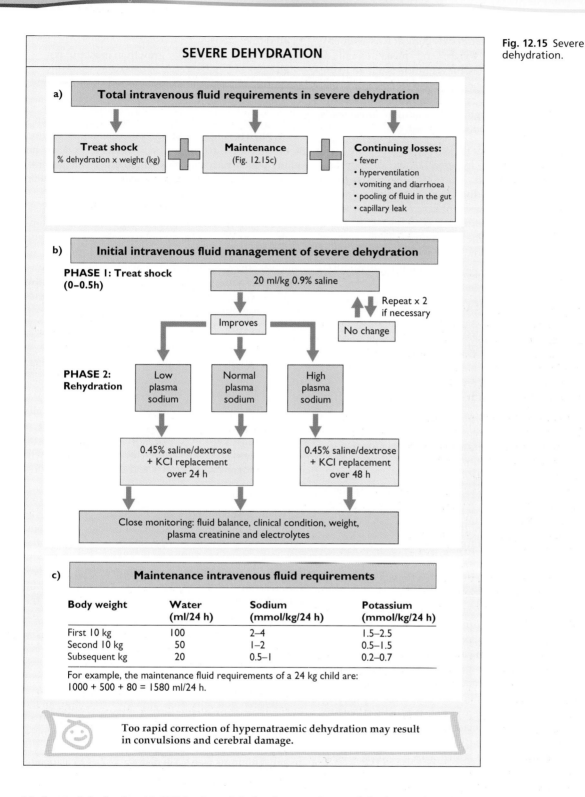

Fig. 12.15 Severe dehydration.

SEVERE DEHYDRATION

a) Total intravenous fluid requirements in severe dehydration

Treat shock
% dehydration x weight (kg)

+

Maintenance
(Fig. 12.15c)

+

Continuing losses:
• fever
• hyperventilation
• vomiting and diarrhoea
• pooling of fluid in the gut
• capillary leak

b) Initial intravenous fluid management of severe dehydration

PHASE 1: Treat shock (0–0.5h)

20 ml/kg 0.9% saline

Repeat x 2 if necessary

Improves

No change

PHASE 2: Rehydration

Low plasma sodium

Normal plasma sodium

High plasma sodium

0.45% saline/dextrose + KCl replacement over 24 h

0.45% saline/dextrose + KCl replacement over 48 h

Close monitoring: fluid balance, clinical condition, weight, plasma creatinine and electrolytes

c) Maintenance intravenous fluid requirements

Body weight	Water (ml/24 h)	Sodium (mmol/kg/24 h)	Potassium (mmol/kg/24 h)
First 10 kg	100	2–4	1.5–2.5
Second 10 kg	50	1–2	0.5–1.5
Subsequent kg	20	0.5–1	0.2–0.7

For example, the maintenance fluid requirements of a 24 kg child are:
1000 + 500 + 80 = 1580 ml/24 h.

Too rapid correction of hypernatraemic dehydration may result in convulsions and cerebral damage.

Moderate dehydration (6–10% body weight loss)
These children have clinical signs of dehydration. A 6 h trial of oral rehydration can be instituted, aiming to give 100 ml/kg over this period (orally or by nasogastric tube). If there is no improvement in the child's symptoms and state of hydration, intravenous rehydration should be given.

Severe dehydration (>10% loss of body weight)
Intravenous rehydration is always indicated. Patients who are shocked require immediate resuscitation with plasma volume expansion (Fig. 12.15a). Rehydration is achieved by replacement of the fluid deficit, whilst allowing for maintenance fluid requirement and any ongoing fluid losses (Figs 12.15b and c). Fluid balance

needs to be closely monitored by clinical reassessment, including the child's weight and measurement of plasma electrolytes. Potassium chloride is added to the intravenous infusion once the child is passing urine. Acute renal failure may rarely complicate severe dehydration. Failure to recognise continuing oliguria leads to overhydration and pulmonary oedema.

Hypernatraemic dehydration

The management of hypernatraemic dehydration is particularly difficult. Once circulation has been restored, a too rapid reduction in plasma sodium concentration and osmolality will lead to a shift of water into cerebral cells, resulting in cerebral oedema and possible convulsions. The reduction in plasma sodium should therefore be slow, over 48 h, in order not to exceed a reduction in plasma sodium of 10 mmol/L per 24 h.

Anti-diarrhoea drugs (e.g. loperamide, Lomotil) and anti-emetics

There is no place for medications for the vomiting or diarrhoea of gastroenteritis as they:

- are ineffective
- may prolong the excretion of bacteria in stools
- can be associated with side-effects
- add unnecessarily to cost
- focus attention away from oral rehydration.

Antibiotics are indicated only for specific bacterial or protozoal infections (e.g. cholera, shigellosis, giardiasis).

> **Death in gastroenteritis is caused by dehydration. Its correction is the mainstay of treatment.**

Post-gastroenteritis syndrome

Infrequently, following an episode of gastroenteritis, the introduction of a normal diet results in a return of watery diarrhoea. Temporary lactose intolerance may have developed, which can be confirmed by the presence of non-absorbed sugar in the stools giving a positive Clinitest result. In such circumstances, a return to an oral rehydration solution for 24 h, followed by a further introduction of a normal diet, is usually successful.

Rarely, multiple dietary intolerances may result, such that specialist dietary management is required in the implementation of a diet which excludes cow's milk, disaccharides and gluten. In very severe cases, a period of parenteral nutrition is required to enable the injured small intestinal mucosa to recover sufficiently to absorb luminal nutrients.

MALABSORPTION

Disorders affecting the digestion or absorption of nutrients manifest as:

- abnormal stools
- failure to thrive or poor growth in most but not all cases
- specific nutrient deficiencies, either singly or in combination.

In general, parents know when their children's stools have become abnormal. The true malabsorption stool is difficult to flush down the toilet and has an odour which pervades the whole house. In general, colour is a poor guide to abnormality. Reliable dietetic assessment is important. It is inappropriate to investigate children for malabsorption as a cause of their failure to thrive when dietary energy intake is demonstrably low and other symptoms are absent. Some disorders affecting the small intestinal mucosa or pancreas may lead to the malabsorption of many nutrients (pan-malabsorption), whereas others are highly specific, e.g. zinc malabsorption in acrodermatitis enteropathica.

Coeliac disease

Coeliac disease is an enteropathy in which the gliadin fraction of gluten provokes a damaging immunological response in the proximal small intestinal mucosa. As a result, the rate of migration of absorptive cells moving up the villi (enterocytes) from the crypts is massively increased but is insufficient to compensate for increased cell loss from the villous tips. Villi become progressively shorter and then absent, leaving a flat mucosa.

Overall, the incidence of coeliac disease varies between 1 in 500 and 1 in 3000. It has been particularly high in the west of Ireland but, in common with some parts of Europe, including the UK, the frequency in early childhood is falling. In contrast, the frequency in other European countries, e.g. Sweden, has recently increased. These changes appear to be related to the amount of gluten in the diet in the first year of life and the age at which it is introduced. The overall picture in the UK is unclear. It seems likely that a lower rate in infancy will be reflected in a higher rate in later childhood, i.e. manipulating dietary gluten in infancy postpones rather than prevents the disease.

Children normally present in the first 2 years of life with failure to thrive following the introduction of gluten in cereals. General irritability, abnormal stools, abdominal distension and buttock wasting are the usual symptoms (see Case history 12.2). Occasionally, children present in later childhood with anaemia (iron and/or folate deficiency) or growth failure, with little or no gastrointestinal symptoms.

Diagnosis

The diagnosis requires demonstration of a flat mucosa on jejunal biopsy followed by the resolution of symptoms and catch-up growth upon gluten withdrawal. There is no place for the empirical use of a

CASE HISTORY 12.2

COELIAC DISEASE

This 2-year-old (Fig. 12.16a) had a history of poor growth from 12 months of age. His parents had noticed that he tended to be crotchety and had three or four foul-smelling stools a day. A jejunal biopsy at 2 years of age showed subtotal villous atrophy (Fig. 12.16b) and he was started on a gluten-free diet. Within a few days, his parents commented that his mood had improved and within a month he was a 'different child'. He subsequently exhibited good catch-up growth (Fig. 12.16d).

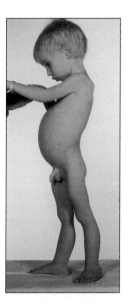

Fig. 12.16a Coeliac disease causing wasting of the buttocks and distended abdomen.

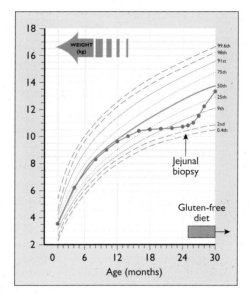

Fig. 12.16d Growth chart showing failure to thrive and response to a gluten-free diet. (Adapted from chart © Child Growth Foundation)

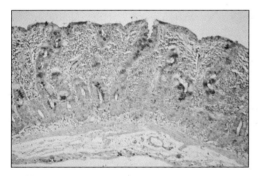

Fig. 12.16b Histology of a jejunal biopsy showing lymphocytic infiltration and villous atrophy confirming coeliac disease.

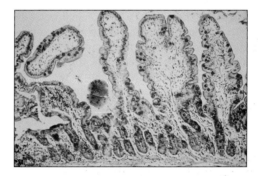

Fig. 12.16c Normal jejunal histology is shown for comparison.

gluten-free diet as a diagnostic test for coeliac disease in the absence of a jejunal biopsy. Serological tests, such as anti-gliadin and anti-endomysial antibodies, are not sufficiently sensitive and specific to replace jejunal biopsy for definitive diagnosis but are useful screening tests.

Management

All products containing wheat, rye and barley are removed from the diet and this results in resolution of symptoms. Supervision by a dietician is essential. In children in whom the initial biopsy or the response to gluten withdrawal is doubtful, or when the disease presents before the age of 2, a gluten challenge is required in later childhood to demonstrate continuing susceptibility of the jejunal mucosa to damage by gluten. The gluten-free diet should be adhered to for life. The incidence of small bowel malignancy in adulthood is increased in coeliac disease although a gluten-free diet probably reduces the risk to normal.

Transient dietary protein intolerances

In contrast to coeliac disease, which requires lifelong gluten withdrawal, there are a number of transient intolerances to dietary proteins. These usually manifest as:

- diarrhoea and/or vomiting with failure to thrive
- eczema
- acute colitis
- migraine
- occasionally, an acute anaphylactic reaction with urticaria, stridor, bronchospasm and shock.

Cow's milk protein is the most commonly incriminated antigen, but intolerance to soya and less frequently to wheat, fish, egg, chicken and rice are also described. When an acute reaction occurs immediately after ingestion, the diagnosis can be readily established. When the reaction is delayed, diagnosis is difficult. Intolerances occur more commonly in infants with IgA deficiency or with a strong family history of atopy.

Although no single laboratory test is diagnostic, affected children may have:

- eosinophilia in the peripheral blood
- positive antibody tests to specific food proteins (RAST tests)
- a high IgE concentration in plasma.

Those children who present with failure to thrive and protracted diarrhoea may require a jejunal biopsy to establish the diagnosis, in particular to differentiate it from coeliac disease. In cow's milk protein intolerance, there is a patchy enteropathy in the jejunal mucosa, usually with prominent eosinophils in the lamina propria. Elimination of the offending antigen results in rapid resolution of symptoms and this, together with their return upon challenge, is the only diagnostic test. The advice of an experienced dietician is essential in the supervision of all exclusion diets in infancy and childhood, to ensure complete antigen exclusion whilst maintaining a nutritionally adequate diet.

In cow's milk protein intolerance, a case in hydrolysate-based formula is preferred to a soya-based feed, as up to 30% of infants will also be (or become) intolerant to soya. Most children outgrow their intolerance by the age of 2 years, which is therefore an appropriate time to conduct a further challenge. Anaphylaxis occurs infrequently, but it is important that the challenge is conducted in hospital, beginning with a skin test followed by the ingestion of increasing amounts of antigen.

Other rare causes of nutrient malabsorption

Abnormal nutrient absorption occurs in blind loops from *small intestinal bacterial contamination*, when there is colonisation of the small intestine by Gram-negative organisms or anaerobes normally found in the colon. *Bile salt deficiency*, from cholestatic disorders or following resection of the distal ileum, leads to substantial malabsorption of fat and fat-soluble vitamins.

Impaired fat transport may occur in the rare disorders of *intestinal lymphangiectasia*, in which there are abnormal lymphatics, and in *a-betalipoproteinaemia*, in which there is a failure to make chylomicrons. The latter disorder presents in childhood with steatorrhoea, acanthocytosis of red blood cells, retinal degeneration and fat-soluble vitamin malabsorption, particularly vitamin E which causes severe neuronal degeneration in later childhood and adolescence. Large oral doses of vitamin E from early childhood are preventive.

In contrast to transient lactose intolerance following diarrhoea, *late-onset lactase deficiency* is the norm in most of the world's population. Lactase is no longer expressed in the small intestine after early childhood in non-Caucasians. Symptoms vary considerably and are not present before 2 or 3 years of age. Northern Europeans and North Americans are unusual in continuing to express lactase throughout life.

Specific transport defects (rare)

There are many such defects, each limited to a specific carrier protein. They are all rare. *Glucose–galactose malabsorption* results in severe, life-threatening diarrhoea from the introduction of milk feeds and affected children are only able to tolerate fructose as their dietary carbohydrate.

Acrodermatitis enteropathica results from a congenital defect in zinc transport in the small intestine. Affected children present in infancy with a symmetrical erythematous rash mainly affecting mucocutaneous junctions around the mouth and anus. Plasma zinc is very low, as are the activities of zinc-dependent enzymes such as alkaline phosphatase in plasma.

TODDLER DIARRHOEA

This condition, also called chronic non-specific diarrhoea, is the commonest cause of persistent loose stools in preschool children. Characteristically, the stools are of varying consistency, sometimes well formed, sometimes explosive and loose. The presence of undigested vegetables in the stools is common, giving rise to the alternative title 'peas and carrots syndrome'. Affected children are well and thriving and there are no precipitating dietary factors.

Toddler diarrhoea probably results from an underlying maturational delay in intestinal motility. Most children have grown out of their symptoms by 5 years of age.

No treatment is usually required. Loperamide used cautiously may be helpful in children with socially disruptive symptoms.

INFLAMMATORY BOWEL DISEASE

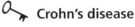 Crohn's disease

Since the 1950s, there has been a marked increase in the incidence of Crohn's disease in all age groups.

It becomes progressively more common throughout childhood. In northern Europe and North America, the overall incidence is about 4 per 100 000. About a quarter of patients with Crohn's disease present in childhood or adolescence.

Crohn's disease is a transmural, focal, sub-acute or chronic inflammatory disease. It affects any part of the gastrointestinal tract from the mouth to the anus, but most commonly the distal ileum and proximal colon. The affected intestine is thickened and adhesions between affected loops are common. Perianal skin tags, fissures and fistulae are also common. The histological hallmark is the presence of non-caseating epitheloid cell granulomata.

Abdominal pain, diarrhoea and growth failure with pubertal delay are the most common presenting features. There may be oral and perianal ulcers. The disease may be insidious in onset, and extraintestinal symptoms such as growth failure, intermittent fever, arthritis, uveitis and erythema nodosum may be present with little or no pointers towards gastrointestinal disease. Some adolescents may present with a clinical picture virtually indistinguishable from anorexia nervosa.

Diagnosis rests upon the demonstration of characteristic abnormalities on barium follow-through (narrowing, fissuring, mucosal irregularities and mural thickening) and at colonoscopy on histology of a biopsy. Acute-phase reactants (e.g. C-reactive protein and ESR) are usually raised and can be useful in monitoring disease severity.

The aims of treatment are to induce remission by suppressing inflammation with steroids or by using an elemental diet for about 6 weeks. Recurrence is common and, with the exception of azathioprine in Crohn's colitis, no medical regimen has been shown to maintain remission. Overnight enteral feeding may be helpful in correcting growth failure. Surgery is necessary for complications of Crohn's disease – obstruction, fistulae, failed medical treatment, growth failure or abscess formation. In general, the long-term prognosis for Crohn's disease beginning in childhood is good and most patients lead normal lives despite occasional recurrent disease.

> **In Crohn's disease, up to one-third of children will experience growth failure and delayed puberty.**

Ulcerative colitis

Ulcerative colitis is a recurrent, inflammatory and ulcerating disease involving the mucous membrane of the colon. Characteristically, the disease presents with rectal bleeding, diarrhoea, colicky pain and weight loss.

The diagnosis is made on the characteristic appearance at colonoscopy and on the histological features,

after exclusion of infective causes of colitis. Extraintestinal complications include erythema nodosum, pyoderma gangrenosum, arthritis and spondylitis. There is an increased incidence of adenocarcinoma of the colon in adults (1 in 200 risk for each year of disease between 10 and 20 years from diagnosis).

Mild attacks are managed with topical steroids when the disease is confined to the rectum and sigmoid colon, or sulphasalazine for more extensive disease. More severe disease requires systemic steroids. Severe fulminating disease is a medical emergency and requires treatment with broad-spectrum antibiotics, intravenous fluids and steroids. One-third of patients require colectomy during the course of their disease. Colectomy is performed for chronic poorly controlled disease, to prevent malignancy in longstanding disease or for severe fulminating disease, sometimes complicated by a toxic megacolon, which fails to respond to intensive medical treatment.

CONSTIPATION

In healthy infants there is a wide range in bowel frequency. Breast-fed infants may not pass stools for several days. In young children, constipation, which is the painful passage of hard, infrequent stools, is common. It often follows an acute febrile illness or a transient superficial anal fissure. Most such cases resolve with mild laxatives and extra fluids. Occasionally, following such events, or perhaps in association with forceful potty training, the use of uncomfortable lavatories on holiday or at school, or psychological family stress, more protracted constipation results. Children may refrain from defaecation for fear of the associated pain. The rectum becomes full and overdistended, and with time the sensation of needing to defaecate is lost. Involuntary soiling usually follows as the full rectum overflows. Children of school age are frequently teased as a result and secondary behavioural problems are common. At this stage, the use of stimulant laxatives without first emptying the rectum completely is likely to make soiling worse.

Examination often reveals an abdominal mass and, on rectal examination, stool is present down to the anal margin. Organic causes of constipation are uncommon, but hypothyroidism, hypercalcaemia, a urinary concentrating defect or Hirschsprung's disease should be considered.

It should be explained to the child and the parents that soiling is involuntary and that recovery of normal rectal size and sensation may take a long time.

For mild cases, where faeces are not palpable per abdomen, dietary fluid and fibre should be increased. Stool softeners (lactulose or docusate) and stimulant laxatives (sodium picosulphate or senna) may be required.

For more severe cases, when the faeces are palpable per abdomen, the first aim of management is to evacuate the overloaded rectum completely. Following

1–2 weeks of stool softeners (lactulose or docusate), large doses of powerful oral laxatives (sodium picosulphate or senna) and high volumes of oral polyethylene glycol solutions (Klean-Prep) are given daily until the stools are liquid. Advice about improving the dietary fluid and food intake is given. This is followed by daily evening doses of a stimulant laxative (e.g. senna), combined with regular postprandial visits to the lavatory, and a star chart is introduced to record and reward progress.

Encouragement by family and health professionals is essential, as relapse is common and psychological support is sometimes required. Occasionally the faecal retention is so severe that evacuation is only possible using enemas or by manual evacuation under an anaesthetic. Care must be taken to avoid distress if enemas or washouts are used. The management of constipation is summarised in Figure 12.17.

Hirschsprung's disease

The absence of ganglion cells from the myenteric and submucosal plexuses of part of the large bowel results in a narrow, contracted segment. The abnormal bowel extends from the rectum for a variable distance proximally, ending in a normally innervated, dilated colon. In 75% of cases, the lesion is confined to the rectosigmoid, but in 10% the entire colon is involved. Presentation is usually in the neonatal period with intestinal obstruction heralded by failure to pass meconium within the first 24 h of life. Abdominal distension and later bile-stained vomiting develop (Fig. 12.18). Rectal examination may reveal a narrowed segment and withdrawal of the examining finger often releases a gush of liquid stool and flatus. Temporary improvement in the obstruction following the dilatation caused by the rectal examination can lead to a delay in diagnosis.

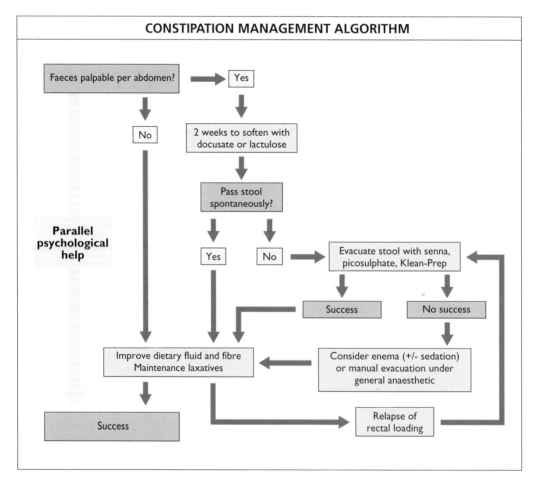

Fig. 12.17 Summary of the management of constipation.

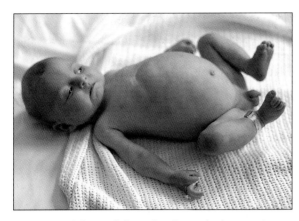

Fig. 12.18 Abdominal distension from Hirschsprung's disease.

Occasionally infants present with severe, life-threatening Hirschsprung's enterocolitis during the first few weeks of life, sometimes due to *Clostridium difficile* infection. In later childhood, presentation is with chronic constipation, usually profound, and associated with abdominal distension but usually without soiling. Growth failure may also be present.

Diagnosis is made by demonstrating the absence of ganglion cells together with the presence of large, acetylcholinesterase-positive nerve trunks on a suction rectal biopsy. Anorectal manometry or barium studies may be useful in giving the surgeon an idea of the length of the aganglionic segment but are unreliable for diagnostic purposes. Management is surgical and usually involves an initial colostomy followed by anastomosing normally innervated bowel to the anus.

FURTHER READING

Hutson J (ed.) 1999 Jones' clinical paediatric surgery. Blackwell Science, Oxford. *Short textbook*

Kelly D A, Booth I W 1997 Pediatric gastroenterology and hepatology. Mosby-Wolfe, London

Walker W A, Durie P R, Hamilton J R, Walker-Smith J A, Watkins J B B C (eds) 2000 Pediatric gastrointestinal disease, 3rd edn. Decker, Ontario. *Comprehensive textbook*

13

Infection and immunity

CHAPTER CONTENTS

- Common childhood infections
- Staphylococcal and streptococcal infections
- Kawasaki's disease
- Meningitis
- Encephalitis/encephalopathy

- Tuberculosis
- Lyme disease
- Tropical infections
- Immunodeficiency disorders
- Immunisation

Infections are the most common cause of acute illness in children. Worldwide, acute respiratory infections, gastroenteritis, measles and malaria, often accompanied by malnutrition, are major causes of death. It has been estimated that each year they are responsible for the deaths of about 8 million children under the age of 5 years.

In developed countries, with improved nutrition, living conditions, sanitation, immunisations, antibiotic therapy and modern medical care, morbidity from infections has declined dramatically, and deaths from infectious diseases are uncommon. However, some infections remain a major problem, e.g. meningococcal

septicaemia, meningitis, malaria and HIV. Some have re-emerged, e.g. tuberculosis. Children with immuno-deficiency, whether congenital or acquired, are also vulnerable to a range of unusual or opportunist pathogens. To facilitate the control of communicable diseases within the community, certain diseases must be notified by doctors to the local public health specialist.

Many of the common childhood infections present with rash and fever. Figure 13.1 shows the different types of rashes and the infections associated with them. The incubation period and length of time affected children should be kept away from nursery or school are shown in Figure 13.2.

Fig. 13.1 Rashes caused by childhood infections.

	Type of lesion	Infection
	Macular/papular/maculopapular Macules – red/pink discrete flat areas, blanch on pressure Papules – solid raised hemispherical lesions, usually tiny, also blanch on pressure	Rubella (macular only), measles, rubella, HHV-6/7, enterovirus Uncommon: scarlet fever, Kawasaki's disease (but remember drug rashes)
	Purpuric/petechial Non-blanching red/purple spots, test with a glass	Meningococcal, enterovirus, Henoch–Schönlein purpura, thrombocytopenia
	Vesicular Raised hemispherical lesions, <0.5 cm diameter, contain clear fluid	Chickenpox, shingles, herpes simplex, hand, foot and mouth disease
	Pustular/bullous Raised hemispherical lesions, >0.5 cm diameter, contain clear or purulent fluid	Impetigo, scalded skin
	Desquamation Dry and flaky loss of surface epidermis, often peripheries	Post-scarlet fever, Kawasaki's disease

Fig. 13.2 Incubation and school exclusion period of common childhood infections.

Illness	Incubation (days)	School/nursery exclusion
Measles	10–14	From onset of coryza until day 5 of rash
Mumps	14–21	Until parotid swelling goes (5–7 days)
Rubella (German measles)	14–21	None
Parvovirus (erythema infectiosum)	4–14	None
Herpes simplex stomatitis	3–5	Until lesions crusted/treated
Chickenpox	10–23	Until day 5 of rash, or until lesions crusted
HHV-6/7 (exanthem subitum)	Not known	None
Enterovirus	3–5	If with diarrhoea
Hand, foot and mouth (Coxsackie)	4–6	None
Scarlet fever	2–4	Until completed 5 days antibiotics
Impetigo	10–15	Until lesions healed/crusted/treated
Scalded skin	Not known	Until lesions healed/treated
Kawasaki's disease	Not known	None

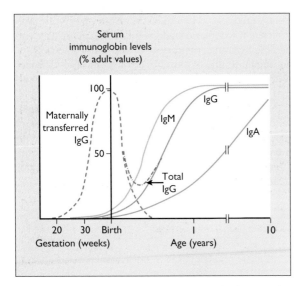

Fig. 13.3 Serum immunoglobulin levels in the fetus and infant. When maternal immunoglobulin levels decline, infants become susceptible to viral infections.

At birth, infants possess all the essential components of the immune system, although these are immature. Circulating immunoglobulins are derived transplacentally from the mother (Fig. 13.3) and decrease during the first few months of life, leaving them susceptible to the common infections.

COMMON CHILDHOOD INFECTIONS

 Measles

Since the introduction of an effective vaccine in 1968, the incidence of measles in England and Wales has declined dramatically, from a peak of 800 000 cases per year in the early 1960s to 3000 cases per year in the 1990s. This has been accompanied by a decline in its complications. However, the mean age of infection has increased, with a significant proportion now over 10 years old, when the disease is often more severe. Most clinical cases currently diagnosed as measles in the UK are caused by other infections (e.g. HHV-6). For epidemiological tracking of infection, serological confirmation of clinical cases of measles should be undertaken by testing either blood or saliva.

Clinical features

These are shown in Figure 13.4. There are a number of serious complications which can occur in previously healthy children:

- *Encephalitis* – occurs in only 1 in 5000, about 8 days after the onset of the illness. Initial symptoms are headache, lethargy and irritability, proceeding to convulsions and ultimately coma. Mortality is 15%. Serious long-term sequelae include seizures, deafness, hemiplegia and severe learning difficulties affecting up to 40% of survivors.

- *Subacute sclerosing panencephalitis (SSPE)* – a rare but devastating illness manifesting, on average, 7 years after measles infection in about 1 in 100 000 cases. Most children who develop SSPE have primary measles infection before 2 years of age. SSPE is caused by a variant of the measles virus which persists in the central nervous system. The disorder presents with loss of neurological function, which progresses over several years to dementia and death. The diagnosis is essentially clinical, supported by finding high levels of measles antibody in both blood and CSF and by characteristic EEG abnormalities. Since the introduction of measles immunisation, it has become extremely rare.

In developing countries, where malnutrition and particularly vitamin A deficiency lead to impaired cell-mediated immunity, measles often follows a protracted course with severe complications. The rash may progress to a dark red/violet colour followed by

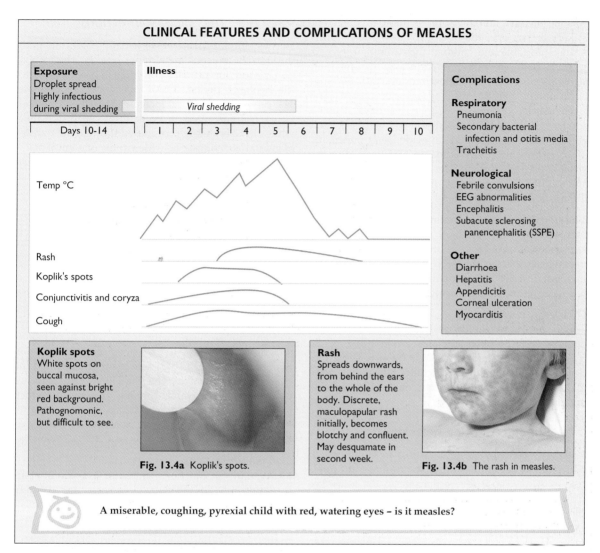

CLINICAL FEATURES AND COMPLICATIONS OF MEASLES

Exposure
Droplet spread
Highly infectious
during viral shedding

Illness

Viral shedding

Days 10-14

1 2 3 4 5 6 7 8 9 10

Temp °C

Rash

Koplik's spots

Conjunctivitis and coryza

Cough

Complications

Respiratory
Pneumonia
Secondary bacterial
  infection and otitis media
Tracheitis

Neurological
Febrile convulsions
EEG abnormalities
Encephalitis
Subacute sclerosing
  panencephalitis (SSPE)

Other
Diarrhoea
Hepatitis
Appendicitis
Corneal ulceration
Myocarditis

Koplik spots
White spots on
buccal mucosa,
seen against bright
red background.
Pathognomonic,
but difficult to see.

Fig. 13.4a Koplik's spots.

Rash
Spreads downwards,
from behind the ears
to the whole of the
body. Discrete,
maculopapular rash
initially, becomes
blotchy and confluent.
May desquamate in
second week.

Fig. 13.4b The rash in measles.

A miserable, coughing, pyrexial child with red, watering eyes – is it measles?

Fig. 13.4 Clinical features and complications of measles.

desquamation and depigmentation, which may last weeks or months. Pre-existing malnutrition is further exacerbated by oral infections and diarrhoea.

Lack of an effective T lymphocyte response in immunocompromised patients makes measles a dangerous illness. A measles interstitial pneumonitis, known as 'giant cell pneumonia', may be fatal in children with malignant disease, even when in remission. These children are also susceptible to a measles encephalopathy.

Treatment

Treatment for measles is symptomatic. Children who are admitted to hospital should be isolated. In immunocompromised patients, the antiviral drug ribavirin may be used. Vitamin A, which may modulate the immune response, should be given in developing countries.

Prevention

Prevention by immunisation is the most successful strategy for reducing the morbidity and mortality of

measles. There is a 10% vaccine failure rate from primary vaccination with MMR (measles, mumps, rubella vaccine) at 12–18 months of age, but immunisation coverage of school-age children in the UK has been improved by the introduction of a preschool booster of MMR.

Mumps

Mumps occurs worldwide, but its incidence has been reduced dramatically with the mumps component of the MMR vaccine. Mumps usually occurs in the winter and spring months. It is spread by droplet infection to the respiratory tract where the virus replicates within epithelial cells. The virus gains access to the parotid glands before further dissemination to other tissues.

Clinical features

The incubation period is 14–21 days. Onset of the illness is with fever, malaise and parotitis, but in up to 30% of cases the infection is subclinical. Only one side may be swollen initially, but bilateral involvement usually occurs over the next few days. The parotitis is uncomfortable and children may complain of earache or pain on eating or drinking. Examination of the parotid duct may show redness and swelling. Occasionally, parotid swelling may be absent. The fever usually disappears within 3–4 days. Plasma amylase levels are often elevated and, when associated with abdominal pain, may be evidence of pancreatic involvement. Infectivity is for up to 7 days after the onset of parotid swelling. The illness is generally mild and self-limiting. Although hearing loss can follow mumps it is usually unilateral and transient.

Viral meningitis and central nervous system involvement

Lymphocytes are seen in the CSF in about 50%, meningeal signs are only seen in 10% and encephalitis in about 1 in 5000. The common clinical features are headache, photophobia, vomiting and neck stiffness.

Orchitis

This is the most feared complication, although it is uncommon in prepubertal males. When it does occur, it is usually unilateral. Although there is some evidence of a reduction in sperm count, infertility is actually extremely unusual. Rarely, oophoritis, mastitis and arthritis may occur.

Rubella (German measles)

Rubella is generally a mild disease in childhood. It occurs in winter and spring. It is an important infection as it can cause severe damage to the fetus (see Ch. 8). The incubation period is 14–21 days. It is spread by the respiratory route, frequently from a known contact. The prodrome is usually mild with a low-grade fever or none at all. The maculopapular rash is often the first sign of infection, appearing initially on the face and then spreading centrifugally to cover the whole body. It fades in 3–5 days. Unlike in adults, the rash is not itchy. Lymphadenopathy, particularly the suboccipital and postauricular nodes, is prominent. Complications are rare in childhood but include arthritis, encephalitis, thrombocytopenia and myocarditis. Clinical differentiation from other viral infections is unreliable. The diagnosis should be confirmed serologically if there is any risk of exposure of a non-immune pregnant woman. There is no effective antiviral treatment. Prevention therefore lies in immunisation.

The human herpesviruses

There are currently eight known human herpesviruses (herpes simplex virus 1 and 2, varicella zoster virus, cytomegalovirus, Epstein–Barr virus, and human herpesviruses 6, 7 and 8). The hallmark of the herpesviruses is that, after primary infection, latency is established and there is long-term persistence of the virus within the host, usually in a dormant state. After certain stimuli, reactivation of infection may occur.

1. Herpes simplex infections

Herpes simplex virus (HSV) usually enters the body through the mucous membranes or skin. The incubation period for primary infection is 3–5 days. After the neonatal period, HSV1 infections predominate. The prevalence of HSV2 increases in early adulthood. HSV1 is transmitted in body fluids such as saliva, while HSV2 is mainly transmitted through the transfer of genital secretions. The wide variety of clinical manifestations are described below. Treatment is with aciclovir, a viral DNA polymerase inhibitor, which may be used to treat severe symptomatic skin, ophthalmic, cerebral and systemic infections.

Asymptomatic

Herpes simplex infections are very common and are mostly asymptomatic.

Gingivostomatitis

This is the most common form of primary HSV illness in children. It usually occurs from 10 months to 3 years of age. There are vesicular lesions on the lips, gums and anterior surfaces of the tongue and hard palate, which often progress to extensive, painful ulceration with bleeding (Fig. 13.5). There is a high fever and the child is very miserable. The illness may persist for up to 2 weeks. Eating and drinking are painful, which may lead to dehydration. Management is symptomatic, but severe disease may necessitate intravenous fluids and aciclovir.

Skin manifestations

Mucocutaneous junctions and damaged skin are particularly prone to infection. 'Cold sores' are recurrent HSV1 lesions on the lip margin.

Eczema herpeticum

In this serious condition, widespread vesicular lesions develop on eczematous skin (Fig. 13.6). This may be complicated by secondary bacterial infection, which may result in septicaemia.

Herpetic whitlows

These are painful, erythematous, oedematous white pustules on the site of broken skin on the fingers. Spread is by autoinoculation from gingivostomatitis and infected adults kissing their children's fingers. In sexually active adolescents, HSV2 may be the cause.

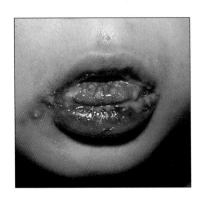

Fig. 13.5 Vesicles with ulceration in gingivostomatitis.

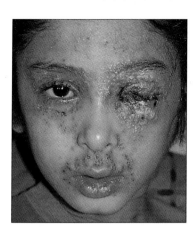

Fig. 13.6 Eczema herpeticum.

Eye disease

Eye disease may cause a blepharitis or conjunctivitis. It may extend to involve the cornea, producing dendritic ulceration. This can lead to corneal scarring and ultimately loss of vision. Any child with herpetic lesions near or involving the eye requires ophthalmic investigation of the cornea by slit lamp examination.

Central nervous system infection
Aseptic meningitis

This is rare in children, but may occur in sexually active adolescents. It is usually a complication of HSV2 infection, occurring within 10 days of a primary infection. It resolves without sequelae.

Encephalitis

By contrast, this is a very serious condition with a mortality of more than 70% if untreated. It may follow either primary or recurrent infection. The clinical features and management are described below.

Neonatal infection (see Ch. 9)

The infection may be focal, affecting the skin or eyes, may cause encephalitis or may be widely disseminated. Its morbidity and mortality are high.

Infection in the immunocompromised host

Infection is severe. Cutaneous lesions may spread to involve adjacent sites, e.g. oesophagitis and proctitis. Pneumonia and disseminated infections involving multiple organs are serious complications.

 ## 2A. Varicella zoster (chickenpox)

Varicella zoster virus (VZV) shares many features with HSV, as both produce a vesicular rash. In contrast to HSV, however, varicella zoster is spread by the respiratory route, progressing via the blood and lymphatics to cause vesicular lesions in the skin. More then 90% of primary VZV infections are clinically symptomatic with a vesicular rash.

Clinical features

These are shown in Figure 13.7. There are a number of rare but serious complications which can occur in previously healthy children:

- *Secondary bacterial infection* with staphylococci, streptococci or other organisms. May lead to further complications such as toxic shock syndrome or necrotising fasciitis. Secondary bacterial infection should be considered where there is onset of a new fever or persistent high fever after the first few days.

- *Encephalitis*. This may be generalised, usually occurring early during the illness. In contrast to the encephalitis caused by HSV, the prognosis is good. Most characteristic is a VZV-associated cerebellitis. This usually occurs within a week of the onset of rash. The child is ataxic with cerebellar signs. It usually resolves over a few days.

- *Purpura fulminans*. This is the consequence of vasculitis in the skin and subcutaneous tissues. It is best known in relation to meningococcal disease and can lead to loss of large areas of skin by necrosis. It may rarely occur after VZV infection due to production of antiviral antibodies which cross-react and inactivate the coagulation factor protein S. There is subsequent dysregulation of fibrinolysis and an increased risk of clotting, most often manifest in the skin.

- *Strokes*. Although very rare, there is an increased incidence of strokes in children after VZV infection, due to either vasculitis or protein S deficiency.

In the immunocompromised, primary varicella infection may result in severe progressive disseminated disease, which has a mortality of up to 20%. The vesicular eruptions persist and frequently become haemorrhagic (Fig. 13.7b). The disease in the neonatal period is described in Chapter 9.

Treatment and prevention

Human varicella zoster immunoglobulin (ZIG) is recommended for high-risk immunosuppressed individuals with deficient T lymphocyte function, following contact with chickenpox. They include:

- bone marrow transplant recipients
- patients with congenital or acquired immune deficiency (e.g. HIV) affecting T cell function
- patients on high doses of steroids or other immunosuppressive drugs within the previous 3 months
- neonates whose mothers develop varicella within 5 days before or 2 days after delivery
- neonates born at less than 30 weeks' gestation who have been exposed to varicella.

Protection from infection with zoster immunoglobulin is not absolute, and depends on how soon after contact with chickenpox it is given. Families should be warned that after zoster immunoglobulin, onset of chickenpox may be delayed and the lesions

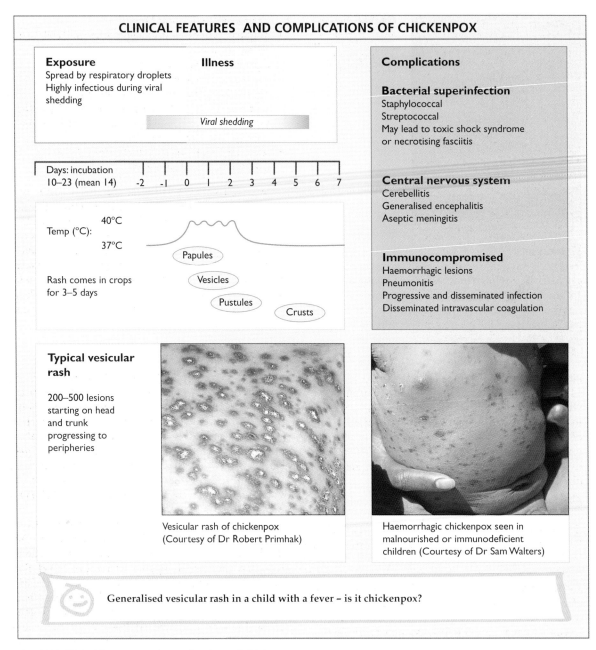

CLINICAL FEATURES AND COMPLICATIONS OF CHICKENPOX

Exposure   **Illness**
Spread by respiratory droplets
Highly infectious during viral
shedding

Viral shedding

Days: incubation
10–23 (mean 14)   -2   -1   0   1   2   3   4   5   6   7

Temp (°C):   40°C
      37°C

Papules

Vesicles

Rash comes in crops
for 3–5 days

Pustules

Crusts

Typical vesicular rash

200–500 lesions starting on head and trunk progressing to peripheries

Vesicular rash of chickenpox
(Courtesy of Dr Robert Primhak)

Haemorrhagic chickenpox seen in malnourished or immunodeficient children (Courtesy of Dr Sam Walters)

Complications

Bacterial superinfection
Staphylococcal
Streptococcal
May lead to toxic shock syndrome
or necrotising fasciitis

Central nervous system
Cerebellitis
Generalised encephalitis
Aseptic meningitis

Immunocompromised
Haemorrhagic lesions
Pneumonitis
Progressive and disseminated infection
Disseminated intravascular coagulation

Generalised vesicular rash in a child with a fever – is it chickenpox?

Fig. 13.7 Clinical features and complications of chickenpox.

may be atypical, so they should seek urgent medical attention if any rash appears. Intravenous aciclovir should be given in severe chickenpox and in the immunocompromised. Trials in the USA have shown some benefit from oral aciclovir in normal children, but the drug is not currently recommended for this in the UK. Adolescents should be treated with aciclovir as they are more likely to develop severe disease. Although an effective varicella vaccine exists, there are concerns that adults may become susceptible to infection when immunity wanes. It is not currently licensed in the UK.

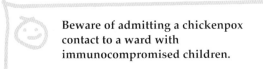

Beware of admitting a chickenpox contact to a ward with immunocompromised children.

2B. Herpes zoster (shingles)

Latent varicella zoster can reactivate, causing a vesicular eruption in the distribution of sensory nerves (shingles). It occurs most commonly in the thoracic region,

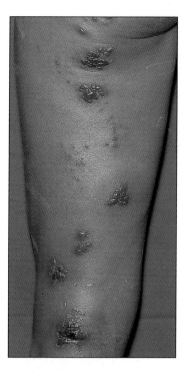

Fig. 13.8 Herpes zoster (shingles) in a child. Distribution is along the S1 dermatome.

Diagnosis is supported by:
- atypical lymphocytes (numerous large T cells seen on blood film)
- a positive Monospot test
- the presence of heterophil antibodies, i.e. antibodies that agglutinate sheep or horse erythrocytes but which are not absorbed by guinea pig kidney extracts – this test is often negative in young children with the disease
- seroconversion with production of IgM and IgG to Epstein–Barr virus antigens.

Symptoms may persist for 1–3 months but ultimately resolve. They are caused by the host immune response to the infection, rather than the virus itself.

Treatment is symptomatic. When the airway is severely compromised, corticosteroids may be considered. In 5% of infected individuals, group A *streptococcus* is grown from the tonsils. This should be treated with penicillin. Ampicillin or amoxicillin may cause a florid maculopapular rash in children infected with EBV and should be avoided.

4. Cytomegalovirus

Cytomegalovirus (CMV) is usually transmitted via saliva, genital secretions or breast milk, and more rarely via blood products, organ transplants and transplacentally. CMV causes mild or subclinical infection in normal hosts. In developed countries, about half of the adult population show serological evidence of past infection. In developing countries, most children have been infected by 2 years of age, often via breast milk. In the immunocompromised and the fetus, CMV is an important pathogen.

As with EBV, CMV may cause a mononucleosis syndrome. Pharyngitis and lymphadenopathy are not usually as prominent as in EBV infections. Patients may have atypical lymphocytes on the blood film but are heterophile antibody-negative. Maternal CMV infection may result in congenital infection (see Ch. 8) which may be present at birth or develop when older. In the immunocompromised host, CMV can cause retinitis, pneumonitis, encephalitis, hepatitis, colitis and oesophagitis. It is a particularly important pathogen following organ transplantation. Organ recipients are closely monitored for evidence of CMV activation by sensitive tests such as polymerase chain reaction (PCR). Interventions used to reduce the risk of transmission of CMV disease are CMV-negative blood for transfusions and anti-CMV drug prophylaxis; also, if possible, CMV-positive organs are not transplanted into CMV-negative recipients.

CMV disease may be treated with ganciclovir or foscarnet, but both have serious side-effects.

5. Human herpesvirus 6 (HHV6)

Most children are infected with HHV6 by the age of 2, usually from the oral secretions of a family

although any dermatome can be affected (Fig. 13.8). Children, unlike adults, rarely suffer neuralgic pain with shingles. Shingles in childhood is more common in those who had primary infection in the first year of life. Recurrent shingles may be a manifestation of underlying immune suppression, e.g. HIV infection. In the immunocompromised, reactivated infection can also disseminate to cause severe disease.

3. Epstein–Barr virus

Epstein–Barr virus (EBV) is the major cause of the infectious mononucleosis syndrome, but it is also involved in the pathogenesis of Burkitt's lymphoma, lymphoproliferative disease in immunocompromised hosts and nasopharyngeal carcinoma. The virus has a particular tropism for B lymphocytes and epithelial cells of the pharynx. Transmission usually occurs by oral contact and the majority of infections are subclinical.

Infectious mononucleosis (glandular fever)

Older children, and occasionally young children, may develop a syndrome with the features of:

- fever
- malaise
- tonsillopharyngitis – often severe, limiting oral ingestion of fluids and food; rarely, breathing may be compromised
- lymphadenopathy – prominent cervical lymph nodes, often with diffuse adenopathy.

Other features include:
- petechiae on the soft palate
- splenomegaly (50%), hepatomegaly (10%)
- a maculopapular rash (5%)
- jaundice.

member. The classic infectious syndrome associated with HHV6 is exanthem subitum (also known as roseola infantum) where there is a high fever with malaise lasting a few days, followed by a generalised macular rash which appears as the fever wanes. Many children have a febrile illness without rash, and some have a subclinical infection. Exanthem subitum is frequently clinically misdiagnosed as measles or rubella and this is why these more significant infections should be confirmed serologically. Another frequent clinical consequence of primary HHV6 infection is that infants seen by a doctor during the febrile stage may be prescribed antibiotics; then, when the rash appears, it is erroneously attributed to an 'allergic' reaction to the drug. Primary HHV6 infection is a common cause of febrile convulsions. It is associated with up to a third of febrile convulsions in the first year of life. HHV6 has rarely been associated with aseptic meningitis, encephalitis, hepatitis, infectious mononucleosis-like syndrome and haematological malignancies.

6. Human herpesvirus 7 (HHV7)

This virus is very closely related to HHV6, causing similar clinical disease, including exanthem subitum and febrile convulsions. Again, most children are infected with HHV7 in the first few years of life.

7. Human herpesvirus 8 (HHV8)

This virus is associated with Kaposi's sarcoma (KS), a tumour which occurs in immunosuppressed patients as well as certain populations in Africa and around the Mediterranean. HHV8 does not appear to be associated with disease in otherwise healthy children. Primary HHV8 infection may be associated with a mild febrile illness and infection is usually transmitted from saliva. Up to 40% of African teenagers have antibodies to HHV8, whereas <5% are seropositive in the UK.

> **Primary HHV6 infection is a common cause of febrile convulsions.**

Parvovirus B19

Parvovirus B19 causes erythema infectiosum or fifth disease (so-named because it was the fifth disease to be described of a group of illnesses with similar rashes), also called slapped cheek syndrome. Infections can occur at any time of the year, although outbreaks are most common during the spring months. Transmission is via respiratory secretions from viraemic patients, by vertical transmission from mother to fetus and by transfusion of contaminated blood products. Parvovirus infects the erythroblastoid red cell precursors in the bone marrow.

Parvovirus causes a range of clinical syndromes:

- asymptomatic infection – common; about 5–10% of preschool children and 65% of adults have antibodies.
- erythema infectiosum – the most common illness, with a viraemic phase of fever, malaise, headache and myalgia followed by a characteristic rash a week later on the face ('slapped cheek'), progressing to a maculopapular, 'lace'-like rash on the trunk and limbs; complications are rare in children, although arthralgia or arthritis is common in adults
- aplastic crisis – the most serious consequence of parvovirus infection; it occurs in children with chronic haemolytic anaemias, where there is an increased rate of red cell turnover (e.g. sickle cell disease or thalassaemia); and in immunodeficient children (e.g. malignancy) who are unable to produce an antibody response to neutralise the infection
- fetal disease – from maternal parvovirus infection may lead to fetal hydrops and death due to severe anaemia, although the majority of infected fetuses will recover.

Enteroviruses

Human enteroviruses, of which there are many (including the Coxsackie viruses, echoviruses and polio viruses), are a common cause of childhood infection. Transmission is primarily by the faecal–oral route. Following replication in the pharynx and gut, the virus spreads to infect other organs. Infections occur most commonly in the summer and autumn. Over 90% of infections are asymptomatic or cause a non-specific febrile illness, but characteristic clinical syndromes exist and are listed below. An effective vaccine is available against the polioviruses.

The following may be caused by enteroviruses:

Asymptomatic or non-specific febrile illness
Over 90% of infections.

Herpangina
Vesicular and ulcerated lesions on the soft palate and uvula causing anorexia, pain on swallowing and fever.

Hand, foot and mouth disease
Painful vesicular lesions on the hands, feet, mouth and tongue. Systemic features are mild. The disease subsides within a few days.

Meningitis/encephalitis
Aseptic meningitis is caused by many of the enteroviruses. There may be a skin rash, which can be petechial and therefore difficult to differentiate clinically from meningococcal infection. Complete recovery can be expected.

Pleurodynia (Bornholm's disease)

An acute illness with fever, pleuritic chest pain and muscle tenderness. There may be a pleural rub but examination is otherwise normal. Recovery is within a few days.

Myocarditis and pericarditis

Heart failure associated with a febrile illness and ECG evidence of myocarditis.

Poliovirus infection

Clinical disease is now very rare, due to successful immunisation programmes. It falls into four main categories:

- >90% are asymptomatic
- 5% have a poliomyelitis 'minor illness' – fever, headache, malaise, sore throat and vomiting occur within 4 days of exposure and recovery is uneventful
- 2% of patients progress to central nervous system involvement with aseptic meningitis; there is stiffness of the back, neck and hamstrings from meningeal irritation
- in <1% of cases, classical paralytic polio occurs about 4 days after the minor illness has subsided – involvement of the anterior horn cells and cerebral cortex leads to varying degrees of paralysis which may recover completely or be permanent; involvement of the muscles of respiration may be fatal.

Infection in the immunocompromised host

Enteroviruses can cause severe disease in immuno-compromised individuals. Echovirus can cause a persistent and sometimes fatal central nervous system infection in agammaglobulinaemic patients. Live attenuated vaccine strains of polio can cause fatal infections in children with severe combined immunodeficiency or agammaglobulinaemia, and in these patients inactivated vaccine should be used.

STAPHYLOCOCCAL AND STREPTOCOCCAL INFECTIONS

Staphylococcal and streptococcal infections are usually caused by direct invasion of the organisms. They may also cause disease by releasing toxins which act as superantigens. Whereas conventional antigens stimulate only a small subset of T cells which have a specific receptor, superantigens bind to a part of the T cell receptor which is shared by many T cells and therefore stimulates massive T cell proliferation and cytokine release. Other diseases are immune-mediated. The wide range of diseases caused by these organisms is shown in Figure 13.9.

Impetigo

This is a localised, highly contagious, staphylococcal and/or streptococcal skin infection, most common in infants and young children. It is more common where there is pre-existing skin disease, e.g. atopic eczema. Lesions are usually on the face, neck and hands and begin as erythematous macules which become vesicular (Fig. 13.10). Rupture of the vesicles with exudation of fluid leads to the characteristic confluent honey-coloured crusted lesions. The lesions are sometimes bullous. Infection is readily spread to adjacent areas and other parts of the body by autoinoculation of the infected exudate. Topical antibiotics (e.g. mupirocin) are effective for mild cases. Systemic antibiotics (e.g. flucloxacillin or erythromycin) are needed for more severe infections. Affected children should not go to nursery or school until the lesions are dry. Nasal carriage is an important source of infection which can be eradicated with a nasal cream containing mupirocin or chlorhexidine and neomycin.

Boils

These are infections of hair follicles or sweat glands, usually caused by *Staphylococcus aureus*. Treatment is with systemic antibiotics and occasionally surgery. Recurrent boils are usually from persistent nasal carriage in the child or family acting as a reservoir for reinfection. Only rarely are they a manifestation of immune deficiency.

Periorbital cellulitis

In periorbital cellulitis there is fever with erythema, tenderness and oedema of the eyelid (Fig. 13.11). It is almost always unilateral. In young, unimmunised children it may also be caused by a *Haemophilus influenzae* b infection, which may also cause infection at other sites, e.g. meningitis. It may follow local trauma to the skin. In older children, it may spread from a paranasal sinus infection or dental abscess. Periorbital cellulitis should be treated promptly with intravenous antibiotics to prevent posterior spread of the infection to become an orbital cellulitis. In orbital cellulitis, there is proptosis, painful or limited ocular movement and reduced visual acuity. It may be complicated by abscess formation, meningitis or cavernous sinus thrombosis. Where orbital cellulitis is suspected, a CT scan should be performed to assess the posterior spread of infection and a lumbar puncture may be required to exclude meningitis.

Scalded skin syndrome

This is caused by an exfoliative staphylococcal toxin which causes separation of the epidermal skin through the granular cell layers. It affects infants and young children, who develop fever and malaise and may have a purulent, crusting, localised infection around the eyes, nose and mouth with subsequent widespread erythema and tenderness of the skin. Areas of epidermis separate on gentle pressure (Nikolsky's sign), leaving denuded areas of skin (Fig. 13.12) which subsequently dry and heal without scarring. Management is with an intravenous antistaphylococcal antibiotic and monitoring of fluid balance.

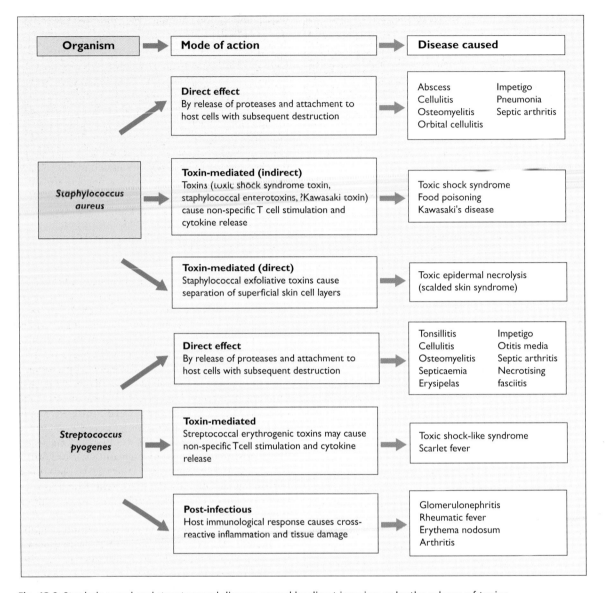

Organism	Mode of action	Disease caused
Staphylococcus aureus	**Direct effect** By release of proteases and attachment to host cells with subsequent destruction	Abscess Impetigo Cellulitis Pneumonia Osteomyelitis Septic arthritis Orbital cellulitis
	Toxin-mediated (indirect) Toxins (toxic shock syndrome toxin, staphylococcal enterotoxins, ?Kawasaki toxin) cause non-specific T cell stimulation and cytokine release	Toxic shock syndrome Food poisoning Kawasaki's disease
	Toxin-mediated (direct) Staphylococcal exfoliative toxins cause separation of superficial skin cell layers	Toxic epidermal necrolysis (scalded skin syndrome)
Streptococcus pyogenes	**Direct effect** By release of proteases and attachment to host cells with subsequent destruction	Tonsillitis Impetigo Cellulitis Otitis media Osteomyelitis Septic arthritis Septicaemia Necrotising Erysipelas fasciitis
	Toxin-mediated Streptococcal erythrogenic toxins may cause non-specific T cell stimulation and cytokine release	Toxic shock-like syndrome Scarlet fever
	Post-infectious Host immunological response causes cross-reactive inflammation and tissue damage	Glomerulonephritis Rheumatic fever Erythema nodosum Arthritis

Fig. 13.9 Staphylococcal and streptococcal disease caused by direct invasion or by the release of toxins. Immune-mediated disease may also follow streptococcal infections.

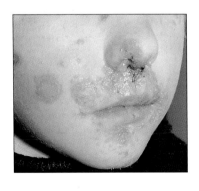

Fig. 13.10 Impetigo showing characteristic confluent honey-coloured crusted lesions. (Courtesy of Dr Paul Hutchins.)

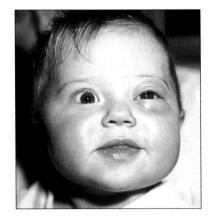

Fig. 13.11 Periorbital cellulitis. It should be treated promptly with intravenous antibiotics to prevent spread into the orbit.

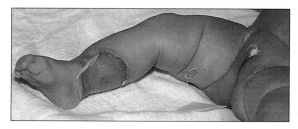

Fig. 13.12 Staphylococcal scalded skin syndrome. Its appearance must not be mistaken for a scald from non-accidental injury.

Necrotising fasciitis/necrotising cellulitis

This is a severe subcutaneous infection often involving tissue planes from the skin down to fascia and muscle. The skin surface involved may enlarge rapidly, leaving poorly perfused necrotic areas of tissue, usually at the centre. There is severe pain and systemic illness which may require intensive care. The invading organism may be *Staphylococcus* or group A *Streptococcus*, with or without another synergistic anaerobic organism. Intravenous antibiotic therapy alone is not sufficient to treat this condition. Without surgical intervention and debridement of necrotic tissue, the infection will continue to spread. Clinical suspicion of necrotising fasciitis warrants urgent surgical consultation and intervention.

Toxic shock syndrome

Toxin-producing staphylococci and streptococci can produce this syndrome. The toxin, released from infection at any site, including small abrasions, acts as a superantigen. It causes a systemic illness with high fever, a diffuse macular rash, hypotension and shock. There may be redness of the mucous membranes (Fig. 13.13), vomiting or diarrhoea, severe myalgia, altered consciousness, thrombocytopenia, coagulopathy, and abnormal hepatic and renal function. About 1–2 weeks after the onset of the illness, there is desquamation of the palms, soles, fingers and toes. Intensive care support is required to manage the shock. Areas of infection should be surgically debrided. Intravenous immunoglobulin may be given to neutralise circulating toxin.

KAWASAKI'S DISEASE (ACUTE FEBRILE MUCOCUTANEOUS SYNDROME)

Although uncommon, Kawasaki's disease is an important diagnosis to make, as aneurysms of the coronary arteries are an important and potential complication. Prompt treatment reduces their incidence.

Kawasaki's disease mainly affects children of 6 months to 4 years old, with a peak at the end of the first year. The disease is much more common in

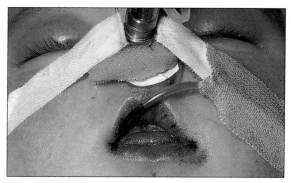

Fig. 13.13 A child with toxic shock syndrome receiving intensive care, including artificial ventilation via a nasotracheal tube. The lips are red and the eyelids are oedematous from capillary leak. (Courtesy of Professor Mike Levin.)

children of Japanese and, to a lesser extent, Afro-Caribbean ethnicity than it is in Caucasians. Young infants tend to be more severely affected than older children. The cause is unknown, but the many clinical and immunological similarities with the staphylococcal and streptococcal toxic shock syndromes have led to the suggestion that it is also caused by a bacterial toxin acting as a superantigen. The diagnosis is made on clinical findings (Fig. 13.14). The disease is a vasculitis affecting the small and medium-sized vessels. It affects the coronary arteries in about one-third of affected children within the first 6 weeks of the illness. This can lead to aneurysms which are best visualised on echocardiography (see Case history 13.1). Subsequent narrowing of the vessels from scar formation can result in myocardial ischaemia and sudden death. Mortality is 1–2%.

Prompt treatment with intravenous immunoglobulin given within the first 10 days has been shown to lower the risk of coronary artery aneurysms. Aspirin is used to reduce the risk of thrombosis. It is given at a high anti-inflammatory dose until the fever subsides and continued at a low anti-platelet dose when there is an abnormality of the coronary arteries. When the platelet count is very high, anti-platelet aggregation agents may also be used to reduce the risk of coronary thrombosis. Children suspected of the disease but who do not have all the clinical features should still be considered for treatment.

 Prolonged fever – is it Kawasaki's disease?

MENINGITIS

Meningitis occurs when there is inflammation of the meninges covering the brain. This can be confirmed by finding inflammatory cells in the cerebrospinal fluid (CSF). Viral infections are the most common

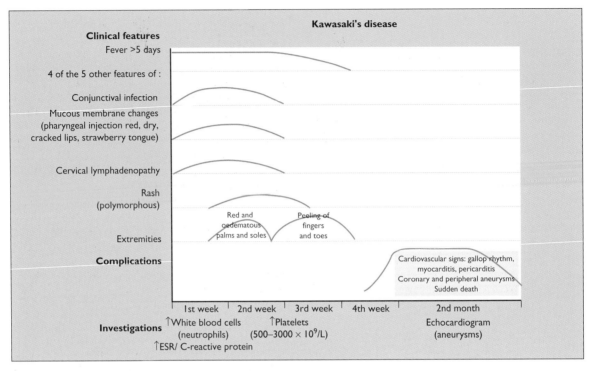

Fig. 13.14 Clinical features and investigations in Kawasaki's disease.

CASE HISTORY 13.1

KAWASAKI'S DISEASE

This 3-year-old boy had developed a high fever of 3 days' duration. Examination showed a mild conjunctivitis, a rash and cervical lymphadenopathy. A viral infection was diagnosed and his mother was reassured. Four days later she presented to her local hospital. The child's condition was unchanged, but he was noted to have cracked red lips (Fig. 13.15a). He was admitted for observation as he appeared unwell and was not eating. A full septic screen, including a lumbar puncture, was performed and antibiotics started. A urine infection was suspected as there were 50–100 WBC/mm^3 in the urine sample, although culture proved to be negative. After a further 5 days, he was still febrile and irritable and the antibiotics were changed after a repeat blood count, blood and urine culture. He remained febrile and irritable. Four days later, the neutrophil count was 15×10^9/L, platelet count 800×10^9/L and ESR (erythrocyte sedimentation rate) 125. Sixteen days into the illness, there was peeling of the skin of the fingers and toes (Fig. 13.15b) and Kawasaki's disease was suspected. An echocardiogram showed aneurysms of the coronary arteries. He was treated with intravenous immunoglobulins, following which his clinical condition improved and he became afebrile. Delayed diagnosis meant that the potential benefit from immunoglobulin therapy in preventing coronary artery aneurysms was missed.

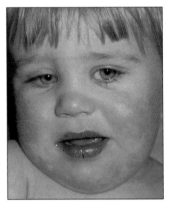

Fig. 13.15a Red, cracked lips and conjunctival inflammation.

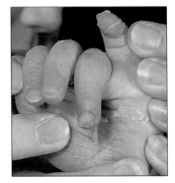

Fig. 13.15b Peeling of the fingers, which developed on the 15th day of the illness.

cause of meningitis, and most are self-resolving. Bacterial meningitis may have severe consequences. Other causes of non-infectious meningitis include malignancy and autoimmune diseases.

Bacterial meningitis

Over 80% of patients with bacterial meningitis in the UK are younger than 16 years old. Bacterial meningitis remains a serious infection in children, with a 5–10% mortality. Over 10% of survivors are left with long-term neurological impairment.

Pathophysiology
Bacterial infection of the meninges usually follows bacteraemia. It is now thought that much of the damage caused by meningeal infection results from the host response to infection and not from the organism itself. The release of inflammatory mediators and activated leucocytes, together with endothelial damage, leads to cerebral oedema, raised intracranial pressure and decreased cerebral blood flow.

Organisms
The organisms which commonly cause bacterial meningitis vary according to the child's age (Fig. 13.16).

Presentation
The clinical features are listed in Figure 13.17. The early signs and symptoms of meningitis are non-specific, which makes early diagnosis difficult. Infants and young children may present with any combination of fever, poor feeding, vomiting, irritability, lethargy, drowsiness, seizures or reduced consciousness. A bulging fontanelle, neck stiffness and the infant lying with an arched back (opisthotonus) are late signs. Children old enough to talk are likely to describe the classical meningitis symptoms of headache, neck stiffness and photophobia. Neck stiffness may also be seen in some children with tonsillitis and cervical lymphadenopathy. As children with meningitis may also be septicaemic, signs of shock, such as tachycardia, poor capillary refill, oliguria and hypotension, should be sought. Purpura in a febrile child of any age should be assumed to be due to meningococcal sepsis, even if the child does not appear unduly ill at the time; meningitis may or may not be present.

Fig. 13.16 Organisms causing bacterial meningitis according to age.

Neonatal–3 months	Group B *Streptococcus*
	E. coli and other coliforms
	Listeria monocytogenes
1 month–6 years	*Neisseria meningitidis*
	Streptococcus pneumoniae
	Haemophilus influenzae
>6 years	*Neisseria meningitidis*
	Streptococcus pneumoniae

Investigations
The essential investigations are listed in Figure 13.17. A lumbar puncture is performed to obtain CSF to confirm the diagnosis, identify the organism responsible, and its antibiotic sensitivity. If any of the contra-indications listed in Figure 13.17 are present, a lumbar puncture should not be performed, as under these circumstances the procedure carries a risk of coning of the cerebellum through the foramen magnum. If necessary, a lumbar puncture can be performed once the child's condition has stabilised. Although by this stage the organism will rarely be grown, the cytological and biochemical abnormalities of bacterial meningitis will still be present for severel days after starting treatment. Even without a lumbar puncture, bacteriological diagnosis can be achieved, in at least 50% of cases, from the blood by culture, rapid antigen screen or PCR. A throat swab should also be taken. Scrapings from a purpuric skin lesion may also be cultured. A serological diagnosis can be made on convalescent serum 4–6 weeks after the presenting illness.

Management
It is imperative that there is no delay in the administration of antibiotics and supportive therapy in a child with meningitis. The choice of antibiotics will depend on the likely pathogen. A third-generation cephalosporin, e.g. cefotaxime or ceftriaxone, is the preferred choice to cover the most common bacterial causes. Although still rare in the UK, pneumococcal resistance to penicillin and cephalosporins is increasing rapidly in certain parts of the world. Whilst waiting for the sensitivity of pneumococcal cultures, rifampicin or vancomycin should be added. Ampicillin with chloramphenicol is an alternative in certain countries where third generation cephalosporins are not available, but resistance to these drugs means that they cannot be relied upon when used as single agents. Below 3 months of age, ampicillin should be included to cover *Listeria monocytogenes* infection. The length of the course of antibiotics given depends on the causative organism and the clinical progress of the patient. Dexamethasone administered with the antibiotics reduces the risk of long-term complications such as deafness.

Cerebral complications
- *Hearing loss.* Inflammatory damage to the cochlear hair cells may lead to deafness. All children who have had meningitis should have an audiological assessment at follow-up.
- *Local vasculitis.* This may lead to cranial nerve palsies or other focal lesions.
- *Local cerebral infarction.* This may result in focal or multifocal seizures which may subsequently lead to epilepsy.
- *Subdural effusion.* Particularly associated with *Haemophilus influenzae* and pneumococcal meningitis. This is confirmed by CT scan. Most resolve spontaneously.

ASSESSMENT AND INVESTIGATION OF MENINGITIS/ENCEPHALITIS

History
Fever
Headache
Photophobia
Lethargy
Poor feeding/vomiting
Irritability
Hypotonia
Drowsiness
Loss of consciousness
Seizures

Examination
Fever
Purpuric rash (meningococcal disease)
Neck stiffness (not always present in infants)
Positive Brudzinski's/Kernig's signs
Signs of shock
Focal neurological signs
Altered conscious level
Papilloedema (rare)

Investigations
Full blood count and differential count
Blood glucose and blood gas (for acidosis)
Coagulation screen, C-reactive protein
Urea and electrolytes, liver function tests
Culture of blood, throat swab, urine, stool for bacteria and viruses
Rapid antigen test for meningitis organisms (can be done on blood, CSF, or urine)
Lumbar puncture for CSF unless contraindicated (see below for tests on CSF)
Serum for comparison of convalescent titres
PCR of blood and CSF for possible organisms
If TB suspected: chest X-ray, Mantoux test, gastric washings or sputum, early morning urines
Consider CT/MRI brain scan and EEG

For optimal results, collect diagnostic samples as early as possible.

Signs associated with neck stiffness
Brudzinski's sign – flexion of the neck with the child supine causes flexion of the knees and hips

Kernig's sign – with the child lying supine and with the hips and knees flexed, there is back pain on extensionof the knee

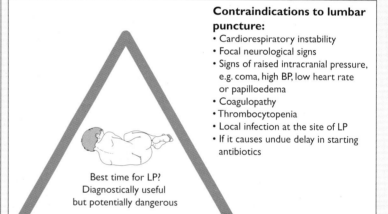

Best time for LP?
Diagnostically useful but potentially dangerous

Contraindications to lumbar puncture:
• Cardiorespiratory instability
• Focal neurological signs
• Signs of raised intracranial pressure, e.g. coma, high BP, low heart rate or papilloedema
• Coagulopathy
• Thrombocytopenia
• Local infection at the site of LP
• If it causes undue delay in starting antibiotics

Typical changes in the CSF in meningitis or encephalitis, beyond the neonatal period

	Aetiology	Appearance	White blood cells	Protein	Glucose
Normal	—	Clear	0–5/mm³	0.15–0.4 g/L	≥50% of blood
Meningitis	Bacterial	Turbid	Polymorphs:↑↑	↑↑	↓↓
	Viral	Clear	Lymphocytes:↑ (initially may be polymorphs)	Normal/↑	Normal/↓
	Tuberculosis	Turbid/clear/ viscous	Lymphocytes:↑	↑↑↑	↓↓↓
Encephalitis	Viral/unknown	Clear	Normal/↑ lymphocytes	Normal/↑	Normal/↓

Fig. 13.17 Assessment and investigation of meningitis and encephalitis.

MENINGOCOCCAL SEPTICAEMIA

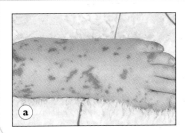
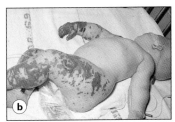

Fig. 13.18 Rash of meningococcal infection. (a) Characteristic purpuric skin lesions, irregular in size and outline and with a necrotic centre. (b) The lesions may be extensive, when it is called 'purpura fulminans'.

CASE HISTORY 13.2

MENINGOCOCCAL SEPTICAEMIA AND MENINGITIS

This 7-month-old boy presented with a 12-h history of lethargy and a spreading purpuric rash. In hospital, he required immediate resuscitation and transfer to a paediatric intensive care unit for multi-organ failure (Fig. 13.19a). The gross oedema is from leak of capillary fluid into the tissues. He required colloid and inotropic support and peritoneal dialysis for renal failure. He made a full recovery (Fig. 13.19b).

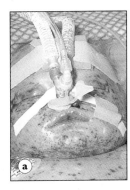
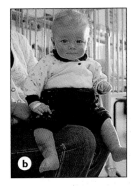

Fig. 13.19 (a) A boy with meningococcal septicaemia receiving intensive care. (b) After full recovery.

- *Hydrocephalus*. May result from impaired resorption of CSF. A ventricular shunt may be required.
- *Cerebral abscess*. The child's clinical condition deteriorates with the emergence of signs of a space-occupying lesion. The temperature will continue to fluctuate. It is confirmed on CT scan. Drainage of the abscess is required.

Prophylaxis
Prophylactic treatment with rifampicin is given to all household contacts for meningococcal meningitis and for young children in the household for *Haemophilus influenzae* infection. It is not required for the patient if he has received a third-generation cephalosporin as this will eradicate nasopharyngeal carriage. Household contacts of patients who have had group C meningococcal meningitis should be vaccinated with the meningococcal group C vaccine.

Specific causes
Meningococcal infection
In the UK, *Neisseria meningitidis* (meningococcus) is the most common cause of meningitis and its incidence has increased over the last 5 years. There have been winter peaks and small outbreaks. In countries where it remains endemic, larger outbreaks occur. Meningococcal infection is a disease that strikes fear into both parents and doctors as it can kill previously healthy children within hours. While meningitis is the main clinical form of infection with this organism, meningococcal septicaemia carries a worse prognosis (Case history 13.2). Of the three main causes of bacterial meningitis, meningococcal has the lowest risk of long-term neurological sequelae, with most survivors recovering fully. The septicaemia is accompanied by a purpuric rash which may start anywhere on the body and then spread. The rash may or may not be present with meningococcal meningitis. Characteristic lesions are non-blanching on palpation, irregular in size and outline and have a necrotic centre (Fig. 13.18a, b). Any febrile child who develops a purpuric rash should be treated immediately, at home or in the general practitioner's surgery, with systemic antibiotics such as penicillin before urgent admission to hospital. Although there are vaccines against groups A and C *meningococcus*, there is no effective vaccine for group B *meningococcus*, which accounts for more than half of the isolates in the UK.

 Meningococcal septicaemia can kill children in hours.

A febrile child with a purpuric rash should be given systemic antibiotics immediately and transferred urgently to hospital.

Haemophilus meningitis

Before the introduction of Hib vaccine, *H. influenzae* type B was the second most common cause of meningitis in the UK and the most common in the USA. Immunisation has been highly effective and this is now a rare cause of meningitis.

Pneumococcal meningitis

While this organism was responsible for only 10% of meningitis before Hib vaccine was introduced, its prominence has now increased. It is associated with a high mortality (10%) and morbidity, with more than 30% of survivors having neurological impairment.

Partially treated bacterial meningitis

Children are frequently given oral antibiotics for a non-specific febrile illness. If they have early meningitis, this partial treatment with antibiotics may cause diagnostic problems. CSF examination shows a raised number of white cells, but cultures are usually negative. Rapid antigen screen or PCR is sometimes helpful in these circumstances. Where the diagnosis is suspected clinically, a full course of antibiotics should be given.

Tuberculous meningitis

Tuberculous meningitis is rare in the UK. The onset of the illness is often insidious, over 2–3 weeks. Meningism may be minimal. There may be a history of TB contact. Most, but not all, affected children have a positive Mantoux test and abnormal chest X-ray. The acid-fast bacilli may be identified on Ziehl–Nielsen or auromine staining of the CSF or in early morning urine samples or gastric aspirates. As there are few organisms, they are easily missed. PCR may aid diagnosis. The mycobacteria may take 2–3 months to culture, but ascertainment of the sensitivities of the organism is important as multi-drug resistance is increasing. Treatment should be started empirically, when the CSF shows the features suggestive of TB meningitis. The disease is associated with a high mortality and morbidity, especially when treatment is only started after reduced consciousness or when focal neurological signs are present. Depending on the condition of the patient, three or four anti-tuberculous drugs will be required for 2 months (e.g. rifampicin, pyrazinamide, isoniazid +/– amikacin or streptomycin). In total, a year of treatment is given. Dexamethasone should be given for the first month at least, to decrease the risk of long-term sequelae.

Viral meningitis

Overall, two-thirds of CNS infections are viral. Causes include enteroviruses, Epstein–Barr virus, adenoviruses and mumps. Mumps meningitis is now rare in the UK due to wide uptake of MMR vaccine. The illness is usually much less severe than bacterial meningitis and a full recovery can be anticipated. Diagnosis of viral meningitis can be confirmed by culture or PCR of CSF; culture of stool, urine, or throat swabs; and serology.

Uncommon pathogens and other causes

Where the clinical course is atypical or there is failure to respond to antibiotic and supportive therapy, unusual organisms, e.g. *Mycoplasma* or *Borrelia burgdorferi* (Lyme disease), or fungal infections need to be considered. Uncommon pathogens are particularly likely in children who are immunocompromised. Rarely, recurrent bacterial meningitis may occur in the immuno-deficient or in children with congenital abnormalities of the ears or meninges which facilitate bacterial access. Aseptic meningitis may be seen in malignancy or autoimmune disorders.

ENCEPHALITIS/ENCEPHALOPATHY

Whereas in meningitis there is inflammation of the meninges, in encephalitis there is inflammation of the brain substance, although the meninges are often also affected. Encephalitis may be caused by:

- direct invasion of the cerebrum by a neurotoxic virus
- delayed brain swelling following a disordered neuroimmunological response to an antigen, usually a virus (post-infectious encephalopathy), e.g. following chickenpox
- slow virus infection such as HIV infection or subacute sclerosing panencephalitis (SSPE) following measles.

In encephalopathy from a non-infectious cause, e.g. a metabolic abnormality, the clinical features may be similar to an infectious encephalitis.

The clinical features and investigation of encephalitis are described in Figure 13.17. Most children present with fever, altered consciousness and often seizures. Initially, it is not possible to clinically differentiate encephalitis from meningitis, and treatment for both should be started. The underlying causative organisms are only detected in up to 50%. In the UK, the most frequent causes of encephalitis are enteroviruses, respiratory viruses and herpesviruses (e.g. varicella and HHV-6). Worldwide, microorganisms causing encephalitis include *Mycoplasma*, *Borrelia burgdorfii* (Lyme disease), *Bartonella henselae* (cat scratch disease), rickettsial infections (e.g. Rocky mountain spotted fever) and the arboviruses.

Herpes simplex virus (HSV) is a very rare cause of childhood encephalitis but it may have devastating long-term consequences. All children with encephalitis should therefore be treated initially with aciclovir to cover this possibility. Most affected children do not have outward signs of herpes infection, such as cold sores, gingivostomatitis or skin lesions. The PCR of the CSF may be positive for HSV. As HSV encephalitis is a

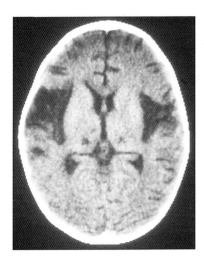

Fig. 13.20 Herpes simplex encephalitis. The CT scan shows gross atrophy from loss of neural tissue in the temporoparietal regions.

destructive infection, the EEG and CT/MRI scan may show focal changes, particularly within the temporal lobes (Fig. 13.20). These tests may initially give non-specific results and require to be repeated after a few days if the child is not improving. Later confirmation of the diagnosis may be made from HSV antibody production in the CSF. Proven cases of HSV encephalitis or cases where there is a high index of suspicion should be treated with intravenous aciclovir for 3 weeks, as relapses have occurred after shorter courses of treatment. Untreated, the mortality rate from HSV encephalitis is over 70% and survivors usually have severe neurological sequelae.

Neonatal meningitis
See Chapter 9.

TUBERCULOSIS

The decline in the incidence and mortality from tuberculosis (TB) in developed countries was hailed as an example of how public health measures and antimicrobial therapy can dramatically modify a disease. However, TB is again becoming a public health problem partly through its increasing incidence in patients with HIV infection and the emergence of multi-resistant strains.

With the decline in TB from infected dairy cattle, the spread is usually by the respiratory route. Close proximity, infectious load and underlying immuno-deficiency enhance the risk of transmission. Children are usually infected by adults within the same household. Child-to-child transmission is rare.

Clinical features
These are outlined in Figure 13.21.

Diagnosis
Diagnosing TB in children is even more difficult than in adults. The clinical features of the disease, which include prolonged fever, malaise, anorexia, weight loss and focal signs of infection, may be the only clues and empirical treatment may be necessary. Children

usually swallow sputum, so gastric washings on three consecutive mornings are required to visualise or culture acid-fast bacilli originating from the lung. To obtain these, a nasogastric tube is passed and secretions are rinsed out of the stomach with saline on three consecutive mornings before food. Urine, lymph node, CSF and radiological examinations should also be performed where appropriate. Although it is difficult to culture TB from children, the presence of multi-drug-resistant strains makes it important to try to grow the organism so that antibiotic sensitivity can be assessed. Heaf tests are used for screening for TB, but in individuals suspected of having the disease, a Mantoux test is usually used. In a Mantoux test, 10 units of purified protein derivative of tuberculin (0.1 ml of 1:1000) are given intradermally and read after 48–72 h; 1 unit is only used when there is a likelihood of a hypersensitivity reaction, e.g. in a child with erythema nodosum. Induration of greater than 10 mm is positive. When interpreting the result, consideration needs to be given to the child's age, any previous BCG and relative anergy due to immunosuppression or malnutrition.

Treatment
Triple therapy with rifampicin, isoniazid and pyrazinamide is the recommended initial combination. This is decreased to the two drugs rifampicin and isoniazid after 2 months and by this time antibiotic sensitivities are often known. Asymptomatic children who are Mantoux-positive and therefore infected should also be treated (e.g. with rifampicin and isoniazid for 3 months) as this will decrease the risk of reactivation of infection later in life.

Prevention and contact tracing
BCG immunisation has been shown to be helpful in preventing or modifying TB in the UK. However, its usefulness worldwide in preventing the disease is controversial. In the UK, BCG is recommended at birth for high-risk groups (communities with a relatively high prevalence of TB, i.e. Asian or African origin or TB in a family member in the previous 5 years) and routinely for all tuberculin-negative children between 10 and 14 years. BCG should not be given to HIV-positive or other immunosuppressed children due to the potential risk of dissemination.

As most children are infected from a household contact, it is essential to screen other family members for the disease. Children who are exposed to smear-positive individuals (where organisms are visualised on sputum) should be assessed for evidence of asymptomatic infection. Mantoux-negative children over 5 years should receive BCG immunisation and some clinicians suggest that those who are Mantoux-negative and less than 5 years should receive chemoprophylaxis (e.g. rifampicin and isoniazid for 3 months). If at the end of this time they remain Mantoux-negative they should also receive BCG immunisation. Again, the aim of treatment is to decrease the risk of reactivation of TB infection later in life.

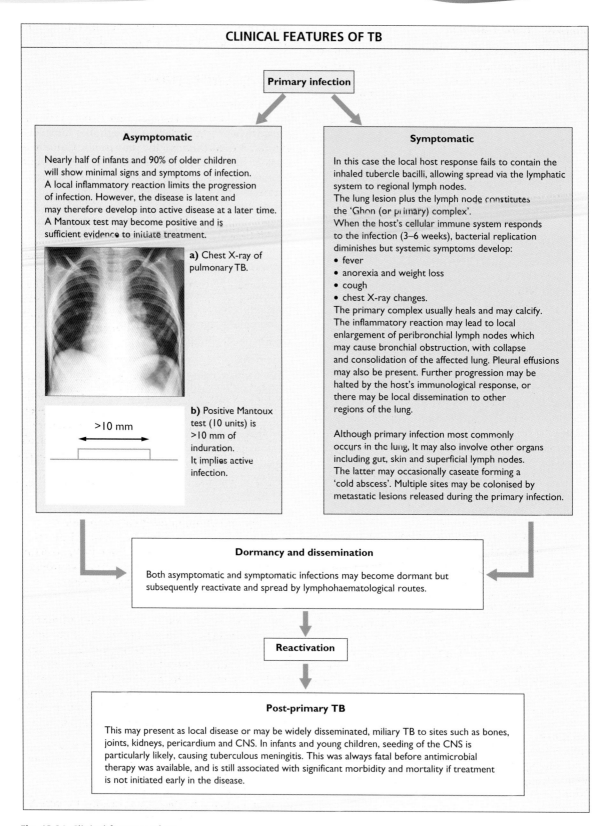

Fig. 13.21 Clinical features of TB.

Atypical mycobacteria

There are numerous mycobacteria found in the environment. Immunocompetent individuals rarely suffer from diseases caused by these organisms. They occasionally cause persistent lymphadenopathy in children, which is usually treated surgically. These organisms, however, may cause disseminated infection in immunocompromised individuals. *Mycobacterium avium intracellulare* (MAI) infections are particularly common in patients with advanced HIV disease. These organisms do not respond well to treatment and require a cocktail of antituberculous drugs.

LYME DISEASE

This disease, caused by the spirochaete *Borrelia burgdorferi*, was first recognised in 1975 in a cluster of children with arthritis in Lyme, Connecticut. Some cases have been reported in the UK. *Borrelia burgdorferi* is transmitted by the hard tick, which has a range of hosts but favours deer and moose. Infections occur most commonly in the summer months in susceptible persons in rural settings.

Clinical features

Following an incubation period of 4–20 days, an erythematous macule at the site of the tick bite enlarges to cause the classical skin lesion known as erythema migrans, a painless red expanding lesion with a bright red outer spreading edge. During early disease, the skin lesion is often accompanied by fever, headache, malaise, myalgia, arthralgia and lymphadenopathy. Usually these features fluctuate over several weeks and then resolve. Dissemination of infection in the early stages is rare and may lead to cranial nerve palsies, meningitis, arthritis or carditis.

The late stage of Lyme disease occurs after weeks to months with neurological, cardiac and joint manifestations. Neurological disease includes meningoencephalitis and cranial (particularly facial nerve) and peripheral neuropathies. Cardiac disease includes myocarditis and heart block. Joint disease occurs in about 50% and varies from brief migratory arthralgia to acute asymmetric mono- and oligoarthritis of the large joints. Recurrent attacks of arthritis are common. In 10%, chronic erosive joint disease occurs months to years after the initial attack.

Diagnosis

This is based on clinical and epidemiological features and serology. Serology may be negative in early disease, so repeat titres after 2–4 weeks are advised. Isolation of the organism is difficult.

Treatment

The drug of choice for early uncomplicated cases over 8 years of age is doxycycline, and for younger children, amoxicillin. Intravenous treatment with ceftriaxone is required for carditis or neurological disease.

TROPICAL INFECTIONS

When approaching an unwell child returning from the tropics, tropical infections must be considered, although it is important to remember that these children are still susceptible to the usual range of infections found in temperate climes. The most common or most serious imported infections are outlined in Figure 13.22.

IMMUNODEFICIENCY DISORDERS

Immunodeficiencies may be primary or secondary. In primary disorders there is an intrinsic defect in the immune system. Secondary immune deficiency is more common and may occur with malignant disease, immunosuppressive therapy, HIV infection, malnutrition, splenectomy, nephrotic syndrome and many bacterial and viral infections.

Clinical features

Many of the primary immunodeficiencies (Fig. 13.23) are inherited as X-linked or autosomal recessive disorders. There may be a family history of parental consanguinity and unexplained death, particularly in boys. Children with an immunodeficiency will usually have a history of infections which are recurrent, persistent or unusual (Fig. 13.24). There may also be evidence of a protein-losing enteropathy and failure to thrive.

Investigation of immunological competence

This is directed towards the most likely cause (Fig. 13.25). Investigations can quantify the essential components of the immune system and also provide a functional assessment of immunocompetence.

Treatment

The recent discovery of the genetic basis of many of the primary immunodeficiencies is likely to have a profound impact on future management. It is hoped that, in the future, gene therapy, in which a normally functioning gene is transfected into defective progenitor cells, may become a feasible treatment for many conditions. Until such corrective therapy becomes available, management will continue to comprise:

* antibiotic prophylaxis to prevent infection, e.g. cotrimoxazole to prevent *Pneumocystis carinii* pneumonia
* appropriate antibiotics to treat infection
* immunoglobulin replacement therapy for defects in antibody function or production
* bone marrow transplantation for severe immunodeficiency.

AN APPROACH TO THE FEBRILE CHILD RETURNING FROM THE TROPICS

History
All places visited and duration of stay. Immunisation, malaria prophylaxis. History of food, drink (infected water), accommodation (exposure to vectors), contacts, swimming (infected rivers and lakes).

Examination
Particular reference to: fever, jaundice, anaemia, enlarged liver or spleen

Non-tropical causes of fever
Consider non-tropical causes of fever in childhood – urinary tract infection, upper and lower respiratory tract infections, gastroenteritis, septicaemia, meningitis, osteomyelitis, hepatitis, viral infections including the childhood exanthems.

Tropical infections

Malaria

40% of the world's population live in an area where the female *Anopheles* mosquito transmits malaria. Over 1 million children die in Africa each year predominantly from *Plasmodium falciparum* malaria. The clinical features include fever (often not cyclical), diarrhoea, vomiting, flu-like symptoms, jaundice, anaemia and thrombocytopenia. Whilst typically the onset is 7–10 days after inoculation, infections can present many months later. Children are particularly susceptible to severe anaemia and the gravest form of the disease, cerebral malaria. The infection is diagnosed by examination of a thick film. The species (*falciparum, vivax, ovale* or *malariae*) is confirmed on a thin film. Repeated blood films may be necessary.

Quinine is required in nearly all cases seen in the UK because of the emergence of chloroquine-resistant strains worldwide, and primaquine is given (after a G6PD screen) for *Plasmodium vivax* and *ovale* infection to prevent relapse. Travellers to endemic areas should always seek up-to-date information on malaria prevention. Prophylaxis reduces but does not eliminate the risk of infection. Prevention of mosquito bites with repellants and bed nets is also important.

Typhoid

A child with worsening fever, headaches, cough, abdominal pain, anorexia, malaise and myalgia may be suffering from infection with *Salmonella typhi* or *paratyphi*. Gastrointestinal symptoms (diarrhoea or constipation) may not appear until the second week. Splenomegaly, bradycardia and rose-coloured spots on the trunk may be present. The serious complications of this disease include gastrointestinal perforation, myocarditis, hepatitis and nephritis. The recent increase in multi-resistant strains, particularly from the Indian subcontinent, means that treatment with cotrimoxazole, chloramphenicol or ampicillin may be inadequate. A third-generation cephalosporin or ciprofloxacin is usually effective.

Dengue fever

This viral infection is widespread in the tropics, and it is transmitted by mosquitoes. The primary infection is characterised by a fine erythematous rash, myalgia, arthralgia and high fever. After resolution of the fever, a secondary rash with desquamation may occur. Dengue haemorrhagic fever, also known as dengue shock syndrome, occurs when a previously infected child has a subsequent infection with a serologically different strain of the virus. Unfortunately, the partially effective host immune response serves to augment the severity of the infection. The child presents with severe capillary leak syndrome leading to hypotension as well as haemorrhagic manifestations. With fluid resuscitation, most children will recover fully. A patient with this condition is not infectious as direct person-to-person spread does not occur.

Gastroenteritis and dysentery

Gastroenteritis frequently accompanies foreign travel. 'Traveller's diarrhoea' is commonly caused by a change in gut flora, viruses including rotavirus and by *E. coli*. It rarely needs more than attention to rehydration. Fever accompanied by loose stools with blood or mucus suggests dysentery caused by *Shigella, Salmonella, Campylobacter* or *Entamoeba histolytica*. Blood cultures and stool cultures should be taken and appropriate antibiotics started.

Viral haemorrhagic fevers

Causes include the Lassa, Marburg, Ebola and Crimean–Congo viruses. These infections are imported, although Hantavirus has recently been isolated from within the UK. These are highly contagious, often lethal, infections. If suspected, strict isolation procedures should be initiated for any symptomatic patient who has returned from an endemic area within the 21-day incubation period of these infections. Specialist advice should be sought.

Fig. 13.22 An approach to the febrile child returning from the tropics.

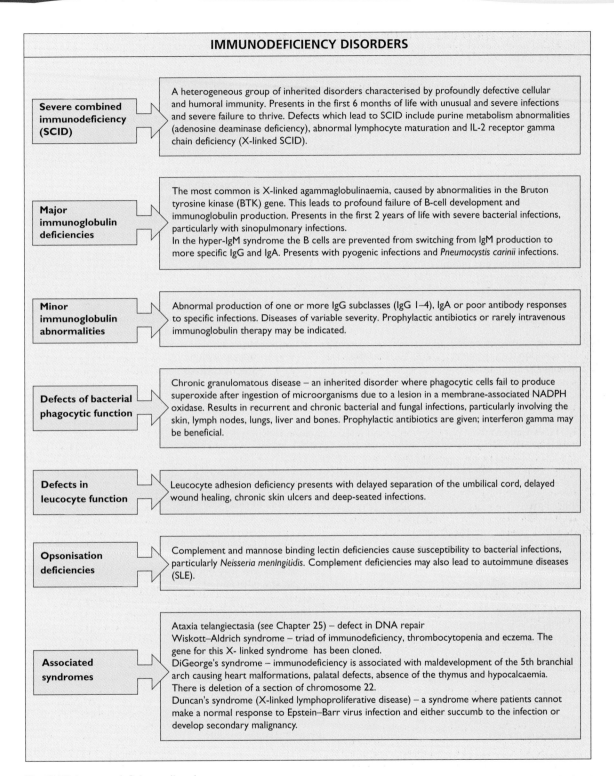

IMMUNODEFICIENCY DISORDERS

Severe combined immunodeficiency (SCID)
A heterogeneous group of inherited disorders characterised by profoundly defective cellular and humoral immunity. Presents in the first 6 months of life with unusual and severe infections and severe failure to thrive. Defects which lead to SCID include purine metabolism abnormalities (adenosine deaminase deficiency), abnormal lymphocyte maturation and IL-2 receptor gamma chain deficiency (X-linked SCID).

Major immunoglobulin deficiencies
The most common is X-linked agammaglobulinaemia, caused by abnormalities in the Bruton tyrosine kinase (BTK) gene. This leads to profound failure of B-cell development and immunoglobulin production. Presents in the first 2 years of life with severe bacterial infections, particularly with sinopulmonary infections.
In the hyper-IgM syndrome the B cells are prevented from switching from IgM production to more specific IgG and IgA. Presents with pyogenic infections and *Pneumocystis carinii* infections.

Minor immunoglobulin abnormalities
Abnormal production of one or more IgG subclasses (IgG 1–4), IgA or poor antibody responses to specific infections. Diseases of variable severity. Prophylactic antibiotics or rarely intravenous immunoglobulin therapy may be indicated.

Defects of bacterial phagocytic function
Chronic granulomatous disease – an inherited disorder where phagocytic cells fail to produce superoxide after ingestion of microorganisms due to a lesion in a membrane-associated NADPH oxidase. Results in recurrent and chronic bacterial and fungal infections, particularly involving the skin, lymph nodes, lungs, liver and bones. Prophylactic antibiotics are given; interferon gamma may be beneficial.

Defects in leucocyte function
Leucocyte adhesion deficiency presents with delayed separation of the umbilical cord, delayed wound healing, chronic skin ulcers and deep-seated infections.

Opsonisation deficiencies
Complement and mannose binding lectin deficiencies cause susceptibility to bacterial infections, particularly *Neisseria meningitidis*. Complement deficiencies may also lead to autoimmune diseases (SLE).

Associated syndromes
Ataxia telangiectasia (*see* Chapter 25) – defect in DNA repair
Wiskott–Aldrich syndrome – triad of immunodeficiency, thrombocytopenia and eczema. The gene for this X- linked syndrome has been cloned.
DiGeorge's syndrome – immunodeficiency is associated with maldevelopment of the 5th branchial arch causing heart malformations, palatal defects, absence of the thymus and hypocalcaemia. There is deletion of a section of chromosome 22.
Duncan's syndrome (X-linked lymphoproliferative disease) – a syndrome where patients cannot make a normal response to Epstein–Barr virus infection and either succumb to the infection or develop secondary malignancy.

Fig. 13.23 Immunodeficiency disorders.

Fig. 13.24 Specific defects in the components of the immune system lead to particular types of infection. (Only the most common/important are listed.)

Immune defect	Infectious susceptibility	
Antibody/humoral (B lymphocytes)	Bacteria	*Pneumococcus* *Staphylococcus, Streptococcus, Haemophilus influenzae, Moraxella catarrhalis*
	Viruses	Enteroviruses
Cellular immunity (T lymphocytes)	Bacteria	*Mycobacterium, Listeria*
	Viruses	CMV, VZV, HSV, EBV, measles, respiratory viruses
	Fungi	*Candida, Aspergillus, Pneumocystis carinii*
Combined cellular and humoral (T and B lymphocytes)	Bacteria Viruses Fungi	All of above
Neutrophils	Bacteria	Gram-positive, Gram-negative
	Fungi	*Aspergillus, Candida*
Opsonisation (complement, mannose binding lectin)	Bacteria	*Neisseria meningitidis, Staphylococcus*

Fig. 13.25 Some of the more commonly used tests of immune function in children.

Test	Function
Full blood count	Number of white blood cells, and differential count of neutrophils, lymphocytes, platelets
Blood film	Morphology of cells
Lymphocytes	
Lymphocyte subsets	Determines the number of T and B cells, monocytes and natural killer cells
Immunoglobulins	Level of IgG, IgM, IgA and IgE and IgG subclasses
Specific immunoglobulin	Tests the ability to mount an appropriate antibody response to known antigens, e.g. vaccine responses
T cell proliferation in response to mitogens and antigens, e.g. phytohaemagglutin and *Candida*	Functional test of cell-mediated immunity
Tests of purine and pyrimadine metabolism	Abnormal in some forms of severe combined immunodeficiency
Chromosomal fragility test	Test for ataxia telangiectasia
Neutrophils	
Nitroblue tetrazolium test (NBT)	Abnormal response in chronic granulomatous disease
Surface adhesion molecules (CD18)	Test for leucocyte adhesion deficiency
Tests of chemotaxis	Test of leucocyte motility
Complement	
Individual complement components	Reduced in complement deficiency states and other diseases
Total haemolytic complement	Functional test for complement
Identification of genetic polymorphisms	Specific abnormal genes have been identified for a number of conditions (e.g. Wiskott–Aldrich syndrome, Bruton's agammaglobulinaemia, DiGeorge's syndrome, severe combined immunodeficiency, Mannose binding (lectin) deficiency, Duncan's syndrome)

HIV infection

The major route of HIV transmission to children is vertically from mother to child, usually intrapartum, but also intrauterine or via breast-feeding. Mothers who are most likely to transmit HIV to their infants are those with a greater load of HIV virus and more advanced disease. Where mothers breast-feed, 25–40% of infants become infected with HIV. In Europe and the USA, where mothers can avoid breast-feeding, only around 15% of infants are infected. Worldwide, the majority of women are infected heterosexually, with only a small minority of women infected by intravenous drug use. The virus is also rarely transmitted to children by infected blood products and contaminated needles.

In children over 18 months old, HIV infection is diagnosed by detecting antibodies to the virus. As infants born to infected mothers will have circulating maternal HIV antibodies, the test is unreliable before this age and their status will be indeterminate. The most sensitive test for HIV in infants is by detection of the viral genome by PCR. Other less sensitive tests in infants include HIV culture, p24 antigen, elevated immunoglobulins, low CD4 T cell count for age and clinical features of infection.

Reduction of vertical transmission of HIV
Vertical transmission of HIV can now be reduced to less than 2% by the use of a number of interventions, including:

- avoidance of breast-feeding
- use of antenatal, perinatal and postnatal antiretroviral drugs to reduce viral load, e.g. zidovudine or nevirapine
- avoidance of labour and contact with the birth canal by elective caesarean section delivery.

Unfortunately this effective combination of interventions is not available to the majority of women with HIV.

HIV-infected children
Infected children may remain asymptomatic for months or years before progressing to severe disease and immunodeficiency (or an AIDS diagnosis). Clinical presentation varies with the degree of immunosuppression. Children with mild immunosuppression may have lymphadenopathy or parotitis; if moderate, they may have recurrent bacterial infections, candidiasis, chronic diarrhoea and lymphocytic interstitial pneumonitis (LIP) (Fig. 13.26). This lymphocytic infiltration of the lungs may be caused by a response to the HIV infection itself, or it may be related to EBV infection in these children.

Severe AIDS diagnoses include opportunist infections, e.g. *Pneumocystis carinii* infection, severe failure to thrive, encephalopathy (Fig. 13.27) and malignancy, which is rare in children. More than one clinical

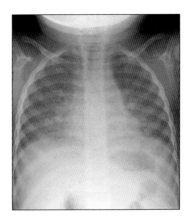

Fig. 13.26
Lymphocytic interstitial pneumonitis (LIP) in a child with HIV infection. There is diffuse reticulonodular shadowing with hilar lymphadenopathy.

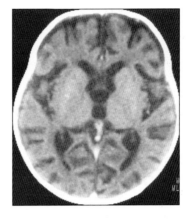

Fig. 13.27 A CT scan in a child with HIV encephalopathy showing diffuse increase in CSF spaces from cerebral atrophy and volume loss.

feature is often present. An unusual constellation of symptoms, especially if due to an infectious cause, should alert the clinician to consider HIV infection.

Treatment
Prophylaxis against primary pneumocystis pneumonia (PCP) with cotrimoxazole is prescribed for infants who are HIV-infected, for infants whose infection status is not yet determined and for older children with low CD4 counts.

Infants of indeterminate status and infected infants should be immunised according to the normal immunisation schedule, except for BCG. This should not be given due to the risk of dissemination. Infants born to HIV-infected mothers should only be given BCG when they are known to be HIV-negative. There is a theoretical risk of infection of immunocompromised care givers if oral polio vaccine is given to a baby, so advice about handwashing should be given. An alternative is to use inactivated (Salk) polio vaccine.

The two most important criteria which predict long-term morbidity and mortality from HIV infection are the plasma HIV viral load and the CD4 count. A child who has symptomatic HIV disease is likely to have a reduced CD4 count for age and a high viral load. Asymptomatic or mildly symptomatic children require regular monitoring of viral load and CD4 count. Deleterious changes in these parameters may mean that these children will require antiretroviral therapy. As with HIV-infected adults, combination antiretroviral therapy is most effective in suppressing viral replication and maintaining health in children. Adherence to antiretroviral therapy regimens is onerous and required long-term; this can be very difficult for families to cope with. Short and long-term side-effects of therapy can also be problematic. There are three families of antiretroviral therapy currently available for children:

- the nuceoside analoge reverse transcriptase inhibitors (NRTIs) (e.g. zidovudine, didanosine, lamivudine)
- the non-nuceoside reverse transcriptase inhibitors (NNRTIs) (e.g. nevirapine, efavirenz)
- the protease inhibitors (PIs) (e.g. ritonavir, indinavir, nelfinavir).

Current regimens for children starting antiretroviral therapy include two NRTIs with either an NNRTI or a PI. In view of rapid new drug developments, the advice of a specialist should be sought before prescribing for children. More active antiretroviral therapy means that most children are now surviving into their teenage years, which brings new challenges in the management of this chronic disease.

Social, psychological and family support

Providing coordinated medical, psychological and social support for all family members is an important part of managing children and families with HIV. A coordinated service for parents and children helps to streamline therapy for the family and reduce the number of hospital visits. The multidisciplinary team can help the family cope with complicated issues, including adherence to treatment, when and what to tell children, confidentiality, schooling and planning for the future.

Antenatal interventions and avoidance of breast-feeding can reduce the risk of transmission of HIV from mother to child to less than 2%.

IMMUNISATION

Immunisation is one of the most effective and economic public health measures to improve the health of both children and adults (Fig. 13.28). The most notable success has been the worldwide eradication of smallpox achieved in 1979, but the prevalence of many other diseases has been dramatically reduced by immunisation programmes (Fig. 13.29). The World Health Organization (WHO) aimed to eradicate poliomyelitis from the world by the year 2000 which was almost achieved. In many countries, the immunisation uptake rate exceeds 90%. If this could be extended worldwide, the deaths of several millions of young children would be prevented.

Differences exist in the composition and scheduling of immunisation programmes in different countries, and schedules are in continuous evolution as new vaccines become available. The current UK and USA schedules are shown in Figure 13.30. In many developing countries, immunisation coverage is not optimal, but WHO is making major efforts to help countries to improve the dissemination and uptake of vaccination.

Fig. 13.28 Immunisations available for children.

Routine immunisations in the UK/USA	Diphtheria (T), tetanus (T), pertussis (I) Poliomyelitis – oral (L), parenteral (I) *Haemophilus influenzae* b (S) Conjugated meningococcus C (S) (UK only) Measles (L), mumps (L), rubella (L) Hepatitis B (USA only) Varicella (USA only) Conjugated pneumococcus (S) (USA only)
Immunisations available for children at risk	TB (BCG) (L) Hepatitis A and B (S) *Meningococcus* (serogroups A, C, Y, WI35) (S) *Pneumococcus* (S) Influenza (S)
Immunisations available for children travelling abroad	Typhoid – oral (L), parenteral (I) Cholera (I) Yellow fever (L) Rabies (I) Japanese encephalitis (I), tick-borne encephalitis (I)

L, live attenuated; I, inactivated; T, toxoid; S, subunit.

Complications and contraindications

Following vaccination, there may be swelling and discomfort at the injection site and a mild fever and malaise. Some vaccines, such as measles and rubella, may be followed by a mild form of the disease. More serious reactions, including anaphylaxis, may occur but are very rare. Local guidelines about vaccination and its contraindications should be followed. Vaccination should be postponed if the child has an acute illness; however, a minor infection without fever or systemic upset is not a contraindication. If there is a personal or family history of febrile convulsions, advice on fever prevention should be given. Live vaccines should not be given to children with impaired immune responsiveness (except in children with HIV infection in whom MMR vaccine can be given).

Following pertussis vaccination, convulsions and encephalopathy are rare complications, but publicity in the UK in the 1970s surrounding this risk resulted in a marked fall in vaccine uptake and was followed by several whooping cough epidemics (see Fig. 13.29). It is now recognised that in many instances the complications were falsely attributed to the vaccine and that the neurological complications from the illness itself

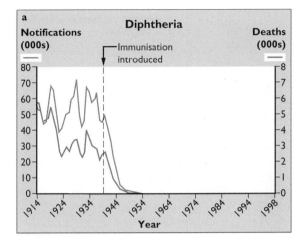

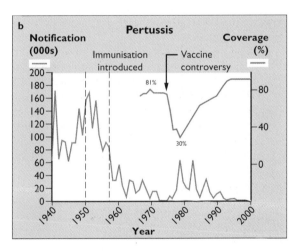

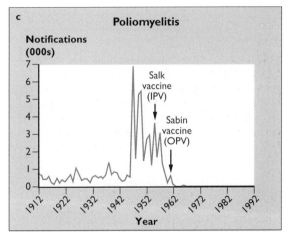

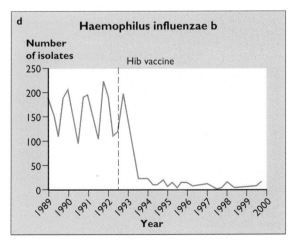

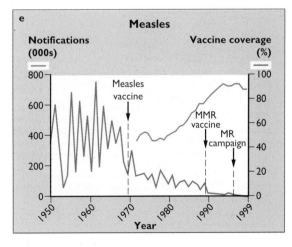

Fig. 13.29 Effect of immunisation on the number of notifications in England and Wales. (a) Diphtheria. (b) Pertussis. (c) Poliomyelitis. (d) *Haemophilus influenzae* b. (e) Measles. (Courtesy of PHLS Communicable Disease Surveillance Centre, Department of Health and Office for Health Statistics.)

IMMUNISATION

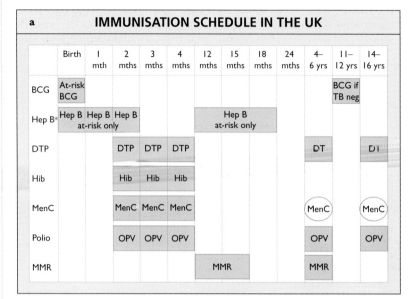

a IMMUNISATION SCHEDULE IN THE UK

	Birth	1 mth	2 mths	3 mths	4 mths	12 mths	15 mths	18 mths	24 mths	4–6 yrs	11–12 yrs	14–16 yrs
BCG	At-risk BCG										BCG if TB neg	
Hep B*	Hep B	Hep B at-risk only	Hep B			Hep B at-risk only						
DTP			DTP	DTP	DTP					DT		DT
Hib			Hib	Hib	Hib							
MenC			MenC	MenC	MenC					MenC		MenC
Polio			OPV	OPV	OPV					OPV		OPV
MMR							MMR			MMR		

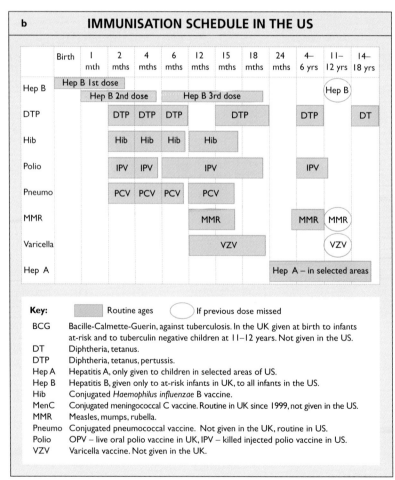

b IMMUNISATION SCHEDULE IN THE US

	Birth	1 mth	2 mths	4 mths	6 mths	12 mths	15 mths	18 mths	24 mths	4–6 yrs	11–12 yrs	14–18 yrs
Hep B	Hep B 1st dose	Hep B 2nd dose			Hep B 3rd dose						Hep B	
DTP			DTP	DTP	DTP		DTP			DTP		DT
Hib			Hib	Hib	Hib	Hib						
Polio			IPV	IPV		IPV				IPV		
Pneumo			PCV	PCV	PCV	PCV						
MMR						MMR				MMR	MMR	
Varicella						VZV					VZV	
Hep A										Hep A – in selected areas		

Key: ▢ Routine ages ◯ If previous dose missed

BCG — Bacille-Calmette-Guerin, against tuberculosis. In the UK given at birth to infants at-risk and to tuberculin negative children at 11–12 years. Not given in the US.
DT — Diphtheria, tetanus.
DTP — Diphtheria, tetanus, pertussis.
Hep A — Hepatitis A, only given to children in selected areas of US.
Hep B — Hepatitis B, given only to at-risk infants in UK, to all infants in the US.
Hib — Conjugated *Haemophilus influenzae* B vaccine.
MenC — Conjugated meningococcal C vaccine. Routine in UK since 1999, not given in the US.
MMR — Measles, mumps, rubella.
Pneumo — Conjugated pneumococcal vaccine. Not given in the UK, routine in US.
Polio — OPV – live oral polio vaccine in UK, IPV – killed injected polio vaccine in US.
VZV — Varicella vaccine. Not given in the UK.

Fig. 13.30 Immunisation schedules: (a) UK, 2000; (b) USA, 2000. Box denotes usual/first time(s) for vaccine doses. Oval denotes later times when missed doses may be caught up.

are considerably more frequent than after the vaccine. The only contraindication to pertussis vaccination is if the child has experienced a severe local or general reaction to a preceding dose. If there is an evolving neurological problem, immunisation should be deferred until the condition is stable.

The MMR vaccine is contraindicated in children who are allergic to neomycin or kanamycin, which may be present in small quantities in the vaccine. Children with a history of anaphylaxis to egg (in which the virus for the vaccine is grown) can be immunised but only under medical supervision.

FURTHER READING

American Academy of Pediatrics 1999 Report of the committee on infectious diseases. 'Red Book', 25th edn. AAP, Illinois. *Useful manual on paediatric infection and immunisation in the USA*
Davies E G, Elliman D A C, Hart C A, Nicoll A, Rudd P T 1996 Manual of childhood infections. W B Saunders, London
Department of Health 1996 Immunisation against infectious disease (green book). HMSO, London.
Feigin R D, Cherry J D 1998 Textbook of pediatric infectious diseases, 4th edn. Saunders, Philadelphia. *Large comprehensive textbook*

Internet sites for updates on immunisation and current information on infectious diseases
www.CDC.gov – Centres for Disease Control, Atlanta, USA
www.aap.org – American Academy of Pediatrics
www.phls.co.uk – Public Health Laboratory Service, UK
www.who.org – World Health Organization
www.unaids.org – wordwide information on HIV

14

Respiratory disorders

Respiratory disorders are important as:

- they account for 50% of consultations with general practitioners for acute illness in young children and a third of consultations in older children
- respiratory illness leads to 20–35% of acute paediatric admissions to hospital, some of which are life-threatening
- asthma is the most common chronic illness of childhood in the UK
- cystic fibrosis is the most common inherited disorder in Caucasians causing chronic disease.

RESPIRATORY INFECTIONS

These are the most frequent infections of childhood. The preschool child has, on average, six to eight respiratory infections a year. Most are mild self-limiting illnesses of the upper respiratory tract (ear, nose, throat) but some, such as bronchiolitis or pneumonia, are potentially life-threatening.

Pathogens

Viruses cause 80–90% of childhood respiratory infections. The most important are the respiratory syncytial virus (RSV), rhinoviruses, parainfluenza, influenza and adenoviruses. An individual virus can cause several different patterns of illness, e.g. RSV can cause bronchiolitis, croup, pneumonia or a common cold.

The important bacterial pathogens of the respiratory tract are *Streptococcus pneumoniae* (pneumococcus) and other streptococci, *Haemophilus influenzae*, *Bordetella pertussis*, which causes whooping cough, and *Mycoplasma pneumoniae*. Dual infections, with two viral pathogens, or a viral and bacterial pathogen, are more common than previously recognised. *Mycobacterium tuberculosis* remains an important pathogen. Some pathogens cause predictable epidemics, such as RSV bronchiolitis every winter, whereas others, e.g. *Pneumococcus*, show little seasonal variation.

Host and environmental factors

An increased risk of respiratory infection is associated with:

- poor socioeconomic status (such as overcrowded, damp housing and poor nutrition)
- large family size
- parental, especially maternal smoking
- boys more than girls
- prematurity – especially those who required artificial ventilation or prolonged oxygen therapy
- congenital abnormalities of the heart or lungs
- rarely, immune deficiency – either congenital (e.g. agammaglobulinaemia) or acquired (e.g. as a result of therapy for malignant disease or from HIV infection).

The child's age influences the prevalence and severity of infections (Fig. 14.1). It is in infancy that serious respiratory illness requiring hospital admission

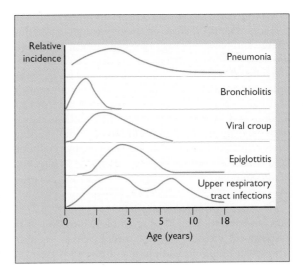

Fig. 14.1 Age distribution of acute respiratory infections in children.

is most common and the risk of death is greatest. There is an increased frequency of infections when the child or older siblings start nursery or school. Repeated upper respiratory tract infection is common and rarely indicates underlying disease.

Classification of respiratory infections

Respiratory infections are classified according to the level of the respiratory tree most involved:

- upper respiratory tract infection
- laryngeal/tracheal infection
- bronchitis
- bronchiolitis
- pneumonia.

 ## Upper respiratory tract infection (URTI)

Approximately 80% of respiratory infections involve only the nose, throat, ears or sinuses. The term URTI embraces a number of different conditions.

- common cold (coryza)
- sore throat (pharyngitis, including tonsillitis)
- acute otitis media
- sinusitis (relatively uncommon).

The commonest presentation is a child with a combination of a painful throat, fever, nasal discharge and blockage, and earache. Cough may be troublesome. URTIs may cause:

- difficulty in feeding in infants as their noses are blocked and this obstructs breathing
- febrile convulsions
- acute exacerbations of asthma.

In infants, hospital admission may be required to exclude a more serious infection, to ensure feeding is adequate, or for parental reassurance.

The common cold (coryza)

This is the commonest infection of childhood. Classical features include a clear or mucopurulent nasal discharge and nasal blockage. The commonest pathogens are viruses – rhinoviruses (of which there are over 100 different serotypes), coronaviruses and RSV. Health education to advise parents that colds are self-limiting and have no specific curative treatment may reduce anxiety and save unnecessary visits to doctors. Fever and pain are best treated with paracetamol or ibuprofen. Antibiotics are of no benefit as the common cold is viral in origin and secondary bacterial infection is uncommon.

Sore throat (pharyngitis)

Sore throats are usually due to viral infection with respiratory viruses (mostly adenoviruses, enteroviruses and rhinoviruses). In the older child, group A β-haemolytic *Streptococcus* is a common pathogen. The pharynx and soft palate are inflamed and local lymph nodes are enlarged and tender.

Tonsillitis

This is a form of pharyngitis where there is intense inflammation of the tonsils, often with a purulent exudate. Group A β-haemolytic *Streptococci* and the Epstein–Barr virus (in infectious mononucleosis) are common pathogens.

Although viruses are the commonest cause of pharyngitis or tonsillitis, especially in preschool children, it is not possible to distinguish clinically between viral and bacterial causes. Marked constitutional disturbance, such as headache, apathy and abdominal pain, tonsillar exudate and cervical lymphadenopathy, is more common with bacterial infection.

Antibiotics (often penicillin, or erythromycin if there is penicillin allergy) are often prescribed for severe pharyngitis and tonsillitis even though only a third are caused by bacteria. They may hasten recovery from streptococcal infection, but 10 days of treatment is required to eradicate the organism to prevent rheumatic fever, although this is now exceedingly rare in the UK. Some doctors restrict the use of antibiotics to those children with positive streptococcal cultures from throat swabs. Amoxicillin is best avoided as it may cause a widespread maculopapular rash if the tonsillitis is due to infectious mononucleosis.

> It is not possible to distinguish clinically between viral and bacterial tonsillitis.

Acute infection of the middle ear (acute otitis media)

Acute otitis media is common; 20% of children under 4 years old are affected at least once a year. There is pain in the ear and fever. The child is irritable and may pull at the affected ear. Every child with a fever must have the tympanic membranes examined (Fig. 14.2a–d). In acute otitis media, the tympanic membrane is seen to be bright red and bulging with loss of the normal light reflection. Occasionally there is acute perforation of the eardrum with pus visible in the external canal. Pathogens include viruses, *Pneumococcus*, group A β-haemolytic *Streptococcus*, *H. influenzae* and *Moraxella catarrhalis*. Serious complications such as mastoiditis and meningitis are now uncommon. Pain should be treated with paracetamol. Although many cases of acute otitis media resolve spontaneously within 24 h, an antibiotic is usually given to shorten the duration of pain and reduce the risk of complications (see p. 49). Amoxicillin is widely used, but augmentin (amoxicillin with clavulanic acid) is a reasonable alternative in view of the increasing proportion of beta-lactamase-producing *H. influenzae* and *M. catarrhalis*. Decongestants are often given to help Eustachian tube drainage, but their efficacy is unproven.

Recurrent ear infections can lead to chronic secretory otitis media (glue ear), the most common cause of

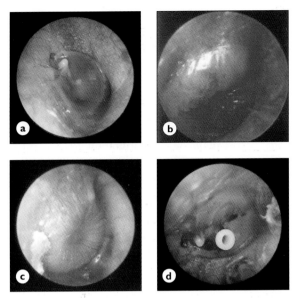

Fig. 14.2 Appearance of the eardrum. (a) Normal.
(b) Acute otitis media. (c) Chronic secretory otitis media.
(d) Grommet. ((a) and (d) courtesy of Mr N. Shah &
Mr N. Tolley, (b) and (c) from Stafford N D, Youngs R
Colour Guide ENT, Churchill Livingstone Edinburgh, 1999,
with permission.)

conductive hearing loss in children. This can interfere with normal speech development and result in learning difficulties in school. This condition also causes earache due to pressure changes resulting from obstruction to the Eustachian tube.

Sinusitis

Infection of the paranasal sinuses may occur with viral URTIs. Occasionally there is secondary bacterial infection, with pain, swelling and tenderness over the cheek from infection of the maxillary sinus. As the frontal sinuses do not develop until late childhood, frontal sinusitis is uncommon in the first decade of life. Antibiotics and analgesia are used for acute sinusitis.

Tonsillectomy and adenoidectomy

Children with recurrent URTIs are often referred for removal of their tonsils and adenoids, one of the commonest operations performed in children. Many children have large tonsils but this in itself is not an indication for tonsillectomy as they shrink spontaneously in late childhood.

The indications for tonsillectomy are controversial but include:

- recurrent tonsillitis (as opposed to recurrent URTIs), particularly if interfering with the child's development or schooling, despite adequate antibiotic treatment
- a peritonsillar abscess (quinsy)
- obstructive sleep apnoea.

Like the tonsils, adenoids increase in size until about the age of 7 years and then gradually regress. They may narrow the posterior nasal space sufficiently to justify adenoidectomy if they cause:

- Chronic secretory otitis media and hearing loss from Eustachian tube malfunction. These children may also benefit from the insertion of ventilation tubes (grommets) into the tympanic membrane, although there is also debate about the benefit of this procedure.
- Upper airway obstruction leading to snoring and mouth breathing and hypoxaemia during sleep. More seriously, obstructive sleep apnoea may develop, when the child snores loudly, breathes 'heavily' and may struggle for breath, and stops breathing for 30–45 s whilst asleep. Sleep disturbance can lead to daytime somnolence and, in severe cases, pulmonary hypertension, failure to thrive and developmental delay. Adenotonsillectomy is usually curative (Fig. 14.3a,b).

Laryngeal and tracheal infections

The mucosal inflammation and swelling produced by laryngeal and tracheal infections can rapidly cause life-threatening obstruction of the airway in young children. Several conditions can cause acute upper airways obstruction (Fig. 14.4). They are characterised by:

- stridor, a rasping sound heard predominantly on inspiration

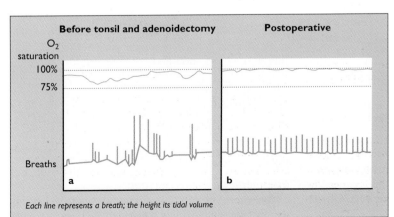

Fig. 14.3 Extract from cardiorespiratory monitoring in a child with obstructive sleep apnoea. (a) Irregular breathing with periodic pauses associated with oxygen desaturation. (b) Post-adenotonsillectomy, the breathing is regular and the desaturation has resolved. (Courtesy of Dr Parviz Habibi.)

Each line represents a breath; the height its tidal volume

Fig. 14.4 Differential diagnosis of acute upper airways obstruction.

Croup
Viral laryngotracheitis (very common)
Recurrent or spasmodic croup (common)
Bacterial tracheitis (rare)

Rare causes
Epiglottitis
Inhalation of smoke and hot air in fires
Trauma to the throat
Retropharyngeal abscess
Laryngeal foreign body
Angioedema
Infectious mononucleosis
Measles
Diphtheria
Acute-on-chronic stridor, e.g. from a floppy larynx
  (laryngomalacia)

Basic management of acute upper airways obstruction:

- **Don't examine the throat!**
- **Reduce anxiety by staff being calm, confident and well organised.**
- **Observe carefully for signs of hypoxia or deterioration.**
- **If respiratory failure develops from increasing airways obstruction, exhaustion or secretions blocking the airway, urgent tracheal intubation is required.**

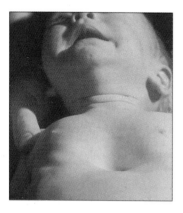

Fig. 14.5 The degree of subcostal, intercostal and sternal recession is a more useful indicator of severity of upper airways obstruction than the respiratory rate (© Boehringer Ingelheim International GmbH).

- hoarseness due to inflammation of the vocal cords
- a barking cough like a sea lion
- a variable degree of dyspnoea.

The severity of upper airways obstruction is best assessed clinically by:

- the degree of sternal and subcostal recession (Fig. 14.5)
- respiratory rate
- heart rate
- increasing agitation
- drowsiness, tiredness, exhaustion
- central cyanosis indicating severe hypoxaemia and the need for urgent intervention – the measurement of oxygen saturation by pulse oximetry is the most reliable objective measure of hypoxaemia.

Total obstruction of the upper airway may be precipitated by examination of the throat using a spatula. One must avoid looking at the throat of a child with upper airways obstruction unless full resuscitation equipment and personnel are at hand.

Viral croup

Viral croup accounts for over 95% of laryngotracheal infections. Parainfluenza viruses are the commonest cause, but other viruses, such as RSV and influenza, can produce a similar clinical picture. There is mucosal inflammation and increased secretions affecting the larynx, trachea and bronchi, but it is the oedema of the subglottic area that is potentially dangerous in young children because it may result in critical narrowing of the trachea. Croup occurs from 6 months to 6 years of age but the peak incidence is in the second year of life. The typical features are of a barking cough, harsh stridor and hoarseness usually preceded by fever and coryza. The symptoms often start, and are worse, at night.

The child with mild viral croup can usually be managed at home. When the upper airway obstruction is mild, the stridor and chest recession disappear when the child is at rest. The parents need to observe the child closely for the signs of increasing severity. The decision to manage the child at home or in hospital is influenced by the severity of the illness, time of day, ease of access to hospital, the age of the child (with a low threshold admission for those <12 months old) and parental understanding and confidence about the disorder.

Inhalation of warm moist air is widely used but is of unproven benefit. Both oral dexamethasone and nebulised steroids (budesonide) have been shown to be effective in reducing the severity and duration of viral croup. Nebulised adrenaline can provide transient improvement in severe upper airways obstruction, but close observation and cardiorespiratory monitoring should be performed when it is administered. Children with the clinical features of severe croup, or an oxygen saturation of less than 93% in air, should be given warm humidified oxygen by face mask and closely monitored. Less than 2% of children admitted with croup require tracheal intubation. This figure has fallen since the introduction of steroid therapy.

Spasmodic or recurrent croup

Some young children suddenly develop a barking cough and stridor at night without preceding respiratory tract symptoms. These children appear to have hyper-reactive upper airways and some will develop asthma or other atopic illnesses such as hay fever or eczema.

Bacterial tracheitis (pseudomembranous croup)

This rare but dangerous condition is usually caused by infection with *Staphylococcus aureus* or *H. influenzae*. The clinical picture is similar to severe viral croup

except that the child has a high fever, appears toxic and has rapidly progressive airways obstruction. At tracheal intubation copious thick secretions are found.

 ### Acute epiglottitis

Acute epiglottitis is a life-threatening emergency due to respiratory obstruction. It is caused by *H. influenzae* type b. In the UK and many other countries, the introduction of universal Hib immunisation in infancy has led to a decrease of over 99% in the incidence of epiglottitis and other invasive *H. influenzae* type b infection. There is intense swelling of the epiglottis and surrounding tissues associated with septicaemia. Epiglottitis is most common in children aged 1–6 years but affects all age groups. It is important to distinguish between epiglottitis and viral croup (Fig. 14.6) as they require quite different treatment.

The onset of epiglottitis is often very acute (see Case history 14.1), with:

- high fever in an ill, toxic-looking child
- an intensely painful throat that prevents the child from speaking or swallowing; saliva drools down the chin
- soft inspiratory stridor and rapidly increasing respiratory difficulty over hours
- the child sits immobile, upright, with an open mouth to optimise the airway.

Fig. 14.6 Clinical features of viral laryngotracheitis (croup) and epiglottitis.

	Croup	Epiglottitis
Onset	Over days	Over hours
Preceding coryza	Yes	No
Cough	Severe, barking	Absent or slight
Able to drink	Yes	No
Drooling saliva	No	Yes
Appearance	Unwell	Toxic, very ill
Fever	<38.5°C	>38.5°C
Stridor	Harsh, rasping	Soft, whispering
Voice, cry	Hoarse	Muffled, reluctant to speak

CASE HISTORY 14.1

ACUTE EPIGLOTTIS

This 5-year-old girl developed a severe sore throat, drooling of saliva, a high fever and increasing difficulty breathing over 8 h (Fig. 14.7a) Epiglottitis was diagnosed and her airway was guaranteed with a nasotracheal tube. Antibiotics were started immediately (Fig. 14.7b, c). She made a full recovery.

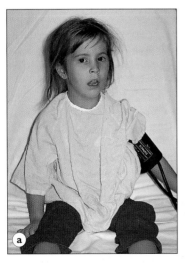 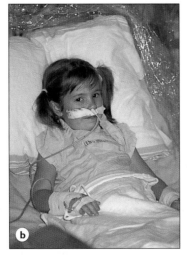 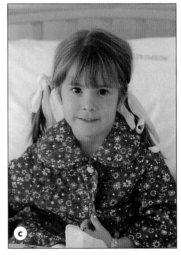

Fig. 14.7 Acute epiglottitis. (a) At presentation. (b) At 14 h, with nasotracheal and nasogastric tubes and an indwelling cannula for intravenous antibiotics. (c) At 36 h, following removal of the nasotracheal and nasogastric tubes.

In contrast to viral croup, cough is minimal or absent. Attempts to lie the child down or examine the throat with a spatula or perform a lateral neck X-ray must not be undertaken as they can precipitate total airway obstruction and death.

Once the diagnosis of epiglottitis has been made, urgent hospital admission and treatment are required. A senior anaesthetist, paediatrician and ENT surgeon should be summoned to the accident and emergency department and treatment initiated without delay. The child should be transferred directly to the intensive care unit or an anaesthetic room, and must be accompanied by senior medical staff in case respiratory obstruction occurs. The child should be intubated under controlled conditions with a general anaesthetic. Rarely, this is impossible and urgent tracheostomy is life-saving. Only after the airway is secured should blood be taken for culture and intravenous antibiotics started. A second- or third-generation cephalosporin (e.g. ceftriaxone or cefotaxime) is suitable. The tracheal tube can usually be removed after 24 h and antibiotics given for 3–5 days. With appropriate treatment, most children recover completely within 2–3 days. As with other serious *H. influenzae* infections, prophylaxis with rifampicin is offered to close household contacts.

> **Minutes count in acute epiglottitis.**

Bronchitis

There is controversy about the term bronchitis in childhood. Whilst some inflammation of the bronchi producing a mixture of wheeze and coarse crackles is often a feature of respiratory infections, bronchitis in children is very different from the chronic bronchitis of adults. In acute bronchitis in children, cough and fever are the main symptoms. The cough may persist for about 2 weeks, or longer with pertussis or *Mycoplasma* infections. There is no evidence that antibiotics, cough suppressants or expectorants speed recovery.

There is also disagreement over the use of the term 'wheezy bronchitis'. Many authorities define this as a presentation of asthma, while others consider that the bronchial inflammation and smooth muscle spasm are related to the effect of the particular infectious organisms affecting infants rather than to the child's permanent predisposition to bronchial hyperreactivity. If there is 'recurrent bronchitis' with hyperinflation of the chest or wheeze, the child probably has asthma and appropriate therapy should be given.

Whooping cough (pertussis)

This is a specific and highly infectious form of bronchitis, caused by *Bordetella pertussis*. It is endemic, with epidemics every 4 years. After 2–3 days of coryza, the child develops a characteristic paroxysmal or spasmodic cough followed by a characteristic inspiratory whoop. The spasms of cough are often worse at night and may culminate in vomiting. During a paroxysm, the child goes red or blue in the face, and mucus flows from the nose and mouth. The whoop at the end of a spasm may be absent in infants. Epistaxes and subconjunctival haemorrhages can occur after vigorous coughing. Symptoms may persist for 10–12 weeks.

Complications of pertussis, such as pneumonia, convulsions and bronchiectasis, are uncommon, but there is still a significant mortality, particularly in infants in whom the infection can cause apnoea and sudden death. Infants and young children suffering severe spasms of cough or cyanotic attacks should be admitted to hospital.

The organism can be identified early in the disease from culture of a per-nasal swab. Characteristically, there is a marked lymphocytosis (>15 000 cells/mm^3). Although erythromycin eradicates the organism and its early use may reduce family spread, there is no specific treatment that reduces the duration of the illness. Siblings, parents and school contacts may develop a similar cough. Immunisation reduces the risk of an individual developing pertussis by 80–90% but does not guarantee protection. The level of protection declines steadily during childhood.

Bronchiolitis

Bronchiolitis is the commonest serious respiratory infection of infancy: 2–3% of all infants are admitted to hospital with the disease each year during annual winter epidemics; 90% are aged 1–9 months (bronchiolitis is rare after 1 year of age). Respiratory syncitial virus (RSV) is the pathogen in 75–80% cases.

Clinical features

Coryzal symptoms precede a dry cough and increasing breathlessness. Wheezing is often, but not always, present. Feeding difficulty associated with increasing dyspnoea is often the reason for admission to hospital. Recurrent apnoea is a serious complication, especially in young infants. Infants born prematurely who develop bronchopulmonary dysplasia and infants with congenital heart disease are most at risk from this disease. The characteristic findings on examination (Fig. 14.8) are:

- sharp, dry cough
- tachypnoea
- subcostal and intercostal recession
- hyperinflation of the chest
  — sternum prominent
  — liver displaced downwards
- fine end-inspiratory crackles
- high-pitched wheezes – expiratory > inspiratory
- tachycardia
- cyanosis or pallor.

Investigations

RSV can be identified rapidly on nasopharyngeal secretions demonstrating binding of a fluorescent

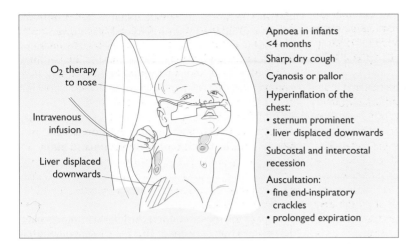

Fig. 14.8 Clinical features of severe bronchiolitis in an infant.

O₂ therapy to nose

Intravenous infusion

Liver displaced downwards

Apnoea in infants <4 months

Sharp, dry cough

Cyanosis or pallor

Hyperinflation of the chest:
• sternum prominent
• liver displaced downwards

Subcostal and intercostal recession

Auscultation:
• fine end-inspiratory crackles
• prolonged expiration

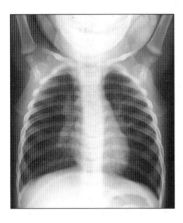

Fig. 14.9 In acute bronchiolitis, the chest X-ray shows hyperinflation of the lungs with flattening of the diaphragm, horizontal ribs and increased hilar bronchial markings.

antibody. The chest X-ray shows hyperinflation of the lungs due to small airways obstruction and air trapping (Fig. 14.9). Blood gas analysis, which is required in only the most severe cases, shows lowered arterial oxygen and raised CO₂ tension.

Management

This is supportive. Humidified oxygen is delivered via nasal cannulae or into a headbox; the concentration required is determined by pulse oximetry. The child is monitored for apnoea. Mist, antibiotics and steroids are not helpful. Nebulised bronchodilators, such as salbutamol or ipratropium, though often used, have not been shown to reduce the severity or duration of the illness. The antiviral drug ribavirin only marginally shortens viral excretion and clinical symptoms, and should be considered only for infants with underlying cardiopulmonary disorders or immune deficiency. Fluids may need to be given by nasogastric tube or intravenously. Mechanical ventilation is required in about 2% of infants admitted to hospital.

Prognosis

Most infants recover from the acute infection within 2 weeks. However, as many as half will have recurrent episodes of cough and wheeze over the next 3–5 years.

Rarely, the illness is very severe and results in permanent damage to the airways (*bronchiolitis obliterans*). This is most likely if adenovirus, rather than RSV, is the pathogen.

Prevention

A monoclonal antibody to RSV (Palivizumab, given monthly by intramuscular injection) reduces the number of hospital admissions in high-risk (mainly preterm) infants. Its use is limited by cost and the need for repeated injections.

Pneumonia

A wide range of pathogens cause pneumonia in childhood and different organisms affect different age groups.

The *newborn* is infected by organisms from the mother's genital tract. The commonest is the group B β-haemolytic *Streptococcus*. Other pathogens are *E. coli* and other Gram-negative bacilli.

In *infancy*, respiratory viruses, particularly RSV, are the most frequent cause but bacterial infection from *Strep. pneumoniae* and *H. influenzae* are also important, although the latter organism has become uncommon. *Chlamydia trachomatis* (which is also a cause of neonatal conjunctivitis) is occasionally the pathogen. *Staphylococcus aureus* is uncommon but causes severe infection.

As *children* become older, viruses become less frequent pathogens and bacterial infection more prominent. *Mycoplasma pneumoniae* is a common cause of pneumonia in school-age children. Tuberculosis should be considered at all ages.

Clinical features

These are fever, cough, breathlessness and lethargy following an upper respiratory infection. Breathing is rapid and shallow, giving the impression that the child is afraid to breathe deeply. There may be grunting on expiration. Pleuritic chest pain, neck stiffness and abdominal pain may be present if there is pleural inflammation. Classical signs of consolidation with

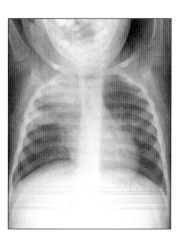

Fig. 14.10 Consolidation of the right upper lobe. Lobar consolidation is a feature of pneumococcal pneumonia.

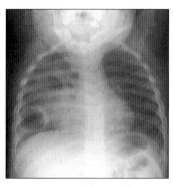

Fig. 14.11 Multiple cavities containing fluid and air in staphylococcal pneumonia.

dullness on percussion, decreased breath sounds and bronchial breathing are often absent, particularly in infants, and a chest X-ray is needed. The chest X-ray may show lobar consolidation (Fig. 14.10), widespread bronchopneumonia or, less commonly, cavitation of the lung (Fig. 14.11). For reasons that are not understood, infected pleural effusions (empyema) are becoming more common in children with pneumonia, especially when *Pneumococcus* is the pathogen. Blood culture, nasopharyngeal aspirates for viral isolation and a full blood count should also be performed in children needing hospitalisation. It is usually not possible to obtain sputum from children.

Management

It is not possible to differentiate reliably between bacterial or viral pneumonia on clinical or radiological grounds, so all children diagnosed as having pneumonia should be given antibiotics as the pathogen is rarely known when treatment is started. The choice of antibiotic is determined by the child's age, severity of illness and appearance of the chest X-ray. If intravenous therapy is required, activity against pneumococci, *H. influenzae* and *Staph. aureus* can be achieved with a cephalosporin (e.g. cefotaxime). Oral antibiotics (e.g. co-amoxiclav or a second-generation cephalosporin such as cefaclor) are given for less severe infections. If *M. pneumoniae* or *Ch. trachomatis* pneumonia is suspected, erythromycin is given. Physiotherapy and an adequate fluid intake are important and oxygen

may be required in severe pneumonia. Empyema requires drainage by an intercostal chest drain or by surgery. If a child has recurrent or persistent pneumonia, investigations to exclude an underlying condition such as cystic fibrosis or immunodeficiency are indicated (see chronic lung infection).

> **Consider pneumonia in children with neck stiffness or acute abdominal pain.**

ASTHMA

Asthma is the most common chronic respiratory disorder in children, affecting 10–15% of schoolchildren. There has been a real increase in the prevalence of asthma in the community. The reasons for this are unclear. In childhood, asthma is twice as common in males as in females, but by adolescence the ratio is equal.

Asthma is responsible for 10–20% of all acute medical admissions to paediatric wards in children aged 1–16 years. Hospital admissions for asthma increased dramatically in the UK between 1970 and 1992, sevenfold for children less than 4 years old and threefold in those aged 5–14 years. In the last few years, there has been a reduction in the number of hospital admissions. In most children, the symptoms of asthma are readily controlled, but it is an important cause of school absenteeism, restricted activity and anxiety for the child and family. There are still 15–20 deaths from asthma in children each year in the UK.

Pathophysiology

We now have a better understanding of the pathophysiology of asthma (Fig. 14.12). A combination of a genetic predisposition and environmental influences (e.g. exposure to housedust mite or cigarette smoke) results in chronic inflammation of the bronchial mucosa and airway hyperreactivity. This inflammatory process involves several different cells (eosinophils, neutrophils, lymphocytes, mast cells) and many different mediators and cytokines. Exposure of the sensitized airway to a number of trigger factors results in bronchoconstriction, mucosal oedema and excessive mucus production, which in turn lead to airway narrowing and the typical clinical features of asthma.

Atopy

The term 'atopy' is not clearly defined but describes a group of disorders that tend to coexist in individuals and their families (Fig. 14.13). One-third of children with asthma have eczema at some time in their lives. One-half have symptoms of allergic rhinitis – recurrent or persistent obstruction of the nostrils with sniffing, sneezing and nasal discharge. There may be accompanying redness and swelling of the eyes (allergic conjunctivitis). These symptoms may occur only in the summer when the grass pollen count is high (hay fever) or throughout the year (perennial rhinitis). Most atopic

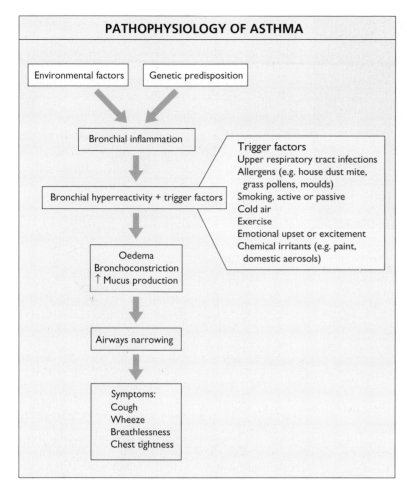

PATHOPHYSIOLOGY OF ASTHMA

Environmental factors

Genetic predisposition

↓

Bronchial inflammation

↓

Bronchial hyperreactivity + trigger factors

Trigger factors
Upper respiratory tract infections
Allergens (e.g. house dust mite,
   grass pollens, moulds)
Smoking, active or passive
Cold air
Exercise
Emotional upset or excitement
Chemical irritants (e.g. paint,
   domestic aerosols)

↓

Oedema
Bronchoconstriction
↑ Mucus production

↓

Airways narrowing

↓

Symptoms:
Cough
Wheeze
Breathlessness
Chest tightness

Fig. 14.12 Pathophysiology of asthma.

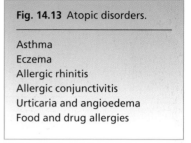

Fig. 14.13 Atopic disorders.

Asthma
Eczema
Allergic rhinitis
Allergic conjunctivitis
Urticaria and angioedema
Food and drug allergies

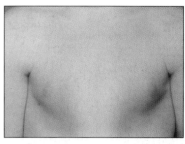

Fig. 14.14 Pectus carinatum ('pigeon chest') deformity is usually associated with chronic airways obstruction, such as asthma. The depressions at the base of the thorax associated with the muscular insertion of the diaphragm are called Harrison's sulcus.

patients have positive skin tests to common allergens (such as housedust mite, pollens and animal danders), eosinophilia and raised serum level of IgE.

Diagnosis

The diagnosis of asthma is primarily clinical and depends on eliciting a history of the typical symptoms of recurrent wheeze, cough and breathlessness. In the preschool child, the main symptom may be a troublesome nocturnal cough. The frequency and severity of symptoms vary enormously, from the child who has infrequent attacks once or twice a year to the child who is rarely free of debilitating symptoms. The diagnosis is supported by a history of characteristic trigger factors and a personal or family history of atopic disease, although the absence of a family history of atopy does not exclude the diagnosis.

The severity of asthma can be assessed by asking:

- How frequent are the symptoms?
- How is it affecting the child's life?
- How much school has been missed in the last 6 months?
- Can he play sport normally?
- How often is sleep disturbed?
- What is the longest symptom-free period?

Examination of the chest is usually normal between attacks. In long-standing airways obstruction there may be hyperinflation of the chest and generalised expiratory wheeze with a prolonged expiratory phase. A chest deformity accompanied by Harrison's sulci or pectus carinatum (pigeon chest) usually indicates long-standing airways obstruction (Fig. 14.14). Eczema may be present and there may be pale bogginess of the nasal mucosa from allergic rhinitis. Growth is normal unless the asthma is very severe. The presence of finger clubbing or the production of discoloured sputum indicates another underlying pathology such as cystic fibrosis or congenital heart disease.

Investigations

Usually the diagnosis is clear from the history and examination and no investigations are needed. Skin tests are usually positive, indicating atopy, and may help to identify a specific allergen, but their role in diagnosis remains controversial. Similarly, a chest X-ray will often show hyperinflation but rarely influences management. In infants, a chest X-ray is helpful to exclude congenital abnormalities. Most children over the age of 5 years can use a peak flow meter; their peak expiratory flow rate (PEFR) should be compared with that predicted for their height and their best

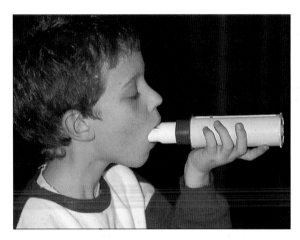

Fig. 14.15 Measurement of the peak expiratory flow rate (PEFR) provides a simple objective measurement of the severity of airflow obstruction in asthma. Normal values of PEFR are related to height.

Fig. 14.16 Causes of recurrent wheeze in infancy.

Asthma
Following RSV bronchiolitis
Recurrent viral infections
Recurrent aspiration of feeds
Ex-preterm infant
Cystic fibrosis
Maternal smoking
Cow's milk protein intolerance
Inhaled foreign body
Congenital abnormality of lung, airway or heart
Idiopathic

Fig. 14.17 Drugs in asthma.

Type of drug	Drug
Short-acting bronchodilators (relievers)	
β_2-bronchodilator	Salbutamol
	Terbutaline
Anticholinergic bronchodilator	Ipratropium bromide
Preventative/prophylactic treatment	
Inhaled steroids	Budesonide
	Beclometasone
	Fluticasone
Long-acting β_2-bronchodilators	Salmeterol, Formoterol
Sodium cromoglicate	
Methylxanthines	Theophylline
Leukotriene inhibitors	Montelukast
	Zafirlukast
Oral steroids	Prednisolone

All are given by inhalation, except prednisolone, leukotriene modulators and theophylline preparations.

---

performance (Fig. 14.15 and Appendix). If necessary, the presence of reversible airways obstruction can be demonstrated by measuring the PEFR before and 15 min after inhalation of a bronchodilator or a period of vigorous exercise. Bronchial challenge tests (histamine or cold air) are used to demonstrate bronchial hyperreactivity in research studies but not in everyday clinical practice.

Differential diagnosis

Asthma is still underdiagnosed and undertreated. Many children are labelled as having recurrent chest infections or wheezy bronchitis and receive inappropriate or inadequate treatment. However, there is also increasing concern that asthma is diagnosed too readily in any child with recurrent cough. The diagnosis is more difficult in the infant or toddler where many other conditions can cause wheeze and breathlessness (Fig. 14.16). It is now recognised that there are several different clinical patterns of asthma (phenotypes) in early childhood, with different relationships to atopy, previous viral infections, parental smoking and different prognoses.

Management

The aim is to allow the child to lead as normal a life as possible. This should be achieved with as little medication and disruption to the family's life as possible. The drug treatment of asthma can be divided into maintenance therapy to control symptoms and the management of acute exacerbations (Fig. 14.17). Their use is determined by the type of asthma experienced by the child (Fig. 14.18a).

Maintenance therapy

The two main groups of drugs used for maintenance therapy are **bronchodilators** (relievers), which give short-term symptomatic relief, and **prophylactic drugs** (preventers) which reduce bronchial inflammation and hyperreactivity (Fig. 14.17).

- *Short-acting bronchodilator therapy (relievers)*. These relievers, e.g. salbutamol or terbutaline, should be given by inhalation. They have a rapid onset of action with few side-effects. Ipratropium bromide, an anticholinergic bronchodilator, is sometimes given to infants when other bronchodilators are found to be ineffective or to children with severe symptoms not controlled by high-dose inhaled steroids.

- *Prophylactic therapy (preventers)*. Prophylactic drugs are effective only if taken regularly. Inhaled steroids are the most effective inhaled prophylactic therapy. They have no clinically significant side-effects when given in low doses. They can produce systemic side-effects, including impaired growth, adrenal

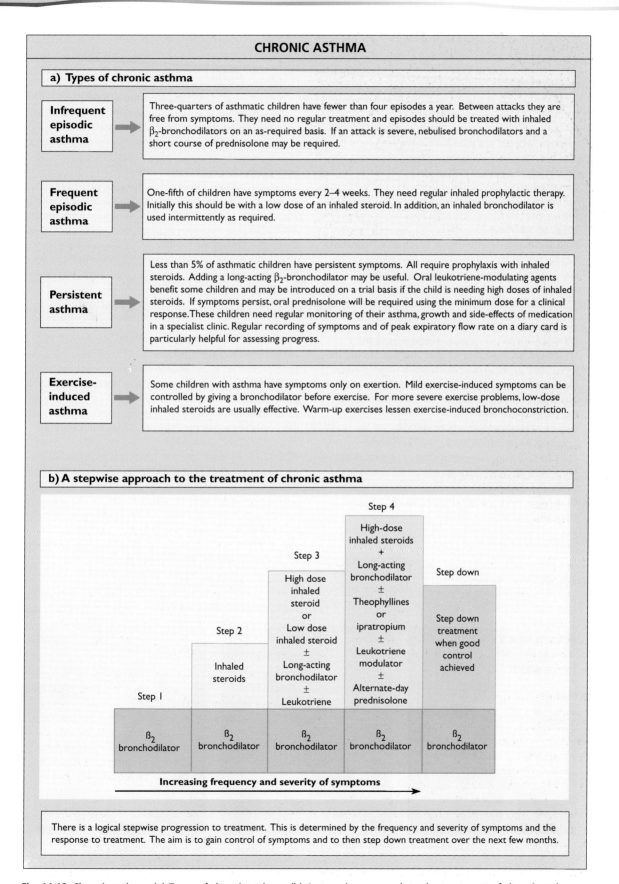

CHRONIC ASTHMA

a) Types of chronic asthma

Infrequent episodic asthma
Three-quarters of asthmatic children have fewer than four episodes a year. Between attacks they are free from symptoms. They need no regular treatment and episodes should be treated with inhaled β_2-bronchodilators on an as-required basis. If an attack is severe, nebulised bronchodilators and a short course of prednisolone may be required.

Frequent episodic asthma
One-fifth of children have symptoms every 2–4 weeks. They need regular inhaled prophylactic therapy. Initially this should be with a low dose of an inhaled steroid. In addition, an inhaled bronchodilator is used intermittently as required.

Persistent asthma
Less than 5% of asthmatic children have persistent symptoms. All require prophylaxis with inhaled steroids. Adding a long-acting β_2-bronchodilator may be useful. Oral leukotriene-modulating agents benefit some children and may be introduced on a trial basis if the child is needing high doses of inhaled steroids. If symptoms persist, oral prednisolone will be required using the minimum dose for a clinical response. These children need regular monitoring of their asthma, growth and side-effects of medication in a specialist clinic. Regular recording of symptoms and of peak expiratory flow rate on a diary card is particularly helpful for assessing progress.

Exercise-induced asthma
Some children with asthma have symptoms only on exertion. Mild exercise-induced symptoms can be controlled by giving a bronchodilator before exercise. For more severe exercise problems, low-dose inhaled steroids are usually effective. Warm-up exercises lessen exercise-induced bronchoconstriction.

b) A stepwise approach to the treatment of chronic asthma

Step 4
High-dose inhaled steroids
+
Long-acting bronchodilator
±
Theophyllines
or
ipratropium
±
Leukotriene modulator
±
Alternate-day prednisolone

Step 3
High dose inhaled steroid
or
Low dose inhaled steroid
±
Long-acting bronchodilator
±
Leukotriene

Step 2
Inhaled steroids

Step 1
β_2 bronchodilator

Step down
Step down treatment when good control achieved

β_2 bronchodilator | β_2 bronchodilator | β_2 bronchodilator | β_2 bronchodilator | β_2 bronchodilator

Increasing frequency and severity of symptoms

There is a logical stepwise progression to treatment. This is determined by the frequency and severity of symptoms and the response to treatment. The aim is to gain control of symptoms and to then step down treatment over the next few months.

Fig. 14.18 Chronic asthma. (a) Types of chronic asthma. (b) A stepwise approach to the treatment of chronic asthma.

suppression and altered bone metabolism, when high doses are used. Oral prednisolone, usually given on alternate days to minimise the adverse effect on height, is required only in severe persistent asthma where other treatment has failed. Sodium cromoglicate, which stabilises the mast cell and is exceptionally free of side-effects, is now seldom used, as inhaled steroids have been shown to be much more effective. Long-acting β_2-agonists are prophylactic agents which, if given regularly, have a steroid-sparing effect. They are particularly effective for nocturnal or exercise-induced symptoms. Slow-release oral theophylline may also be useful as an adjuvant to inhaled steroids. However, it has a high incidence of side-effects (vomiting, insomnia, headaches, poor concentration) and blood levels need to be monitored, so is now rarely used in children. Leukotriene modulators may be helpful add-on therapy when inhaled steroids fail to control symptoms. Antibiotics are of no value in the absence of a bacterial infection. Cough medicines and decongestants are unhelpful. Antihistamines, e.g. loratadine and nasal steroids, are useful in the treatment of allergic rhinitis, and this may improve the control of coexisting asthma.

Non-pharmacological measures

Although many children's asthma is precipitated or worsened by specific allergens, complete avoidance of the allergen is difficult. The value of many commonly used allergen avoidance measures such as regular dusting, removal of feather or woollen bedding and wrapping of mattresses in plastic to reduce the level of housedust mites is unproven, as even low levels

CHOOSING THE CORRECT INHALER

Many children fail to gain the benefit of their treatment because they cannot use the inhaler they have been given. The child's age is often the best guide as to whether it will be possible to use a particular device. Of all the inhalers available, the pressurised metered-dose inhaler (MDI) requires the greatest coordination and is the least efficient. MDIs alone should not be used in children. Dry-powder inhalers, e.g. terbutaline sulphate (Bricanyl Turbohaler) and salbutamol (Ventolin Accuhaler), require less coordination than MDIs and are suitable for school-age children (Fig. 14.19). Using an MDI through a spacer device such as the Nebuhaler or Volumatic increases the proportion of the drug reaching the airways, reduces impaction of drug on the throat and requires less coordination. In children below the age of 2 years, a soft face mask can be attached to the spacer (Fig. 14.20). Spacers are very effective at delivering bronchodilators and inhaled steroids to the preschool child. Children who need inhaled therapy, but who are unable to use any of these devices or require high doses, may need a nebuliser for drug delivery at home (Fig. 14.21), but this is rarely necessary with expert guidance. Because of the worldwide ban on chlorofluorocarbons (CFCs) as a propellant, these old MDIs will be phased out by 2003. They will be replaced by MDIs containing hydrofluoro-alkaline (HFA), which does not damage the ozone layer of the atmosphere. HFA containing MDIs may be more effective than the old ones.

> **The correct way to use an inhaler must be demonstrated and the child's ability to use it checked.**

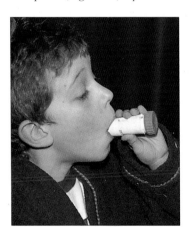

Fig. 14.19 4–10 years old: dry-powder inhaler as shown or metered dose inhaler with spacer.

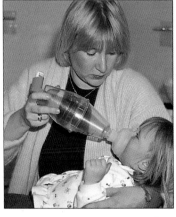

Fig. 14.20 <4 years old: metered dose inhaler with spacer. Use a mask if <2 years old.

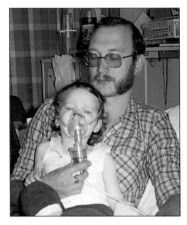

Fig. 14.21 Nebulisers deliver high-dose therapy and are used in severe acute attacks.

may be sufficient to provoke symptoms. Pets present a difficult problem. Whilst some children react immediately and obviously to exposure to a pet, in others there is chronic bronchial hyperreactivity which is difficult to attribute to the pet. A trial period of several months without the pet cat or dog can be considered but may cause family upset. A thorough cleaning of carpets and furniture to remove danders and banning the pet from bedrooms can be recommended. Parents should be advised about the harmful effects of cigarette smoking in the house. Parental cigarette smoking markedly increases the frequency and severity of symptoms of childhood asthma. Although exercise improves general fitness, there is no evidence that physical training improves asthma itself.

Acute asthma

With each acute attack, the duration of symptoms, the treatment already given and the course of previous attacks should be noted. It can be difficult to assess the severity of an acute asthma:

- Wheeze and respiratory rate are poor indicators of severity.
- Contraction of the sternomastoids, chest recession and pulse rate are better guides.
- The presence of marked pulsus paradoxus (the difference between systolic pressure on inspiration and expiration) indicates significant airways obstruction in children but is difficult to measure accurately.
- If breathlessness interferes with talking, the attack is severe.
- Cyanosis is a late sign, indicating life-threatening asthma.

In the assessment of severity:
- Arterial oxygen saturation should be measured with a pulse oximeter in all children presenting to hospital with acute asthma.
- Measurement of the peak expiratory flow rate should be routine in school-age children.

The features of a severe and life-threatening acute attack are shown in Figure 14.22.

Fig. 14.22 Features of severe and life-threatening acute asthma.

Severe
Too breathless to talk or feed
Respirations >50/min
Pulse >140/min
Peak flow <50% predicted or best value

Life-threatening
Peak flow <33% predicted or best value
Fatigue, agitation, drowsiness
Cyanosis, silent chest or poor respiratory effort

Criteria for hospital admission

Children require hospital admission if, after high-dose inhaled bronchodilator therapy, they:

- have not responded adequately clinically
- are exhausted
- still have a marked reduction in their predicted (or usual) peak flow rate
- have a reduced oxygen saturation (<92% in air).

A chest X-ray is indicated only if there is severe dyspnoea or unusual features (e.g. asymmetry of chest signs suggesting pneumothorax, lobar collapse) or signs of severe infection. In children, arterial blood gases are only indicated in life-threatening or refractory cases.

Treatment

Acute breathlessness is frightening for both the child and the parents. Calm and skilful management (Fig. 14.23) is the key to their reassurance. High-dose inhaled bronchodilators, steroids and oxygen form the foundation of therapy of severe acute asthma.

As soon as the diagnosis has been made, the child should be given a β_2 bronchodilator. For severe exacerbations, high-dose 'burst' therapy should be given with three doses given back-to-back. In the past, high doses of bronchodilators were always given by nebulisers. Recent evidence indicates that 5–10 puffs of bronchodilator from a pressurised aerosol given one puff at a time through a spacer is equally effective. The addition of nebulised ipratropium to the initial therapy in severe asthma has been shown to be beneficial. Oxygen is given when there is any evidence of arterial oxygen desaturation. A short course (2–5 days) of oral prednisolone expedites recovery from severe acute asthma.

Intravenous therapy has a role in the minority of children who fail to respond adequately to inhaled

Fig. 14.23 Summary of the treatment of acute severe or life-threatening asthma.

Immediate treatment
Oxygen via a face mask
Salbutamol (5 mg) or terbutaline (5 mg) via oxygen-driven nebuliser (half dose if <5 years old) – three back-to-back nebulisers
Ipratropium nebulised 250 μg
Oral prednisolone (1–2 mg/kg; maximum dose 40 mg)

Life-threatening features
Intravenous aminophylline (5 mg/kg, over 20 min, then continuously 1 mg/kg per h) or salbutamol (15 μg/kg over 10 min)
Intravenous hydrocortisone (100 mg q.i.d.)

Subsequent management
Oxygen if S_aO_2 <94%
Repeat β_2-agonist 1–4 hourly
Monitor peak flow and oxygen saturation

bronchodilator. Aminophylline is usually used for this purpose, but there is increasing evidence of the greater efficacy of intravenous salbutamol. For intravenous aminophylline, a loading dose is given over 20 min, followed by continuous infusion. Seizures, severe vomiting and fatal cardiac arrhythmias may follow a rapid infusion. If the child is already on oral theophylline, the loading dose should be omitted. With both aminophylline and salbutamol, the ECG should be monitored and blood electrolytes checked. Antibiotics are only given if there are clinical features of bacterial infection. Occasionally, these measures are insufficient and artificial ventilation is required.

After an acute exacerbation, the nature of the precipitant should be considered and the child's maintenance treatment and inhaler technique should be reviewed and altered if inadequate. Structured discharge planning can reduce the readmission rate for acute asthma. Follow-up arrangements should be made to monitor progress by the general practitioner or, for the more problematic patients, by a paediatrician.

Patient education

In order for families to make rational decisions, they need to know:

- when drugs should be used (regularly or 'as required')
- how to use the drug (inhaler technique)
- what each drug does (relief vs. prevention)
- how often and how much can be used (frequency and dosage)
- what to do if asthma worsens (management of acute attacks).

The child and parents need to know that increasing cough, wheeze and breathlessness and difficulty in walking, talking and sleeping, or decreasing relief from bronchodilators all indicate poorly controlled asthma. Some asthmatics find it difficult to perceive gradual deterioration – measurement of peak flow rate at home allows earlier recognition. Parents need to know when to start steroids at home and what dose to give. A personalised, written, self-management plan from the doctor reduces confusion, improves compliance and reduces hospital admissions. Information booklets about asthma for children and parents are useful, but are not a replacement for individual explanation. Nurse specialists have an important role in patient education.

RECURRENT COUGH

Cough is the most common symptom of respiratory disease and indicates irritation of nerve receptors in the pharynx, larynx, trachea or large bronchi. While recurrent cough may simply indicate that the child is having recurrent respiratory infections, other causes need to be considered (Fig. 14.24).

Asthma is the commonest cause of recurrent cough in childhood. Although there is usually associated

Fig. 14.24 Causes of recurrent or persistent cough.

Recurrent respiratory infections
Asthma
Allergic rhinitis
Infection (e.g. pertussis, RSV, *Mycoplasma*)
Recurrent aspiration (+/– gastro-oesophageal reflux)
Cigarette smoking (active or passive)
Inhaled foreign body
Suppurative lung diseases (e.g. cystic fibrosis or ciliary dyskinesia)
Tuberculosis
Habit cough

wheeze and breathlessness triggered by characteristic factors, in the preschool child a troublesome night-time cough may sometimes be the only symptom. Many children have a persistent nasal discharge due to allergic rhinitis; their nocturnal cough may be due to their postnasal drip or may be caused by coexisting asthma. A trial of therapy with a bronchodilator or topical nasal steroid may be required to make the diagnosis.

Certain infections (e.g. pertussis, RSV and *Mycoplasma* infection) can cause a cough that persists for weeks or months, long after the infective organism has disappeared. Persistent cough after an acute infection may indicate cystic fibrosis or unresolved lobar collapse, which will be seen on a chest X-ray. In any child with a severe, persistent cough, TB should be excluded with a chest X-ray and tuberculin skin (Mantoux) test.

Aspiration of feeds may cause coughing and wheeze. This may be caused by gastro-oesophageal reflux in infants or as a result of swallowing disorders, e.g. in children with cerebral palsy.

Some older children and adolescents develop a barking, unproductive, habit cough after an infection or an asthma attack. The cough characteristically disappears during sleep. Reassurance and explanation after a thorough examination are usually effective.

The importance of parental smoking on children is generally underestimated. If both parents smoke, young children are twice as likely to have recurrent cough and wheeze than in non-smoking households. In the older child, active smoking is common – 10% of 13-year-olds and 21% of 15-year-olds smoke regularly.

CHRONIC LUNG INFECTION

Children with recurrent pneumonia or who produce purulent sputum may have bronchiectasis, which is permanent dilatation of the bronchi. It can be localised or present throughout the lung. Cystic fibrosis, primary ciliary dyskinesia and immunodeficiency must be considered. Bronchiectasis following severe pneumonia, particularly tuberculosis, pertussis or measles, has now become uncommon. Nevertheless, as it can

FOREIGN BODY INHALATION

A previously well 3-year-old boy presented with a 5-day history of severe cough and wheeze. His symptoms developed after choking on some peanuts. A chest X-ray revealed a hyperlucent right lung (Fig. 14.25). Bronchoscopy was performed and revealed a peanut wedged in the right main bronchus.

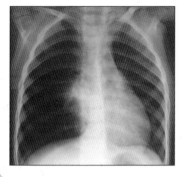

Fig. 14.25 Hyperlucency of the right lung and mediastinal shift to the left. (Courtesy of Dr Abbas Khakoo.)

follow pneumonia, it is prudent to do a repeat chest X-ray 4–6 weeks after an acute pneumonia to ensure that any collapse or consolidation has resolved, particularly if cough persists.

Tuberculosis remains an important cause of chronic lung infection and all children with a persistent productive cough should have a chest X-ray and tuberculin skin test. Marked hilar or paratracheal lymphadenopathy is highly suggestive of tuberculosis.

Failure of pneumonia to resolve may also indicate an underlying inhaled foreign body (e.g. peanut), in which case a bronchoscopy should be carried out to remove the object (see Case history 14.2). Persistent infection also occurs where there is a congenital abnormality of the lungs, such as congenital cysts or a sequestrated lobe.

The microcilia of the respiratory epithelium are an important defence against infection. Children with primary ciliary dyskinesia, in which there are abnormalities of ciliary structure or function, have recurrent infection of the upper and lower respiratory tract. They characteristically have recurrent productive cough, a purulent nasal discharge and chronic ear infections; 50% also have dextrocardia and situs inversus (Kartagener's syndrome). Ciliary structure can be assessed by electron microscopy of nasal mucosal brushings.

Children with immunodeficiency may develop severe, unusual or recurrent chest infections. The immune deficiency may be secondary to an illness, e.g. malignant disease or its treatment with chemotherapy. Less commonly it is due to HIV infection or a primary immune deficiency.

CYSTIC FIBROSIS

Cystic fibrosis (CF) is the commonest cause of chronic suppurative lung disease in Caucasians. In the past, CF led to death in early childhood from progressive bronchiectasis and respiratory failure, but with improved antibiotic and nutritional therapy, survival into mid-adult life can now be expected for most patients.

CF is an autosomal recessive disease. In Caucasians the carrier rate is 1 in 25, with 1 in 2500 affected births. The disease is much less common in other ethnic groups. A gene located on chromosome 7 codes for the protein called cystic fibrosis transmembrane regulator (CFTR), which is defective in CF. CFTR is a cyclic AMP-dependent chloride channel blocker. Over 800 different gene mutations have been discovered in CF, but the ΔF508 mutation is found in 78% of cases in the UK. Identification of the gene mutation involved within a family allows prenatal diagnosis and carrier detection in the wider family.

In CF, the abnormal ion transport across the epithelial cells of the exocrine glands of the respiratory tract and pancreas results in increased viscosity of secretions. Abnormal function of the sweat glands results in excessive concentrations of sodium and chloride in the sweat (80–125 mmol/L in cystic fibrosis, 10–14 mmol/L in normal children). This forms the basis of the essential diagnostic procedure, the sweat test, in which sweating is stimulated by pilocarpine iontophoresis. The sweat is collected into a special capillary tube or absorbed onto a weighed piece of filter paper. Diagnostic errors are common if there is an inadequate volume of sweat collected, so two tests with an adequate volume of sweat should be performed by experienced staff. Thick and viscid mucus is not the only basis of the pathogenesis of CF. Abnormality of the CFTR also affects inflammatory processes and defence against infection.

Clinical features
Most children with CF present with malabsorption and failure to thrive from birth, accompanied by recurrent or persistent chest infections (Fig. 14.26). In the lungs, viscid mucus in the smaller airways predisposes to chronic infection, initially with *Staph. aureus* and *H. influenzae* and subsequently with *Pseudomonas* species. This leads to damage of the bronchial wall, bronchiectasis and abscess formation (Fig. 14.27). The child has a persistent, loose cough productive of purulent sputum. On examination there is hyperinflation of the chest due to air trapping, coarse crepitations or expiratory rhonchi. With established disease, there is finger clubbing.

About 10–20% of CF infants present in the neonatal period with meconium ileus, in which inspissated meconium causes intestinal obstruction with vomiting, abdominal distension and failure to pass meconium in the first few days of life. Over 90% of children with CF have malabsorption and steatorrhoea due to insufficiency of the pancreatic exocrine enzymes (lipase, amylase and proteases). This leads to failure to

Fig. 14.26 Clinical features of cystic fibrosis.

Infancy
Meconium ileus in newborn period
Prolonged neonatal jaundice
Failure to thrive
Recurrent chest infections
Malabsorption, steatorrhoea

Young child
Bronchiectasis
Rectal prolapse
Nasal polyp
Sinusitis

Older child and adolescent
Diabetes mellitus (often not insulin-dependent)
Cirrhosis and portal hypertension
Distal intestinal obstruction (DIOS, meconium ileus
  equivalent)
Pneumothorax or recurrent haemoptysis
Aspergillosis
Sterility in males
Increasing psychological problems

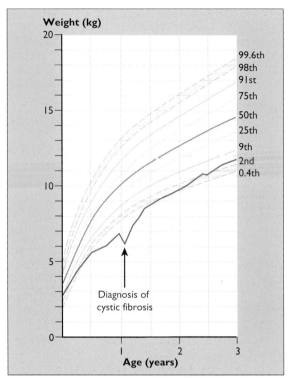

Fig. 14.28 Growth chart of a child with cough and recurrent wheeze. Only when the diagnosis of cystic fibrosis was made and appropriate treatment started did he gain weight. (Adapted from growth chart © Child Growth Foundation.)

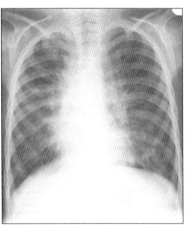

Fig. 14.27
A chest X ray in cystic fibrosis showing hyperexpansion, marked peribronchial shadowing, bronchial wall thickening and ring shadows.

thrive (Fig. 14.28) in spite of a voracious appetite. They may pass large, pale, very offensive and greasy stools several times a day.

Management

The effective management of CF requires a multidisciplinary team approach, including paediatricians, physiotherapists, dieticians, nursing staff, the primary care team, teachers and, most importantly, the child and parents. All patients with CF should be periodically reviewed in a specialist centre. The condition cannot be cured. The principal aims of therapy are to prevent progression of the lung disease and to maintain adequate nutrition and growth.

Respiratory management

Children should have physiotherapy at least twice a day, depending on the amount of sputum they produce.

Parents are taught to perform chest percussion and postural drainage at home to reduce the accumulation of secretions. Older patients can carry out their own physiotherapy using self-percussion and deep breathing exercises. Physical exercise should be encouraged, as it helps to strengthen chest muscles and avoids reaccumulation of secretions.

Persistent bacterial chest infection is the major problem. Most centres recommend continuous oral antibiotics with prompt and vigorous intravenous therapy for acute exacerbations to limit lung damage. Nebulised antibiotics are used in patients colonised with *Pseudomonas*. Acute exacerbations are treated with intermittent intravenous antibiotic therapy. To facilitate this, a central venous catheter with a subcutaneous port of access (e.g. Portacath) is often implanted. This allows the antibiotics to be given at home, provided there is appropriate community support. Up to one-third of children have reversible airways obstruction and may benefit from bronchodilators or inhaled steroids. Mucolytics are expensive and of uncertain benefit.

Nutritional management

Dietary status should be assessed regularly. Pancreatic insufficiency is treated with oral enteric-coated pancreatic supplements taken with all meals and snacks. Dosage is adjusted according to clinical response.

A high-calorie diet is essential not only to compensate for malabsorption but because the energy requirement of children with CF is 30–40% above normal. To achieve this, overnight feeding via a gastrostomy is increasingly used. Fat-soluble vitamin supplements are routinely given.

Teenagers and adults

Most CF sufferers now survive into adult life. The improved survival rate has been accompanied by a change in a range of problems seen. In addition to recurrent chest infections, other late complications include pneumothorax, haemoptysis, diabetes and liver disease. In distal intestinal obstruction syndrome (meconium ileus equivalent), viscid mucofaeculent material obstructs the bowel. Most adolescents have persistent *Pseudomonas* infection. Some become colonised with a particularly virulent organism, *Burkholderia cepacia*, which is often accompanied by a marked decline in lung function. Spread is from person to person; to limit transmission, CF patents are segregated and advised not to socialise with other CF sufferers.

Males are usually infertile due to abnormalities of the vas deferens. Women have reduced fertility but many have had successful pregnancies. They should be cautioned that their breast milk has a high sodium concentration.

The psychological repercussions on the affected child and family of a chronic and ultimately fatal illness which requires regular physiotherapy and drugs, frequent hospital admissions and absences from school are considerable. The team should provide psychological and emotional support. Adolescents have particular needs which must receive special consideration.

Heart–lung transplantation has been successful in patients with CF in terminal respiratory failure, but is available to only a minority. Gene therapy (see p. 94) is currently being assessed but is unlikely to be of practical value in the foreseeable future.

Screening

Screening of all newborn infants for CF is now possible, but the benefits remain controversial and it is not routinely performed throughout the UK. Immunoreactive trypsin (IRT) is raised in CF patients and can be measured in routine blood taken for biochemical screening of all babies (Guthrie test). A positive test requires confirmation with a sweat test and counselling of parents. As with all screening tests, the false-positive and false-negative rates are important in determining whether a mass programme is likely to be worthwhile. Identifying cases in the neonatal period allows the early introduction of prophylactic antibiotics and prompt recognition and treatment of any respiratory infections. It also allows early nutritional management, which will avoid the child failing to thrive. It also enables early genetic counselling for the parents about the 1 in 4 risk of recurrence and the possibility of prenatal diagnosis in future pregnancies.

Cystic fibrosis should be considered in any child with recurrent chest infections, loose stools and failure to thrive.

FURTHER READING

British Thoracic Society 1997 The British guidelines on asthma management. Thorax, 52 (Suppl.): S1–21.
Couriel J M 1998 Respiratory infections in children. In: Ellis M (ed) Infections of the respiratory tract. Cambridge University Press, Cambridge. *Review chapter*
Couriel J, Child F 1999 Paediatric asthma – an interactive CD-Rom. Royal Society of Medicine Press, London
Silverman M 2001 Childhood asthma and other wheezing disorders. Chapman Hall, London
Taussig L, Landau L 1999 Textbook of pediatric respiratory medicine. Mosby, St Louis. *Definitive textbook*

15

Cardiac disorders

Whereas heart disease in adults is mostly acquired in origin, in children it is mostly congenital. The exception is rheumatic heart disease, which is rare in developed countries but remains a major cause of heart disease in some developing countries.

Congenital heart disease is the most common single group of structural malformations in infants:

- 6–8 per 1000 live-born infants have significant malformations
- some abnormality of the cardiovascular system, e.g. a bicuspid aortic valve, is present in 10–20 per 1000 live births
- about 1 in 10 stillborn infants have a cardiac anomaly.

The eight most common anomalies account for over 80% of all lesions (Fig. 15.1), but:

- about 10–15% have complex lesions with more than one cardiac abnormality
- about 10–15% also have a non-cardiac abnormality.

Until relatively recently, the investigation of congenital heart lesions involved invasive catheter studies and the outcome for most serious lesions was poor. This situation has been transformed and now:

- antenatal ultrasound increasingly offers early diagnosis
- most structural defects are diagnosed non-invasively by echocardiography
- even complex defects can often be corrected completely at the initial operation, e.g. transposition of the great arteries.
- an increasing number of defects are treated non-invasively, e.g. patent ductus arteriosus
- the overall infant cardiac surgical mortality has been reduced from approximately 20% in 1970 to 5% in 1999.

Fig. 15.1 The eight most common congenital heart lesions.

Non-cyanotic
Ventricular septal defect (VSD) 32%
Patent ductus arteriosus (PDA) 12%
Pulmonary stenosis 8%
Atrial septal defect (ASD) 6%
Coarctation of the aorta 6%
Aortic stenosis 5%

Cyanotic
Tetralogy of Fallot 6%
Transposition of the great arteries 5%

AETIOLOGY

Little is known about the aetiology of congenital heart disease. A small proportion are related to external teratogens (Fig. 15.2). About 8% are associated with major chromosomal abnormalities (Fig. 15.3), but recently more subtle chromosomal abnormalities have been identified, e.g. abnormalities of chromosome 22 have been detected in many patients with aortic arch abnormalities. The less obvious, polygenic abnormalities probably explain why family members of affected individuals have a slightly increased incidence of congenital heart disease.

Congenital heart disease is the most common group of structural malformations in children.

Fig. 15.2 Some cardiovascular teratogens.

Teratogen	Cardiac abnormalities	Frequency
Maternal disorders		
Rubella	Peripheral pulmonary stenosis, PDA	30–35%
Systemic lupus erythematosus (SLE)	Complete heart block (anti-Ro antibody)	35%
Alcoholism (fetal alcohol syndrome)	ASD, VSD, Tetralogy of Fallot	25%
Diabetes	Incidence increased overall	2%
Drugs		
Warfarin	Pulmonary valve stenosis, PDA	5%

ASD, atrial septal defect; PDA, patent ductus arteriosus; VSD, ventricular septal defect.

Fig. 15.3 Chromosomal abnormalities and congenital heart disease.

Chromosomal abnormality	Incidence	Type
Down's syndrome (trisomy 21)	40%	Atrioventricular septal defect (40%), VSD (30%), ASD (10%), Tetralogy of Fallot (6%)
Edwards' syndrome (trisomy 18)	60–80%	Complex
Patau's syndrome (trisomy 13)	60–80%	Complex
Turner's syndrome (45XO)	15%	Aortic valve stenosis, coarctation of the aorta
Chromome 22 microdeletion	—	Aortic arch anomalies

CIRCULATORY CHANGES AT BIRTH

In the fetus, the left atrial pressure is low, as relatively little blood returns from the lungs. The pressure in the right atrium is higher than in the left, as it receives all the systemic venous return including blood from the placenta. The flap valve of the foramen ovale is held open, blood flows across the atrial septum into the left atrium and then into the left ventricle, which in turn pumps it to the upper body (Fig. 15.4).

With the first breaths, resistance to pulmonary blood flow falls and the volume of blood flowing through the lungs increases sixfold. This results in a rise in the left atrial pressure. Meanwhile, the volume of blood returning to the right atrium falls as the placenta is excluded from the circulation. The change in the pressure difference causes the flap valve of the foramen ovale to be closed. The ductus arteriosus, which connects the pulmonary artery to the aorta in fetal life, will normally close within the first few hours or days. Some babies with congenital heart lesions rely on blood flow through the duct (duct-dependent circulation). Their clinical condition will deteriorate dramatically when the duct closes.

PRESENTATION

Congenital heart disease may present with:

- antenatal cardiac ultrasound diagnosis
- detection of a heart murmur
- cyanosis
- heart failure
- shock.

Antenatal diagnosis

The four-chamber view of the heart has become a routine part of the fetal anomaly scan widely performed in the UK between 18 and 20 weeks' gestation. It allows the detection of hypoplasia of the right or left side of the heart. Interpretation requires high-quality equipment and is highly operator-dependent. More detailed

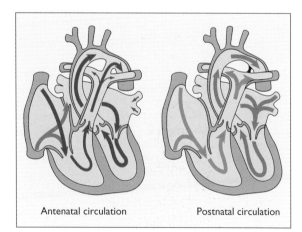

Fig. 15.4 Changes in the circulation from the fetus to the newborn. When congenital heart lesions rely on blood flow through the duct (a duct-dependent circulation), there will be dramatic deterioration in the clinical condition when the duct closes.

Antenatal circulation   Postnatal circulation

fetal echocardiography is performed at tertiary referral centres for high-risk pregnancies, e.g. a previous child with heart disease or if a cardiac abnormality has been identified on routine scanning. Most, but not all, complex abnormalities can be diagnosed. This detailed echocardiography allows the parents to be reassured or counselled appropriately and, if the pregnancy is continued, postnatal management can be planned.

Heart murmurs

The most common presentation of congenital heart disease is with a heart murmur. However, the vast majority of children with murmurs have a normal heart. They have an 'innocent murmur', which can be heard at some time in almost 30% of children. It is obviously important to be able to distinguish an innocent murmur from a pathological one. There are two types of innocent murmur:

- Ejection murmur – generated in the ventricle, outflow tracts or great vessels on either side of the heart by turbulent blood flow. They are not associated with any structural abnormality.
- Venous hum – from turbulent blood flow in the head and neck veins. It is a continuous low-pitched rumble heard beneath either clavicle. It may increase on inspiration and will be louder after exercise. It may be mistaken for a patent ductus arteriosus, but can be distinguished by its disappearance on lying flat or with compression of the jugular veins on the ipsilateral side.

Hallmarks of an innocent ejection murmur are:
- soft blowing systolic murmur (usually from the right side pulmonary outflow in the second left interspace) or short 'buzzing' murmur (usually from the left side of the heart – aortic blood flow – in the fourth left interspace)
- localised to left sternal edge
- no diastolic component
- no radiation
- normal heart sounds with no added sounds
- no parasternal thrill
- asymptomatic patient.

During a febrile illness, innocent murmurs are often heard because of increased cardiac output.

Differentiating between innocent and significant murmurs can be difficult. If a murmur is thought to be significant, or if there is uncertainty about whether it is innocent, the child should be seen by an experienced paediatrician to decide about referral to a paediatric cardiologist for echocardiography. A chest X-ray and ECG occasionally help with the diagnosis.

Many newborn infants with potential shunts have neither symptoms nor a murmur at birth, as the pulmonary vascular resistance is still high. Therefore conditions such as a ventricular septal defect or patent ductus arteriosus may only become apparent at several weeks of age when the pulmonary vascular resistance falls.

Cyanosis

Peripheral cyanosis (blueness of the hands and feet) may occur when a child is cold or unwell from any cause. This should be distinguished from central cyanosis, seen on the tongue, which is associated with a fall in arterial blood oxygen tension. It can be recognised clinically if the concentration of reduced haemoglobin in the blood exceeds 5 g/dl, so it is less pronounced if the child is anaemic. Persistent arterial desaturation in an otherwise well infant is nearly always a sign of structural heart disease. An exception to this is persistent pulmonary hypertension of the newborn (persistent fetal circulation), when there may be profound cyanosis due to failure of the pulmonary vascular resistance to fall after birth. In infants with respiratory distress, cyanosis may be due to respiratory disease or polycythaemia.

In the neonatal period, cardiac cyanosis may be caused by (Fig. 15.5):

- Reduced pulmonary blood flow – infants may have a duct-dependent pulmonary circulation that relies on blood flowing from left to right across the ductus arteriosus (e.g. see Fig. 15.6). They become severely cyanosed when the duct closes shortly after birth. Maintenance of ductal patency is the key to the early survival of these children. This is achieved with intravenous prostaglandin (E), while monitoring for potential side-effects – apnoea, jitteriness and seizures, flushing, vasodilatation and hypotension.

Fig. 15.5 Causes of neonatal cyanosis.

Reduced or duct-dependent pulmonary circulation
Tetralogy of Fallot (severe)
Pulmonary atresia
Tricuspid atresia

Abnormal mixing
Transposition of the great arteries
Total anomalous pulmonary venous drainage

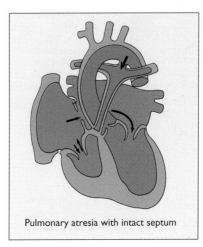

Pulmonary atresia with intact septum

Fig. 15.6 The pulmonary circulation is maintained by blood flowing left to right across the duct – an example of a duct-dependent pulmonary circulation.

- Abnormal mixing of systemic venous and pulmonary venous blood – most infants present with cyanosis in the first day or two of life. In transposition of the great arteries, the systemic and pulmonary circulations are in parallel but there must be some mixing of blood between the two circulations.

The diagnosis of cyanotic congenital heart disease can be confirmed by the nitrogen washout test if detailed echocardiography is not readily available. The infant is placed in 100% oxygen for 10 min. If the right radial arterial Po_2 remains low (<15 kPa, 113 mmHg) after this time, a diagnosis of 'cyanotic' congenital heart disease can be made if lung disease and persistent pulmonary hypertension of the newborn (persistent fetal circulation) have been excluded. Alternatively, if the oxygen saturation on a pulse oximeter is less than 85%, cyanotic congenital heart disease is likely, but this is a less sensitive indicator.

 Heart failure

Heart failure is difficult to define but in children is best summarised as a clinical syndrome.

Symptoms
- Breathlessness (particularly on feeding or exertion)
- Sweating
- Poor feeding
- Recurrent chest infections.

Signs
- Poor weight gain or 'failure to thrive'
- Tachypnoea
- Tachycardia
- Heart murmur, gallop rhythm
- Enlarged heart
- Hepatomegaly
- Cool peripheries.

Heart failure in the neonatal period (Fig. 15.7) usually results from left heart obstruction e.g. coarctation of the aorta. If the obstructive lesion is very severe then arterial perfusion may be predominantly by right-to-left flow of blood via the arterial duct, so-called duct-dependent systemic circulation (e.g. see Fig. 15.8).

Fig. 15.7 Causes of heart failure.

1. Neonates – obstructed (duct-dependent) systemic circulation
Hypoplastic left heart syndrome
Critical aortic valve stenosis
Severe coarctation of the aorta
Interruption of the aortic arch

2. Infants
Ventricular septal defect
Atrioventricular septal defect
Large patent ductus arteriosus

CASE HISTORY 15.1

SHOCK

A 3-day-old baby had been discharged home the day after delivery following a normal routine examination. He suddenly collapsed and was rushed to hospital. He was pale, with grey lips.

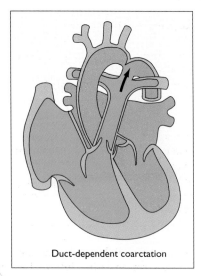

Fig. 15.8 The systemic circulation is maintained by blood flowing right to left across the ductus arteriosus – a duct-dependent systemic circulation.

Duct-dependent coarctation

The right brachial pulse could just be felt, the femoral pulses were impalpable. Blood gases showed a severe metabolic acidosis. He was ventilated and treated with volume support, inotropes and sodium bicarbonate. Blood cultures were taken, a suprapubic aspiration of urine performed and antibiotics started for possible sepsis. Blood and urine samples were taken for an amino acid screen and urine for organic acids. As the femoral pulses remained impalpable, a prostaglandin infusion was started. Within 2 hours he was pink and well perfused and the acidosis had almost resolved. Severe coarctation of the aorta (Fig. 15.8) was diagnosed on echocardiography. He had developed shock from left heart outflow tract obstruction once the arterial duct had closed.

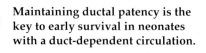

Maintaining ductal patency is the key to early survival in neonates with a duct-dependent circulation.

CASE HISTORY 15.2

HEART FAILURE

A 5-week-old female infant was referred to hospital because of wheezing, poor feeding and poor weight gain during the previous 2 weeks. Before this, she had been well. Her routine neonatal examination had been normal. She was tachypnoeic (50–60 breaths/min) and there was some sternal and intercostal recession. The pulses were normal. There was a thrill, a loud pansystolic murmur at the lower left sternal edge and a slightly accentuated pulmonary component to the second heart sound. There were scattered wheezes. The liver was enlarged, palpable at 4 cm below the costal margin. The ECG was unremarkable. The chest X-ray showed cardiomegaly and increased pulmonary vascular markings. An echocardiogram showed a moderate-sized ventricular septal defect (VSD) (Fig. 15.9). Treatment was with diuretics. The VSD closed spontaneously at 11 months.

This infant developed heart failure from a VSD presenting at several weeks of age when the pulmonary resistance fell, causing increased left-to-right shunting of blood.

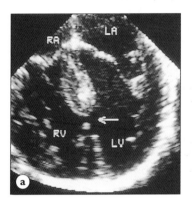
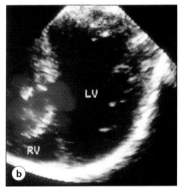
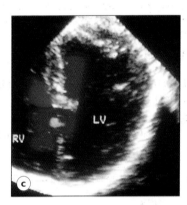

Fig. 15.9 (a) Echocardiogram showing a medium-sized muscular ventricular septal defect (arrow). (b) The colour Doppler shows a left-to-right shunt (blue) during systole. (c) There is also a small right-to-left shunt (red) during diastole (RA, right atrium; LA, left atrium; RV, right ventricle; LV, left ventricle).

Closure of the duct under these circumstances rapidly leads to severe acidosis, collapse and death unless ductal patency is restored (Case history 15.1).

Beyond the neonatal period, progressive heart failure is most likely due to a left-to-right shunt (Case history 15.2). During the first few weeks of life, as the pulmonary vascular resistance falls, there is a progressive increase in pulmonary blood flow. Symptoms of heart failure will increase up to the age of about 6 months, but may subsequently improve as the pulmonary vascular resistance rises in response to the left-to-right shunt. If left untreated, some of these children may develop Eisenmenger's syndrome, which is irreversibly raised pulmonary vascular resistance resulting from chronically raised pulmonary arterial pressure and flow. If this develops, the only surgical option is a heart–lung transplant.

DIAGNOSIS

If congenital heart disease is suspected, a chest X-ray and ECG (Fig. 15.10) should be performed. Although rarely diagnostic, they may be helpful in establishing

Fig. 15.10 ECGs in children.

Important features
Arrythmias
Superior QRS axis (negative deflection in AVF) (Fig. 15.11e)
Right ventricular hypertrophy (upright T wave in V_1, over 1 month of age) (Fig. 15.12d)
Left ventricular strain (inverted T wave in V_6) (Fig. 15.17d)

Pitfalls
P wave morphology is rarely helpful in children
Partial right bundle branch block – most are normal children, although it is common in ASD
Left ventricular hypertrophy is difficult to define

ASD, atrial septal defect.

that there is an abnormality of the cardiovascular system and as a baseline for assessing future changes. Echocardiography, combined with Doppler ultrasound, enables almost all causes of congenital heart disease to be diagnosed. Cardiac catheterisation is seldom required to make the diagnosis and is now reserved for haemodynamic measurements and therapy.

> **A normal chest X-ray and ECG does not exclude congenital heart disease.**

NON-CYANOTIC CONGENITAL HEART DISEASE

Atrial septal defect

There are two main types of atrial septal defect (ASD):

- ostium secundum (Fig. 15.11a)
- ostium primum (Fig. 15.11b).

Both present with similar symptoms and signs, but their anatomy is quite different. The ostium secundum defect is a deficiency of the foramen ovale and the surrounding atrial septum. The ostium primum defect is a deficiency of the atrioventricular septum and is characterised by:

- an inter-atrial communication between the bottom end of the atrial septum and the atrioventricular valves
- an abnormal atrioventricular junction
- abnormal atrioventricular valves (a trileaflet left atrioventricular valve is its hallmark).

Clinical features
Symptoms
- None (commonly)
- Recurrent chest infections/wheeze
- Heart failure
- Arrhythmias (fourth decade onwards).

ATRIAL SEPTAL DEFECT

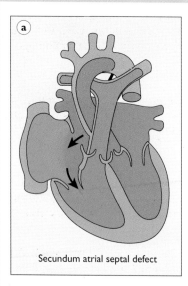

Secundum atrial septal defect

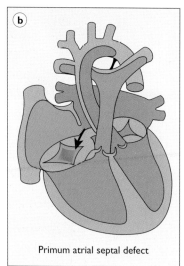

Primum atrial septal defect

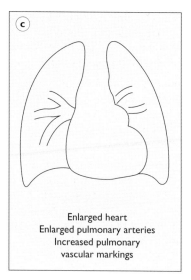

Enlarged heart
Enlarged pulmonary arteries
Increased pulmonary
vascular markings

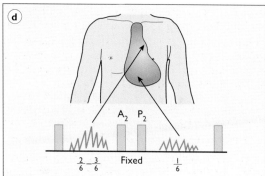

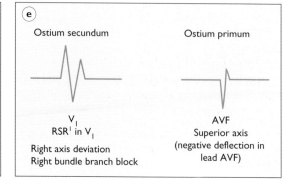

Ostium secundum

V$_1$
RSR^1 in V$_1$

Right axis deviation
Right bundle branch block

Ostium primum

AVF
Superior axis
(negative deflection in
lead AVF)

Fig. 15.11 (a) The ostium secundum atrial septal defect (ASD) is a deficiency of the foramen ovale and surrounding atrial septum. (b) The ostium primum ASD is a deficiency of the atrioventricular septum. (c) Murmur. (d) Chest X-ray. (e) ECG.

Physical signs (Fig. 15.11c)
- A fixed and widely split second heart sound – due to the right ventricular stroke volume being equal in both inspiration and expiration
- An ejection systolic murmur best heard in the third left intercostal space – due to increased flow across the right ventricular outflow tract because of the left-to-right shunt
- A rumbling mid-diastolic murmur best heard at the lower left sternal edge – due to increased flow across the tricuspid valve, because of the left-to-right shunt at atrial level.

Investigations
Chest X-ray (Fig. 15.11d)
May show cardiomegaly, an enlarged pulmonary artery and increased pulmonary vascular markings, all non-specific features.

ECG (Fig. 15.11e)
May provide a strong diagnostic clue. With an ostium secundum ASD, there will be sinus rhythm with right axis deviation due to right ventricular enlargement. Right ventricular hypertrophy is uncommon. Partial or complete right bundle branch block is common but may occur in normal children. When there is a primum ASD, the most characteristic feature is the presence of left axis deviation, a so-called 'superior' QRS axis.

Cross-sectional echocardiography
Will delineate the anatomy, although in some older teenagers and adults transoesophageal echocardiography may be required to demonstrate the atrial septum with precision.

Management
All children with symptoms and most with evidence of right atrial and right ventricular volume overload will be offered surgery or, for secundum defects, closure with an 'umbrella' device inserted percutaneously. Surgical closure is usually electively performed in the fourth or fifth year of life, with the intention of preventing right heart failure and arrhythmias in later life. This is a controversial issue – it has become routine to close nearly all ASDs but there are few data supporting its effectiveness particularly with increasing age.

Ventricular septal defects

Ventricular septal defects (VSDs) are common, accounting for 32% of all cases of congenital heart disease. There are two main types:

- perimembranous (adjacent to the tricuspid valve)
- muscular (completely surrounded by muscle) (Fig. 15.12a).

Presentation is usually early, with a loud murmur heard during routine clinical examination, but there may be symptoms of heart failure. Most will close spontaneously during the first few years of life, with fewer than 10% requiring surgical closure.

Clinical features
Symptoms
- Asymptomatic
- Heart failure with breathlessness and failure to thrive
- Recurrent chest infections
- Cyanosis (due to pulmonary vascular disease – now rare)
- Endocarditis (late).

Physical signs (Fig. 15.12b)
- Parasternal thrill
- Heart murmur at lower left sternal edge
  — loud pansystolic murmur when a small defect
  — unimpressive ejection murmur from flow across the pulmonary valve when a large defect
- Variable pulmonary component of second sound
  — normal when small defect
  — loud when large defect with pulmonary hypertension
- Tachypnoea, tachycardia and enlarged liver from heart failure.

Investigations
Chest X-ray (Fig. 15.12c)
Normal in small defects. With large defects, may be abnormal with cardiomegaly, enlarged pulmonary arteries, increased pulmonary vascular markings and pulmonary oedema.

ECG (Fig. 15.12d)
Also varies from normal to grossly abnormal. The most important abnormality is the presence of right ventricular hypertrophy, which always requires further investigation.

Echocardiography
Almost invariably demonstrates the precise anatomy of the defect. It should also be possible to assess its haemodynamic effects using Doppler ultrasound.

Management
Drug therapy for heart failure is only required for children with symptoms. Commonly used diuretics are furosemide (frusemide) or a thiazide and spironolactone. More recently, angiotensin-converting enzyme (ACE) inhibitors have been used in conjunction with diuretics. There is little evidence to suggest that digoxin is useful, and it is now less widely prescribed than in the past. There are two main reasons for performing surgery within the first year of life:

- severe symptoms with failure to thrive
- pulmonary hypertension with possible progression to pulmonary vascular disease.

In children with a large left-to-right shunt, increased pulmonary blood flow and pulmonary hypertension will ultimately lead to irreversible damage of the pulmonary capillary vascular bed. This pulmonary vascular disease usually becomes established in the second year of life, but Eisenmenger's syndrome, with cyanosis due to intracardiac shunting from right to

VENTRICULAR SEPTAL DEFECT

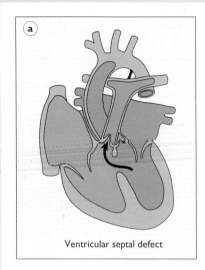

Ventricular septal defect

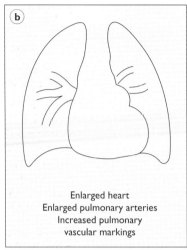

Enlarged heart
Enlarged pulmonary arteries
Increased pulmonary
vascular markings

Fig. 15.12 (a) Ventricular septal defect showing a left-to-right shunt. (b) Murmur. (c) Chest X-ray. (d) ECG.

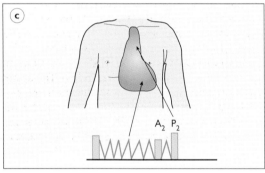

A₂ P₂

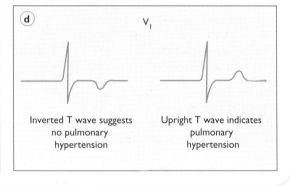

V₁

Inverted T wave suggests
no pulmonary
hypertension

Upright T wave indicates
pulmonary
hypertension

left, rarely evolves until the second decade (Fig. 15.13). It is therefore of critical importance to be able to recognise the development of pulmonary hypertension during infancy. The clinical hallmarks of pulmonary hypertension are:

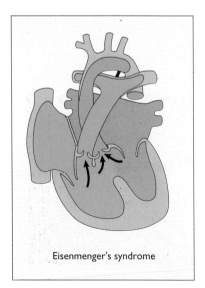

Fig. 15.13 Eisenmenger's syndrome with right-to-left shunting from pulmonary vascular disease following increased pulmonary blood flow and pulmonary hypertension.

Eisenmenger's syndrome

- a loud pulmonary component to the second heart sound
- right ventricular hypertrophy on ECG.

In general, a child with a long, loud pansystolic murmur and a normal pulmonary component to the second heart sound will not require surgery, even if symptomatic early in life. Even if asymptomatic, surgery will be required for any child with an unimpressive murmur but a loud pulmonary component to the second heart sound, implying a raised pulmonary arterial diastolic pressure.

> **Symptoms of heart failure from a VSD may initially resolve because of the development of pulmonary hypertension rather than the success of drug therapy.**

Atrioventricular septal defects

This is a special form of ventricular septal defect (Fig. 15.14) most commonly seen in children with Down's syndrome. There are many different forms,

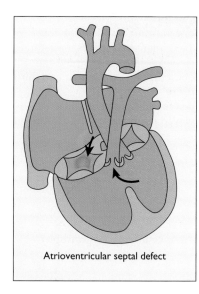

Fig. 15.14
Atrioventricular
septal defect.

Atrioventricular septal defect

All children with a VSD must be
given antibiotic prophylaxis to
prevent bacterial endocarditis.

Patent ductus arteriosus

The ductus arteriosus connects the pulmonary artery
to the descending aorta. Failure to close shortly after
birth frequently occurs in preterm neonates. In older
children, it is due to a defect in the constrictor mechanism of the duct. The flow of blood across a patent
ductus arteriosus (PDA) is from the aorta to the pulmonary artery (i.e. left to right), following the fall in
pulmonary vascular resistance after birth.

Clinical features

In preterm infants, a PDA may be suspected by detecting a bounding pulse (due to increased pulse pressure)
and a systolic murmur at the left sternal edge. When
severe, the resulting heart failure may make it difficult
to wean the infant from artificial ventilation.

Most older children present with a continuous murmur beneath the left clavicle (Fig. 15.15a). The murmur
continues into diastole because the pressure in the
pulmonary artery is lower than that in the aorta
throughout the cardiac cycle. The pulse pressure is
increased, causing a collapsing pulse. Symptoms are

ranging from a primum-type ASD to a complete atrioventricular septal defect (AVSD) with a coexisting
large VSD and a single common atrioventricular valve.
In these children, assessment and management are
the same as for VSD, although surgical correction is
more hazardous because of the complexity of the intracardiac repair. Children with Down's syndrome are
particularly liable to develop pulmonary hypertension
and AVSDs must be corrected early in infancy.

PATENT DUCTUS ARTERIOSUS

Fig. 15.15 Patent ductus arteriosus. (a) Murmur. (b) Chest X-ray. (c) ECG.
(d) A patent ductus arteriosus visualised on angiography. (e) A coil used to
close small ducts. It is passed through a catheter via the femoral vein
(f) Angiogram to show coil in the duct. (PT, pulmonary trunk; AO, aorta).

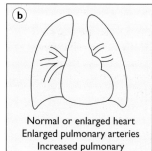

(a) A_2 P_2

(c) **ECG**
- Usually normal
- Left ventricular hypertrophy
  with large left-to-right shunt
- Right ventricular hypertrophy
  with pulmonary hypertension

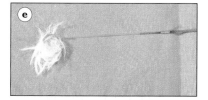
(e)

(b)
Normal or enlarged heart
Enlarged pulmonary arteries
Increased pulmonary
vasculature

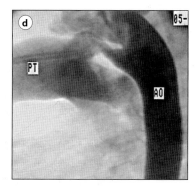
(d) PT AO

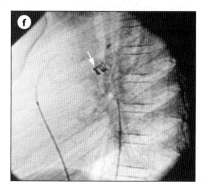
(f)

rare, but when the duct is large there will be increased pulmonary blood flow with heart failure and even pulmonary hypertension.

Investigations

The findings on chest X-ray (Fig. 15.15b) and ECG (Fig. 15.15c) with a large symptomatic PDA will be indistinguishable from those seen in a patient with a large VSD. However, the duct should be readily identified with cross-sectional echocardiography assisted by Doppler ultrasound.

Management

In most preterm infants, the duct will ultimately close, but, if symptomatic, treatment with fluid restriction, diuretics, indomethacin (a prostaglandin synthetase inhibitor) or surgical ligation may be required. In the young child with an asymptomatic PDA, closure is recommended to abolish the lifelong risk of bacterial endocarditis. Surgical ligation was previously the method of choice but it is now possible to close most ducts by transvenous occlusion with a coil device (Fig. 15.15d–f).

Pulmonary valve stenosis

Clinical features

Most children with pulmonary valve stenosis (Fig. 15.16a) are asymptomatic. It is diagnosed clinically. A small number of neonates with critical pulmonary stenosis have a duct-dependent pulmonary circulation and present in the first few days of life.

Physical signs (Fig. 15.16b)
- An ejection systolic murmur best heard in the second and third left intercostal spaces, radiating to the back
- An ejection click best heard in the second and third left intercostal spaces
- When severe, a prolonged right ventricular impulse, with delayed pulmonary valve closure on auscultation.

Investigations

Chest X-ray (Fig. 15.16c)
May show post-stenotic dilatation of the pulmonary artery.

ECG (Fig. 15.16d)
Shows evidence of right ventricular hypertrophy.

Management

Although most children are asymptomatic, progressive right ventricular hypertrophy and reduced exercise tolerance eventually occur. When the pressure gradient across the pulmonary valve becomes markedly increased (greater than about 50 mmHg), intervention will be required. Transvenous balloon dilatation is the treatment of choice in most children.

Aortic valve stenosis

Aortic valve stenosis (Fig. 15.17a) may not be an isolated lesion. It is often associated with mitral valve stenosis and coarctation of the aorta, and their presence should always be excluded.

PULMONARY VALVE STENOSIS

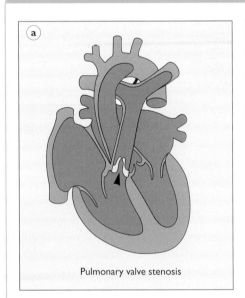

Pulmonary valve stenosis

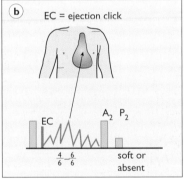

EC = ejection click

EC

A₂ P₂

soft or absent

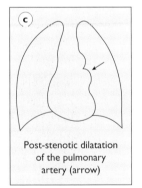

Post-stenotic dilatation of the pulmonary artery (arrow)

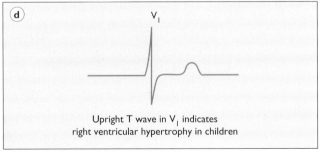

Upright T wave in V₁ indicates right ventricular hypertrophy in children

Fig. 15.16 (a) Pulmonary valve stenosis. (b) Murmur. (c) Chest X-ray. (d) ECG.

Clinical features

Symptoms are more common than in pulmonary valve stenosis. In the neonatal period, there may be a duct-dependent systemic circulation or severe heart failure. In later life, most children with mild or moderate stenosis present with an asymptomatic murmur. Those with severe stenosis may present with reduced exercise tolerance, chest pain on exertion or syncope.

Physical signs (Fig. 15.17b)

- small volume, slow rising, plateau-type pulses
- carotid thrill
- ejection systolic murmur maximal in the aortic area and radiating to the neck
- delayed and soft aortic second sound
- apical ejection click.

Investigations

Chest X-ray (Fig. 15.17c)
There may be a prominent left ventricle with post-stenotic dilatation of the ascending aorta.

ECG (Fig. 15.17d)
There may be left ventricular hypertrophy.

Management

In neonates, balloon valvotomy, avoiding the need for surgery, is frequently performed but it is less widely accepted than in pulmonary stenosis. This is because of concern about arterial damage and occlusion following percutaneous insertion of a large balloon through the femoral artery and the risk of severe aortic incompetence due to disruption of the aortic valve.

In older children, regular clinical and echocardiographic assessment is required in order to assess when to intervene. Children with symptoms on exercise or who have a high resting pressure gradient (more than 50–60 mmHg) across the aortic valve will undergo either balloon or surgical valvotomy. Balloon dilatation in this age group is generally safe and uncomplicated.

Most neonates and children with significant aortic valve stenosis requiring treatment in the first few years of life will eventually require aortic valve replacement. Early treatment is therefore palliative and directed towards delaying this for as long as possible.

Coarctation of the aorta

Coarctation of the aorta (Fig. 15.18a) is often associated with other lesions, the most common being a bicuspid aortic valve and ventricular septal defect.

Clinical features

In the neonatal period, severe coarctation presents with a duct-dependent systemic circulation, and circulatory collapse occurs on closure of the duct. If less severe, it may present with symptoms of heart failure or with a heart murmur between the shoulder blades (Fig. 15.18b). In older children or adults, coarctation may present with hypertension. The key to the clinical diagnosis is the recognition of weak or absent femoral pulses. The blood pressure in the arms will be markedly higher than in the legs. Palpation of the femoral pulses must be performed routinely during the cardiovascular examination of any child.

AORTIC VALVE STENOSIS

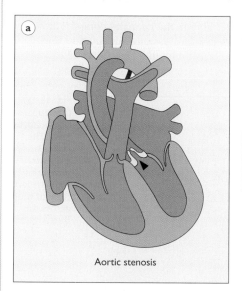

Aortic stenosis

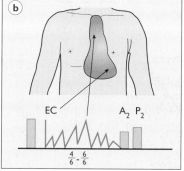

EC   A$_2$ P$_2$

$\frac{4}{6} - \frac{6}{6}$

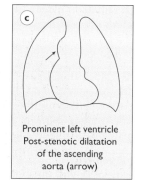

Prominent left ventricle
Post-stenotic dilatation
of the ascending
aorta (arrow)

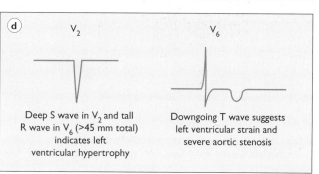

V$_2$ V$_6$

Deep S wave in V$_2$ and tall
R wave in V$_6$ (>45 mm total)
indicates left
ventricular hypertrophy

Downgoing T wave suggests
left ventricular strain and
severe aortic stenosis

Fig. 15.17 (a) Aortic valve stenosis. (b) Murmur. (c) Chest X-ray. (d) ECG.

COARCTATION OF THE AORTA

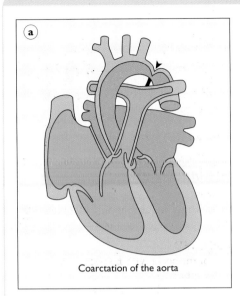

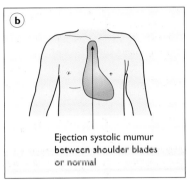

Ejection systolic mumur between shoulder blades or normal

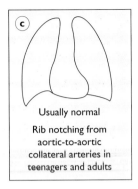

Usually normal

Rib notching from aortic-to-aortic collateral arteries in teenagers and adults

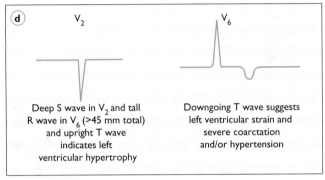

V_2

Deep S wave in V_2 and tall R wave in V_6 (>45 mm total) and upright T wave indicates left ventricular hypertrophy

V_6

Downgoing T wave suggests left ventricular strain and severe coarctation and/or hypertension

Coarctation of the aorta

Fig. 15.18 (a) Coarctation of the aorta. There is narrowing of the aorta distal to the left subclavian artery adjacent to the insertion of the arterial duct. (b) Murmur. (c) Chest X-ray. (d) ECG.

Investigations

Chest X-ray (Fig. 15.18c)

This is usually normal but may show cardiomegaly and increased vascular markings in children with heart failure. In older children there may also be 'rib-notching' due to the development of large collateral intercostal arteries running under the ribs posteriorly to bypass the obstruction.

ECG

In the neonatal period, this shows right ventricular hypertrophy because the right ventricle is supplying the descending aorta in fetal life. In older children, there will be left ventricular hypertrophy (Fig. 15.18d).

Management

The majority will undergo surgery. There are several different operations, the most common being resection with end-to-end anastomosis and the subclavian flap procedure, when the left subclavian artery is transected and used as a flap to relieve the coarctation just distal to it. This is performed via a left thoracotomy and, although the left arm pulses are lost, the arm develops normally. There is a small incidence (approximately 5–10%) of re-coarctation after surgery, but the mortality is now low (less than 2%). Balloon dilatation, avoiding the need for surgery, is performed at some centres but its exact role remains uncertain. If re-stenosis occurs after operation, balloon dilatation is the treatment of choice.

Interruption of the aortic arch

This is a severe form of coarctation with no connection between the aorta proximal and distal to the arterial duct. A VSD is usually present. Presentation is almost invariably in the neonatal period with features of a duct-dependent systemic circulation (Fig. 15.19). Complete correction with closure of the VSD and

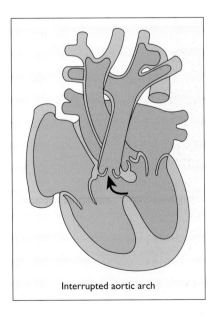

Interrupted aortic arch

Fig. 15.19 Interruption of the aortic arch. The lower body circulation is maintained by right-to-left flow of blood across the duct.

repair of the aortic arch is usually performed within the first few days of life. The risk of death is higher than that for simple coarctation of the aorta, being in the order of 10–20%. There is an association with DiGeorge's syndrome (absence of thymus, palatal defects, immunodeficiency and hypocalcaemia).

Hypoplastic left heart syndrome

In this condition there is underdevelopment of the entire left side of the heart (Fig. 15.20). The mitral valve is small or atretic, the left ventricle is diminutive and there is usually aortic valve atresia. The ascending aorta is very small, and there is almost invariably coarctation of the aorta or interruption of the aortic arch.

Clinical features

These are the sickest of all neonates presenting with a duct-dependent systemic circulation. There is no flow through the left side of the heart, so ductal constriction leads to profound acidosis and rapid cardiovascular collapse. There is weakness or absence of all peripheral pulses, in contrast to weak femoral pulses in coarctation of the aorta. The infant will fail the nitrogen washout test by remaining desaturated in oxygen, as there is common mixing of pulmonary venous and systemic venous blood at atrial level. As in all suspected duct-dependent lesions, prostaglandin must be commenced and the diagnosis established urgently by echocardiography.

Management

This condition has previously been considered inoperable, but two surgical approaches are now possible. One comprises a series of difficult and demanding operations, the effect of which is palliative (Norwood's procedure), and the other is neonatal heart transplantation, but few donor organs are available in neonates.

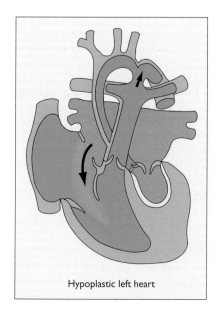

Fig. 15.20 Hypoplastic left heart syndrome. The entire left side of the heart is underdeveloped.

Hypoplastic left heart

CYANOTIC CONGENITAL HEART DISEASE

In congenital heart disease there are two causes of cyanosis:

- decreased pulmonary blood flow with a right-to-left shunt, e.g. Tetralogy of Fallot
- abnormal mixing of systemic and pulmonary venous return, e.g. transposition of the great arteries and tricuspid atresia.

Tetralogy of Fallot

This is the most common cause of cyanotic congenital heart disease (Fig. 15.21a).

Clinical features

In Tetralogy of Fallot, as implied by the name, there are four cardinal anatomical features:

- a large outlet VSD
- overriding of the aorta with respect to the ventricular septum
- right ventricular outflow tract obstruction (infundibular and valvular pulmonary stenosis)
- right ventricular hypertrophy.

Symptoms
A few children present with severe cyanosis in the first few days of life with a duct-dependent pulmonary circulation, but most are diagnosed in the first month or two of life following the identification of a murmur. Cyanosis at this stage may not be obvious. The classical description of severe cyanosis, hypercyanotic spells and squatting on exercise developing in late infancy is now rare. However, it is important to recognise hypercyanotic spells, as they may lead to myocardial infarction, cerebrovascular accidents and even death if left untreated. They are characterised by a rapid increase in cyanosis, usually associated with irritability or inconsolable crying, because of severe hypoxia, and breathlessness and pallor because of tissue acidosis.

Signs
Clubbing of the fingers and toes may develop in older children. A long, loud ejection systolic murmur is best heard in the third left intercostal space, usually with a single second heart sound (Fig. 15.21b). With increasing right ventricular outflow tract obstruction, which is predominantly muscular and below the pulmonary valve, the murmur will shorten and cyanosis will increase. During a hypercyanotic spell, the murmur will be very short or inaudible.

Investigations
Chest X-ray (Fig. 15.21c)
This will show a relatively small heart, possibly with an uptilted apex due to right ventricular hypertrophy. There may be a right-sided aortic arch, but characteristically there is a pulmonary artery 'bay', a concavity on the left heart border where the convex-shaped main pulmonary artery and right ventricular outflow tract are normally profiled. There may also be decreased

TETRALOGY OF FALLOT

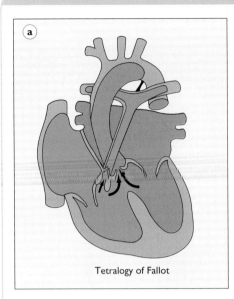

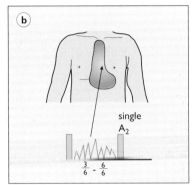

single
A₂

$$\frac{3}{6} - \frac{6}{6}$$

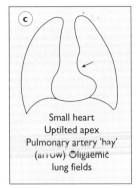

Small heart
Uptilted apex
Pulmonary artery 'bay'
(arrow) Oligaemic
lung fields

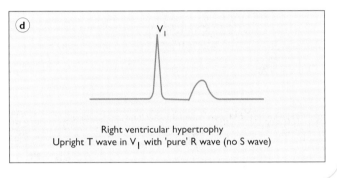

Right ventricular hypertrophy
Upright T wave in V₁ with 'pure' R wave (no S wave)

Fig. 15.21 (a) Tetralogy of Fallot. The right ventricular outflow tract obstruction results in blood flowing from right to left across the ventricular septal defect. (b) Murmur. (c) Chest X-ray. (d) ECG.

pulmonary vascular markings reflecting reduced pulmonary blood flow.

ECG (Fig. 15.19d)
This will show right axis deviation and right ventricular hypertrophy.

Echocardiography
This will demonstrate the cardinal features, but cardiac catheterisation may be required to show the detailed anatomy of the pulmonary arteries, which may be small or stenosed.

Management
Hypercyanotic spells are usually self-limiting and followed by a period of sleep. If prolonged (beyond about 15 min), they require prompt treatment with:

- sedation and pain relief (morphine is excellent)
- intravenous propranolol, which probably works both as a peripheral vasoconstrictor and by relieving the subpulmonary muscular obstruction that is the cause of reduced pulmonary blood flow
- bicarbonate to correct acidosis
- muscle paralysis and artificial ventilation in order to reduce metabolic oxygen demand.

Infants who become symptomatic in the first few months of age require palliative surgery to increase pulmonary blood flow. This is usually done by surgical placement of an artificial tube between the subclavian artery and the pulmonary artery (a modified

Blalock–Taussig shunt) or sometimes by balloon dilatation of the right ventricular outflow tract. Corrective surgery is now usually performed at around 6 months of age. It involves closing the VSD and relieving right ventricular outflow tract obstruction with an artificial patch which sometimes extends across the pulmonary valve. The operative risk is approximately 2–5%. Most are free from significant symptoms in childhood.

Transposition of the great arteries

In transposition of the great arteries, there are two parallel circulations – the systemic venous return passes from the right atrium into the right ventricle and then into the aorta, and there is a separate circulation of pulmonary venous blood returning to the left atrium via the left ventricle and back into the pulmonary arteries (Fig. 15.22a). If there is no mixing of blood between the two circulations then this condition is incompatible with life. Fortunately, there are a number of naturally occurring associated anomalies, e.g. VSD, ASD and patent ductus, as well as therapeutic interventions which can achieve this.

Clinical features
Symptoms
Cyanosis is the predominant symptom. It may be profound and life-threatening; a P_{O_2} of 1–3 kPa is not unusual. These children usually present within the first day or two of life when spontaneous closure of the

TRANSPOSITION OF THE GREAT ARTERIES

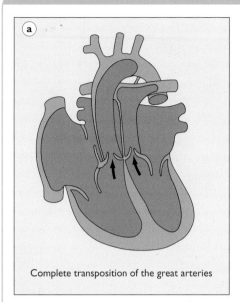

Complete transposition of the great arteries

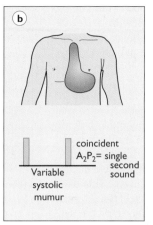

Variable systolic mumur

coincident A_2P_2 = single second sound

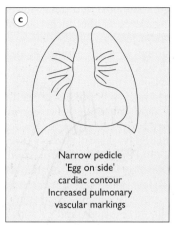

Narrow pedicle
'Egg on side'
cardiac contour
Increased pulmonary
vascular markings

d **ECG**
Usually normal neonatal pattern

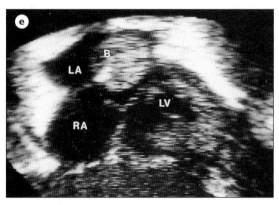

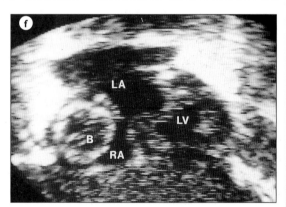

Fig. 15.22 (a) Transposition of the great arteries. There must be mixing of blood between the two circulations for this to be compatible with life. (b) Murmur. (c) Chest X-ray. (d) ECG. (e,f) Echocardiogram showing balloon atrial septostomy in transposition of the great arteries. A balloon (about 2 ml) is pulled through the atrial septum from the left atrium (e) across the atrial septum to the right atrium (f) in order to increase the size of the atrial septum (B, balloon; LA, left atrium; RA, right atrium; LV, left ventricle).

ductus arteriosus leads to a marked reduction in mixing of the desaturated and saturated blood. Cyanosis will be less severe and presentation delayed if there is more mixing of blood from associated anomalies, e.g. a VSD.

Physical signs (Fig. 15.22b)
There will always be cyanosis and, in the occasional child presenting after the first year of life, there may be finger clubbing. The remainder of the cardiovascular examination will vary depending on the associated abnormalities. The second heart sound is often closely split or single. There may be a systolic murmur, due to increased flow or stenosis within the left ventricular (pulmonary) outflow tract, but there may be no murmur.

Investigations
Chest X-ray (Fig. 15.22c)
This may reveal the classic findings of a narrow upper mediastinum with an 'egg on side' appearance of the cardiac shadow (due to the anteroposterior relationship of the great vessels and hypertrophied right ventricule, respectively). Increased pulmonary vascular markings are common.

ECG (Fig. 15.22d)
This is rarely helpful in establishing the diagnosis, as it is usually normal.

Echocardiography
This is essential to demonstrate the abnormal arterial connections and associated abnormalities.

Management

In the sick cyanosed neonate, the key is to improve mixing of saturated and desaturated blood. Maintaining the patency of the ductus arteriosus with a prostaglandin infusion is mandatory. A balloon atrial septostomy is a life-saving procedure which is now virtually routine in children with all forms of transposition of the great arteries (Fig. 15.20e,f). It was first performed by Rashkind in the USA, and was one of the most important advances in treating congenital heart disease. A catheter, with an expandable balloon at its tip, is passed through the umbilical or femoral vein and then on through the right atrium and foramen ovale. The balloon is inflated within the left atrium and then pulled through the atrial septum. This tears the atrial septum, renders the flap valve of the foramen ovale incompetent, and so allows mixing of the systemic and pulmonary venous blood within the atrium.

All patients with transposition of the great arteries will ultimately require some form of surgery. Until the 1980s, a 'corrective' operation was performed by placing a baffle within the atrium to divert the systemic venous blood towards the left ventricle and then on to the pulmonary artery, thus allowing the pulmonary venous blood to pass into the right ventricle and then on to the aorta (the Mustard of Senning procedure). This 'physiological' correction was usually performed at about 9 months of age and had a low early risk. Long-term concerns regarding the ability of the right ventricle to perform as a systemic pump, as well as late problems with stenosis of the intra-atrial baffle and frequent atrial dysrhythmias, have led to the widespread introduction of the arterial switch procedure, so-called anatomical correction. In this operation, performed in the first few weeks of life, the pulmonary artery and aorta are transected above the arterial valves and switched over. In addition, the coronary arteries have to be transferred across to the new aorta. Thus the left ventricle acts as the systemic ventricle, pumping fully oxygenated blood into the aorta, and the right ventricle assumes its more normal role of pumping blood to the lungs. This is a technically demanding operation, and the surgical risk was initially high. However, with increasing experience, the risk has fallen and the long-term prospects are thought to be much better than those of the atrial redirection procedure.

Tricuspid atresia

In tricuspid atresia (Fig. 15.23), only the left ventricle is effective, the right being small and non-functional.

Clinical features

There is 'common mixing' of systemic and pulmonary venous return in the left atrium. Presentation is with cyanosis in the newborn period.

Management

Early palliation is required:

- a Blalock–Taussig shunt in most children

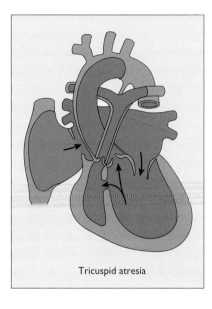

Fig. 15.23 In tricuspid atresia, there is only one effective ventricle because of complete absence of the tricuspid valve.

Tricuspid atresia

- pulmonary artery banding, to reduce pulmonary blood flow may be required.

Completely corrective surgery is not possible as there is only one effective functioning ventricle. The Fontan operation is a form of palliation which connects the right atrium directly to the pulmonary arteries and closes the ASD. Thus the left ventricle drives blood around the body and systemic venous pressure supplies blood to the lungs. The Fontan operation results in a less than ideal functional outcome, but has the advantages of relieving cyanosis and removing the long-term volume load on the single functional ventricle. Many of the children lead normal, or near-normal, lives. These operations were first performed in the early 1970s, so the late outcome is unknown but a significant number of hearts progressively fail in adult life.

CARE FOLLOWING CARDIAC SURGERY

Most children recover rapidly following cardiac surgery and are back at nursery or school within a month. Almost all will require antibiotic prophylaxis against bacterial endocarditis. Exercise tolerance will be variable and most children can be allowed to find their own limits. Restricted exercise is advised only for children with severe residual aortic stenosis and ventricular dysfunction.

Most of the children are followed up in specialist cardiac clinics. Most lead normal, unrestricted lives, but any change in symptoms, e.g. decreasing exercise tolerance or palpitations, requires further investigation. An increasing number of adolescents and young adults require revision of surgery performed in early life. The most common reason for this is replacement of artificial valves and relief of post-surgical suture line stenosis, e.g. re-coarctation or pulmonary artery stenosis.

CARDIAC ARRHYTHMIAS

Sinus arrythmia is normal in children and is detectable as a cyclical change in heart rate with respiration. There is acceleration during inspiration and slowing on expiration (the heart rate changing by up to 30 beats/min).

Supraventricular re-entry tachycardia

This is the most common childhood arrhythmia. The heart rate is rapid, between 250 and 300 beats/min. It can cause poor cardiac output and pulmonary oedema. It typically presents with symptoms of heart failure in the neonate or young infant. It is a cause of hydrops fetalis and intrauterine death. The term re-entry tachycardia is used because a circuit of conduction is set up, with premature activation of the atrium via an accessory pathway. There is rarely a structural heart problem, but an echocardiogram should be performed.

Investigation

The ECG will generally show a narrow complex tachycardia of 250–300 beats/min (Fig. 15.24). It may be possible to discern a P wave after the QRS complex due to retrograde activation of the atrium via the accessory pathway. If heart failure is severe, there may be changes suggestive of myocardial ischaemia, with T wave inversion in the lateral precordial leads. When in sinus rhythm, a short P–R interval may be discernible. In the Wolff–Parkinson–White (WPW) syndrome, the early antegrade activation of the ventricle via the pathway results in a short P–R interval and a delta wave.

Management

In the severely ill child, prompt restoration of sinus rhythm is the key to improvement. This is achieved by:

- Circulatory and respiratory support   tissue acidosis is corrected, positive pressure ventilation if required.
- Vagal stimulating manoeuvres – carotid sinus massage or an ice pack on the face should be tried and is successful in about 80%.
- Intravenous adenosine – the treatment of choice. This is safe and effective, inducing atrioventricular block after rapid bolus injection. It terminates the tachycardia by breaking the re-entry circuit that is set up between the atrioventricular node and accessory pathway. It is given incrementally in increasing doses (up to a maximum of 0.5 mg/kg)
- Electrical cardioversion with a synchronised DC shock (0.5–2 J/kg bodyweight) if adenosine fails.

Once sinus rhythm is restored, maintenance therapy will be required Digoxin can be used when there is no overt pre-excitation wave (delta wave) on the resting ECG. Alternatively, flecainide is highly effective but, as with digoxin, blood levels need to be closely monitored. Even though the resting ECG may remain abnormal, 90% of children will have no further attacks after infancy. Treatment is therefore stopped at 1 year of age. Those who relapse thereafter are usually treated with percutaneous radiofrequency ablation of the accessory pathway.

Congenital complete heart block

This is a rare condition (Fig. 15.25) which is usually related to the presence of *anti-Ro* antibodies in maternal serum. These mothers will have either manifest or latent connective tissue disorders. Subsequent pregnancies are often affected. This antibody appears to prevent normal development of the electrical conduction system in the developing heart, with atrophy and fibrosis of the atrioventricular node. It may cause fetal hydrops, death *in utero* and heart failure in the neonatal period. However, most remain symptom-free for many years, but a few become symptomatic with pre-syncope or syncope. All children with symptoms require insertion of an endocardial or epicardial pacemaker.

Other arrhythmias

Prolonged QT syndrome may be associated with sudden loss of consciousness during exercise, stress or emotion, usually in late childhood. It may be mistakenly diagnosed as epilepsy. If unrecognised, sudden death from ventricular tachycardia may occur. It may be autosomal dominant or autosomal recessive accompanied by deafness. Prolongation of the QT interval on ECG has been associated with the drug cisapride, which was used to treat gastro-oesophageal reflux.

Atrial fibrillation, atrial flutter, ectopic atrial tachycardia, ventricular tachycardia and ventricular fibrillation occur in children, but all are rare. They are most often seen in children who have undergone surgery for complex congenital heart disease, and in general their treatment is similar to that of adults.

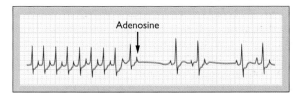

Fig. 15.24 Rhythm strip showing supraventricular re-entry tachycardia, in which there is a narrow complex tachycardia (<120 ms or three small squares) of 250–300 beats/min, and response to treatment with adenosine.

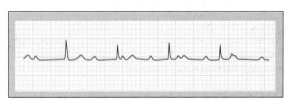

Fig. 15.25 ECG of congenital complete heart block. The P waves and QRS complexes are dissociated.

RHEUMATIC FEVER

Worldwide, this remains the most important cause of heart disease in children. Improvements in sanitation, social factors, the more liberal use of antibiotics and changes in streptococcal virulence have led to its virtual disappearance in developed countries. In susceptible individuals, there is an abnormal immune response to a preceding infection with group A β-haemolytic *streptococcus*. It mainly affects children aged 5–15 years.

Clinical features

After a latent interval of 2–6 weeks following a pharyngeal infection, polyarthritis, mild fever and malaise develop. The clinical features and diagnostic criteria are shown in Figure 15.26.

Chronic rheumatic heart disease

The most common form of long-term damage from scarring and fibrosis of the valve tissue of the heart is mitral stenosis. If there have been repeated attacks of rheumatic fever with carditis, this may occur as early as the second decade of life, but usually symptoms do not develop until later adult life. Although the mitral valve is the most frequently affected, aortic, tricuspid and, rarely, pulmonary valve disease may occur.

Management

The acute episode is usually treated with bed rest and anti-inflammatory agents. While there is evidence of active myocarditis (echocardiographic changes with a raised ESR), bed rest and limitation of exercise are

JONES CRITERIA FOR DIAGNOSIS OF RHEUMATIC FEVER

Required to make the diagnosis

Two major, or one major and two minor, criteria plus supportive evidence of preceding group A streptococcal infection (markedly raised ASO titre or other streptococcal antibodies, or group A *streptococcus* on throat culture)

Major manifestations

Pancarditis (50%)
Endocarditis
- significant murmur
- valvular dysfunction

Myocarditis
- may lead to heart failure and death

Pericarditis
- pericardial friction rub
- pericardial effusion
- tamponade

Polyarthritis (80%)
Ankles, knees and wrists
Exquisite tenderness, moderate redness and swelling
'Flitting', lasting <1 week in a joint, but migrating to other joints over 1–2 months

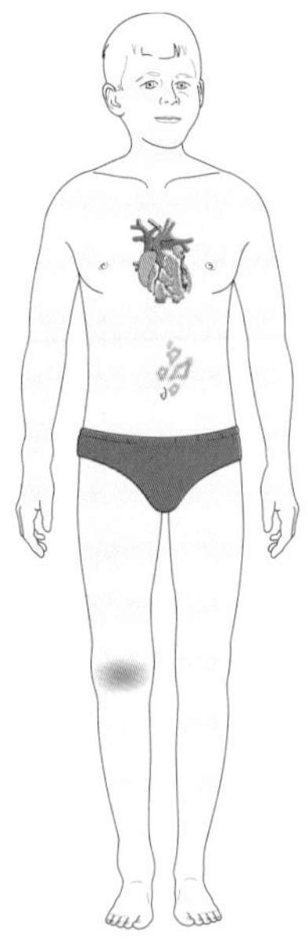

Sydenham's chorea (10%)
2–6 months after the streptococcal infection
Involuntary movements and emotional lability for 3–6 months

Erythema marginatum (<5%)
Uncommon, early manifestation
Rash on trunk and limbs
Pink macules spread outwards, causing pink border with fading centre. Borders may unite to give a map-like outline

Subcutaneous nodules (rare)
Painless, pea-sized, hard
Mainly on extensor surfaces

Minor manifestations

Fever
Polyarthralgia
History of rheumatic fever
Raised acute-phase reactants: ESR, C-reactive protein, leucocytosis
Prolonged P–R interval on ECG

Fig. 15.26 Jones criteria for diagnosis of rheumatic fever.

essential. Aspirin is very effective at suppressing the inflammatory response of the joints and heart. It needs to be given in high dosage and serum levels monitored. If the fever and inflammation do not resolve rapidly, corticosteroids will be required. Symptomatic heart failure is treated with diuretics and ACE inhibitors, and significant pericardial effusions will require pericardiocentesis. Antistreptococcal antibiotics may be given if there is any evidence of persisting infection.

Following resolution of the acute episode, recurrence should be prevented. Monthly injections of benzathine penicillin is the most effective prophylaxis. Alternatively, the penicillin can be given orally every day, but compliance may be a problem. Oral erythromycin can be substituted in those sensitive to penicillin. The length of treatment is controversial. Most recommend treatment to the age of 18 or 21 years, but, more recently, lifelong prophylaxis has been advocated. The severity of eventual rheumatic valvular disease relates to the number of childhood episodes of rheumatic fever.

INFECTIVE ENDOCARDITIS

All children of any age with congenital heart disease, including neonates, are at risk of infective endocarditis. The risk is highest when there is a turbulent jet of blood, as with a VSD, coarctation of the aorta and patent ductus arteriosus or if prosthetic material has been inserted at surgery. It may be difficult to diagnose, but should be suspected in any child or adult with a sustained fever, malaise, raised ESR, unexplained anaemia or haematuria. The presence of the classical peripheral stigmata of infective endocarditis should not be relied upon.

Clinical signs
- Fever
- Anaemia and pallor
- Splinter haemorrhages
- Clubbing (late)
- Necrotic skin lesions (Fig. 15.27)
- Changing cardiac signs
- Splenomegaly
- Neurological signs from cerebral infarction
- Retinal infarcts
- Arthritis/arthralgia
- Haematuria (microscopic).

Diagnosis
Multiple blood cultures should be taken before antibiotics are started. Detailed cross-sectional echocardiography may confirm the diagnosis by identification of vegetations but can never exclude it. The vegetations consist of fibrin and platelets and contain infecting organisms. Acute-phase reactants are raised and can be useful to monitor response to treatment.

The most common causative organism is α-haemolytic *streptococcus* (*streptococcus viridans*). Bacterial

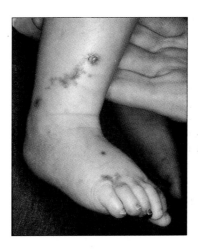

Fig. 15.27 Widespread infected emboli and infarcts in a child with bacterial endocarditis. The tip of the third toe is gangrenous.

endocarditis is usually treated with high-dose penicillin in combination with an aminoglycoside, giving 6 weeks of intravenous therapy and checking that the serum level of the antibiotic will kill the organism. If there is infected prosthetic material, e.g. prosthetic valves, VSD patches or shunts, there is less chance of complete eradication and surgical removal may be required.

Prophylaxis
The most important factor in prophylaxis against endocarditis is good dental hygiene, and this should be strongly encouraged in all children with congenital heart disease. Antibiotic prophylaxis will be required for:

- dental treatment, however trivial
- surgery which is likely to be associated with bacteraemia (e.g. appendicectomy, ENT surgery).

 Antibiotic prophylaxis is essential for dental and surgical treatment in almost all children with congenital heart disease.

MYOCARDITIS/CARDIOMYOPATHY

Dilated cardiomyopathy (a large, poorly contracting heart) may be inherited, or may result from a direct viral infection of the myocardium. It is rare but should be suspected in any child with an enlarged heart and heart failure who has previously been well. The diagnosis is readily made on echocardiography. Treatment is symptomatic with diuretics. The role of steroids and immunoglobulin infusion is controversial. It usually improves spontaneously, but some children ultimately require heart transplantation. Other cardiomyopathies (hypertrophic/restrictive) are rare in childhood and are usually related to a systemic disease (e.g. Hurler's, Pompe's or Noonan's syndromes).

FURTHER READING

Anderson R, Baker E, McCartney F, Rigby M, Shinebourne E, Tynon M 2001 Paediatric cardiology, 2nd edn. Churchill Livingstone, Edinburgh
Archer N, Burch M 1998 Paediatric cardiology. Chapman and Hall, London
Jordan S C, Scott O 1989 Heart disease in paediatrics. Butterworth/Heinemann, Oxford

The anatomical illustrations used in this chapter are based on artwork provided by Dr Yen Ho, Royal Brompton National Heart & Lung Hospital, London, UK.

16

Kidney and urinary tract

The spectrum of renal disease in children differs from that in adults:

- many structural abnormalities of the kidneys and urinary tract are identified on antenatal ultrasound screening
- urinary tract infection, vesicoureteric reflux and urinary obstruction have the potential to damage the growing kidney
- nephrotic syndrome is usually steroid-sensitive and only rarely leads to chronic renal failure
- dialysis and transplantation are more difficult, but recent advances enable even neonates to be treated.

Assessment of the kidneys and urinary tract

Renal blood flow in the fetus is very low. The glomerular filtration rate (GFR) at 28 weeks' gestation is only 25% of that at term. Over the first 2 weeks of life the GFR doubles, increasing sixfold from birth to a year of age when the adult rate (120 ml/min per 1.73 m^2) is achieved. The assessment of renal function in children is listed in Figure 16.1 and the radiological investigations of the kidneys and urinary tract in Figure 16.2.

ANTENATAL DIAGNOSIS OF URINARY TRACT ANOMALIES

Antenatal ultrasound scanning has markedly altered the presentation of congenital abnormalities of the kidneys and urinary tract. In the past, these were identified only when symptoms developed during childhood or adult life. Abnormalities can be identified in approximately 1 in 400 fetuses and are important as they may:

- be associated with abnormal renal development or function

Fig. 16.1 Assessment of renal function in children.

Plasma creatinine concentration
Rises progressively throughout childhood according to height and muscle bulk. Plasma creatinine does not rise until renal function has fallen to less than half normal

Glomerular filtration rate (GFR)
In suspected renal failure, a rough estimate of GFR can be obtained using the formula:

$$\frac{\text{height (cm)} \times 40}{\text{plasma creatinine } (\mu mol/L)}$$

More accurate measurement of GFR is by measuring the clearance from the plasma of a substance that is freely filtered at the glomerulus and is not secreted or reabsorbed by the tubules (e.g. inulin, chromium EDTA). The need for repeated blood tests limits its use in children.

Creatinine clearance
Rarely measured in children because of the difficulties in collecting a complete, timed urine sample

- predispose to postnatal infection
- involve urinary obstruction which requires surgical treatment.

The early detection and treatment of urinary tract anomalies provide an exciting opportunity of minimising or preventing renal damage. A disadvantage is that mild abnormalities are also detected which do not require treatment or resolve spontaneously but engender unnecessary investigation, treatment and parental anxiety.

Fig. 16.2 Radiological investigation of the kidneys and urinary tract.

Ultrasound
Provides a non-invasive anatomical assessment of the whole urinary tract. It is now the standard imaging procedure of the kidneys and urinary tract, but it does not give information about function and its accuracy is operator-dependent.

Functional scanning
Radioisotopes give a lower radiation dose than conventional X-rays and allow comparison of individual kidney function. Good images cannot be obtained until several weeks of age.

Static nuclear medicine scanning
This uses an isotope-labelled substance (e.g. DMSA) that is incorporated into the functioning renal tissue. It is particularly good for the detection of renal scars.

Dynamic nuclear medicine scanning
This uses an isotope-labelled substance (e.g. MAG 3, DTPA) that is excreted by glomerular filtration, and gives information on blood flow, renal function and drainage. It is particularly useful for detecting urinary obstruction. It can also be used to detect vesicoureteric reflux in the older child who can cooperate by stopping and starting micturition on command (indirect cystography).

Micturating cystourethrography (MCUG)
Filling the bladder with contrast via a urethral catheter outlines the bladder and is used to identify vesicoureteric reflux. Urethral obstruction is demonstrated on views during voiding without the catheter. As infection may be introduced on catheterisation, prophylactic antibiotics are given. Other disadvantages are that catheterisation is unpleasant and the radiation dose is high, particularly to the gonads. Using radioisotope scanning lowers the radiation dose but will not identify urethral obstruction.

Intavenous urography (IVU)
This is rarely indicated in children unless detailed anatomy of the calyces or ureter is required.

Anomalies detectable on antenatal ultrasound screening

Absence of both kidneys (renal agenesis) results in Potter's syndrome (Fig. 16.3). A *multicystic kidney* results from the failure of union of the ureteric bud (which forms the ureter, pelvis, calyces and collecting ducts) with the nephrogenic mesenchyme. It is a non-functioning structure with large fluid-filled cysts with no renal tissue and no connection with the bladder (Fig. 16.4). If the multicystic kidneys are bilateral, there will not be any renal function and it will result in Potter's syndrome. Other causes of large cystic kidneys are autosomal recessive infantile polycystic kidney disease, autosomal dominant adult-type polycystic disease and tuberous sclerosis. In contrast to a multicystic kidney, in these disorders some or normal renal function is maintained.

Abnormal caudal migration may result in a *pelvic kidney* or a *horseshoe kidney* (Fig. 16.4b). The abnormal position may predispose to infection or obstruction to urinary drainage.

Premature division of the ureteric bud gives rise to a *duplex system*, which can vary from simply a bifid renal pelvis to complete division with two ureters. These ureters frequently have an abnormal drainage so that the ureter from the lower pole moiety often refluxes, whereas the upper pole ureter may drain ectopically into the urethra or vagina or may prolapse into the bladder (ureterocele) and obstruct urine flow (Fig. 16.4c).

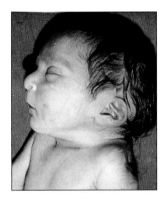

Fig. 16.3 Potter's syndrome. Intrauterine compression of the fetus from oligohydramnios caused by lack of fetal urine causes a characteristic facies, large and low-set ears, lung hypoplasia and postural deformities including severe talipes. The infant may be stillborn or die soon after birth from respiratory failure.

Failure of fusion of the infraumbilical midline structures results in exposed bladder mucosa (bladder extrophy) or absent abdominal musculature with a large bladder and dilated ureters (megacystis-megaureters) and cryptorchidism, the *prune belly syndrome* (Fig. 16.5).

Obstruction to urine flow may occur at the pelviureteric or vesicoureteric junction, at the bladder neck (e.g. due to disruption of the nerve supply, *neuropathic bladder*) or at the posterior urethra in a boy due to mucosal folds or a membrane, known as a posterior urethral valve. The consequences of obstruction to urine flow are shown in Figure 16.6. At worst, this results in a *dysplastic kidney* which is small, poorly functioning and may contain cysts and aberrant embryonic tissue such as cartilage and hair. Renal dysplasia can also occur in association with severe intrauterine vesicoureteric reflux or in isolation.

SOME ANOMALIES OF THE URINARY TRACT

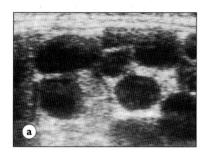

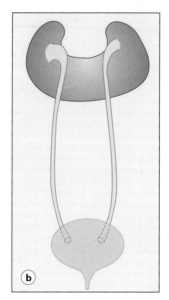

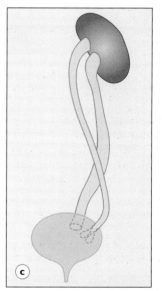

Fig. 16.4 Some anomalies of the urinary tract detectable on antenatal ultrasound: (a) multicystic kidney; (b) horseshoe kidney; (c) duplex kidney showing ureterocele of upper moiety and reflux into lower pole moiety.

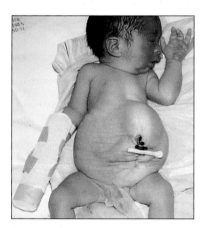

Fig. 16.5 Prune belly syndrome. The name arises from the wrinkled appearance of the abdomen. It is associated with a large bladder, dilated ureters and cryptorchidism. (Courtesy of Dr Jane Deal.)

Antenatal treatment

The male fetus with a posterior urethral valve may develop severe urinary outflow obstruction resulting in progressive bilateral hydronephrosis, poor renal growth and declining liquor volume. Intrauterine bladder drainage procedures are currently under evaluation. They must be undertaken early to prevent severe renal damage. Early delivery is rarely indicated.

Postnatal management

An example of a protocol for infants with antenatally diagnosed anomalies is shown in Figure 16.7. Prophylactic antibiotics should be started at birth to prevent urinary tract infection and an ultrasound performed within the first week of life. As the newborn kidney has a low GFR, urine flow is low and mild outflow obstruction may not be evident. The scan should therefore be

repeated several weeks later. Bilateral hydronephrosis in a male infant warrants urgent further investigation to exclude a posterior urethral valve, which always requires surgery (see Case history 16.1).

URINARY TRACT INFECTION

Three per cent of girls and 1% of boys have a symptomatic urinary tract infection (UTI) before the age of 11 years, and 50% of them have a recurrence within a year. All children should be thoroughly assessed and investigated following their first UTI as:

- up to half have a structural abnormality of their urinary tract
- a UTI may damage the growing kidney by forming a scar, predisposing to hypertension and to chronic renal failure if the scarring is bilateral.

Clinical features

Presentation of UTI varies with age (Fig. 16.9). In the newborn, symptoms are non-specific and septicaemia may develop rapidly. The classical symptoms of dysuria, frequency and loin pain are rarely seen in infants. Beyond infancy, dysuria without a fever is often due to vulvitis in girls or balanitis in boys rather than a UTI. Symptoms suggestive of a UTI may also occur following sexual abuse.

Collection of urine samples

It is essential that UTIs are diagnosed accurately. Contamination of a urine specimen may lead to a false-positive diagnosis which will commit the child to

URINARY TRACT OBSTRUCTION

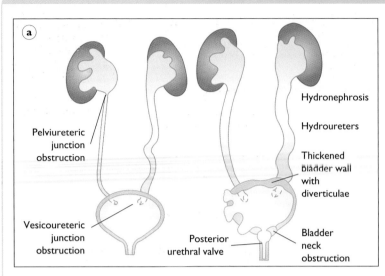

Pelviureteric junction obstruction

Vesicoureteric junction obstruction

Posterior urethral valve

Hydronephrosis

Hydroureters

Thickened bladder wall with diverticulae

Bladder neck obstruction

Fig. 16.6a Obstruction to urine flow results in dilatation of the urinary tract proximal to the site of obstruction. Obstruction may be at the pelviureteric or vesicoureteric junction (left), the bladder neck or urethra (right).

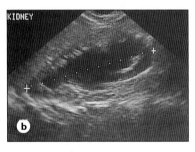

Fig. 16.6b An ultrasound showing a dilated renal pelvis from pelviureteric junction obstruction.

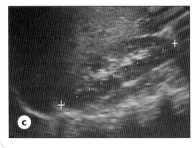

Fig. 16.6c A normal ultrasound of the kidney is shown for comparison.

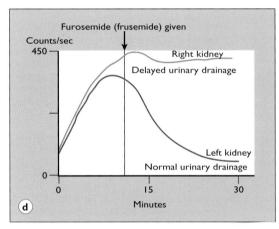

Fig. 16.6d Graph from dynamic nuclear medicine scan (MAG 3) showing delayed excretion from a pelviureteric junction obstruction.

unnecessary investigations. For the child in nappies, urine can be collected by:

- a 'clean-catch' sample into a waiting sterile pot when the nappy is removed; this is easier in boys
- an adhesive plastic bag applied to the perineum after careful washing, although there may be contamination from the skin
- suprapubic aspiration (SPA), the method of choice in the severely ill infant under 1 year old requiring urgent diagnosis and treatment and in those where previous samples have suggested contamination (Fig. 16.10); catheter samples are used as an alternative in some centres.

In the older child, urine can be obtained by collecting a midstream sample. Careful cleaning and collection are necessary, as contamination with both white cells and bacteria can occur from under the foreskin in boys, and from reflux of urine into the vagina during voiding in girls.

Diagnosis

Ideally, the urine sample should be microscoped and cultured straight away. If not, it should be refrigerated to prevent the overgrowth of contaminating bacteria. Alternatively, delay in culture can be circumvented by the use of boric acid or dipslides. Microscopy will demonstrate pyuria, which is virtually always present with a UTI, and organisms may be identified. However, the presence of urinary white cells alone are not a reliable feature of a UTI, as white cells may be present in febrile children without a UTI and in

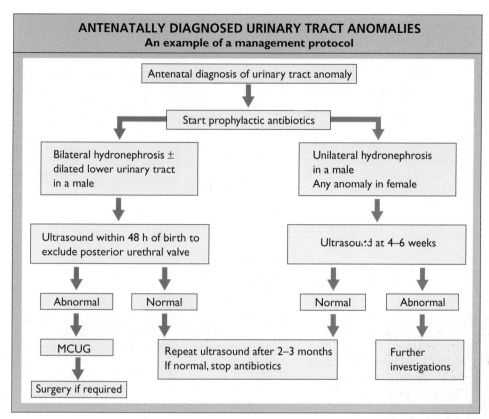

Fig. 16.7 An example of a protocol for the management of infants with antenatally diagnosed urinary tract anomalies (MCUG, micturating cystourethrogram).

CASE HISTORY 16.1

POSTERIOR URETHRAL VALVE

Bilateral hydronephrosis was noted on antenatal ultrasound at 20 weeks' gestation in a male fetus. There was poor renal growth, progressive hydronephrosis and decreasing volume of amniotic fluid (Fig. 16.8a) on repeated scans. After birth, prophylactic antibiotics were started. An urgent ultrasound showed bilateral hydronephrosis with small dysplastic kidneys. The bladder and ureters were grossly distended. The plasma creatinine was raised. A micturating cystourethrogram (MCUG) (Fig. 16.8b) showed vesicoureteric reflux, a dilated posterior urethra and a posterior urethral valve which was treated endoscopically. Renal function initially

improved but then progressed to chronic renal failure. He had a renal transplant at 10 years of age.

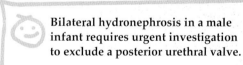

Bilateral hydronephrosis in a male infant requires urgent investigation to exclude a posterior urethral valve.

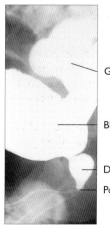

Fig. 16.8b Micturating cystourethrogram (MCUG) in the same patient.

Gross vesicoureteric reflux

Bladder with trabeculated wall

Dilated posterior urethra
Posterior urethral valve

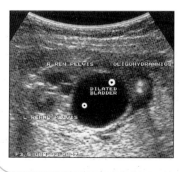

Fig. 16.8a Antenatal ultrasound scan in an infant with urinary outflow obstruction from a posterior urethral valve. (Courtesy of Mr Karl Murphy.)

Fig. 16.9 Presentation of UTI in infancy and childhood.

Infancy	Childhood
Fever	Dysuria and frequency
Lethargy or irritability	Fever with or without rigors
Vomiting, diarrhoea	Lethargy and anorexia
Poor feeding/failure to thrive	Vomiting, diarrhoea
	Abdominal or loin pain
Prolonged neonatal jaundice	Febrile convulsion (not to be confused with rigors)
Septicaemia	Recurrence of enuresis
Febrile convulsion (>6 months)	

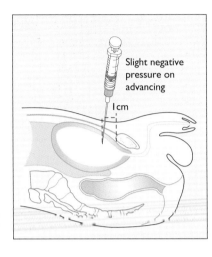

Fig. 16.10 Suprapubic aspiration. In an infant, the bladder extends into the abdomen. Negative pressure is applied to the syringe while advancing the needle until urine appears. This should avoid puncture of the rectum.

children with balanitis or vulvovaginitis. Positive testing of the urine with sticks for nitrite and white cell esterase is also suggestive of infection but there may be false-negative results.

A bacterial culture of >10^5 colony-forming units of a single organism per ml in a properly collected specimen gives a 90% probability of infection. If the same result is found in a second sample, the probability rises to 95%. A growth of mixed organisms in the absence of white blood cells usually represents contamination, but if there is doubt, another sample should be collected.

Bacterial and host factors that predispose to infection

Infecting organism

UTI is usually the result of bowel flora entering the urinary tract via the urethra. The commonest organism to do this is *E. coli*, followed by *Proteus* and *Pseudomonas*. The virulence of *E. coli* varies with its cell wall antigens and possession of endotoxin. *Proteus* infection is more common in boys, possibly because of its presence under the prepuce. *Proteus* infection predisposes to the formation of phosphate stones. *Pseudomonas* infection often indicates that there is some structural abnormality in the urinary tract affecting drainage.

Incomplete bladder emptying

Contributing factors in some children are:

- infrequent voiding, resulting in bladder enlargement
- vulvitis
- hurried micturition
- obstruction by a loaded rectum from constipation
- neuropathic bladder.

Vesicoureteric reflux

Vesicoureteric reflux is a developmental anomaly of the vesicoureteric junctions. The ureters are displaced laterally and enter directly into the bladder rather than at an angle, with a shortened intramural course.

Severe cases may be associated with renal dysplasia. It is familial, with at least a 10% chance of occurring in first-degree relatives. It may also occur with bladder pathology, e.g. a neuropathic bladder or urethral obstruction, or temporarily after a UTI. Its severity varies from reflux into the lower end of the ureter during micturition to the severest form with reflux during bladder filling and voiding, with a distended ureter, renal pelvis and clubbed calyces (Fig. 16.11). With growth, reflux resolves in 10% each year.

Reflux with associated ureteric dilatation is important, as:

- urine returning to the bladder from the ureters after voiding results in incomplete bladder emptying, which encourages infection
- the kidneys may become infected (pyelonephritis), particularly if there is intrarenal reflux
- bladder voiding pressure is transmitted to the renal papillae; this may contribute to renal damage if voiding pressures are high.

Infection may destroy renal tissue, leaving a scar, resulting in a shrunken, poorly functioning segment of kidney. If scarring is bilateral and severe, chronic renal failure may develop. Renal scars may produce increased quantities of renin, leading to hypertension. The risk for this is around 10% in childhood.

Management

Prompt treatment reduces the risk of renal scarring. Most children can be treated with oral antibiotics (e.g. co-amoxiclav for 5 days, or for 10 days if the child was systemically unwell), adjusting the choice of antibiotic according to sensitivity on urine culture. All infants, and any child who is severely ill, require intravenous antibiotic therapy (e.g. cefotaxime or ampicillin and an aminoglycoside such as gentamicin, monitoring its serum levels) until the temperature has settled, when oral treatment is substituted. The urine should be recultured to ensure that infection has been eradicated.

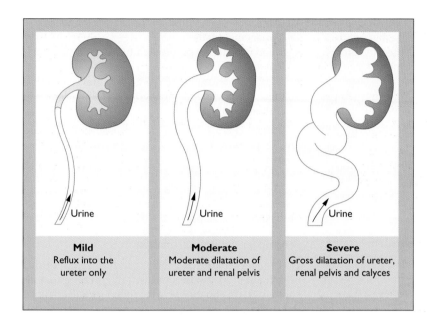

Fig. 16.11 Spectrum of severity of vesicoureteric reflux during a micturating cystourethrogram (MCUG).

Mild	Moderate	Severe
Reflux into the ureter only	Moderate dilatation of ureter and renal pelvis	Gross dilatation of ureter, renal pelvis and calyces

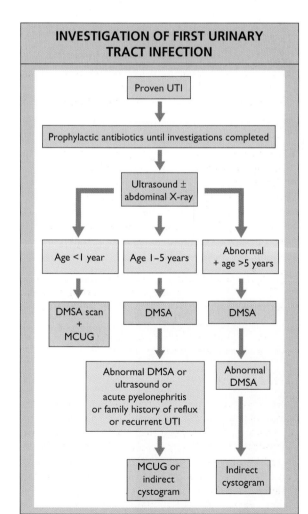

INVESTIGATION OF FIRST URINARY TRACT INFECTION

Proven UTI → Prophylactic antibiotics until investigations completed → Ultrasound ± abdominal X-ray

- Age <1 year → DMSA scan + MCUG
- Age 1–5 years → DMSA → Abnormal DMSA or ultrasound or acute pyelonephritis or family history of reflux or recurrent UTI → MCUG or indirect cystogram
- Abnormal + age >5 years → DMSA → Abnormal DMSA → Indirect cystogram

Fig. 16.12 An example of a protocol for the investigation of a first UTI.

All children should be investigated following their first confirmed UTI. The aim is to identify:

- serious structural abnormalities and urinary obstruction
- renal scars
- vesicoureteric reflux.

The investigations used are:
- a preliminary ultrasound to identify serious structural abnormalities and to detect bladder dysfunction (incomplete bladder emptying)
- an abdominal X-ray – ordered selectively to identify renal stones if this is suggested in the history or to identify occult spinal abnormalities if bladder emptying is abnormal
- static radioisotope scanning (e.g. DMSA scan to identify renal scars
- cystography (direct, i.e. MCUG, or indirect, e.g. MAG 3) to identify reflux.

The number of investigations should be kept to a minimum, particularly direct cystography which is unpleasant for the child and has a relatively high radiation dose. It can be replaced by indirect cystography when the child can void on request.

Infants less than 1 year old are fully investigated, as the incidence of abnormalities is highest at this age and the rapidly growing kidney is most susceptible to damage. With increasing age, renal scars and reflux become less common, and investigations are performed selectively. A suggested scheme of investigations is outlined in Figure 16.12, although protocols differ between centres.

The initial ultrasound of the kidneys and urinary tract should be performed promptly. Cystography and functional scans should be deferred for about 3 months after a UTI to avoid missing a newly developed scar and because of false-positive results due to transient reflux or inflammation (see Case history 16.2). Recurrence of infection can be prevented by prophylactic antibiotic therapy while awaiting the results of the investigations.

Several simple measures can be taken to try to prevent recurrence of UTI:

- high fluid intake to produce a high urine output
- regular voiding
- complete bladder emptying using double micturition to empty any residual or refluxed urine returning to the bladder
- avoidance of constipation
- good perineal hygiene.

Follow-up of children with recurrent UTIs, renal scarring or reflux

These children require:

- urine culture to be checked with non-specific illnesses in case it is caused by a UTI
- long-term low-dose antibiotic prophylaxis – trimethoprim (2 mg/kg at night) is used most often, but nitrofuranion or nalidixic acid may be given
- circumcision in boys to be considered as there is some evidence that it reduces the incidence of urinary tract infection

- surgical reimplantation of the ureters if medical management fails
- blood pressure to be checked twice a year if renal scarring is present
- regular assessment of renal growth and function if there is bilateral scarring because of the risk of chronic renal failure.

If there is renal scarring, an ultrasound is repeated after 2 years to check for renal growth. If there are further symptomatic UTIs, investigations are required to determine whether there are new scars or continuing reflux. Once reflux has resolved, or if the child has been asymptomatic for at least a year, antibiotic prophylaxis can be stopped.

Asymptomatic bacteriuria

Occasionally bacteriuria may be discovered during investigation of another problem in an asymptomatic child. Although treatment with antibiotics will eradicate the bacteriuria, recurrence is common. Asymptomatic bacteriuria does not need treatment as it does not cause renal damage.

> **All children need investigation after a first urinary tract infection.**

CASE HISTORY 16.2

URINARY TRACT INFECTION

A 2-month-old infant stopped feeding and had a high, intermittent fever. She was referred to hospital, where she had an infection screen. Urine examination showed >100 white blood cells, >10^5 E. coli/ml. She was treated with intravenous antibiotics. An ultrasound showed a small right kidney with a dilated renal pelvis and a dilated ureter. She was started on prophylactic antibiotics. A DMSA scan (Fig. 16.13) performed 3 months later confirmed bilateral renal scarring, with the right kidney contributing only 17% of renal function. The MCUG (Fig. 16.14) showed bilateral vesicoureteric reflux. At 5 years of age, the reflux had resolved and antibiotic prophylaxis was stopped. Her blood pressure and renal growth and function continue to be monitored.

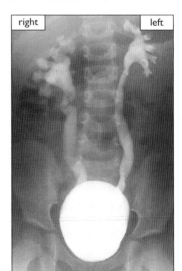

Fig. 16.14 Micturating cystourethrogram showing bilateral vesicoureteric reflux with ureteric dilatation and dilated, clubbed calyces on the right.

Fig. 16.13 DMSA scan showing a small scarred right kidney and scars at the upper and lower poles of the left kidney.

ENURESIS

Primary nocturnal enuresis

This is considered on page 320.

Daytime enuresis

This is a lack of bladder control during the day in a child old enough to be continent. Nocturnal enuresis is also usually present. It may be caused by:

- lack of attention to bladder sensation, a manifestation of a developmental or psychogenic problem which may be secondary to stress or part of a general behavioural problem
- detrusor instability (uncoordinated bladder contractions)
- bladder neck weakness
- a neurogenic bladder
- a urinary tract infection
- constipation
- an ectopic ureter.

Examination may reveal evidence of a neurogenic bladder, i.e. the bladder may be distended, there may be abnormal perineal sensation and anal tone or abnormal leg reflexes and gait. A midline spinal lesion may be present. Girls who are dry at night but wet on getting up are likely to have pooling of urine from an ectopic ureter opening into the vagina.

A urine is checked for microscopy, culture and sensitivity. Other investigations are performed if indicated. An ultrasound may show bladder pathology, with incomplete bladder emptying after passing urine or thickening of the bladder wall. Urodynamic studies may be required. An X-ray of the spine may reveal a vertebral anomaly. An MRI scan will be required to show any tethering of spinal nerve roots.

Affected children may benefit from star charts, bladder training and pelvic floor exercises. Constipation should be treated. A small portable alarm with a pad in the pants, which is activated by urine, can be used when there is lack of attention to bladder sensation. Anticholinergic or adrenergic drugs (e.g. oxybutynin to damp down bladder contractions or ephedrine to increase tone at the bladder neck) may be helpful if other measures fail.

Secondary enuresis

The loss of previously achieved urinary continence may be due to:

- emotional upset, the commonest cause
- UTI
- polyuria from an osmotic diuresis in diabetes mellitus or a renal concentrating disorder, e.g. sickle cell disease or chronic renal failure.

Investigation should include:
- checking a urine sample for infection, glycosuria and proteinuria

- assessment of urinary concentrating ability by measuring the osmolality of an early morning urine sample
- ultrasound of the renal tract.

PROTEINURIA

Proteinuria may be detected on urine 'dipstick' testing either incidentally in an asymptomatic child or when checked in a symptomatic child. Transient proteinuria may occur during febrile illnesses or after exercise and does not require investigation. Persistent proteinuria can be quantified by a 24-h urine, a timed collection (protein excretion should not exceed 4 mg/h per m^2) or, more usefully in younger children, by measuring the urine protein/creatinine ratio in an early morning sample (protein should not exceed 20 mg/mmol of creatinine).

A common cause is orthostatic proteinuria, where proteinuria is only found when the child is upright, i.e. during the day. It can be diagnosed by measuring the urine protein/creatinine ratio in early morning and daytime urine specimens. Renal function is normal and the prognosis is good. Other causes of proteinuria are listed in Figure 16.15.

Nephrotic syndrome

In nephrotic syndrome, heavy proteinuria results in a low plasma albumin and oedema. The cause of the condition is unknown, but a few cases are secondary to systemic diseases such as Henoch–Schönlein purpura (HSP), vasculitis (e.g. systemic lupus erythematosus, SLE), infections (e.g. malaria) or allergens (e.g. bee sting).

Clinical signs of the nephrotic syndrome are:
- periorbital oedema (particularly on waking), the earliest sign (Fig. 16.16)
- scrotal, leg and ankle oedema (Fig. 16.17)
- ascites
- breathlessness due to pleural effusions and abdominal distension.

The initial investigations are listed in Figure 16.18.

Fig. 16.15 Causes of proteinuria.

Orthostatic proteinuria
Glomerular abnormalities
  Minimal change disease
  Glomerulonephritis
  Abnormal glomerular basement membrane
    (familial nephritides)
Increased glomerular perfusion pressure
Reduced renal mass
Hypertension
Tubular proteinuria

NEPHROTIC SYNDROME

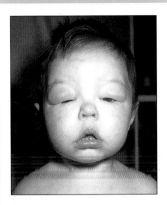

Fig. 16.16 Facial oedema in nephrotic syndrome.

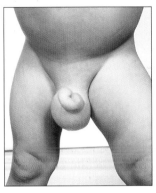

Fig. 16.17 Gross oedema of the scrotum and legs as well as abdominal distension from ascites.

Fig. 16.18 Investigations performed at presentation of nephrotic syndrome.

Urine protein – on test strips ('Dipstick')
Full blood count and ESR
Urea, electrolytes, creatinine, albumin
Complement levels – C3, C4
Antistreptolysin O titre and throat swab
Urine microscopy and culture
Urinary sodium concentration
Hepatitis B antigen

Steroid-sensitive nephrotic syndrome

In over 90% of children with nephrotic syndrome, the proteinuria resolves with corticosteroid therapy (steroid-sensitive nephrotic syndrome). These children do not progress to renal failure. It is commoner in boys and in atopic families. It is often precipitated by respiratory infections. Features suggesting steroid-sensitive nephrotic syndrome are:

- age between 1 and 10 years
- no macroscopic haematuria
- normal blood pressure
- normal complement levels
- normal renal function.

Management

At clinical presentation, treatment is begun with daily oral corticosteroids (60 mg/m² per day) unless there are atypical features. The average time for the urine to become free of protein is 10 days. After 4 weeks the dose is reduced to 40 mg/m² on alternate days for 4 weeks and then stopped. Children who do not respond to 4 weeks of corticosteroid therapy or have atypical features may have a more sinister diagnosis and require a renal biopsy. Renal histology in steroid-sensitive nephrotic syndrome is usually normal on light microscopy but podocyte fusion is seen on electron microscopy. For this reason it is called minimal change disease. In most of these children, the protein leak is mainly of low-molecular-weight proteins and is referred to as selective proteinuria, although this is no longer measured routinely as it does not reliably predict steroid responsiveness.

The child with nephrotic syndrome is susceptible to several serious complications at presentation or relapse:

- *Hypovolaemia*. During the initial phase of oedema formation the intravascular compartment may become volume-depleted. The child who becomes hypovolaemic characteristically complains of abdominal pain and may feel faint. There is peripheral vasoconstriction and urinary sodium retention. A low urinary sodium (<20 mmol/L) and a high packed cell volume are indications of hypovolaemia, which requires urgent treatment with intravenous albumin (4.5%), as the child is at risk of vascular thrombosis and shock.

Increasing peripheral oedema, assessed clinically and by daily weight, may cause striae, discomfort and respiratory compromise. If severe, this needs treatment with intravenous albumin and diuretics. Care must be taken with the use of colloid, as it may precipitate pulmonary oedema and hypertension from fluid overload, and also with diuretics, which may cause or worsen hypovolaemia.

- *Thrombosis*. A hypercoagulable state, due to urinary losses of antithrombin, increased synthesis of clotting factors and increased blood viscosity from the raised haematocrit, predisposes to thrombosis.

- *Infection*. Urinary loss of immunoglobulins contributes to the increased susceptibility to infection, particularly with *Pneumococcus*. Peritonitis may occur. Penicillin prophylaxis should be given to all children while they have hypoalbuminaemia.

- *Hypercholesterolaemia*. This correlates inversely with the serum albumin, but the cause of the hyperlipidaemia is not fully understood.

Prognosis

This is summarised in Figure 16.19. Relapses are identified by parents on urine testing. The side-effects of corticosteroid therapy may be reduced by an alternate-day regimen. If relapses are frequent or if a high maintenance dose is required, involvement of a paediatric nephrologist is advisable as other drug

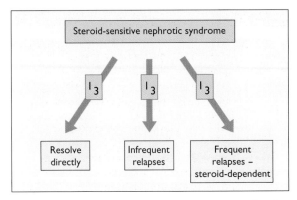

Fig. 16.19 Clinical course in steroid-responsive nephrotic syndrome.

therapy may be considered. Levamisole, an immuno-modulator, may maintain remission. Cyclophosphamide maintains remission in 75% of cases for 1 year, and 50% at 5 years, but its toxicity restricts its use to the most severely affected children. Cyclosporin A maintains remission while it is being taken, but relapse often occurs when it is stopped. Renal biopsy is necessary before starting cyclosporin A because of its nephrotoxicity.

Steroid-resistant nephrotic syndrome (Fig. 16.20)
These children should be managed by a paediatric nephrologist. Management of the oedema is by diuretic therapy, salt restriction and captopril, an ACE inhibitor, which may reduce proteinuria.

Congenital nephrotic syndrome
Congenital nephrotic syndrome presents in the first 3 months of life. It is rare. It is associated with early end-stage renal failure and a high mortality. When renal failure develops, nephrectomy and dialysis are instituted until the child is large enough for transplantation.

An oedematous child – test for proteinuria to diagnose nephrotic syndrome.

HAEMATURIA

Urine which is red in colour or tests positive for haemoglobin on test strips (dipstick) should be examined under the microscope to confirm haematuria (>10 red blood cells per high-power field). Glomerular haematuria is suggested by brown urine, the presence of deformed red cells (which occurs as they pass through the basement membrane) and casts, and is often accompanied by proteinuria. Lower urinary tract haematuria is usually red, occurs at the end of the urinary stream, is not accompanied by proteinuria and is unusual in children.

Urinary tract infection is the most common cause of haematuria (Fig. 16.21). The history and examination may suggest the diagnosis, e.g. a family history of stone formation or nephritis or a history of trauma. A plan of investigation is outlined in Figure 16.22. A renal biopsy is indicated if:

- there is recurrent macroscopic haematuria
- a familial nephritis is suspected
- renal function is abnormal
- the complement levels are persistently abnormal
- there is proteinuria.

Acute nephritis

Acute nephritis in childhood usually follows a streptococcal sore throat or skin infection. Streptococcal nephritis remains a common condition in the developing world, but has become uncommon and mild in the UK, although there has been a recent increase in its incidence. Other less common causes of acute nephritis are listed in Figure 16.23. In acute nephritis, increased glomerular cellularity restricts glomerular blood flow and therefore filtration is decreased. This leads to:

- decreased urine output and volume overload
- hypertension, which may cause seizures
- oedema, characteristically around the eyes
- haematuria and proteinuria.

Management is by attention to water and electrolyte balance and the use of diuretics when necessary. Rarely, there may be a rapid deterioration in renal

Fig. 16.20 Steroid-resistant nephrotic syndrome.

Cause	Specific features	Prognosis
Focal segmental glomerulosclerosis	Most common Familial or idiopathic	30% progress to end-stage renal failure in 5 years; 20% respond to cyclophosphamide, vincristine or cyclosporin
Mesangiocapillary glomerulonephritis (membranoproliferative glomerulonephritis)	More common in older children Haematuria and low complement level present	Decline in renal function over many years
Membranous nephropathy	Associated with hepatitis B	Most remit spontaneously within 5 years May precede SLE

HAEMATURIA

Fig. 16.21 Causes of haematuria.

Non-glomerular
Infection (bacterial, viral, TB, schistosomiasis)
Trauma to genitalia, urinary tract or kidneys
Stones
Tumours
Sickle cell disease
Bleeding disorders
Renal vein thrombosis
Hypercalciuria

Glomerular
Acute glomerulonephritis
Chronic glomerulonephritis
IgA nephropathy
Familial nephritis
Thin basement membrane disease

Fig. 16.22 Investigation of haematuria.

All patients
Urine microscopy (with phase contrast) and culture
Protein and calcium excretion
Kidney and urinary tract ultrasound and abdominal
    X-ray
Plasma urea, electrolytes, creatinine, calcium,
    phosphate, albumin
Full blood count, platelets, clotting screen,
    sickle cell screen

If suggestive of glomerular haematuria
ESR complement levels and anti-DNA binding
Throat swab and antistreptolysin O titre
Hepatitis B antigen
Renal biopsy if indicated
Test mother's urine for blood ⎫ if Alport's
Hearing test   ⎭ syndrome suspected

Fig. 16.23 Causes of acute nephritis.

Post-infectious (including *streptococcus*)
Vasculitis (Henoch–Schönlein purpura or, rarely,
    SLE, Wegener's granulomatosis, microscopic
    polyarteritis, polyarteritis nodosa)
IgA nephropathy and mesangiocapillary
    glomerulonephritis
Anti-glomerular basement membrane disease
    (Goodpasture's syndrome) – very rare

---

function (rapidly progressive glomerulonephritis). This may occur with any cause of acute nephritis, but is uncommon when the cause is post-streptococcal; it is characteristic of anti-glomerular basement membrane disease. If left untreated, irreversible renal failure will occur over weeks or months, so renal biopsy and treatment with immunosuppression must be undertaken promptly.

Post-streptococcal nephritis

This is diagnosed by a raised ASO titre and low complement C3 levels that return to normal after 3–4 weeks. Long-term prognosis is good.

Henoch–Schönlein purpura

Henoch–Schönlein purpura is the combination of:

- characteristic skin rash
- arthralgia
- periarticular oedema
- abdominal pain
- glomerulonephritis.

It usually occurs between the ages of 3 and 10 years, is twice as common in boys, peaks during the winter months and is often preceded by an upper respiratory infection. It is postulated that genetic predisposition and antigen exposure increase circulating IgA levels and disrupt IgG synthesis. The IgA and IgG interact to produce complexes that activate complement and are deposited in affected organs, precipitating an inflammatory response with vasculitis.

Clinical findings (Fig. 16.24)
At presentation, affected children often have a fever. The *rash* is the most obvious feature. It is symmetrically distributed over the buttocks, the extensor surfaces of the arms and legs, and the ankles. The trunk is spared unless lesions are induced by trauma. The rash may initially be urticarial, rapidly becoming maculopapular and purpuric, is characteristically palpable and may recur over several weeks. The rash is the first clinical feature in about 50% and is the cornerstone of the diagnosis, which is clinical.

Joint pain occurs in two-thirds of patients, particularly of the knees and ankles. There is *periarticular oedema*. Long-term damage to the joints does not occur, and symptoms usually resolve before the rash goes.

Colicky abdominal pain occurs in many children and, if severe, can be treated with corticosteroids. Gastrointestinal petechiae can cause haematemesis and melaena. Intussusception can occur and can be particularly difficult to diagnose under these circumstances. Ileus, protein-losing enteropathy, orchitis and occasionally central nervous system involvement are rare complications.

Renal involvement is common, but is rarely the first symptom. Over 80% have microscopic or macroscopic

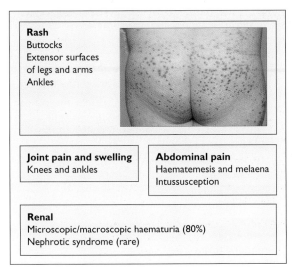

Rash
Buttocks
Extensor surfaces
of legs and arms
Ankles

Joint pain and swelling
Knees and ankles

Abdominal pain
Haematemesis and melaena
Intussusception

Renal
Microscopic/macroscopic haematuria (80%)
Nephrotic syndrome (rare)

Fig. 16.24 Main clinical manifestations of Henoch–Schönlein purpura. (Photo courtesy of Dr Michael Markiewicz.)

Fig. 16.25 Causes of palpable kidneys.

Unilateral
Multicystic kidney
Compensatory hypertrophy
Obstructed hydronephrosis
Renal tumour (Wilms's tumour)
Renal vein thrombosis

Bilateral
Autosomal recessive (infantile) polycystic kidneys
Autosomal dominant (adult) polycystic kidneys
Tuberous sclerosis
Renal vein thrombosis

haematuria or mild proteinuria. These children usually make a complete recovery. If proteinuria is more severe, nephrotic syndrome may result. Risk factors for progressive renal disease are heavy proteinuria, oedema, hypertension and deteriorating renal function, when a renal biopsy will determine if treatment is necessary. All children with renal involvement are followed for a year to detect those with persisting urinary abnormalities (5–10%). Follow-up is necessary as hypertension and declining renal function may develop after an interval of several years.

IgA nephropathy

This may present with episodes of macroscopic haematuria, commonly in association with upper respiratory tract infections. Histological findings and management are as for Henoch–Schönlein purpura, which may be a variant of the same pathological process but not restricted to the kidney.

Familial nephritis

The commonest familial nephritis is Alport's syndrome. This is usually an X-linked recessive disorder that progresses to end-stage renal failure by early adult life in males and is associated with nerve deafness and ocular defects. The mother may have haematuria.

Vasculitis

The commonest vasculitis to involve the kidney is Henoch–Schönlein purpura. However, renal involvement may occur in SLE, which presents in teenage girls, and rarer vasculitides such as polyarteritis nodosa, microscopic polyarteritis and Wegener's granulomatosis. Characteristic symptoms are fever, malaise, weight loss, skin rash and arthropathy. Many autoantibodies occur in SLE, but anti-double-stranded DNA antibodies with low complement levels are characteristic. Haematuria and proteinuria are indications for renal biopsy, as immunosuppression is likely to be necessary and its intensity will depend on the severity of renal involvement. Antineutrophil cytoplasm antibodies may be present in other vasculitides. Renal arteriography, to demonstrate the presence of aneurysms, will diagnose polyarteritis nodosa.

RENAL MASSES

An abdominal mass identified on palpating the abdomen should be investigated promptly by ultrasound scan (Fig. 16.25). Bilaterally enlarged kidneys in early life are most frequently due to autosomal recessive polycystic kidney disease, which is associated with hypertension, hepatic fibrosis and progression to chronic renal failure. This form of polycystic kidney disease must be distinguished from the autosomal dominant adult-type polycystic kidney disease, which has a more benign prognosis.

RENAL CALCULI

Renal stones are uncommon in childhood. When they occur, predisposing causes must be sought:

- urinary tract infection
- structural anomalies of the urinary tract
- metabolic abnormalities.

The commonest are phosphate stones associated with infection, especially with *Proteus*. Calcium-containing stones occur in idiopathic hypercalciuria, the most common metabolic abnormality, and with increased urinary urate and oxalate excretion. Deposition of calcium in the parenchyma (nephrocalcinosis) may occur with hypercalciuria, hyperoxaluria and distal renal tubular acidosis. Nephrocalcinosis may be a complication of frusemide therapy in the neonate. Cystine and xanthine stones are rare.

Presentation may be with haematuria, loin or abdominal pain, UTI or passage of a stone.

Stones that are not passed spontaneously should be removed, by either lithotripsy or surgery, and any predisposing structural anomaly repaired. A high fluid intake is recommended in all affected children. If the cause is a metabolic abnormality, specific therapy may be possible.

RENAL TUBULAR DISORDERS

Abnormalities of renal tubular function may occur at any point along the length of the nephron and affect any of the substances handled by it.

Generalised proximal tubular dysfunction (Fanconi syndrome)

The cardinal features are excessive urinary loss of amino acids, glucose, phosphate, bicarbonate, sodium, calcium, potassium and urate. The causes are listed in Figure 16.26. Fanconi syndrome should be considered in a child presenting with:

- polydipsia and polyuria
- salt depletion and dehydration
- hyperchloraemic metabolic acidosis
- rickets and osteoporosis
- failure to thrive/poor growth.

Specific transport defects
(See Fig. 16.27).

ACUTE RENAL FAILURE

Acute renal failure is a sudden reduction in renal function. Oliguria (<0.5 ml/kg per h) is usually present. It can be classified as (Fig. 16.28):

- prerenal – the commonest cause in children
- renal – there is salt and water retention; blood, protein and casts are often present in the urine; and there may be symptoms specific to an accompanying disease (e.g. Henoch–Schönlein purpura)
- postrenal – from urinary obstruction.

Acute-on-chronic renal failure is suggested by the child having growth failure, anaemia and disordered bone mineralisation (renal osteodystrophy).

Management
Children with acute renal failure should have their circulation and fluid balance meticulously monitored. Investigation by ultrasound scan will identify obstruction of the urinary tract, the small kidneys of chronic renal failure, or large, bright kidneys with loss of cortical medullary differentiation typical of an acute process.

Prerenal failure
This is suggested by hypovolaemia. The urinary sodium concentration is very low as the body tries to retain fluid. The hypovolaemia needs to be urgently corrected with fluid replacement and circulatory support if acute tubular necrosis is to be avoided.

Fig. 16.26 Causes of Fanconi syndrome.

Idiopathic
Secondary to inborn errors of metabolism
Cystinosis (an autosomal recessive disorder causing intracellular accumulation of cystine)
Glycogen storage disorders
Lower's syndrome (oculocerebrorenal dystrophy)
Galactosaemia
Fructose intolerance
Tyrosinaemia
Wilson's disease

Acquired
Heavy metals
Drugs and toxins
Vitamin D deficiency

Renal failure
If there is circulatory overload, restriction of fluid intake and challenge with a diuretic may increase urine output sufficiently to allow gradual correction of sodium and water balance. A high-calorie, low-protein feed will decrease catabolism, uraemia and hyperkalaemia. Emergency management of metabolic acidosis, hyperkalaemia and hyperphosphataemia is shown in Figure 16.29. If the cause of renal failure is not obvious, a renal biopsy should be performed to identify rapidly progressive glomerulonephritis, as this needs immediate treatment with immunosuppression.

Postrenal failure
This requires assessment of the site of obstruction and relief by nephrostomy or bladder catheterisation. Surgery can be performed once fluid volume and electrolyte abnormalities have been corrected.

Dialysis in acute renal failure is indicated when there is:

- failure of conservative management
- hyperkalaemia
- severe hypo- or hypernatraemia
- pulmonary oedema or hypertension
- severe acidosis
- multisystem failure.

Peritoneal dialysis is the most common choice for children as it is easier to perform than haemodialysis. If plasma exchange is part of treatment, haemodialysis is used. If there is cardiac decompensation or hypercatabolism, continuous arteriovenous or venovenous haemofiltration or dialysis provides gentle, continuous dialysis and fluid removal.

Acute renal failure in childhood generally carries a good prognosis for renal recovery unless complicating a life-threatening condition, e.g. severe infection, following cardiac surgery or multisystem failure.

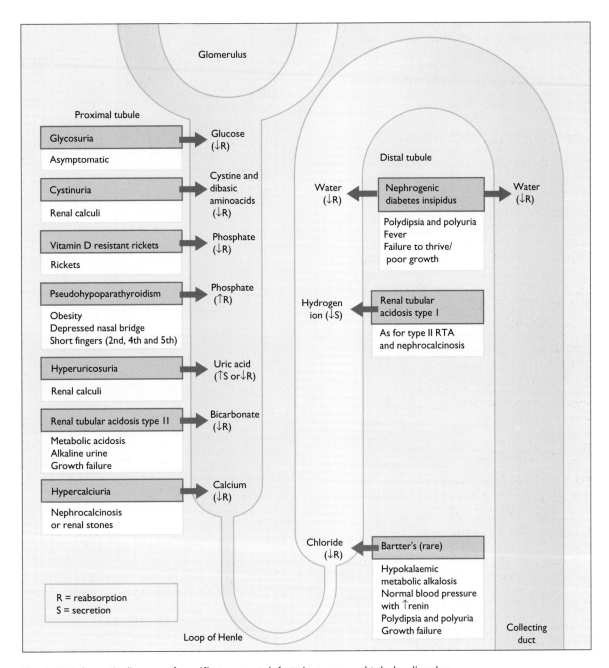

Fig. 16.27 Schematic diagram of specific transport defects in some renal tubular disorders.

Haemolytic uraemic syndrome

Haemolytic uraemic syndrome (HUS) is a triad of acute renal failure, microangiopathic haemolytic anaemia and thrombocytopenia. It is the most common renal cause of acute renal failure in childhood. The disorder is thought to be due to activation of neutrophils which damage vascular endothelium. Typical HUS is secondary to gastrointestinal infection with verocytotoxin-producing *E. coli* O157:H7 or, less often, *Shigella*. It follows a prodrome of bloody diarrhoea. Although the platelet count is reduced, the clotting is normal (unlike in disseminated intravascular coagulation, DIC). Other organs such as the brain, pancreas and heart may also be involved.

With early supportive therapy, including dialysis, the typical diarrhoea-associated HUS usually has a good prognosis, although follow-up is necessary as there may be persistent proteinuria and the development of hypertension and declining renal function in subsequent years. In contrast, atypical HUS has no diarrhoeal prodrome, may be familial and frequently relapses. It has a high risk of hypertension and chronic renal failure and has a high mortality. Children with

> **Fig. 16.28** Causes of acute renal failure.
>
> | Prerenal | Renal | Postrenal |
> |---|---|---|
> | Hypovolaemia | Vascular | Obstruction |
> | Gastroenteritis | Haemolytic uraemic syndrome (HUS) | Congenital |
> | Burns | Vasculitis | Acquired |
> | Sepsis | Embolus | |
> | Haemorrhage | Renal vein thrombosis | |
> | Nephrotic syndrome | Tubular | |
> | Circulatory failure | Acute tubular necrosis (ATN) | |
> | | Ischaemic | |
> | | Toxic | |
> | | Obstructive | |
> | | Glomerular | |
> | | Glomerulonephritis | |
> | | Interstitial | |
> | | Interstitial nephritis | |
> | | Pyelonephritis | |
> | | Acute-on-chronic renal failure | |

> **Fig. 16.29** Metabolic abnormalities in acute renal failure and their therapy.
>
> | Metabolic abnormality | Treatment |
> |---|---|
> | Metabolic acidosis | Sodium bicarbonate |
> | Hyperphosphataemia | Calcium carbonate |
> | Hyperkalaemia | Calcium exchange resin |
> | | Salbutamol |
> | | Glucose and insulin |
> | | Dialysis |

> **Fig. 16.30** Causes of hypertension.
>
> **Renin-dependent**
>   Renal parenchymal disease
>   Renovascular, e.g. renal artery stenosis
>   Renal tumours
> **Coarctation of the aorta**
> **Catecholamine excess**
>   Phaeochromocytoma
>   Neuroblastoma
> **Endocrine causes**
>   Congenital adrenal hyperplasia
>   Cushing's syndrome or corticosteroid therapy
> **Essential hypertension**

intracerebral involvement or with atypical HUS may be treated with prostacyclin or plasma exchange, but the efficacy is unproven.

Haemolytic uraemic syndrome (HUS) – the triad of:
- acute renal failure
- haemolytic anaemia
- thrombocytopenia.

HYPERTENSION

Symptomatic hypertension in children is usually secondary and of renal origin. Most often, this is due to renal parenchymal disease from scarring following reflux nephropathy. Coarctation of the aorta is another important cause in children. Other causes are rare (Fig. 16.30).

Presentation includes vomiting, headaches, facial palsy, hypertensive retinopathy, convulsions or proteinuria. Failure to thrive and cardiac failure are the most common features in infants. Phaeochromocytoma may cause paroxysmal palpitations and sweating.

Some causes are correctable, e.g. nephrectomy for unilateral scarring, angioplasty for renal artery stenosis, surgical repair of coarctation of the aorta, resection of a phaeochromocytoma, but in most cases medical treatment is necessary with antihypertensive drugs.

Early detection of hypertension is important. Any child with renal scarring should have his blood pressure checked twice a year throughout life. Children with a family history of essential hypertension should be encouraged to restrict their salt intake, avoid obesity and have their blood pressure checked regularly.

CHRONIC RENAL FAILURE

Chronic renal failure is much less common in children than in adults, with an incidence of only 10 per million of the child population entering end-stage renal failure each year. Congenital and familial causes are more common in childhood than are acquired diseases (Fig. 16.31).

Fig. 16.31 Causes of chronic renal failure.

Structural malformations	40%
Glomerulonephritis	25%
Hereditary nephropathies	20%
Systemic diseases	10%
Miscellaneous/unknown	5%

Clinical features

Chronic renal failure presents with:

- anorexia and lethargy
- polydipsia and polyuria
- failure to thrive/growth failure
- bony deformities from renal osteodystrophy (renal rickets)
- hypertension
- acute-on-chronic renal failure (precipitated by infection or dehydration)
- incidental finding of proteinuria.

Many children with chronic renal failure have had their renal disease detected before birth by antenatal ultrasound or have previously identified renal disease. Symptoms rarely develop before renal function falls to less than two-thirds of normal.

Management

The aims of management are to prevent the symptoms and metabolic abnormalities of chronic renal failure, to allow normal growth and development and to preserve residual renal function. The management of these children should be supervised by a specialist paediatric nephrology centre.

Diet

Anorexia and vomiting are common. Improving nutrition using calorie supplements and nasogastric or gastrostomy feeding is often necessary to prevent growth failure. Protein intake should be sufficient to maintain growth and a normal albumin, whilst preventing the accumulation of toxic metabolic by-products.

Prevention of renal osteodystrophy

Phosphate retention and hypocalcaemia due to decreased activation of vitamin D result in secondary hyperparathyroidism, osteitis fibrosa and osteomalacia. Phosphate restriction by decreasing the dietary intake of milk products, calcium carbonate as a phosphate binder, and activated vitamin D supplements help to prevent renal osteodystrophy.

Control of salt and water balance and acidosis

Many children with chronic renal failure caused by congenital structural malformations and renal dysplasia have an obligatory loss of salt and water. They need salt supplements and free access to water. Treatment with bicarbonate supplements is necessary to prevent acidosis.

Anaemia

Reduced production of erythropoietin and circulation of metabolites that are toxic to bone marrow result in anaemia. This responds well to the administration of recombinant human erythropoietin.

Hormonal abnormalities

Many hormonal abnormalities occur in chronic renal failure. Most importantly, there is growth hormone resistance with high growth hormone levels but poor growth. Recombinant human growth hormone has been shown to be effective in improving growth for up to 5 years of treatment, but whether it improves final height remains unknown. Many children with chronic renal failure have delayed puberty and a subnormal pubertal growth spurt.

Dialysis and transplantation

It is now possible for all children, no matter how small, to enter renal replacement therapy programmes when end-stage renal failure is reached. The optimum management is by renal transplantation. Technically this is difficult in very small children, but infants weighing 10 kg have been successfully transplanted. Kidneys obtained from parents or relatives have a higher success rate than cadaveric donor kidneys, which are matched as far as possible to the recipient's HLA type. Patient survival is high and first-year graft survival is around 80%, although technical difficulties reduce this rate in very young recipients and with small donor kidneys. Graft losses from both acute and chronic rejection or recurrent disease mean that the 5-year graft survival is reduced to 70% and some children need re-transplantation. Current immunosuppression is with combinations of prednisolone, azathioprine and cyclosporin A.

Ideally a child is transplanted before dialysis is required, but if this is not possible, a period of dialysis may be necessary. Peritoneal dialysis, either by cycling overnight using a machine (continuous cycling peritoneal dialysis) or by manual exchanges over 24 h (continuous ambulatory peritoneal dialysis), is preferable to haemodialysis as it can be done by the parents at home and is therefore less disruptive to family life and the child's schooling.

FURTHER READING

Barratt T M, Avner E D, Harmon W E 1999 Pediatric nephrology. Williams & Wilkins, Baltimore. *A comprehensive textbook*
Garin et al 1998 Primary vesicoureteric reflux; review of current concepts. Pediatric Nephrology 12: 249–256
Poslethwaite R J 1994 Clinical paediatric nephrology. Butterworth-Heinemann, Oxford. *Short textbook*

17

Genitalia

Most abnormalities of the genitalia in male infants are due to abnormal embryogenesis.

INGUINOSCROTAL DISORDERS

Embryology

The testis is formed from the urogenital ridge on the posterior abdominal wall close to the developing kidney. Gonadal induction to form a testis is regulated by genes on the Y chromosome. During gestation, the testis migrates down towards the inguinal canal, guided by mesenchymal tissue known as the gubernaculum, probably under the influence of anti-Mullerian hormone (Fig. 17.1a).

Inguinoscrotal descent of the testis requires the release of testosterone from the fetal testis. A tongue of peritoneum, the processus vaginalis, precedes the

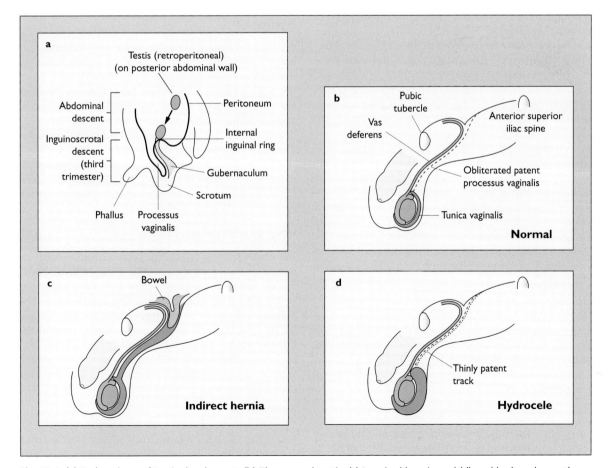

Fig. 17.1 (a) Embryology of testicular descent. (b) The normal testis. (c) Inguinal hernia and (d) and hydrocele are the result of incomplete obliteration of the processus vaginalis.

INGUINAL HERNIA IN INFANTS

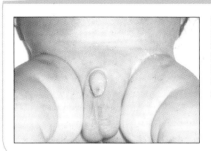

Fig. 17.2 Left inguinal hernia in an infant. The left groin is only slightly swollen.

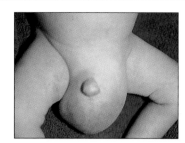

Fig. 17.3 Bilateral inguinal hernias in a preterm infant. Inguinal hernia is primarily a groin swelling; only when it is large does it extend into the scrotum.

migrating testis through the inguinal canal. This peritoneal extension normally becomes obliterated after birth, but failure of this process may lead to the development of an inguinal hernia or hydrocele (Fig. 17.1b–d).

Inguinal hernia

Inguinal hernias in children are almost always indirect and due to a patent processus vaginalis. They are much more frequent in boys and are particularly common in premature infants. Hernias are more common on the right side. At least 1 in 50 boys will develop an inguinal hernia.

Inguinal hernias usually present as an intermittent swelling in the groin or scrotum on crying or straining. Unless the hernia is observed as an inguinal swelling (Figs 17.2 and 17.3), diagnosis relies on the history and the identification of thickening of the spermatic cord (or round ligament in girls). The groin swelling may become visible on raising the intra-abdominal pressure by gently pressing on the abdomen or asking the child to cough.

An inguinal hernia in an infant may present as an irreducible lump in the groin or scrotum. The lump is firm and tender. The infant may be unwell with irritability and vomiting. Most 'irreducible' hernias can be successfully reduced following sustained gentle compression and opioid analgesia. Surgery is delayed for 24–48 h to allow resolution of oedema. If reduction is impossible, emergency surgery is required because of the risk of strangulation of bowel and damage to the testis.

Surgery

The operation is carried out via an inguinal skin crease incision and involves ligation and division of the hernial sac (processus vaginalis). Except in small infants, this can usually be undertaken as a day-case procedure, provided there is appropriate anaesthetic and surgical support.

 Inguinal hernias in infants should be repaired promptly to avoid the risk of strangulation.

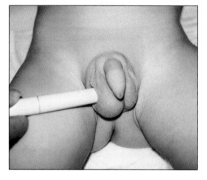

Fig. 17.4 Right-sided hydrocele. This scrotal swelling often has a bluish discoloration and will transilluminate in a darkened room.

Hydrocele

A patent processus vaginalis, which is sufficiently narrow to prevent the formation of an inguinal hernia, may still allow peritoneal fluid to track down around the testis to form a hydrocele (Fig. 17.4). Hydroceles are asymptomatic scrotal swellings, often bilateral, and sometimes with a bluish discoloration. They may be tense or lax but are non-tender and transilluminate. The majority resolve spontaneously as the processus continues to obliterate, but surgery is required in children older than 18 months. A hydrocele of the cord forms a non-tender mobile swelling in the spermatic cord.

Undescended testis

An undescended testis has been arrested along its normal pathway of descent (Fig. 17.5). At birth, about 5% of full-term male infants will have a unilateral or bilateral undescended testis (cryptorchidism). The incidence is higher in preterm infants because testicular descent through the inguinal canal occurs in the third trimester. Testicular descent may continue during early infancy and by 3 months of age the overall rate of cryptorchidism in boys is 1.5%, with little change thereafter.

Examination

This should be carried out in a warm room, with warm hands and a relaxed child. The testes can then be brought down into a palpable position by gently massaging the contents of the inguinal canal towards the scrotum.

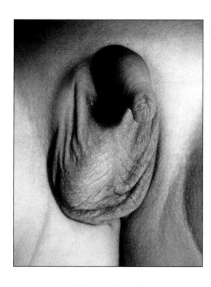

Fig. 17.5 A left undescended testis with an empty hemiscrotum.

Classification
Retractile
The testis can be manipulated into the bottom of the scrotum without tension, but subsequently retracts into the inguinal region, pulled up by the cremasteric muscle. The testis has usually been found in the scrotum at a neonatal check. With age, the testis resides permanently in the scrotum. Follow-up is advisable as, rarely, the testis subsequently ascends into the inguinal canal.

Palpable
The testis can be palpated in the groin but cannot be manipulated into the scrotum. Occasionally, a testis is ectopic, when it lies outside its normal line of descent and may then be found in the perineum or femoral triangle.

Impalpable
No testis can be felt on careful examination. The testis may be in the inguinal canal, intra-abdominal or absent.

Investigations
Useful investigations include:

- ultrasound – this has a role in identifying testes in the inguinal canal in obese boys
- hormonal – for bilateral impalpable testes, the presence of testicular tissue can be confirmed by recording a rise in serum testosterone in response to intramuscular injections of human chorionic gonadotrophin (HCG); these boys may require specialist endocrine review
- laparoscopy – the investigation of choice for the impalpable testis to determine if it is intra-abdominal or absent.

Management
Surgical placement of the testis in the scrotum (*orchidopexy*) is undertaken for several reasons:

- *Fertility* – to optimise spermatogenesis, the testis needs to be in the scrotum below body temperature. The timing of orchidopexy is controversial, but evidence suggests that early orchidopexy during the second year of life may optimise reproductive potential. Fertility after orchidopexy for a unilateral undescended testis is close to normal, but men with a history of bilaterally impalpable testes are usually sterile.
- *Malignancy* – undescended testes have histological abnormalities and an increased risk of malignancy. The greatest risk is for testes which are intra-abdominal. The risk is greater for bilateral undescended testes. There is some evidence that early orchidopexy for a unilaterally undescended testis reduces the risk to nearly the same as a normal testis.
- *Cosmetic and psychological* – if one testis proves to be absent, a prosthesis can be used but this is best delayed until a larger adult-sized prosthesis can be inserted.

Surgery
Most boys with an undescended testis undergo an orchidopexy via an inguinal incision. The testis is mobilised, preserving the vas deferens and testicular vessels, the associated patent processus vaginalis is ligated and divided, and the testis is placed in a scrotal pouch. The operation is usually performed as a day-case procedure. Orchidectomy is often advised for a unilateral intra-abdominal testis which cannot be corrected by simple orchidopexy, because of the future risk of malignancy. Microvascular orchidopexy or staged orchidopexy are two of the options available to preserve the testis in rarer cases of bilateral intra-abdominal testes, when the testicular vessels are too short to allow a single-stage procedure. Although intra-abdominal testes have profoundly defective spermatogenesis, they are capable of producing male hormones.

Varicocele

Varicosities of the testicular veins may develop in boys around puberty. They are usually on the left side and there is an association with subfertility. Treatment is indicated for symptoms (dragging, aching) and, in later life, for infertility. Obliteration of the testicular veins can be achieved by surgery, laparoscopic techniques or radiological embolisation. The role of such interventions in asymptomatic boys is uncertain.

The acute scrotum
Torsion of the testis

Testicular torsion is most common in adolescents but may occur at any age, including the perinatal period (Fig. 17.6). The pain is not always centred on the scrotum but may be in the groin or lower abdomen. There may be a history of previous self-limiting episodes. Torsion of the testis must be relieved within 6–12 h of the onset of symptoms for there to be a good chance of testicular viability. Surgical exploration is mandatory

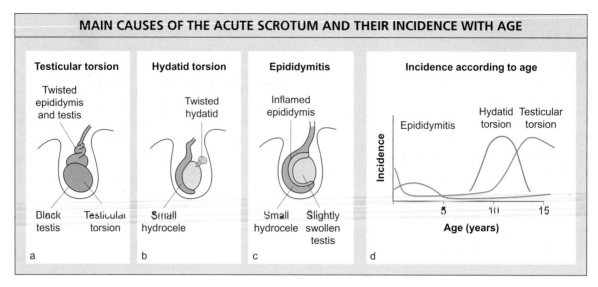

MAIN CAUSES OF THE ACUTE SCROTUM AND THEIR INCIDENCE WITH AGE

Fig. 17.6 Commoner causes of the acute scrotum and their incidence according to age. (a) Testicular torsion. (b) Hydatid torsion. (c) Epididymitis. (d) Incidence in relation to age.

unless torsion can be excluded. Fixation of the contralateral testis is essential because there may be an anatomical predisposition to torsion (e.g. the bell clapper testis). An undescended testis is at increased risk of torsion. Expert Doppler ultrasound looking at flow in the testicular blood vessels may allow the differentiation of torsion of the testis from epididymitis.

Torsion of testicular appendage

A hydatid of Morgagni is an embryological remnant found on the upper pole of the testis. Torsion of this appendage characteristically affects boys just prior to puberty. This may be because of rapid enlargement of the hydatid in response to gonadotrophins. The pain may increase over 1 or 2 days and occasionally the torted hydatid can be seen or felt (the blue dot sign). Surgical exploration and excision of the appendage leads to rapid resolution of the problem.

Other causes

Viral or bacterial epididymo-orchitis or epididymitis may cause an acute scrotum in infants and toddlers, and scrotal exploration is often necessary to confirm the diagnosis. If an associated urinary tract infection is present, antibiotic treatment and full investigation of the urinary tract will be required. Other conditions which may cause scrotal symptoms and signs are idiopathic scrotal oedema (usually painless, bilateral scrotal swelling and redness in a pre-school child) or an incarcerated inguinal hernia.

Torsion of the testis is an emergency and must always be considered in a boy with an acutely painful scrotum.

ABNORMALITIES OF THE PENIS

Hypospadias

In the male fetus, urethral tubularisation occurs in a proximal to distal direction under the influence of fetal testosterone. Failure to complete this process leaves the urethral opening proximal to the normal meatus on the glans and this is termed hypospadias (Fig. 17.7). This is a common congenital anomaly, affecting about 1 in every 300 boys.

Hypospadias consists of:
- A ventral urethral meatus – in most cases the urethra opens on or adjacent to the glans penis, but in severe cases the opening may be on the penile shaft or in the perineum.
- A hooded dorsal foreskin – the foreskin has failed to fuse ventrally (Fig. 17.8).
- Chordee – a ventral curvature of the shaft of the penis, most apparent on erection. This is only marked in the more severe forms of hypospadias (Fig. 17.9).

Glanular hypospadias may be a cosmetic concern. Coronal and more proximal varieties may cause major functional problems. With more severe varieties of hypospadias, additional genitourinary anomalies should be excluded and sometimes it is necessary to consider ambiguous genitalia and intersex disorders.

Surgery

Correction is often undertaken before 2 years of age, often as a single-stage operation. The aims of surgery are to produce:

- a terminal urethral meatus so that the boy can stand to micturate
- a straight erection
- a penis that looks normal.

HYPOSPADIAS

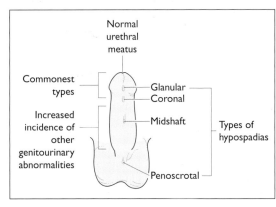

Fig. 17.7 Varieties of hypospadias.

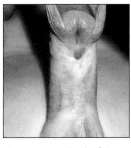

Fig. 17.8 Penile shaft hypospadias with dorsal hooded foreskin.

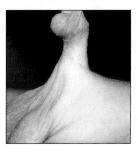

Fig. 17.9 In lateral view, the ventral curvature of the penis (chordee) can be seen.

> **Infants with hypospadias must not be circumcised, as the foreskin is often needed for later reconstructive surgery.**

Circumcision

At birth, the foreskin is adherent to the surface of the glans penis. These adhesions separate spontaneously with time, allowing the foreskin to become more mobile and eventually retractile. At 1 year of age, approximately 50% of boys have a *non-retractile foreskin*, but by 4 years this has declined to 10%, and by 16 years to only 1%. A non-retractile foreskin often leads to ballooning on micturition, which is physiological. Gentle retraction of the foreskin at bathtimes helps to maintain hygiene, but forcible retraction of a healthy non-retractile foreskin should be avoided.

Two conditions that require reassurance are preputial adhesions (when the foreskin remains partially adherent to the glans) and the presence of white 'pearls' under the foreskin due to trapped epithelial squames. Both conditions are usually asymptomatic and resolve spontaneously.

Circumcision is one of the earliest recorded operations and remains an important tradition in the Jewish and Muslim religions. Circumcision has been adopted in some Western societies and is still widely practised in the USA, ostensibly for reasons of hygiene, but the practice has been increasingly criticised in recent times. The issue has been hotly debated (see 'Further reading'). Recent evidence suggesting that uncircumcised men are at greater risk of sexually acquired HIV infection than are circumcised men has added further controversy. However, neonatal circumcision is not without risk of significant morbidity.

There are only a few medical indications for circumcision:

- *Phimosis* (Fig. 17.10). This term is often wrongly used to describe a normal, non-retractile foreskin. Genuine phimosis is seen as a whitish scarring of the foreskin and is rare before the age of 5 years. The condition is due to a localised skin disease known as balanitis xerotica obliterans (BXO), which involves the glans penis as well and can cause urethral meatal stenosis.

- *Recurrent balanoposthitis* (Fig. 17.11). A single attack of redness and inflammation of the foreskin, sometimes with a purulent discharge, is common and usually responds rapidly to warm baths and a broad-spectrum antibiotic. Recurrent attacks of

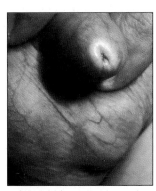

Fig. 17.10 True phimosis.

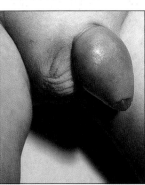

Fig. 17.11 Balanoposthitis.

balanoposthitis (inflammation of the glans and foreskin) are uncommon and circumcision is occasionally indicated.

- *Recurrent urinary tract infections.* The lower incidence of urinary tract infection (UTI) in circumcised male infants suggests that ascending infection is possible from the foreskin. Circumcision may occasionally be appropriate in a small proportion of boys with recurrent UTI and an upper urinary tract abnormality. It may also be helpful in those boys with spina bifida who need to perform clean intermittent urethral catheterisation.

Surgery

Circumcision for medical indications is performed under a general anaesthetic as a day case. During the procedure, a long-acting local anaesthetic block can be given to reduce postoperative pain. Circumcision is not a trivial operation. Healing can take up to 10 days, with discomfort for several days. Bleeding and infection are well-recognised complications, but more serious hazards, such as damage to the glans, may occur if the procedure is not carried out by trained personnel. The procedure also carries the risk of psychological trauma.

Paraphimosis

The foreskin becomes trapped in the retracted position proximal to a swollen glans. The foreskin can usually be reduced, but adequate analgesia (often a general anaesthetic) is needed to achieve this. The problem is not usually recurrent and circumcision is rarely required.

COMMON GENITAL DISORDERS IN GIRLS

Inguinal hernias

These are much less common than in boys. Sometimes the ovary becomes incarcerated in the hernial sac and can be difficult to reduce. Rarely, androgen insensitivity syndrome (testicular feminization) can present as a hernia in a phenotypic female who actually has a male genotype.

Labial adhesions

If the labia minora are adherent in the midline, this may give the appearance of absence of the vagina, except there is a characteristic translucent midline raphe partially or totally occluding the vaginal opening. Asymptomatic adhesions can be left alone and will often lyse spontaneously. If there is perineal soreness or urinary irritation, treatment with an oestrogen cream often dissolves the adhesions. The cream should be applied sparingly and for a brief course to limit absorption. Active separation of the adhesions under anaesthesia is sometimes required.

Vulvovaginitis/vaginal discharge

Vulvovaginitis and vaginal discharge are common in young girls. They may result from infection (bacterial or fungal), specific irritants, poor hygiene or sexual abuse, although none of these factors is present in most cases. Vulvovaginitis may rarely be associated with threadworm infestation. Parents should be advised about hygiene, the avoidance of bubble bath and scented soaps and the use of loose-fitting cotton underwear. Swabs should be taken to identify any pathogens, which can then be specifically treated. Salt baths may be helpful. Oestrogen cream applied sparingly to the vulva may relieve the problem in resistant cases by increasing vaginal resistance to infection. If there are any concerns about sexual abuse, the child should be seen by a paediatrician. Rarely, if the vaginal discharge is persistent or purulent, examination under anaesthesia may be needed to exclude a vaginal foreign body or unusual infections.

FURTHER READING

Atwell J D 1998 Paediatric surgery. Arnold, London
Gordon A, Collin J 1993 Save the normal foreskin. British Medical Journal 306: 1–2
Gough M H 1989 Cryptorchidism. British Journal of Surgery 76: 109–112
Schoen E J 1990 The status of circumcision of newborns. New England Journal of Medicine 322: 1308–1315
Szabo R, Short R V 2000 How does male circumcision protect against HIV infection? British Medical Journal 320: 1592–1594

18

Liver disorders

CHAPTER CONTENTS

- Neonatal liver disease
- Viral hepatitis
- Acute liver failure
- Chronic liver disease
- Cirrhosis and portal hypertension
- Management of children with liver disease
- Liver transplantation

In children:

- persistent neonatal jaundice is the most common presentation of liver disease in the neonatal period
- the earlier in life biliary atresia is diagnosed and treated surgically, the better the prognosis
- the transmission of hepatitis B infection from surface antigen-positive mothers to their babies can usually be prevented by a course of hepatitis B immunisation started at birth
- chronic liver disease (Fig. 18.1), cirrhosis and portal hypertension are uncommon and should be treated in tertiary or national centres
- liver transplantation is an effective therapy for acute or chronic liver failure with greater than 80% 5-year survival.

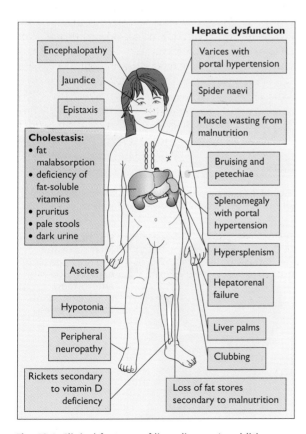

Fig. 18.1 Clinical features of liver disease. In addition, these children may have growth failure and developmental delay.

NEONATAL LIVER DISEASE

Most newborn infants become clinically jaundiced. About 15% are still jaundiced at more than 2 weeks of age, when it is called 'persistent or prolonged neonatal jaundice'. This is usually an unconjugated hyperbilirubinaemia, which resolves shortly afterwards (Fig. 18.2).

Fig. 18.2 Causes of persistent neonatal jaundice.

Unconjugated
Breast milk jaundice
Infection (particularly urinary tract)
Haemolytic anaemia, e.g. G6PD deficiency
Hypothyroidism
High gastrointestinal obstruction
Crigler–Najjar syndrome

Conjugated (>20% of total bilirubin)
Bile duct obstruction
Biliary atresia
Choledochal cyst

Neonatal hepatitis
Congenital infection
Inborn errors of metabolism
  α-1-antitrypsin deficiency
  Galactosaemia
  Tyrosinaemia
Cystic fibrosis
Total parenteral nutrition (TPN) cholestasis

Intrahepatic biliary hypoplasia
Alagille's syndrome

CASE HISTORY 18.1

BILIARY ATRESIA

A term infant was given oral vitamin K shortly after birth. He was breast-fed. He became mildly jaundiced on the third day of life. At 5 weeks of age he presented with poor feeding and vomiting and a history of bruising on his forehead and shoulders. His urine had become dark and stools intermittently pale. He was pale, jaundiced, had several bruises and hepatomegaly. Investigations showed:

- Hb 8.8 g/L
- Platelets 465×10^9/L
- Prothrombin time – grossly prolonged
- Bilirubin 178 μmol/L – 80% conjugated.

The investigation of conjugated hyperbilirubinaemia is shown in Figure 18.3. The TEBIDA radionulide scan showed no excretion at 24 h (Fig. 18.4)

and a liver biopsy suggested biliary atresia (Fig. 18.5). A hepatoportoenterostomy was performed at 6 weeks of age (Fig. 18.6).

In persistent neonatal jaundice, always ask if the stools are pale.

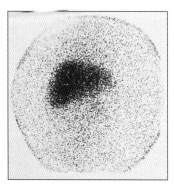

Fig. 18.4 Radioisotope scans (TEBIDA) of liver showing good hepatic uptake of isotope and no excretion into bowel. This scan suggests extrahepatic biliary obstruction or atresia or severe intrahepatic cholestasis.

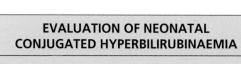

EVALUATION OF NEONATAL CONJUGATED HYPERBILIRUBINAEMIA

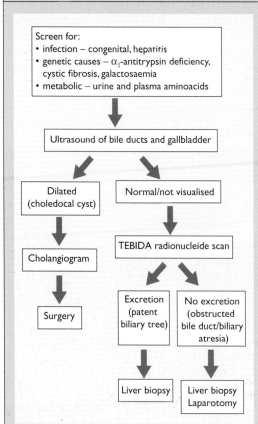

Screen for:
- infection – congenital, hepatitis
- genetic causes – α_1-antitrypsin deficiency, cystic fibrosis, galactosaemia
- metabolic – urine and plasma aminoacids

↓

Ultrasound of bile ducts and gallbladder

↓

Dilated (choledocal cyst) → Cholangiogram → Surgery

Normal/not visualised → TEBIDA radionucleide scan

Excretion (patent biliary tree) → Liver biopsy

No excretion (obstructed bile duct/biliary atresia) → Liver biopsy Laparotomy

Fig. 18.3 Evaluation of neonatal conjugated hyperbilirubinaemia.

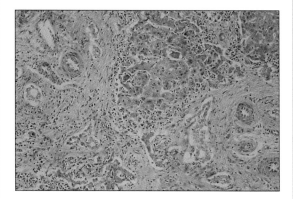

Fig. 18.5 Liver biopsy of biliary atresia showing bands of fibrous tissue with bile duct proliferation.

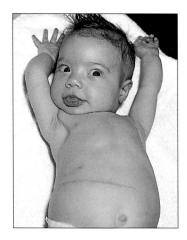

Fig. 18.6 Shortly after successful bile drainage by hepatoporto-enterostomy (Kasai procedure) for biliary atresia.

Persistent neonatal jaundice caused by liver disease is a conjugated hyperbilirubinaemia and is usually accompanied by:

- pale stools
- dark urine
- bleeding tendency
- failure to thrive.

The urgency to diagnose liver disease in the neonatal period as soon as possible is because early diagnosis and management improve the prognosis.

 Persistent neonatal jaundice – is it due to liver disease?

Bile duct obstruction

 ### Biliary atresia

This occurs in 1 in 14 000 live births. It is a progressive disease in which there is destruction or absence of the extrahepatic biliary tree and intrahepatic biliary ducts. This leads to chronic liver failure and death unless surgical intervention is performed. Babies with biliary atresia have a normal birthweight but fail to thrive as the disease progresses. They are jaundiced and from the second day their stools are pale and their urine dark, although both the jaundice and stool colour may fluctuate. Hepatomegaly is present and splenomegaly will develop secondary to portal hypertension.

Standard liver function tests are of little value in the differential diagnosis. A fasting abdominal ultrasound may be normal, or demonstrate a contracted or absent gall bladder. A radioisotope scan with TEBIDA (iminodiacetic acid derivatives) shows good uptake by the liver, but no excretion into the bowel. Liver biopsy demonstrates features of extrahepatic biliary obstruction, i.e. fibrosis and proliferation of bile ductules, although there may be features of neonatal hepatitis. The diagnosis is confirmed at laparotomy by operative cholangiography, which fails to outline a normal biliary tree.

Treatment consists of surgical bypass of the fibrotic ducts, hepatoportoenterostomy (Kasai procedure), in which the jejunum is anastomosed to patent ducts in the cut surface of the porta hepatis. If surgery is performed before the age of 60 days, 80% of children achieve bile drainage. The success rate diminishes with increasing age – hence the need for early diagnosis and treatment. Postoperative complications include cholangitis and fat malabsorption. Even when bile drainage is successful, there is progression to cirrhosis and portal hypertension. If the operation is unsuccessful, liver transplantation has to be considered.

Choledochal cysts

These are cystic dilatations of the extrahepatic biliary system. About 25% present in infancy with cholestasis.

In the older age group, choledochal cysts present with abdominal pain, a palpable mass and jaundice or cholangitis. The diagnosis is established by ultrasound or radionucleide scanning. Treatment is by surgical excision of the cyst with the formation of a roux-en-Y anastomosis to the biliary duct. Future complications include cholangitis and a 2% risk of malignancy, which may develop in any part of the biliary tree.

Neonatal hepatitis

In neonatal hepatitis there is hepatic inflammation. Its causes are listed in Figure 18.2, but often none is identified. In contrast to biliary atresia, these infants may have intrauterine growth restriction and hepatosplenomegaly at birth. Liver biopsy (Fig. 18.7) may be non-specific.

Alpha-1-antitrypsin deficiency

Deficiency of the protease alpha-1-antitrypsin is associated with liver disease in infancy and childhood and emphysema in adults. It is inherited as an autosomal recessive disorder with an incidence of 1 in 2000–4000 in the UK. There are many phenotypes of the protease inhibitor (Pi) which are coded on chromosome 14. Liver disease is associated with the phenotype PiZZ.

The majority of babies present with persistent neonatal jaundice, but some develop bleeding, including intracranial haemorrhage, from vitamin K deficiency, particularly if they are breast-fed. Hepatomegaly is present. Splenomegaly develops with cirrhosis and portal hypertension. The diagnosis is confirmed by estimating the level of α-1-antitrypsin in the plasma and identifying the phenotype. Approximately 30% of children will recover, but the remainder will develop chronic liver disease, some of whom will develop cirrhosis and portal hypertension and require liver transplantation. Pulmonary disease is not significant in childhood. The disorder can be diagnosed antenatally.

Galactosaemia

This very rare disorder has an incidence of 1 in 40 000. The infants develop poor feeding, vomiting, jaundice

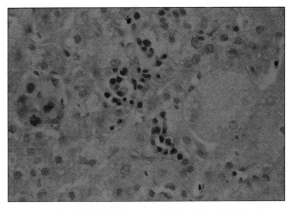

Fig. 18.7 Liver biopsy in neonatal hepatitis showing inflammatory infiltrate throughout the liver, and giant cell and rosette formation of liver cells.

and hepatomegaly when fed milk. Chronic liver failure, cataracts and developmental delay are inevitable if galactosaemia is untreated. A rapidly fatal course with shock, haemorrhage and disseminated intravascular coagulation, often due to Gram-negative sepsis, may occur.

The condition can be screened for in persistent jaundice by detecting galactose, a reducing substance, in the urine. The diagnosis is made by measuring the enzyme galactose-1-phosphate-uridyl transferase in red cells. A galactose-free diet prevents progression of liver disease, but ovarian failure and learning difficulties may occur later.

Other causes
Neonatal hepatitis may be caused by tyrosinaemia, cystic fibrosis, lipid and glycogen storage disorders, peroxisomal disorders, or may be associated with parenteral nutrition.

Intrahepatic biliary hypoplasia
Alagille's syndrome
This is an autosomal dominant condition. Infants have characteristic triangular facies, skeletal abnormalities, peripheral pulmonary stenosis, renal tubular disorders, defects in the eye and intrahepatic biliary hypoplasia with severe pruritus and failure to thrive. Prognosis is variable, with 50% of children surviving into adult life without liver transplantation.

VIRAL HEPATITIS

The clinical features of viral hepatitis include nausea, vomiting, abdominal pain, lethargy and jaundice. Thirty to 50% of children do not develop jaundice. A large tender liver is common and 30% will have splenomegaly. The liver transferases are usually elevated 10-fold. Coagulation is usually normal.

Hepatitis A

Hepatitis A virus (HAV) is an RNA virus which is spread by faecal–oral transmission. The incidence of hepatitis A in childhood has fallen as socioeconomic conditions have improved. Many adults are not immune. Vaccination is required for travellers to endemic areas.

The disease may be asymptomatic, but the majority of children have a mild illness and recover both clinically and biochemically within 2–4 weeks. Some develop prolonged cholestatic hepatitis, which is self-limiting, or fulminant hepatitis. Chronic liver disease does not occur.

The diagnosis can be confirmed by detecting IgM antibody to the virus.

There is no treatment and no evidence that bed rest or change of diet is effective. Close contacts should be given prophylaxis with human normal immunoglobulin (HNIG) or vaccinated within 2 weeks of the onset of the illness.

Hepatitis B

Hepatitis B virus (HBV) is a DNA virus which is an important cause of acute and chronic liver disease worldwide, with the highest incidence and carrier rates in the Far East and sub-Saharan Africa (Fig. 18.8). HBV is transmitted by:

- perinatal transmission from carrier mothers
- blood transfusions, needlestick injuries or biting insects
- renal dialysis
- horizontal spread within families.

Children with HBV may be asymptomatic or have classical features of acute hepatitis. The majority will resolve spontaneously, but 1–2% develop fulminant hepatic failure, while 5–10% become chronic carriers. The diagnosis is made by detecting HBV antigens and antibodies. IgM antibodies to the core antigen (anti-HBc) are positive in acute infection. There is no treatment for acute HBV infection.

Chronic hepatitis B

Infants infected with HBV by vertical transmission from their mothers usually become asymptomatic carriers. Approximately 30–50% of carrier children will develop chronic HBV liver disease, which may progress to cirrhosis in 10%. There is a long-term risk of hepatocellular carcinoma. Treatment for chronic HBV is unsatisfactory. Interferon treatment for chronic hepatitis B is successful in 50% of children infected horizontally and 30% of children infected perinatally, but newer antiviral therapy such as lamivudine may be more effective.

Prevention
Prevention of HBV infection is important. All pregnant women should have antenatal screening for the hepatitis surface antigen (HBsAg). Babies of all

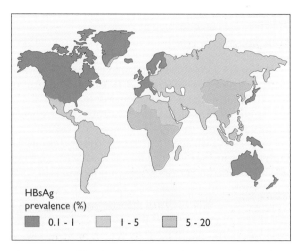

Fig. 18.8 Worldwide prevalence of hepatitis B (HBsAg), showing that it is highest in the Far East and sub-Saharan Africa.

HBsAg-positive mothers should receive a course of hepatitis B vaccination, with hepatitis B immunoglobulin also given if the mother is also hepatitis B e antigen (HBeAg)-positive. Other members of the family should also be vaccinated. There is already evidence from Taiwan that effective neonatal vaccination has reduced the incidence of HBV-related cancer.

Hepatitis C

Hepatitis C virus (HCV) is an RNA virus which was responsible for 90% of post-transfusion hepatitis until screening of donor blood was introduced in 1991. In the UK, about 1 in 2000 donors have HCV antibodies, but the prevalence is higher in southern Europe. The prevalence is high among intravenous drug users. Children at greatest risk are those who have received unscreened blood or blood products, in particular those with haemoglobinopathies or haemophilia. Vertical transmission from infected mothers is rare unless there is co-infection with HIV. It seldom causes an acute infection, but at least 50% develop chronic liver disease, with cirrhosis and hepatocellular carcinoma occurring after a number of years. The combination of interferon and ribavirin therapy in children is being evaluated.

Hepatitis D virus

Hepatitis D virus (HDV) is a defective RNA virus which depends on hepatitis B virus for replication. It occurs as a co-infection with hepatitis B virus or as a superinfection causing an acute exacerbation of chronic hepatitis B virus infection. Cirrhosis develops in 50–70% of those who develop chronic HDV infection.

Hepatitis E virus

This is an RNA virus which is enterally transmitted, usually by contaminated water. Epidemics occur in some developing countries. When a viral aetiology of hepatitis is suspected but not identified, it is known as non-A to G hepatitis.

Epstein–Barr virus

Children with Epstein–Barr virus (EBV) infection are usually asymptomatic. Forty per cent have hepatitis which may become fulminant. Less than 5% are jaundiced.

ACUTE LIVER FAILURE (FULMINANT HEPATITIS)

Acute liver failure in children is uncommon, but has a high mortality. The most common causes in childhood are viral hepatitis non-A to G and metabolic disease (Fig. 18.9). The child may present within hours or weeks with jaundice, encephalopathy, coagulopathy, hypoglycaemia and electrolyte disturbance. Early signs of encephalopathy include alternate periods of

Fig. 18.9 Causes of acute liver failure in children.

Infection	Viral hepatitis A, B, C, non-A to G
Poisons/drugs	Paracetamol, isoniazid, halothane, *Amanita phalloides* (poisonous mushroom)
Metabolic	Wilson's disease, tyrosinaemia
Autoimmune hepatitis	
Reye's syndrome	

irritability and confusion with drowsiness. Older children may be aggressive and unusually difficult. Complications include cerebral oedema, haemorrhage from gastritis or coagulopathy, sepsis and pancreatitis.

Diagnosis

Bilirubin may be normal in the early stages, particularly with metabolic disease. Transaminases are greatly elevated (10–100 times normal), alkaline phosphatase is increased, coagulation is very abnormal and plasma ammonia is elevated. It is essential to monitor the acid–base balance, blood glucose and coagulation times. An EEG will show acute hepatic encephalopathy and a CT scan may demonstrate cerebral oedema.

Management

This includes:

- maintaining the blood glucose (>4 mmol/L) with intravenous dextrose
- preventing sepsis with broad-spectrum antibiotics
- preventing haemorrhage with intravenous vitamin K, fresh frozen plasma and H_2-blockers
- treating cerebral oedema by fluid restriction and mannitol diuresis.

A poor prognosis is likely when the liver begins to shrink in size, if there is a rising bilirubin with falling transaminases, an increasing coagulopathy or progression to coma. Without liver transplantation, 70% of children who progress to coma will die.

Reye's syndrome

Reye's syndrome is an acute non-inflammatory encephalopathy with microvesicular fatty infiltration of the liver. Although the aetiology is unknown, there is a close association with aspirin therapy. Since stopping giving aspirin to children aged less than 12 years, Reye's syndrome has virtually disappeared.

CHRONIC LIVER DISEASE

The causes of chronic liver disease are given in Figure 18.10. The clinical presentation varies from acute hepatitis to the insidious development of hepatosplenomegaly, cirrhosis and portal hypertension with lethargy and malnutrition. The commonest

Fig. 18.10 Causes of chronic liver disease in children.

Chronic hepatitis
  Postviral hepatitis B, C, non-A to G
  Autoimmune hepatitis
  Drugs (nitrofurantoin, non-steroidal
    anti-inflammatory)
  Inflammatory bowel disease
  Primary sclerosing cholangitis (+/– ulcerative colitis)
Wilson's disease (>3 years)
Alpha-1-antitrypsin deficiency
Cystic fibrosis

Secondary to:
  Neonatal liver disease
  Bile duct lesions

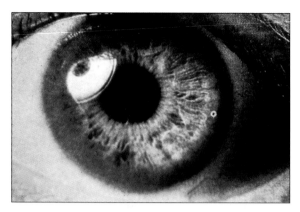

Fig. 18.11 Kayser Fleischer rings from copper in the cornea in a child with Wilson's disease.

causes of chronic hepatitis are postviral hepatitis (B, C or non-A to G) and autoimmune hepatitis, but Wilson's disease should always be excluded. Histology may demonstrate varying degrees of hepatitis, with an inflammatory infiltrate in the portal tracts, which spreads into the liver lobules.

Autoimmune hepatitis

The mean age of presentation is 7–10 years. It is more common in girls. It may present as an acute hepatitis, as fulminant hepatic failure or chronic liver disease with autoimmune features such as skin rash, lupus erythematosus, arthritis, haemolytic anaemia or nephritis. Diagnosis is based on hypergammaglobulinaemia (IgG >20 g/L); positive autoantibodies, e.g. smooth muscle antibodies (SMAs), antinuclear antibodies (ANAs) or liver/kidney microsomal antibodies (LKMs); a low serum complement (C4); and typical histology. Ninety per cent of children will respond to prednisolone and azathioprine.

Cystic fibrosis

Abnormal bile acid concentration and biliary disease is seen in cystic fibrosis as the CFTR is found in biliary epithelial cells. Cirrhosis and portal hypertension develop in 20% of children by mid-adolescence. Early liver disease is difficult to detect by biochemistry, ultrasound or radioisotope scanning. Liver histology includes fatty liver, focal biliary fibrosis or focal nodular cirrhosis. Therapy includes standard supportive and nutritional therapy with ursodeoxycholic acid. Liver transplantation should be considered for those with end-stage liver disease either alone or in combination with a heart–lung transplant.

Wilson's disease

Wilson's disease is an autosomal recessive disorder with an incidence of 1 in 200 000. Many mutations have now been identified (on chromosome 13). The basic genetic defect is a combination of reduced synthesis of caeruloplasmin (the copper-binding protein) and defective excretion of copper in the bile, which leads to an accumulation of copper in the liver, brain, kidney and cornea. Wilson's disease rarely presents in children under the age of 3 years. A hepatic presentation is likely in children less than 12 years. They may present with almost any form of liver disease, including acute hepatitis, fulminant hepatitis, cirrhosis and portal hypertension. Neurological features are common in the second decade and include deterioration in school performance, mood and behaviour change, and extrapyramidal signs such as incoordination, tremor and dysarthria. Renal tubular dysfunction, with vitamin D-resistant rickets, and haemolytic anaemia also occur. Copper accumulation in the cornea (Kayser–Fleischer rings) (Fig. 18.11) are not seen before 7 years of age.

The diagnosis is confirmed by detecting low serum caeruloplasmin, low serum copper, excess urine copper and increased hepatic copper.

Penicillamine reduces hepatic and central nervous system copper and is the drug of choice in combination with zinc to reduce copper absorption. Pyridoxine is given to prevent peripheral neuropathy. Neurological improvement may take up to 12 months of therapy. Thirty per cent of children with Wilson's disease will die from hepatic complications if untreated. Liver transplantation is considered for children with acute liver failure or severe end-stage liver failure.

Congenital hepatic fibrosis

Congenital hepatic fibrosis (CHF) presents in children over 2 years old with hepatosplenomegaly, abdominal distension and portal hypertension. Renal disease may coexist. Congenital hepatic fibrosis differs from cirrhosis in that liver function tests are normal in the early stage. Liver histology shows large bands of hepatic fibrosis containing abnormal bile ductules. The consequent portal hypertension causes bleeding from varices.

CIRRHOSIS AND PORTAL HYPERTENSION

Cirrhosis is the end stage of many forms of liver disease. It is defined pathologically as extensive fibrosis with regenerative nodules. It may be secondary to hepatocellular disease or to chronic bile duct obstruction (biliary cirrhosis). The main pathophysiological effects of cirrhosis are diminished hepatic function and portal hypertension with splenomegaly, varices and ascites (see Fig. 18.1). Hepatocellular carcinoma may develop.

Children with compensated cirrhosis may be asymptomatic if liver function is adequate. They will not be jaundiced and may have normal liver function tests. As the cirrhosis increases, however, the results of deteriorating liver function and portal hypertension become obvious (Fig. 18.12). Physical signs include palmar and plantar erythema and spider naevi, malnutrition and hypotonia. Dilated abdominal veins and splenomegaly suggest portal hypertension, although the liver may be impalpable.

Investigations include:
- screening for the known causes of chronic liver disease (see Fig. 18.10)
- upper gastrointestinal endoscopy to detect the presence of oesophageal varices and/or erosive gastritis
- abdominal ultrasound – may show a shrunken liver and splenomegaly with gastric and oesophageal varices
- liver biopsy – may be difficult because of increased fibrosis but may indicate the aetiology (e.g. alpha-1-antitrypsin granules, copper storage).

As cirrhosis decompensates, biochemical tests may demonstrate an elevation of aminotransferases and alkaline phosphatase. The plasma albumin is low and the prothrombin time is prolonged.

Oesophageal varices

These are an inevitable consequence of portal hypertension and may develop rapidly in children. They are best diagnosed by upper gastrointestinal endoscopy, as a barium swallow may miss small varices. Acute bleeding is treated conservatively with blood transfusions and H_2-blockers (e.g. ranitidine) or omeprazole. If bleeding persists, octreotide infusion, vasopressin analogues, sclerotherapy or band ligation may be effective. Portacaval shunts may preclude liver transplantation, but radiological placement of a stent between the hepatic and portal veins can be used as a temporary measure if transplantation is being considered.

Ascites (Fig. 18.13)

This is a major problem. The cause of ascites is uncertain, but contributory factors are hypoalbuminaemia, sodium retention, renal impairment and fluid redistribution. It is treated by sodium and fluid restriction and diuretics. Additional therapy for refractory ascites includes albumin infusions or paracentesis.

Spontaneous bacterial peritonitis

This should always be considered if there is undiagnosed fever, abdominal pain, tenderness or an unexplained deterioration in hepatic or renal function. A diagnostic paracentesis should be performed and the fluid sent for white cell count and differential and culture. Treatment is with broad-spectrum antibiotics.

Encephalopathy

This is precipitated by gastrointestinal haemorrhage, sepsis, sedatives, renal failure or electrolyte imbalance. It is difficult to diagnose in children as the level of consciousness may vary throughout the day. Infants present with irritability and sleepiness, while older children present with abnormalities in mood, sleep rhythm, intellectual performance and behaviour. Plasma ammonia may be elevated and an EEG is always abnormal.

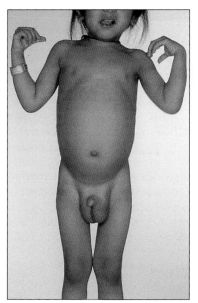

Fig. 18.12 Cirrhosis and portal hypertension. This picture shows:
(i) malnutrition with loss of fat and muscle bulk
(ii) distended abdomen from hepatosplenomegaly and ascites
(iii) scrotal swelling from ascites
(iv) no jaundice despite advanced liver disease.

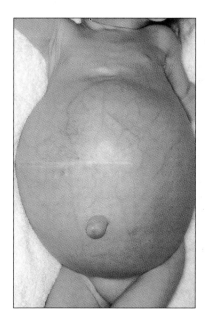

Fig. 18.13 This infant has a grossly distended abdomen from ascites. There are dilated abdominal veins secondary to portal hypertension and an umbilical hernia from increased abdominal pressure. There is a surgical scar.

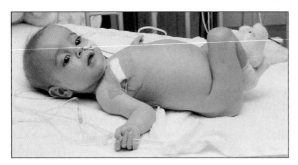

Fig. 18.14 Many infants and children with liver disease need intensive nutritional supplementation. This malnourished infant is having both parenteral nutrition via a central line and continuous nasogastric feeding.

Renal failure

This may be secondary to renal tubular acidosis, acute tubular necrosis or functional renal failure.

MANAGEMENT OF CHILDREN WITH LIVER DISEASE

The management of children with liver disease is supportive, with the emphasis on correction of nutritional abnormalities, prevention of complications and intensive family support.

Nutrition

Malnutrition may be due to protein malnutrition, fat malabsorption, anorexia and fat soluble vitamin deficiency (vitamins A, D, E and K).

Treatment is to provide a high-protein, high-carbohydrate diet with 50% more calories than the recommended dietary allowance. In children with cholestasis, medium-chain triglycerides, which are absorbed by the portal circulation, will provide fat, but 20–40% long-chain triglycerides are required to prevent essential fatty acid deficiency. Many children will require nasogastric tube feeding or parenteral nutrition (Fig. 18.14).

Fat-soluble vitamins

Vitamin K deficiency in liver disease may be due to malabsorption or diminished synthesis. Water-soluble forms of vitamin K are available.

Vitamin A deficiency causes night blindness in adults and retinal changes in infants. It is easily prevented with oral vitamin A.

Vitamin E deficiency causes peripheral neuropathy, haemolysis and ataxia. It is very poorly absorbed in cholestatic conditions and high oral doses are required.

Vitamin D deficiency causes rickets and pathological fractures. It is prevented by using a water-soluble form of vitamin D. Vitamin D-resistant rickets indicates renal tubular acidosis.

Pruritus

Many children with cholestasis have severe pruritus. It is alleviated by phenobarbitone to stimulate bile flow, cholestyramine, which is a bile salt resin, ursodeoxycholic acid, an oral bile acid or evening primrose oil (arachiadonic acid) applied to the skin.

Encephalopathy

In children, encephalopathy is managed by treating the precipitating factor (sepsis, gastrointestinal haemorrhage), by protein restriction or by using oral lactulose to reduce ammonia reabsorption by lowering colonic pH and increasing colonic transit.

LIVER TRANSPLANTATION

Liver transplantation is accepted therapy for acute or chronic end-stage liver failure and has revolutionised the prognosis for these children. Transplantation is also considered for some hepatic malignancy.

The indications for transplantation in chronic liver failure are:

- severe malnutrition unresponsive to intensive nutritional therapy
- recurrent complications (bleeding varices, resistant ascites)
- failure of growth and development
- poor quality of life.

Liver transplant evaluation includes assessment of the vascular anatomy of the liver and exclusion of irreversible disease in other systems. Absolute contraindications include sepsis, untreatable cardiopulmonary disease or cerebrovascular disease.

There is considerable difficulty in obtaining small organs for children. Most children receive part of an adult's liver, which is either reduced to fit the child's abdomen (reduction hepatectomy) or split (shared between an adult and child). Complications posttransplantation include:

- primary non-function of the liver (5%)
- hepatic artery thrombosis (10–20%)
- biliary leaks and strictures (20%)
- rejection (30–60%)
- sepsis, the main cause of death.

In large national centres, the overall 1-year survival is approximately 90%, with an overall 5-year survival of 80%. Most deaths occur in the first 3 months. Children who survive the initial postoperative period usually do well. Long-term studies indicate normal psychosocial development and quality of life in survivors.

FURTHER READING

Booth I W, Kelly D A 1996 Paediatric gastroenterology and hepatology. Mosby-Wolfe, London
Kelly D A 1999 Diseases of the liver and biliary system in childhood. Blackwell Science, Oxford
Mowat A P 1994 Liver disease in childhood, 3rd edn. Butterworth-Heinemann, Oxford

19

Malignant disease

Cancer in children is not common:
- 1 child in 650 develops cancer by 15 years of age
- there are 120–140 new cases per million children aged <15 years per year, about 1400 in the UK.

The types of malignant disease (Fig. 19.1) are very different from those in adults, where carcinomas of the lung, breast, gut and skin predominate. The age at presentation varies with the different types of disease:

- leukaemia affects children at all ages
- neuroblastoma and Wilms' tumour are most frequent in the first 5 years of life
- Hodgkin's disease and bone tumours have their peak incidence in adolescence and early adult life.

The survival rate for many tumours has increased dramatically (Fig. 19.2). However, cancer remains the second most common cause of death in children, after accidents. The overall 5 year survival of children with malignant disease is over 70%, most of whom can be considered cured. This improved life expectancy can be attributed mainly to the introduction of multi-agent chemotherapy and specialist multidisciplinary care. However, for some children, the price of survival is long-term medical or psychosocial difficulties.

In children, leukaemia is the most common malignancy followed by brain tumours.

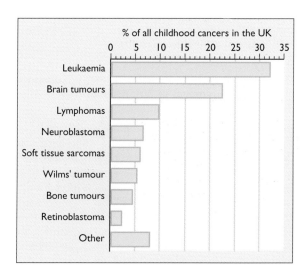

Fig. 19.1 Relative frequency of different types of cancer in children.

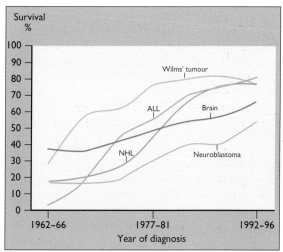

Fig. 19.2 Five-year survival rates showing the considerable improvement over the last 30 years. (ALL, acute lymphoblastic leukaemia; NHL, Non-Hodgkin's lymphoma.)

285

Aetiology

In most cases, the precise aetiology of childhood cancer is unclear, but it is likely to involve an interaction between environmental factors (e.g. radiation, viruses) and host genetic susceptibility (e.g. gene mutation). Most cancers occur as a result of mutations in cellular genes (oncogenes and tumour suppressor genes) which may be either inherited or sporadic. One example of an inherited cancer is bilateral retinoblastoma, which is associated with a deletion on chromosome 13. Several syndromes are associated with an increased risk of cancer in childhood, e.g. Down's syndrome and leukaemia, neurofibromatosis and glioma. Increasingly, modern genetic techniques are being used in a clinical setting to predict prognosis (e.g. amplification of the 'N-*myc*' oncogene associated with a poor prognosis in neuroblastoma) or to confirm an uncertain histological diagnosis (e.g. translocation of chromosomes 11 and 22 in Ewing's sarcoma).

Clinical presentation

Cancer presents with:
- a localised mass
- the consequences of disseminated disease, e.g. bone marrow infiltration, causing systemic ill-health
- the consequences of pressure from a mass on local structures or tissue, e.g. airway obstruction secondary to enlarged lymph nodes.

Investigations

In leukaemia the full blood count is usually abnormal but peripheral blast cells are not always present. Solid tumours are identified and localised on ultrasound, X-rays, CT and MRI scans. Nuclear medicine imaging (e.g. radiolabelled technetium bone scan) may be useful to identify bone or bone marrow disease or tumours of neural crest origin, e.g. neuroblastoma. Tumour marker studies are helpful for neuroblastoma, when there is increased urinary catecholamine excretion (VMA, vanillylmandelic acid) and for germ cell tumours and liver tumours in which there is alphafetoprotein (AFP) production. However, all diagnoses must be confirmed histologically, either by biopsy or by bone marrow aspiration. This may not always be possible for brain tumours. The differentiation between some solid tumours may be difficult by standard microscopy, and further differentiation requires specialised pathology facilities such as immunohistochemistry and electron microscopy.

All diagnoses must be confirmed histologically whenever possible.

Management

Once a tumour has been diagnosed, the parents and child need to be seen and the diagnosis explained to them in a realistic, positive way. Detailed staging to define the extent of the primary and to assess the presence of metastatic disease is essential to plan treatment. Considerable progress has been made in improving outcome by evaluating new treatment regimens through national and international collaborative studies.

Most children with cancer in the UK are initially investigated and treated in regional centres whose development has encouraged work by experienced multidisciplinary teams with facilities for the intensive medical and psychosocial support required. Subsequent management is often shared among the specialist centre, referral hospital and local services within the community to provide the optimum care with the least disruption to the family.

Treatment

Treatment may involve chemotherapy, surgery and radiotherapy.

Chemotherapy
This is used:
- as primary curative treatment, e.g. in acute lymphoblastic leukaemia
- as adjuvant treatment to deal with residual disease and for actual or presumed micrometastases after initial local treatment with surgery, e.g. Wilms' tumour
- to shrink bulky primary or metastatic disease before definitive local treatment with surgery and/or radiotherapy, e.g. sarcomas, neuroblastoma.

Radiotherapy
This retains a role in the treatment of some tumours, but the risk of damage to growth and function of normal tissue is greater in a child than in an adult. The adequate screening of sensitive normal tissues and careful positioning of the patient during treatment raise practical difficulties in children.

Surgery
This is increasingly restricted to primary biopsy for diagnosis and removal of any residual disease after chemotherapy and/or radiotherapy.

High-dose therapy with bone marrow rescue
The limitation of chemotherapy and radiotherapy is the risk of irreversible damage to normal tissues, particularly bone marrow. Bone marrow transplantation can be used as a strategy to treat patients after administering potentially lethal doses of chemotherapy and/or radiation. The source of the bone marrow may be allogeneic (from a compatible donor) or autologous (from the patient himself, harvested beforehand while the marrow is uninvolved or in remission). The harvesting of peripheral blood stem cells from the patient and subsequent reinfusion following high-dose chemotherapy/radiation has provided an acceptable

alternative to autologous bone marrow transplantation. This technique is used most commonly in the treatment of solid tumours whose prognosis is poor using conventional chemotherapy, e.g. neuroblastoma.

Side-effects of chemotherapy

Chemotherapy causes a range of side-effects (Fig. 19.3).

Infection from immunosuppression

Children receiving chemotherapy or wide-field radiation are immunocompromised. Chemotherapy-induced neutropenia places children at risk of septicaemia. Children with fever and neutropenia must be admitted to hospital for cultures and broad-spectrum antibiotics. Some important infections associated with therapy for cancer include *Pneumocystis carinii* pneumonia (especially in children with leukaemia) and disseminated fungal infection (e.g. aspergillosis and candidiasis) and coagulase-negative staphylococcal infections of central venous catheters.

Most common viral infections are no worse in children with cancer than in other children, but measles and varicella zoster may have atypical presentation and be life-threatening. If non-immune, these children are at risk from contact with measles or varicella, although some protection can be afforded by prompt administration of immunoglobulin or zoster immune globulin. Aciclovir is used to treat established varicella infection, but no treatment is available for measles. During chemotherapy and from 6 months to a year subsequently, the use of live vaccines is contraindicated due to depressed immunity.

Bone marrow suppression

Anaemia may require blood transfusions. Thrombocytopenia presents the hazard of bleeding, and considerable blood product support may be required, particularly for children with leukaemia, those undergoing intensive therapy requiring bone marrow transplantation and the more intensive solid tumour protocols.

Gut mucosal damage

Mouth ulcers are common and painful. When severe, they can prevent the child eating adequately. Chemotherapy-induced gut mucosal damage predisposes to Gram-negative infection.

Other side-effects

Many individual drugs have very specific side-effects, e.g. cardiotoxicity with doxorubicin, renal failure and deafness with cisplatin, haemorrhagic cystitis with cyclophosphamide, and neuropathy with vincristine. These require careful monitoring.

 Fever with neutropenia requires hospital admission, cultures and intravenous antibiotics.

Supportive care

Cancer treatment produces frequent, predictable and often severe multisystem side-effects. Supportive care is an important part of management. This includes attention to infection, nutrition, nausea and vomiting. The discomfort of multiple venepunctures for blood sampling and intravenous infusions can be avoided with central venous catheters, although these do carry a risk of infection (Fig. 19.4).

Psychosocial support

The diagnosis of a potentially fatal illness has an enormous and long-lasting impact on the whole family.

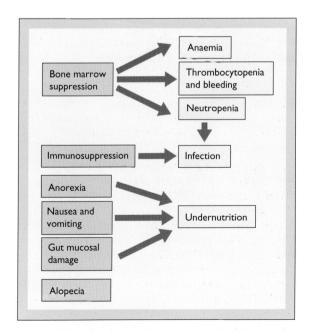

Fig. 19.3 Short-term side-effects of chemotherapy.

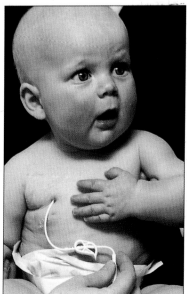

Fig. 19.4 The central venous catheter allows pain-free blood tests and injections for this child on chemotherapy, which has caused the alopecia.

They need the opportunity to discuss the implications and their anxiety, fear, guilt and sadness. Most will benefit from the counselling and practical support provided by health professionals. Help with practical issues, including transport, finances, accommodation and care of siblings, is an early priority. The provision of detailed written material for parents will help them understand their child's disease and treatment. The children themselves and their siblings need an age-appropriate explanation of the disease. Once treatment is established and the disease appears to be under control, families should be encouraged to return to as normal a lifestyle as possible. Early return to school is important and children with cancer should not be allowed to underachieve the expectations previously held for them. It is easy to underestimate the severe stress that persists within families in relation to the uncertainty of the long-term outcome. This often manifests itself as marital problems in parents and behavioural difficulties in both the child and siblings.

Long-term survivors

Currently, it is estimated that almost 1 in 1000 young adults are survivors of childhood cancer. Some will have residual problems as a consequence of the disease or its treatment (Fig. 19.5). All survivors need regular long-term follow-up to provide appropriate treatment or advice. Some will require specific counselling for problems such as poor growth, infertility and sexual dysfunction. The risk of second tumours is small but may rise with increasing survival rates. There is now a need to reduce, whenever possible, the toxicity of treatment to spare the children adverse short- and long-term effects.

Terminal care

When a child relapses, further treatment may be considered. A small number can still be cured and others may have a further significant remission with good quality life. However, for some children a time comes when death is inevitable and the staff and family must make the decision to concentrate on palliative care.

Most parents prefer to care for their terminally ill child at home, but will need practical help and emotional support. Pain control and symptom relief are a serious source of anxiety for parents, but they can often be achieved successfully at home. Health professionals with experience in palliative care for children can work with the family and local health care workers. After the child's death, families should be offered continuing contact with an appropriate member of the team who looked after their child, and be given support through their bereavement.

LEUKAEMIA

Acute lymphoblastic leukaemia (ALL) accounts for 80% of leukaemia in children. Most of the remainder are acute myeloid/acute non-lymphocytic (AML/ANLL) leukaemia. Chronic myeloid leukaemia and other myeloproliferative disorders are rare.

Clinical presentation

Clinical symptoms and signs result from infiltration of the bone marrow or other organs with leukaemic blast cells (Fig. 19.6). In most children, leukaemia presents insidiously over several weeks (see Case history 19.1) with some or all of:

- malaise
- infections
- pallor
- abnormal bruising
- hepatosplenomegaly
- lymphadenopathy
- bone pain.

In some children the illness progresses very rapidly.

In most but not all children, the blood count is abnormal, with low haemoglobin and thrombocytopenia and

---

Fig. 19.5 Problems which may occur following cure of childhood cancer.

Problem	Cause
Specific organ dysfunction	Nephrectomy for Wilms' tumour
	Toxicity from chemotherapy, e.g. renal from cisplatin or ifosfamide, cardiac from doxorubicin or mediastinal radiotherapy
Growth/endocrine problems	Growth hormone deficiency from pituitary irradiation
	Bone growth retardation at sites of irradiation
Infertility	Gonadal irradiation
	Alkylating agent chemotherapy (cyclophosphamide, ifosfamide)
Neuropsychological problems	Cranial irradiation (particularly at age <5 years)
	Brain surgery
Second malignancy	Irradiation
	Alkylating agent chemotherapy
Social/educational disadvantage	Chronic ill health
	Absence from school

evidence of circulating blast cells. Bone marrow examination is essential to confirm the diagnosis and to identify immunological and cytogenetic markers which give useful prognostic information.

Both ALL and AML are classified by morphology. Immunological phenotyping further subclassifies ALL; the common (75%) and T cell (15%) subtypes are the most common. Prognosis and some aspects of clinical

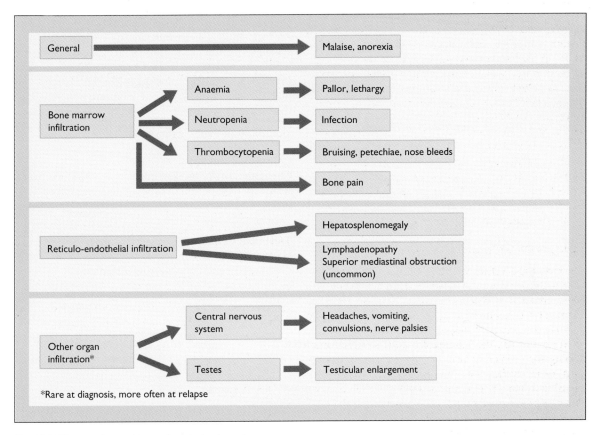

Fig. 19.6 Signs and symptoms of acute leukaemia.

CASE HISTORY 19.1

ACUTE LYMPHOBLASTIC LEUKAEMIA

A 4-year-old girl was generally unwell, feeling lethargic, looking pale and occasionally febrile over a period of 9 weeks. Two courses of antibiotics for recurrent sore throat failed to result in any benefit. Her parents returned to their general practitioner when she developed a rash. Examination showed pallor, petechiae, modest lymphadenopathy and mild hepatosplenomegaly. A full blood count showed:

- Hb 8.3 g/dl
- WBC 15.6×10^9/L
- Platelets 44×10^9/L.

Blast cells were seen on the peripheral blood film. Cerebrospinal fluid (CSF) examination was normal. Bone marrow examination confirmed acute lymphoblastic leukaemia (Fig. 19.7).

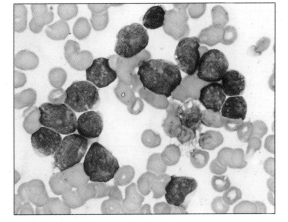

Fig. 19.7 Leukaemic blast cells on a bone marrow smear.

presentation vary according to different subtypes and treatment is adjusted accordingly.

The prognosis in ALL is related to age, tumour load (measured by the white cell count, WBC), speed of response to initial chemotherapy and the presence or absence of specific cytogenetic/molecular genetic abnormalities in tumour cells. High WBC ($>50 \times 10^9/L$), age <1 year or >10 years and persistence of leukaemic blasts in the bone marrow at day 28 of treatment are all important variables in defining treatment intensity. Bone marrow genetic studies are essential at diagnosis.

Treatment of acute lymphoblastic leukaemia
A typical treatment schema is shown in Figure 19.8.

Remission induction
Before starting treatment of the disease, anaemia is corrected with blood transfusion, any infection is treated and adequate hydration and allopurinol are given to protect renal function against the effects of rapid cell lysis. Remission implies eradication of the leukaemic blasts and restoration of normal marrow function. Four weeks of combination chemotherapy is given and current induction schedules achieve remission rates of 95%.

Intensification
Blocks of intensive chemotherapy are given to consolidate remission. They improve cure rates but at the expense of increased toxicity.

Central nervous system (CNS)
Cytotoxic drugs penetrate poorly into the CNS. As leukaemic cells in this site may survive effective systemic treatment, additional treatment with intrathecal chemotherapy is used to prevent CNS relapse. Previously, treatment included cranial radiation or high-dose methotrexate, but there are concerns that these result in adverse neuropsychological effects and they are now omitted from first-line treatment schedules.

Continuing therapy
Chemotherapy of modest intensity is continued over a relatively long period of time, up to 3 years from diagnosis. Co-trimoxazole is given routinely to prevent *Pneumocystis carinii* pneumonia.

Treatment of relapse
High-dose chemotherapy, usually with total body irradiation (TBI) and bone marrow transplantation, is used as an alternative to conventional chemotherapy after a relapse.

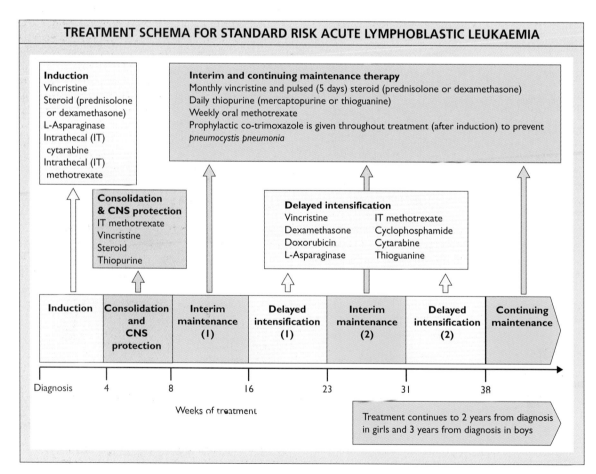

Fig. 19.8 Treatment schema for standard risk acute lymphoblastic leukaemia.

LYMPHOMAS

Lymphoma can be divided into Hodgkin's disease and non-Hodgkin's lymphoma (NHL). NHL is more common in childhood, while Hodgkin's disease is seen more frequently in adolescence.

Non-Hodgkin's lymphoma

Lymphomas are malignancies of the cells of the immune system. A firm distinction between solid and haematological lymphoid malignancy is somewhat artificial as some subtypes of ALL and NHL may represent a continuum of the same disease. In most cases of childhood NHL, the clinical features reflect the pattern of migration of normal lymphoid cells, with lymph nodes being the predominant site of disease.

Presentation will depend on the site of disease. T cell malignancies may present as ALL or NHL, with both being characterised by a mediastinal mass with varying degrees of bone marrow infiltration. B cell malignancies present more commonly as NHL, localised lymph node disease usually in the head and neck or abdomen. Abdominal disease presents with pain, a palpable mass or even intussuception in cases with involvement of the ileum.

Staging must include radiological assessment of all nodal sites (CT or MRI) and examination of the bone marrow and CSF. Treatment is multi-agent chemotherapy, a more intensive course being employed for advanced B cell disease (Fig. 19.9).

Hodgkin's disease

This is relatively uncommon in prepubertal children. It usually presents as painless lymphadenopathy, most frequently in the neck. Lymph nodes are much larger and firmer than the benign lymphadenopathy commonly seen in children. The clinical history is often long, and systemic symptoms (sweating, pruritus, weight loss and fever – the so-called 'B' symptoms) are uncommon, even in more advanced disease.

After diagnostic biopsy, the disease is staged to determine treatment. Intra-abdominal disease is generally assessed radiologically, and staging laparotomy, with biopsies and splenectomy, is no longer performed. Lymphangiography is a technically difficult examination in small children and is rarely required. Combination chemotherapy (possibly with radiotherapy to sites of bulky disease) is the treatment for all except those with localised disease who receive radiotherapy alone. Overall, about 80% of all patients can be cured; even for those with disseminated disease, about 60% can be cured.

BRAIN TUMOURS

In contrast to adults, brain tumours in children are almost always primary and 60% are infratentorial (Fig. 19.10). Signs and symptoms are usually of raised intracranial pressure:

- headache (classically worse on lying down)
- vomiting (especially on waking in the mornings)
- papilloedema
- squint secondary to VIth nerve palsy
- nystagmus
- ataxia
- personality or behaviour change.

The tumour is identified on CT or MRI scan (Fig. 19.11). Lumbar puncture must not be performed in the presence of raised intracranial pressure without neurosurgical advice. Brain tumours present particular diagnostic difficulties as the histological appearance may not be representative of tumour behaviour and biopsy is not always safe. The outcome of treatment is strongly influenced by the anatomical position of the tumour as well as the histological subtype.

The implications of the tumour site, the hazard of surgery and the use of high-dose radiation all combine to place children with brain tumours at particular risk of growth, endocrine and neuropsychological problems. Survivors may present complex difficulties with varying combinations of physical disability, growth failure, sensory loss, seizures and educational problems.

NEUROBLASTOMA

Neuroblastoma arises from neural crest tissue in the adrenal medulla and sympathetic nervous system. It is an unusual tumour in that spontaneous regression sometimes occurs in very young infants. There is a

Fig. 19.9 Principal presentation, treatment and prognosis in non-Hodgkin's lymphoma.

Site	Type	Treatment	Prognosis
Localised – often head and neck, e.g. cervical nodes, oropharynx	Usually of B-cell origin	Short, moderately intensive multi-agent chemotherapy	Good
Intrathoracic – anterior mediastinal mass – pleural effusion	Typical T-cell disease	As for ALL	Approaching that for ALL
Intra-abdominal disease – bulky gut or lymph node masses	Typical advanced B-cell disease	Very intensive multi-agent chemotherapy	Previously very poor; now much improved

BRAIN TUMOURS

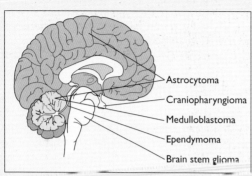

Fig. 19.10 Location of brain tumours

Labels (from figure):
- Astrocytoma
- Craniopharyngioma
- Medulloblastoma
- Ependymoma
- Brain stem glioma

Astrocytoma (40%)
The most common brain tumour type. Juvenile cerebellar astrocytoma is cystic, often slowly growing, and the results of treatment with surgery are excellent. Non-juvenile astrocytoma occurs at all sites but more frequently in the cerebral hemispheres. They vary from relatively benign to highly malignant (*glioblastoma multiforme*) and, despite surgery and radiotherapy, the outlook, particularly for children with high-grade tumours, is poor. The value of chemotherapy in the treatment of astrocytoma is not yet established but may be used more frequently in future.

Medulloblastoma (20%)
Nearly always arises in the midline of the posterior fossa. Presentation is with ataxia as well as headache and vomiting. The tumour may seed through the CNS via the CSF and up to 20% have spinal metastases at diagnosis. Treatment with whole CNS radiation after maximal surgical resection has produced 5-year survival rates of 50%. Chemotherapy has a place in the treatment of children with a higher than average risk of relapse, e.g. after incomplete surgical excision.

Ependymoma (8%)
Mostly occurs in the posterior fossa where it behaves like medulloblastoma, but can also arise in the ventricles or spinal cord.

Brain stem glioma (6%)
Peak incidence is in early childhood. It presents with cranial nerve defects, ataxia and pyramidal tract signs, but frequently without raised intracranial pressure. The diagnosis is often based on clinical findings and CT/MRI scan, as biopsy can be hazardous. The prognosis for this group of children is particularly poor (<20% survival) and radiotherapy is usually only palliative. Chemotherapy has no established role.

Craniopharyngioma (4%)
A developmental tumour arising from the squamous remnant of Rathke's pouch. It is not truly malignant but is locally invasive and grows slowly in the suprasellar region. It presents with raised intracranial pressure, visual field loss and pituitary dysfunction, typically as growth failure. Surgical excision with or without subsequent radiation is required. Although prognosis for survival is good, these children may be visually impaired and often have complex endocrine deficiencies.

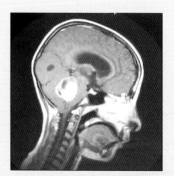

Fig. 19.11 Sagittal MRI scan showing a medulloblastoma in the posterior fossa

Figs 19.10 and 19.11 Location of brain tumours.

Fig. 19.12 Presentation of neuroblastoma.

Common	Less common
Pallor	Paraplegia
Weight loss	Cervical lymphadenopathy
Abdominal mass	Proptosis
Hepatomegaly	Periorbital bruising
Bone pain	Skin nodules
Limp	

disease spectrum from benign ganglioneuroma to malignant neuroblastoma.

It is most common before the age of 5 years. Most children present with an abdominal mass, but the primary can lie anywhere along the sympathetic chain from the neck to the pelvis. Classically, the abdominal primary is of adrenal origin, but at presentation the tumour mass is often large and complex, crossing the midline and enveloping major blood vessels and lymph nodes (Fig. 19.12). Paravertebral tumours may invade through the adjacent intervertebral foramen

NEUROBLASTOMA

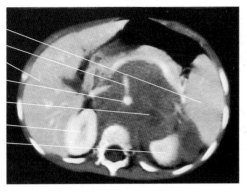

Displaced spleen
Coeliac axis
Liver
Aorta
Neuroblastoma tumour mass
Normal kidney
Displaced kidney

Fig. 19.13 A transverse CT scan of the abdomen showing a very large neuroblastoma tumour mass. Its intimate relationship with the great vessels makes it extremely difficult to resect surgically.

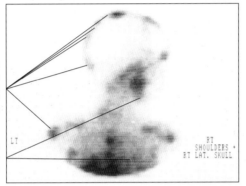

All 'hot' spots in the skeleton are consistent with bone/bone marrow disease

Physiological uptake in salivary glands and myocardium

Fig. 19.14 MIBG (metaiodobenzyl guanidine) scan, a radiolabelled targeting agent specific for neuroblastoma, is used to monitor response to treatment.

and cause spinal cord compression. Over the age of 2 years, clinical symptoms are mostly from metastatic disease, particularly bone pain, bone marrow suppression, weight loss and malaise (Fig. 19.12).

The diagnosis can often be made from characteristic clinical and radiological features (Fig. 19.13) and raised urinary catecholamine (VMA, HVA) levels. Confirmatory biopsy is usually obtained and evidence of metastatic disease detected with bone marrow sampling, bone scan and MIBG (metaiodobenzyl guanidine) scan. MIBG is a radiolabelled tumour-specific agent, which provides a sensitive radioisotope scan to measure disease extent and monitor response to treatment (Fig. 19.14). Its therapeutic use has been explored but has not found an established role.

The most important clinical prognostic features are age and stage of disease at diagnosis. Unfortunately, the majority of children over 1 year present with advanced disease and have a poor prognosis. Increasingly, information about the biological characteristics of neuroblastoma is being used to guide therapy and prognosis. Overexpression of the N-*myc* oncogene and evidence for deletion of material on chromosome 1 (del1p) in tumour cells are associated with poorer prognosis.

The few children with localised primaries without metastatic disease can often be cured with surgery alone. For the majority with advanced disease, chemotherapy has the central role. Children showing a good initial response may benefit from consolidation with high-dose chemotherapy with peripheral blood stem cell rescue. Unfortunately the risk of relapse is high and the prospect for cure for children with metastatic disease is less than 30%

Screening for asymptomatic disease in infants during the first year of life is feasible by detecting raised urinary catecholamines. Most experience with this strategy has been in Japan where over 80% of the infant population are screened. Screening has increased the apparent incidence by detecting some tumours that were destined to regress. There is no conclusive evidence that mortality from the disease has been reduced.

WILMS' TUMOUR (NEPHROBLASTOMA)

Wilms' tumour originates from embryonal renal tissue. There is a Wilms' tumour susceptibility gene which was identified from the rare association between Wilms' tumour and sporadic aniridia which was known to be associated with loss of genetic material from chromosome 11. Over 80% present before 5 years of age. It is very rarely seen after 10 years of age. Most children present with a large abdominal mass, often found incidentally in an otherwise well child (Fig. 19.15). Occasionally, children have chronic symptoms of poor

WILMS' TUMOUR

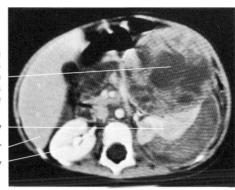

Huge tumour, showing the characteristic mixed tissue densities (cystic and solid). It arises within the kidney and envelopes a remnant of normal renal tissue

Remnant of left kidney

Liver

Normal kidney

Fig. 19.16 Huge Wilms' tumour arising within the left kidney showing characteristic cystic and solid tissue densities.

Fig. 19.15 Presentation of Wilms' tumour.

Common	Uncommon
Abdominal mass	Abdominal pain
	Anorexia
	Haematuria
	Hypertension

appetite and poor weight gain. Haemorrhage into the mass may cause abdominal pain and anaemia. Macroscopic haematuria and severe hypertension are uncommon but important. About 5% have bilateral disease at diagnosis.

Radiological diagnosis from ultrasound or CT (Fig. 19.16) is usually characteristic, showing an intrinsic renal mass distorting the normal structure. Staging information to assess distant metastases (usually in the lung), initial tumour resectability and function of the contralateral kidney is required. The current treatment protocol in the UK compares immediate nephrectomy for patients with resectable tumours with initial chemotherapy followed by delayed nephrectomy. The latter option is offered to all children with very large tumours, metastatic disease and inferior vena cava involvement. All children require chemotherapy, but radiotherapy is restricted to those with more advanced disease.

Overall, the prognosis is good, with more than 80% of all patients cured. The cure rate even for the 15% of patients with metastatic disease at presentation is over 60%, but relapse carries a poor prognosis. Recent clinical trials have shown that it is possible to reduce the intensity of treatment for less advanced disease without compromising survival.

RHABDOMYOSARCOMA

Rhabdomyosarcoma originates from primitive mesenchymal tissue. There is a wide variety of primary sites, resulting in varying presentation and prognosis.

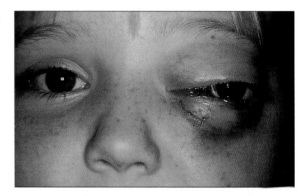

Fig. 19.17 Rhabdomyosarcoma causing proptosis.

Head and neck
These are the most common, causing, for example, proptosis (Fig. 19.17), nasal obstruction and blood-stained nasal discharge.

Genitourinary tumours
These are the next most common, and cause dysuria and urinary obstruction or bloodstained vaginal discharge.

Metastatic disease (lung, liver, bone or bone marrow)
This is present in approximately 15% of patients at diagnosis and is associated with a particularly poor prognosis.

Treatment depends on the site, size and extent of disease. Staging investigations must provide a comprehensive assessment of these factors. The minority (15%) of patients with completely resected local disease require only a short course of chemotherapy to treat presumed micrometastatic disease, and no radiotherapy. The tumour margins are always deceptively ill-defined, and attempts at primary surgical excision are often unsuccessful and should be discouraged unless this can be achieved without mutilation or irreversible organ damage. The majority of patients require aggressive combination chemotherapy and often radiotherapy. Overall cure rates are about 65%.

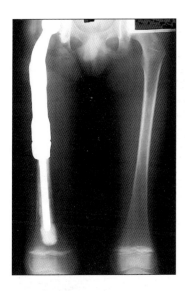

Fig. 19.18 To preserve the leg, an endoprosthetic replacement of the proximal femur has been performed in a boy with Ewing's sarcoma. The prosthesis can be extended for growth.

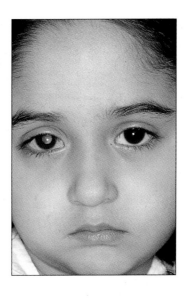

Fig. 19.19 White pupillary reflex in retinoblastoma.

BONE TUMOURS

Malignant bone tumours are uncommon before puberty. Osteogenic sarcoma is more common than Ewing's sarcoma, but Ewing's sarcoma is seen more often in younger children. Both have a male predominance.

The limbs are the most common site. Persistent localised bone pain is a characteristic symptom, usually preceding the detection of a mass. At diagnosis, most patients are well and even metastatic disease (most common in the lungs) is asymptomatic. A bone X-ray shows destruction and variable periosteal new bone formation. In Ewing's sarcoma there is often a substantial soft tissue mass. Initial evaluation must include careful assessment of the primary site to define the extent of the local disease, particularly if limb-saving surgery is contemplated.

Both tumours are difficult to treat, but the prognosis has improved in recent years. In both tumours, treatment involves the use of combination chemotherapy given before surgery. Whenever possible, amputation is avoided by using *en bloc* resection of tumours with endoprosthetic resection (Fig. 19.18). In Ewing's sarcoma, radiotherapy is used in the management of local disease, especially when surgical resection is impossible or incomplete, e.g. in the pelvis or axial skeleton.

RETINOBLASTOMA

Although very rare, retinoblastoma accounts for about 5% of severe visual impairment in children. It may affect one or both eyes. All bilateral tumours are thought to be hereditary, as are about 20% of unilateral cases. The retinoblastoma susceptibility gene has now been identified on chromosome 13. The pattern of inheritance is dominant but with incomplete penetrance. Most cases present within the first 3 years of life. Children from families with the hereditary form of the disease should be screened regularly from birth.

The two most common presentations of unsuspected disease are when a white pupillary reflex is noted to replace the normal red one or with a squint (Fig. 19.19).

The aim of treatment is to cure yet preserve vision. Enucleation of the eye may be necessary for more advanced disease. Treatment with chemotherapy to shrink the tumour followed by local laser treatment to the retina is being used successfully. Radiotherapy may be used in advanced disease, but it is more often reserved for the treatment of recurrence. Most patients are cured, although many are visually impaired. There is a significant risk of second malignancy (especially sarcoma) among survivors of hereditary retinoblastoma.

LIVER TUMOURS

Liver tumours are rare. Primary liver tumours in the newborn are more likely to be benign (haemangioma). Primary malignant liver tumours are mostly hepatoblastoma (65%) or hepatocellular carcinoma (25%). Hepatocellular carcinoma may arise in children with pre-existing liver disease.

Initial presentation is with abdominal distension or with a mass. Pain and jaundice are rare. Investigation with ultrasound or CT scan confirms a large intrinsic liver mass, occasionally with calcification. Elevated serum alphafetoprotein (AFP) is detected in nearly all cases of hepatoblastoma and in some cases of hepatocellular carcinoma. AFP is a sensitive marker for postoperative follow-up, as a rise in the serum level may be the first indication of relapse. Most hepatoblastomas show a good response to chemotherapy (cisplatin and doxorubicin) after which surgical resection can be achieved. Liver transplantation is a possibility for a minority of patients with unresectable disease confined to the liver. The majority of children with hepatoblastoma can now be cured. The prospects for children with hepatocellular carcinoma are less certain.

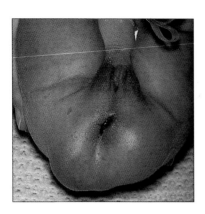

Fig. 19.20
Sacrococcygeal teratoma. These tumours are increasingly detected on antenatal ultrasound screening.

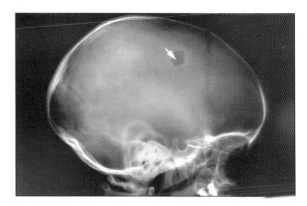

Fig. 19.21 Lytic bone lesions on a skull X-ray in Langerhans cell histiocytosis.

GERM CELL TUMOURS

Germ cell tumours (GCTs) are rare and may be benign or malignant. They arise from the primitive germ cells which migrate from yolk sac endoderm to form gonads in the embryo. Benign tumours are most common in the sacrococcygeal region (Fig. 19.20) and most malignant germ cell tumours are found in the gonads. Serum markers (AFP and β-HCG) are invaluable in confirming the diagnosis and in monitoring response to treatment.

Malignant germ cell tumours are very sensitive to chemotherapy, and a good outcome can be expected for disease at sites other than the brain.

LANGERHANS CELL HISTIOCYTOSIS

Langerhans cell histiocytosis (LCH, previously known as histiocytosis X) is a rare disorder characterised by an abnormal proliferation of histiocytes. It is no longer believed to be a truly malignant condition. However, its sometimes aggressive behaviour and its response to chemotherapy place it within the practice of oncologists. There is a spectrum of the disorder from localised to systemic forms.

Solitary lesions of bone (eosinophilic granuloma)

These may present at any age with pain, swelling or fracture. X-ray reveals a characteristic lytic lesion with a well-defined border. Biopsy is usually necessary and full skeletal survey is required to identify multiple lesions. Curettage, intracavity steroid injection and (in the past) low-dose radiotherapy are all successful forms of treatment. Asymptomatic lesions may not require any treatment.

Multiple bone lesions

These can occur at any site and frequently involve the skull (Fig. 19.21).

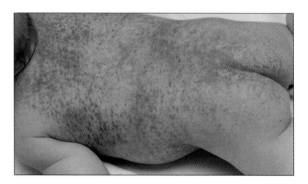

Fig. 19.22 Rash in systemic Langerhans cell histiocytosis. It is often mistaken for seborrhoeic dermatitis or eczema.

Diabetes insipidus

The association of skull disease with proptosis and hypothalamic infiltration causing diabetes insipidus was previously known as Hand–Schüller–Christian disease. Diabetes insipidus can occur with other patterns of presentation and, once established, is not usually reversed by successful treatment of the underlying disease; long-term treatment with desmopressin is usually required.

Systemic LCH

This most aggressive form of LCH (previously known as Letterer–Siwe disease) tends to present in infancy with a seborrhoeic rash (Fig. 19.22) and soft tissue involvement of the gums, ears, lungs, liver, spleen, lymph nodes and bone marrow. The clinical presentation may be characteristic but the diagnosis should be confirmed by biopsy, usually from skin or lymph node. This form of LCH is usually progressive and requires chemotherapy, although spontaneous regression may occur. The prognosis is variable but most patients are cured.

FURTHER READING

Pinkerton C R, Plowman P N, Pearson A D J (eds) 1997 Paediatric oncology. Arnold, London
Pizzo P A, Poplack D G (eds) 1998 Principles & practice of pediatric oncology, 3rd edn. Lippincott, Philadelphia.
    Comprehensive textbook
Voute P A, Kalifa C, Barrett A (eds) 1998 Cancer in children: clinical management, 4th edn. Oxford University Press, Oxford.
    Short textbook

20

Haematological disorders

CHAPTER CONTENTS

- Anaemia
- Haemolytic anaemias

- Bleeding disorders

In the fetus, there is predominantly fetal haemoglobin, HbF. Its oxygen dissociation curve is shifted to the left compared with adult haemoglobin (Fig. 20.1), i.e. it has a higher affinity for oxygen, allowing it to extract and hold on to oxygen, an advantage in the relatively hypoxic environment of the fetus. The haemoglobin concentration is also high; newborn infants have a haemoglobin concentration of 15–23 g/dl. The haemoglobin level increases during the first day of life because of extracellular fluid loss and is exacerbated by delayed clamping of the cord. Thereafter it reaches its minimum at 2–3 months of age, when the lower limit of the normal range is 9.5 g/dl (see Appendix). During this time there is erythroid hypoplasia of the bone marrow. There is also a change from HbF to HbA from late fetal life to 6 months of age. The change of haemoglobin concentration with age is shown in Figure 20.2.

ANAEMIA

Anaemia is defined as a haemoglobin (Hb) level below the normal range for a child of that age and gender. From a year of age until puberty, it is defined as Hb less than 11 g/dl. It can be classified by cause (Fig. 20.3) and according to the size and shape of the red cells.

At birth, severe anaemia is uncommon, but may occur from haemorrhage, from twin to twin, or feto-maternal transfusion, or following placental abruption. Severe anaemia (usually with jaundice) can occur due to haemolysis from rhesus isoimmunisation, although this is now uncommon as anti-D is given to rhesus negative mothers. ABO and other blood group incompatibilities between the mother and infant cause less severe anaemia.

Beyond the neonatal period, by far the commonest cause of anaemia is dietary iron deficiency, which

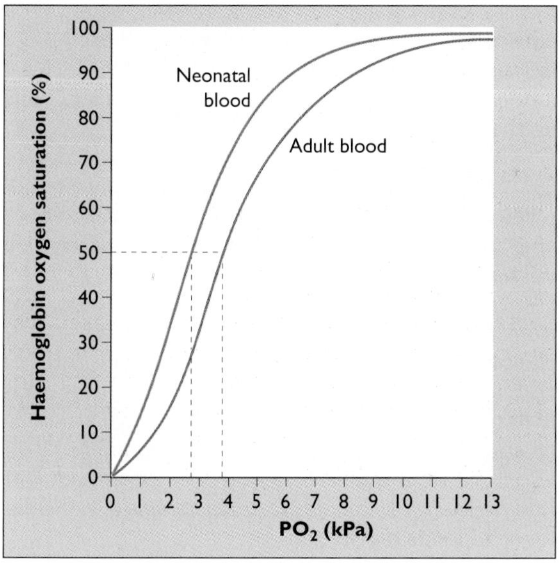

Fig. 20.1 Oxygen dissociation curve showing the left shift of fetal haemoglobin compared with adult haemoglobin. Fetal haemoglobin has a higher affinity for oxygen.

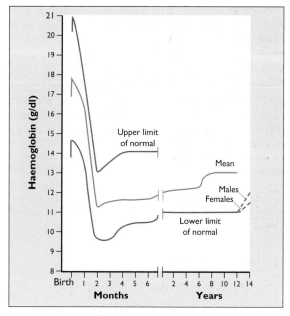

Fig. 20.2 Changes in haemoglobin concentration with age, showing that the haemoglobin is high at birth and falls to its lowest level at 2–3 months of age.

297

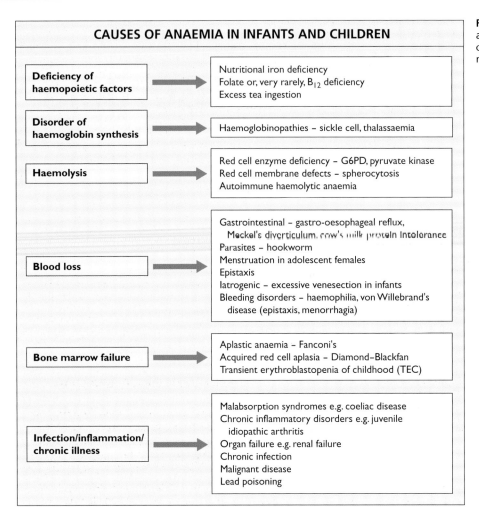

Fig. 20.3 Causes of anaemia in infants and children beyond the neonatal period.

CAUSES OF ANAEMIA IN INFANTS AND CHILDREN

Deficiency of haemopoietic factors →
- Nutritional iron deficiency
- Folate or, very rarely, B_{12} deficiency
- Excess tea ingestion

Disorder of haemoglobin synthesis →
- Haemoglobinopathies – sickle cell, thalassaemia

Haemolysis →
- Red cell enzyme deficiency – G6PD, pyruvate kinase
- Red cell membrane defects – spherocytosis
- Autoimmune haemolytic anaemia

Blood loss →
- Gastrointestinal – gastro-oesophageal reflux, Meckel's diverticulum, cow's milk protein intolerance
- Parasites – hookworm
- Menstruation in adolescent females
- Epistaxis
- Iatrogenic – excessive venesection in infants
- Bleeding disorders – haemophilia, von Willebrand's disease (epistaxis, menorrhagia)

Bone marrow failure →
- Aplastic anaemia – Fanconi's
- Acquired red cell aplasia – Diamond–Blackfan
- Transient erythroblastopenia of childhood (TEC)

Infection/inflammation/ chronic illness →
- Malabsorption syndromes e.g. coeliac disease
- Chronic inflammatory disorders e.g. juvenile idiopathic arthritis
- Organ failure e.g. renal failure
- Chronic infection
- Malignant disease
- Lead poisoning

is found in up to 18% of white children and 33% of immigrant populations in deprived inner city areas in developed countries, and is even more common in developing countries. Iron deficiency is also seen in preterm infants because of their reduced iron stores as well as their greater increase in blood volume accompanying growth compared with full-term infants. They are liable to outstrip their reserves of iron by 4–8 weeks of age.

Blood loss is a much less common cause of anaemia in children than in adults, although repeated blood sampling of sick newborn infants often necessitates replacement transfusions. Hookworm is an important cause of anaemia in some countries. In adolescent females, the onset of menarche may be accompanied by the development of iron deficiency anaemia from a combination of increased demands from their growth spurt and menstrual blood loss.

Iron deficiency

Why infants are at particular risk

The fetus absorbs iron from the mother across the placenta. The term infant has adequate reserves for the first 4 months of age, but during the following year is particularly susceptible to developing iron deficiency because of the additional iron required for the increase in blood volume accompanying growth and to build up the child's iron stores (Fig. 20.4).

Although milk has a relatively low iron content, 50% of the available iron is absorbed from breast milk, whereas only 10% is absorbed from cow's milk. This is one of the main reasons why unmodified cow's milk is not recommended for infants until a year of age. In the UK, infant formula is supplemented with iron. Iron from cereals is absorbed poorly (about 1%) and, to compensate for this, cereals for infants are fortified with iron. Iron deficiency will result from undue delay in the introduction of mixed feeding beyond 3–6 months of age or a diet poor in iron-rich food (Fig. 20.5). Excessive milk intake in toddlers is associated with iron deficiency as there is insufficient space in the diet for solid foods rich in iron.

About 10–15% of dietary iron is absorbed. Iron absorption from food is increased when eaten in combination with food rich in vitamin C (fresh fruit and vegetables) and is inhibited by tannin in tea. The considerable dietary iron requirements of young

IRON REQUIREMENTS DURING CHILDHOOD

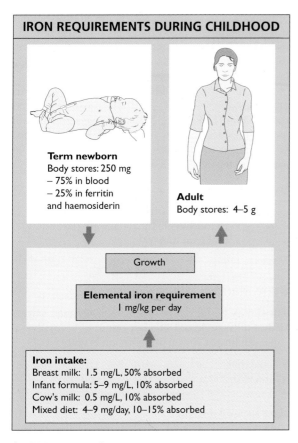

Term newborn
Body stores: 250 mg
– 75% in blood
– 25% in ferritin
and haemosiderin

Adult
Body stores: 4–5 g

Growth

Elemental iron requirement
1 mg/kg per day

Iron intake:
Breast milk: 1.5 mg/L, 50% absorbed
Infant formula: 5–9 mg/L, 10% absorbed
Cow's milk: 0.5 mg/L, 10% absorbed
Mixed diet: 4–9 mg/day, 10–15% absorbed

Fig. 20.4 Iron requirements.

growing children is in marked contrast to the much smaller requirements of adults, who conserve most metabolised iron. A year-old infant requires an intake of iron of about 8 mg/day, which is about the same as his father (9 mg/day) and half that of his mother (15 mg/day). With the infant's much smaller daily food intake, iron deficiency will readily occur from lack of breast-feeding, the delayed introduction of solids or the provision of solids containing little iron, and the early introduction of pasteurised milk instead of continued use of breast-feeding or formula.

Clinical features

Infants and young children are usually asymptomatic until the anaemia becomes marked, when pallor and tiredness are noted. The pallor is most readily detected on the mucosal surfaces of the tongue and mouth and conjunctivae, or by looking at the skin creases in the hands. Clinical assessment is unreliable and iron deficiency anaemia is therefore often found incidentally when blood tests are performed for some other reason.

Pica is a feature of iron deficiency in children. It is the inappropriate eating of non-food materials such as soil, chalk, gravel and foam rubber and may serve as a clue to the diagnosis (see Case history 20.1) – one family had to dismantle their ornamental fireplace because their toddler was picking at and eating the mortar from between the bricks!

Fig. 20.5 Dietary sources of iron.

High in iron
Red meat – beef, lamb
Liver, kidney
Oily fish – pilchards, sardines, etc.

Average iron
Pulses, beans and peas
Fortified breakfast cereals with added vitamin C
Wholemeal products
Dark green vegetables – broccoli, spinach, etc.
Dried fruit – raisins, sultanas
Nuts and seeds – cashews, peanut butter, etc.

Foods to avoid in excess in toddlers
Too much cow's milk
Tea – tannin inhibits iron uptake
High-fibre foods – phytates inhibit iron absorption

CASE HISTORY 20.1

IRON DEFICIENCY ANAEMIA

Anouska, aged 2 years, was noted to look pale when she attended her general practitioner for an upper respiratory tract infection. A blood count showed Hb 5.0 g/dl, MCV 54 fl (normal 72–85 fl) and MCH 16 (normal 24–39 pg). She was drinking 3 pints of cow's milk per day and was a very fussy eater, refusing meat. She had started eating soil when playing in the garden.

Because of the inappropriately large volume of milk she was drinking, she was not sufficiently hungry to eat solid food. Replacing some of the milk with iron-rich food and treatment with oral iron produced a rise in the Hb to 7.5 g/dl within 10 days.

Iron is required for normal brain development. There is evidence that iron deficiency anaemia is associated with behavioural and intellectual deficiencies, which may be reversible with iron therapy. Even children who are not anaemic but who have low iron stores should therefore receive iron supplements. However, not all adverse effects can be reversed by treatment, so it is important to try to prevent iron deficiency in this age group by appropriate nutritional education of parents.

Diagnosis

The diagnosis is confirmed from the blood count and film and the investigations listed in Figure 20.6. Iron deficiency causes a microcytic hypochromic anaemia. Children may have low iron stores without anaemia.

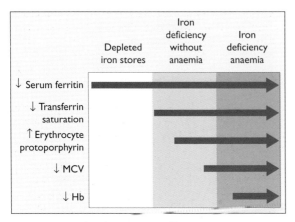

	Depleted iron stores	Iron deficiency without anaemia	Iron deficiency anaemia

↓ Serum ferritin

↓ Transferrin saturation

↑ Erythrocyte protoporphyrin

↓ MCV

↓ Hb

Fig. 20.6 Investigations in iron deficiency. (Adapted from Nathan D G, Oski S H, *Hematology of Infancy and Childhood*, Saunders, Philadelphia, 1993.)

In mild iron deficiency, the haemoglobin, mean corpuscular volume (MCV) and mean corpuscular haemoglobin (MCH) may all be normal. As the deficiency progresses, the MCV and MCH fall until, eventually, anaemia develops. In suspected iron deficiency, the serum ferritin or some other indicator of iron stores should be measured. In some communities there is routine surveillance of young children. There are other less common causes of microcytic anaemia, in particular β- or α-thalassaemia trait. These may be suggested by the racial origin of the child. β-Thalassaemia trait may be confirmed by finding a raised HbA_2 level, but in severe iron deficiency this increase in HbA_2 may be masked and the HbA_2 level needs rechecking when the child is iron-replete (normal ferritin). There is no sure test to diagnose or exclude α-thalassaemia trait other than formal molecular genetic analysis.

Management

For the majority of children who have no symptoms, management involves dietary advice and iron supplementation. Investigation for other causes is advisable if the history or examination suggests a non-dietary cause or if there is failure to respond to therapy in compliant patients. Coeliac disease and Crohn's disease, in particular, should then be considered.

Iron therapy is given orally. Although ferrous sulphate is the most readily absorbed salt and the treatment of choice in adults, the liquid is unpleasant to taste and usually not well tolerated in young children. Good compliance is crucial, so other more palatable medicines are better in this age group. Iron chelates such as Sytron (sodium iron edetate) or Niferex (polysaccharide iron complex) are preferable. They do not stain the teeth. Iron supplementation should be continued for a minimum of 3 months, not only to correct the haemoglobin but also to replenish the iron stores. In severe anaemia, the child should be seen within the first 2 weeks of treatment to ensure a response. With good compliance, the Hb will rise by about 1 g/dl per week and the reticulocyte count will be raised. Failure to respond almost always means the child is not getting the treatment. Blood transfusion should never be necessary for dietary iron deficiency. Even children with a Hb as low as 2–3 g/dl have arrived at this low level over a prolonged period and tolerate it well.

Preterm infants should only be started on iron therapy at several weeks of age. Their iron stores are not depleted until this age and they may be receiving iron in blood transfusions. In addition, the protective effect of lactoferrin from breast-feeding will be reduced by saturating the lactoferrin with iron.

 Treatment of iron deficiency anaemia in toddlers is by dietary advice and oral iron therapy.

Bone marrow failure syndromes

These may be partial or complete. They may start as failure of a single cell line but progress to involve all three cell lines. Clinical presentation is with:

- anaemia
- infection from reduced white cell count
- bruising and bleeding from thrombocytopenia.

Pure red cell aplasia

This can occur as a constitutional abnormality, Diamond–Blackfan syndrome (DBS or DBA). This usually presents in the first few months of life with anaemia. Some affected children are initially responsive to corticosteroids, but many eventually become transfusion-dependent.

An acquired temporary red cell aplasia, transient erythroblastopenia of childhood (TEC), causes anaemia in normal children following a viral infection. Red cell production recovers within 4–6 weeks. A bone marrow examination shows a lack of red cell precursors and the absence of any more sinister underlying cause.

Aplastic anaemia

Aplastic anaemia is a rare condition characterised by a reduction or absence of haemopoietic elements in all cell lines in the bone marrow leading to peripheral blood pancytopenia. While in adults it is usually acquired, in children it usually is idiopathic or one of several 'constitutional' forms with an inherited predisposition.

Fanconi's anaemia

Fanconi's anaemia is the most common inherited form of aplastic anaemia. It is an autosomal recessive condition accompanied by constitutional malformations which include hyperpigmentation, short stature, abnormal radii and thumbs and renal malformations together with developmental delay. These may be evident before the bone marrow failure, which usually occurs at school age.

Cells cultured from the peripheral blood show an increase in spontaneous chromosomal breakages which is reflected in a considerably increased risk of developing acute leukaemia and other malignancies (20%).

Shwachman–Diamond syndrome

These children have a constellation of abnormalities featuring pancreatic exocrine failure, skeletal abnormalities and bone marrow dysfunction. The latter often manifests as mild pancytopenia or isolated neutropenia, eventually progressing to marrow failure. There is a significant risk of leukaemia (up to 25%).

Acquired aplastic anaemia

Acquired aplastic anaemia is uncommon in children. No cause is usually identified, although it may follow the ingestion of drugs (e.g. sulphonamides, chloramphenicol, antithyroid drugs) or infections (hepatitis and Epstein–Barr virus).

Management

Whatever the cause, children with severe aplastic anaemia are likely to die within 6 months without definitive treatment. Treatment is aimed at replacing defective marrow, in particular the stem cells, by bone marrow transplantation, or treatment with immune suppressive therapies, as some forms may be caused by inappropriate immune responses. In idiopathic aplastic anaemia, bone marrow transplants from sibling donors (allografts) can be curative. The efficacy of HLA-matched unrelated donor marrow is being assessed. If no donor is available, immune suppression with antihuman lymphocyte globulin (from either horses or rabbits) together with cyclosporin can produce a response that allows freedom from blood products, but it is usually associated with unpleasant side-effects (serum sickness). If these forms of treatment are ineffective, support with red cell and platelet transfusions is necessary to maintain life, with intravenous antibiotics as indicated for infections. Overwhelming sepsis or haemorrhage are the main causes of death.

HAEMOLYTIC ANAEMIAS

The bone marrow is a very dynamic organ, producing 2 million red blood cells per second, or 173 000 million per day. The life span of a normal red cell is 120 days. In haemolysis, red cell survival may be reduced to a few days. Normal bone marrow production can increase about eightfold, so that haemolysis may occur without anaemia until the bone marrow is no longer able to compensate for premature destruction of red cells.

There are many causes of haemolytic anaemias, which may be inherited or acquired (Fig. 20.7). Inherited defects are the most common, and may be due to:

- metabolic defects – enzyme deficiencies, e.g. G6PD deficiency
- abnormalities in haemoglobin structure and/or function – haemoglobinopathies, e.g. sickle cell disease and thalassaemia
- structural defects – disorders of the red cell membrane, e.g. spherocytosis.

Haemolysis from increased red cell breakdown leads to:

- anaemia
- reticuloendothelial hyperplasia – hepatomegaly and splenomegaly
- elevated unconjugated bilirubin
- excess urinary urobilinogen
- abnormalities of the blood film in some cases, e.g. spherocytes.

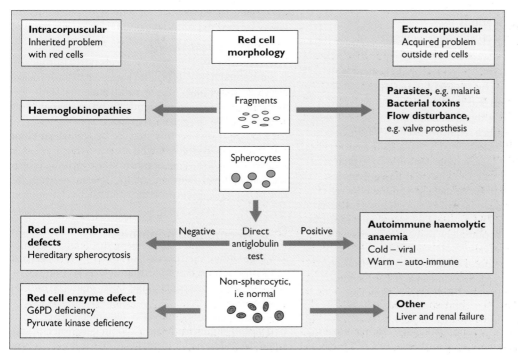

Fig. 20.7 Diagnostic approach to haemolytic anaemias.

Increased red cell production leads to:

- reticulocytosis
- erythroid hyperplasia of the bone marrow, which may cause skeletal deformity of the face and skull, and osteopenia.

Red cell enzyme deficiencies

Glucose-6-phosphate dehydrogenase (G6PD) deficiency

Worldwide, over 100 million people are deficient in glucose-6-phosphate dehydrogenase (G6PD), making it the most common enzyme deficiency. Many different mutations of the gene have been described, leading to different clinical features in different populations.

G6PD is the rate-limiting enzyme of the hexose monophosphate shunt by which red cells generate $NADPH_2$. This maintains glutathione in a reduced state, which is essential for preventing oxidative damage to the cell. Red cells lacking G6PD are susceptible to oxidant-induced haemolysis. The gene for G6PD is located on the X chromosome and so the deficiency mainly affects males. Females who are heterozygotes are usually clinically normal as they have about half the normal G6PD activity. They may be affected either if they are homozygous or, more commonly, when by chance more of the normal X chromosomes than abnormal ones have been inactivated (extreme Lyonisation – the Lyon hypothesis is that, in every XX cell, one of the X chromosomes is inactivated and that this is random). In Mediterranean, Middle Eastern and Oriental populations, affected males have very low or absent enzyme activity in their red cells. Affected Afro-Caribbeans have 10–15% normal enzyme activity. Young red blood cells may have normal enzyme activity whilst older cells are deficient.

Clinical manifestations

G6PD deficiency mostly causes episodes of haemolysis rather than a chronic haemolytic state. It causes:

- *Neonatal jaundice* – onset is usually in the first 3 days of life. This is most common in Mediterranean and Far Eastern variants. Worldwide it is the most common cause of severe neonatal jaundice requiring exchange transfusion.
- *Drug- or infection-induced haemolysis.* Infections are now thought to be a more common precipitating factor than drugs. Intravascular haemolysis is associated with fever, malaise and the passage of dark urine, as it contains haemoglobin as well as urobilinogen. The haemoglobin level falls rapidly. Exposure to naphthalene in mothballs may also induce haemolysis.
- *Favism.* Ingestion of broad beans can cause acute haemolysis in Mediterranean and Far Eastern variants but is not seen in Afro-Caribbeans.

Diagnosis

G6PD deficiency only rarely causes chronic anaemia. Specific enzyme assays are available for G6PD activity.

Fig. 20.8 Drugs which may cause haemolysis in G6PD deficiency.
(Adapted from Beutler E, Glucose-6-phosphate dehydrogenase deficiency, New England Journal of Medicine 1991 **324**:169–174.

Antimalarials
Primaquine

Antibiotics
Some sulphonamides, e.g. co-trimoxazole
Nitrofurantoin
Nalidixic acid
Ciprofloxacin

Others
Dapsone
Naphthalene (mothballs)

During a haemolytic crisis, G6PD levels may be misleadingly elevated due to the higher enzyme concentration in reticulocytes, which are produced in increased numbers in response to the destruction of mature red cells. A repeat assay is then required in the steady state to confirm the diagnosis.

Management

The parents of a child with G6PD deficiency should be given advice about what to watch for in acute infections (jaundice, pallor and dark urine) and provided with a list of drugs to avoid (Fig. 20.8). Many drugs which were thought to induce haemolysis (e.g. aspirin, chloroquine and vitamin K) are now regarded as safe in therapeutic dosage. Eating fava beans should be avoided by affected children of Mediterranean origin. In acute haemolysis, blood transfusion may be required. In Afro-Caribbeans, haemolysis is usually self-limiting, as the newly formed red cells have normal enzyme activity.

Pyruvate kinase deficiency

This is much rarer and mainly affects north Europeans. It is inherited as an autosomal recessive disorder. Most affected individuals run a mild anaemia with few symptoms. The anaemia tends to be exacerbated by infections. The diagnosis requires a specific assay of the enzyme. Splenectomy may be beneficial for some severely affected children who are persistently anaemic and who develop signs of marrow hyperplasia (skeletal deformities). Removal of the spleen reduces the rate of haemolysis because the spleen actively removes abnormal red cells.

Haemoglobinopathies

These are inherited disorders of haemoglobin structure or its production. The molecular defects accounting for most of these disorders have been characterised by gene analysis.

Human haemoglobin is a tetramer consisting of two globin chains from the α-globin gene (on chromosome 16) and two globin chains from the β-globin gene

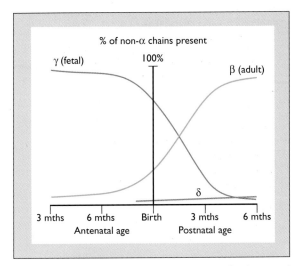

Fig. 20.9 Changes in haemoglobin chains in the fetus and infancy.

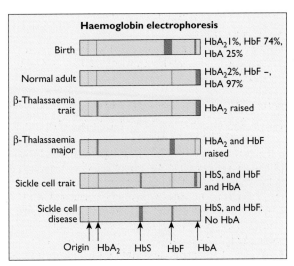

Fig. 20.10 Patterns of haemoglobin electrophoresis showing the types of haemoglobin at birth, in adults and in a range of haemoglobinopathies.

(on chromosome 11). The tetramer constitution varies according to age. In late pregnancy, fetal haemoglobin (HbF) which consists of Hb$\alpha_2\gamma_2$ accounts for 70–90%. The production of β-chains in adult HbA starts from the second trimester and rapidly increases after birth when HbF production is suppressed (Fig. 20.9). By 1 year of age, HbF is normally less than 2%. As most clinically important haemoglobinopathies (other than α-thalassaemia) result from abnormalities of β-chain synthesis, clinical manifestations are usually delayed until after 6 months of age. Diagnosis of these conditions is based on the clinical picture (including racial origin) and confirmed by the pattern of haemoglobin electrophoresis, often with quantitation of the different components (Fig. 20.10).

As many of these conditions occur in particular ethnic groups, selective pre and postnatal screening may offer early recognition of affected individuals. In some parts of the UK, postnatal screening for haemoglobinopathies is performed on the blood sample taken for biochemical screening (Guthrie test). This means that the diagnosis is made before affected children develop any clinical manifestations.

Prenatal diagnosis can be offered for most forms of haemoglobinopathies. Genetic counselling can enable parents to make informed decisions and is especially relevant where an affected individual is likely to have major medical problems (e.g. β-thalassaemia major).

Sickle cell disease

Sickle cell disease (HbS), the homozygous state (SS), results from inheritance of two β-globin genes in which there is a single amino acid substitution (glutamine for valine) on codon 6 of the β-chain. Inheritance of a single mutation results in sickle trait, in which approximately 40% of the haemoglobin is HbS. This does not result in any clinical problems and is not a disease in itself. As the heterozygous state is thought to offer protection against malaria, sickle cell disease is most common in people of black tropical African descent, but is also seen in people from the Mediterranean, Middle East and parts of India.

Pathogenesis

In HbSS, the haemoglobin molecule becomes deformed (insoluble) in the deoxygenated state. Rigid tubular spiral bodies are formed which deform the red cells into a sickle shape. Irreversibly sickled red cells have a reduced life span and may be trapped in the microcirculation, resulting in thrombosis and therefore ischaemia. This is exacerbated by low oxygen tension, dehydration and cold.

The clinical manifestations of sickle cell disease (Fig. 20.11) vary widely between different individuals. Disease severity is also dependent upon the inheritance of other coexisting haemoglobinopathies, e.g. HbS/β°-thalassaemia results in severe disease, HbS/β⁺-thalassaemia in mild disease. Disease severity is greatly reduced by a high HbF level (common in Arab variants).

Management
Acute painful crises
Adequate hydration, oxygenation and warmth need to be ensured. Infection may precipitate painful or haemolytic crises and needs to be treated vigorously.

Analgesia is required for pain. If severe, opiates are required and can be given most effectively using a patient-controlled infusion in older children or a nurse-controlled infusion for younger children.

Other crises
Blood transfusion may be required during aplastic, sequestration or haemolytic crises for a sudden, marked fall in the haemoglobin. Exchange transfusion reduces the proportion of sickle cells without unduly raising the

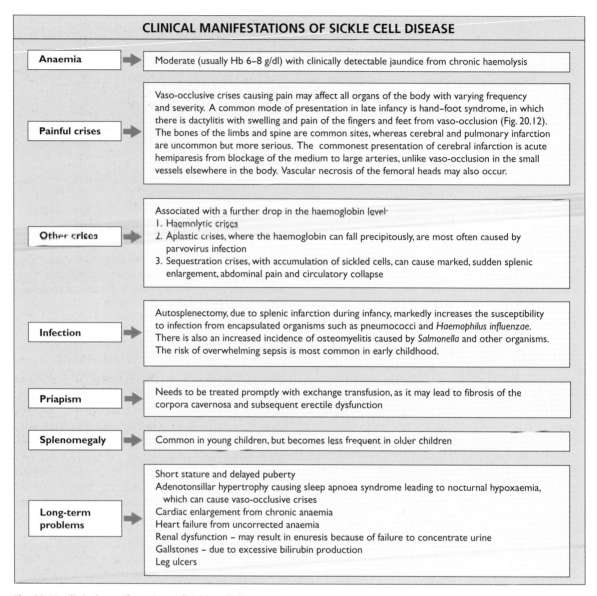

CLINICAL MANIFESTATIONS OF SICKLE CELL DISEASE

Anaemia → Moderate (usually Hb 6–8 g/dl) with clinically detectable jaundice from chronic haemolysis

Painful crises → Vaso-occlusive crises causing pain may affect all organs of the body with varying frequency and severity. A common mode of presentation in late infancy is hand–foot syndrome, in which there is dactylitis with swelling and pain of the fingers and feet from vaso-occlusion (Fig. 20.12). The bones of the limbs and spine are common sites, whereas cerebral and pulmonary infarction are uncommon but more serious. The commonest presentation of cerebral infarction is acute hemiparesis from blockage of the medium to large arteries, unlike vaso-occlusion in the small vessels elsewhere in the body. Vascular necrosis of the femoral heads may also occur.

Other crises → Associated with a further drop in the haemoglobin level:
1. Haemolytic crises
2. Aplastic crises, where the haemoglobin can fall precipitously, are most often caused by parvovirus infection
3. Sequestration crises, with accumulation of sickled cells, can cause marked, sudden splenic enlargement, abdominal pain and circulatory collapse

Infection → Autosplenectomy, due to splenic infarction during infancy, markedly increases the susceptibility to infection from encapsulated organisms such as pneumococci and *Haemophilus influenzae*. There is also an increased incidence of osteomyelitis caused by *Salmonella* and other organisms. The risk of overwhelming sepsis is most common in early childhood.

Priapism → Needs to be treated promptly with exchange transfusion, as it may lead to fibrosis of the corpora cavernosa and subsequent erectile dysfunction

Splenomegaly → Common in young children, but becomes less frequent in older children

Long-term problems → Short stature and delayed puberty
Adenotonsillar hypertrophy causing sleep apnoea syndrome leading to nocturnal hypoxaemia, which can cause vaso-occlusive crises
Cardiac enlargement from chronic anaemia
Heart failure from uncorrected anaemia
Renal dysfunction – may result in enuresis because of failure to concentrate urine
Gallstones – due to excessive bilirubin production
Leg ulcers

Fig. 20.11 Clinical manifestations of sickle cell disease.

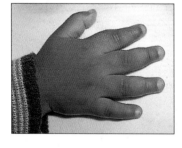

Fig. 20.12 Swelling of the fingers from dactylitis (the hand –foot syndrome) is a common mode of presentation of sickle cell disease in late infancy.

haemoglobin level and is indicated for cerebral and pulmonary infarction (see Case history 20.2) and priapism.

Long term
HbS is a low affinity haemoglobin, which delivers oxygen efficiently, so chronic steady-state anaemia is not an indication for giving blood transfusions.

Vaso-occlusive crises will be prevented if the proportion of HbS is less than 30%. This can be achieved by exchange transfusion followed by regular top-up transfusions. However, regular blood transfusion is often associated with alloimmunisation and is only used following a neurological complication or for multiple, severe crises. Ideally, before any transfusion occurs, the child's blood should be genotyped, i.e. a more extended range of blood group antigens determined (not just ABO and Rh but also Kell and other antigens). Blood or exchange transfusion may be required before major surgery. Allogeneic bone marrow transplantation has been performed in a few patients with severe disease, but there is controversy about this form of therapy and to whom it should be offered. Suitable candidates would be those who experience multiple painful crises or have an abnormal cerebral

CASE HISTORY 20.2

ACUTE SICKLE CHEST SYNDROME

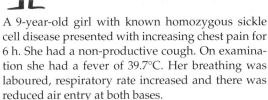

A 9-year-old girl with known homozygous sickle cell disease presented with increasing chest pain for 6 h. She had a non-productive cough. On examination she had a fever of 39.7°C. Her breathing was laboured, respiratory rate increased and there was reduced air entry at both bases.

Investigations

- Haemoglobin 6 g/dl, WBC 14×10^9/L, platelets 350×10^9/L
- Chest X-ray – see Figure 20.18
- Oxygen saturation – 89% in air
- Arterial P_{O_2} – 9.3 kPa (70 mmHg) breathing face mask oxygen
- Blood cultures were taken and viral titres performed.

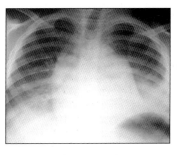

Fig. 20.13 Chest X-ray in acute sickle chest syndrome showing bilateral lower zone consolidation. (Courtesy of Dr Parviz Habibi.)

A diagnosis of acute sickle chest syndrome was made, a potentially fatal condition. She was given oxygen by CPAP (continuous positive airways pressure). An exchange transfusion was performed. Broad-spectrum antibiotics were commenced. She responded well to treatment.

circulation. Treatment with hydroxyurea, which raises the HbF level, has been successful in some cases, but the long-term effects of this antimetabolite are not yet known.

Sickle cell disease carries a greatly increased risk of pneumococcal infection due to progressive splenic dysfunction, so penicillin prophylaxis should be taken throughout life. Affected children should receive the standard course of Hib (*Haemophilus influenzae* type b) and meningococcal C vaccine. Pneumococcal vaccine should be given at about 2 years of age; it does not induce a good antibody response prior to this. Affected children should also be given daily folic acid to compensate for the increased demands due to red blood cell breakdown.

About 85% of those affected survive to the age of 20 years. The main risk of death is in the first 3 years of life, most commonly from infection. Identification of affected infants from screening prenatally or in the neonatal period alerts parents to potential complications and allows prophylaxis against infection to be started promptly.

The risk of bacterial infection is markedly increased in sickle cell disease.

Sickle cell trait (AS)

The heterozygote with sickle cell trait is asymptomatic and rarely has problems except under conditions of low oxygen tension. General anaesthesia does not constitute a risk in this population as long as they have been identified and hypoxia avoided.

Sickle cell-haemoglobin C (SC) disease

Affected children have inherited HbS from one parent and HbC from the other. They usually have a nearly normal haemoglobin level and fewer painful crises than those with sickle cell disease, but they may develop proliferative retinopathy. Their eyes should be checked periodically.

Thalassaemia

Thalassaemia syndromes are due to inherited defects of globin chain synthesis. There are two main types of thalassaemia:

- α-thalassaemia, in which there is a reduced rate of α-chain synthesis
- β-thalassaemias, which are associated with a deficiency of β-chains.

Alteration in the genes controlling globin chain synthesis leads to a reduction or absence of the particular globin. This results in an excess of the other chain, which precipitates within the red cell membrane, bringing about cell death within the bone marrow (ineffective erythropoiesis) and premature removal of circulating red cells by the spleen.

β-Thalassaemia

β-Thalassaemia occurs most often in people from the Mediterranean and Middle East (Fig. 20.14). Over 150 million people carry a β-thalassaemia gene (β-thalassaemia trait). In the UK, thalassaemia is seen predominantly in those who are Greek Cypriot or from the Indian subcontinent. As there is a deficiency of β-chains, γ-chain synthesis continues beyond the neonatal period, producing an increased proportion of HbF, and δ-chain production increases the amount of

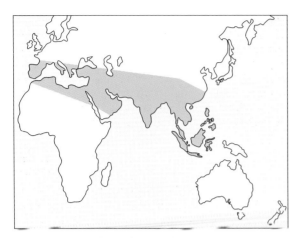

Fig. 20.14 Ethnic origin of patients with thalassaemia.

HbA$_2$. The disease severity of β-thalassaemia depends on the amount of HbA and HbF present:

- *Thalassaemia major* – the child presents with severe anaemia within the first year of life and regular blood transfusions are required.
- *Thalassaemia intermedia* – the clinical manifestations are more variable. The child has inherited two β-globin abnormalities but anaemia is moderate. Blood transfusions may be required to prevent the complications of ineffective erythropoiesis, in particular, skeletal deformity and osteopenia. Each child must be individually assessed.

- *Thalassaemia minor* – asymptomatic carrier; β-thalassaemia trait.

β-Thalassaemia major

Clinical features (Fig. 20.15)
- Severe anaemia and jaundice from about 6 months of age
- Failure to thrive/growth failure
- Extramedullary haemopoiesis, causing bone marrow expansion which leads to the classical facies with maxillary overgrowth (Fig. 20.16) and skull bossing. There is marked hepatosplenomegaly,

Management
The condition is uniformly fatal without regular blood transfusions. The aim is to maintain the haemoglobin concentration above 10 g/dl in order to reduce growth retardation and prevent bone deformation. Children should be genotyped prior to transfusion, and leucocyte-depleted blood (now standard in the UK for all blood transfused from late 1999) is used to minimise transfusion reactions. Repeated blood transfusion causes chronic iron overload and consequent tissue damage. Chelation therapy with subcutaneous desferrioxamine, given regularly as an overnight infusion, promotes urinary iron excretion. Negative iron balance is rarely achieved and compliance is often a problem. The complications of multiple transfusions, particularly iron deposition, in young adults are shown in Figure 20.17.

CLINICAL FEATURES AND COMPLICATIONS OF β-THALASSAEMIA MAJOR

Pallor

Jaundice

Bossing of the skull Maxillary overgrowth

Splenomegaly

Need for repeated blood transfusions
Complications shown in Figure 20.17

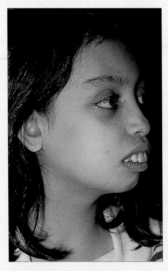

Fig. 20.16 Facies in β-thalassaemia showing maxillary overgrowth and skull bossing.

Fig. 20.17 Complications of multiple blood transfusions.

Iron deposition – the most important
Heart – cardiomyopathy
Liver – cirrhosis
Pancreas – diabetes
Endocrine gland – failure
Skin – hyperpigmentation

Antibody formation – now uncommon
Red cell antibodies
HLA antibodies

Infection – now rare
Hepatitis (blood is now screened for hepatitis B and C)
HIV infection (blood is now screened)
Malaria

Venous access
Multiple infusions and blood samples

Fig. 20.15 Summary of clinical features of β-thalassaemia major.

Bone marrow transplantation is curative but is limited to those children who have an HLA-matched compatible sibling donor. Other areas of research are the development of oral chelating agents, and the possibility of gene modulation.

> β-Thalassaemia major is fatal without regular blood transfusions, but these lead to iron overload.

β-Thalassaemia trait

Heterozygotes are usually asymptomatic. The red cells are usually hypochromic and microcytic. Anaemia is mild or absent, with a disproportionate reduction in MCH (18–22 fl) and MCV (60–70 fl). The red blood cell count is therefore usually increased (>5.5 × 10^{12}/L). The most important diagnostic feature is the raised HbA$_2$ (and in about half there is a mild elevation of HbF level of 1–3%) on haemoglobin electrophoresis. β-Thalassaemia trait can cause confusion with mild iron deficiency and lead to unnecessary iron therapy.

α-Thalassaemia

There are four α-globin genes. The manifestation of the α-thalassaemia syndromes depends on the number of functional genes. α-Thalassaemia genes are particularly common in Asian populations.

The most severe form (four-gene deletion) leads to Hb Barts – tetramers of fetal γ-chains – which does not transport oxygen effectively, therefore causing fetal hydrops and death *in utero*. Hb H (three-gene deletion) leads to moderate chronic haemolysis with production of HbH – tetramers of β-chains. These are unstable, and can be detected in the blood by special staining techniques. One- or two-gene deletions do not cause clinical manifestations but may give rise to hypochromic and microcytic red cells (and hence confusion with iron deficiency). As with all haemoglobinopathies, the correct diagnosis is important for genetic counselling.

Other defects of haemoglobin structure or production

There are many other haemoglobin variants, e.g. HbE, the commonest variant in South-East Asia, which causes a mild, microcytic anaemia. The haemoglobin variants may occur in combinations, which may modify each other, e.g. sickle cell trait together with β-thalassaemia trait clinically resembles sickle cell disease.

Disorders of the red cell membrane

Spherocytosis

Hereditary spherocytosis (HS) is the commonest cause of hereditary haemolysis in the UK. It is caused by abnormalities in one or more of the skeletal proteins of the red cell membrane (spectrin, ankyrin or band 3).

This results in the red cell losing part of its membrane as it passes through the spleen. This reduction in surface to volume ratio causes the cells to become spheroidal. It affects about 1 in 3000 Caucasians with variable severity. It usually has an autosomal dominant inheritance, but in 25% there is no family history and it is caused either by new mutations or by clinically silent mutations in the parents (recessive inheritance).

Clinical features

The disorder is often suspected because of a positive family history. Even within the same family, the clinical manifestations are highly variable. It may be completely asymptomatic. The clinical features include:

- jaundice – usually develops during childhood but may be intermittent; may cause severe haemolytic jaundice in the first few days of life
- anaemia – presents in childhood with mild anaemia (haemoglobin 9–11 g/dl), but the haemoglobin level may fall with an intercurrent infection; many children have 'compensated' haemolysis with a normal haemoglobin
- mild to moderate splenomegaly – depends on the rate of haemolysis; this may be the mode of presentation in the first year of life
- aplastic crisis – uncommon, associated with parvovirus infection
- gallstones – due to increased bilirubin excretion.

Diagnosis

The appearance of the blood film together with a reticulocytosis and raised bilirubin is usually diagnostic, but antibody-induced anaemia is also associated with spherocytes and must be excluded with a direct antiglobulin test in the absence of a family history. Although an osmotic fragility test is often recommended, this is time-consuming and is rarely required. If there is any doubt about the diagnosis, tests for specific membrane proteins can be performed by reference laboratories.

> Parvovirus infection can cause aplastic crises in patients with inherited haemolytic anaemias.

Management

No treatment is required if the disease is mild (i.e. compensated haemolysis, reticulocytosis less than 5%). Folic acid is normally given to compensate for increased demands due to ongoing haemolysis. Occasional blood transfusions may be required for aplastic crises. Splenectomy improves red cell survival but is only indicated for severe disease causing persistent anaemia (e.g. Hb <8 g/dl), marked jaundice or complications (e.g. gallstones). It is preferable to defer this until after 6 years of age because of the risk of overwhelming postsplenectomy infection, particularly with encapsulated bacteria. Before splenectomy, the

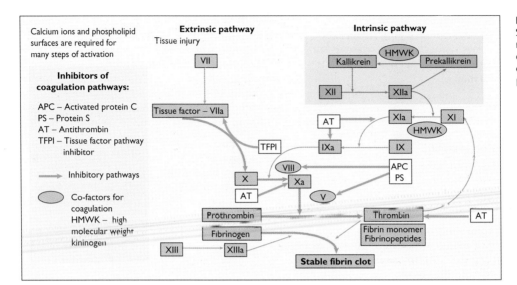

Fig. 20.18 Schematic representation of the coagulation pathway.

Fig. 20.19 Helpful clinical features in evaluating bleeding disorders.

Age of onset
Uncomplicated previous surgery (especially tonsillectomy) or dental extraction suggests the bleeding tendency is acquired rather than inherited

Positive family history
Some congenital bleeding disorders have a sex-linked inheritance. A detailed family tree including the sex of affected family members needs to be determined

Site and type of bleeding
Mucous membrane bleeding and skin haemorrhage – characteristic of platelet disorders or von Willebrand's disease
Bleeding into muscles or into joints – characteristic of severe clotting factor deficiencies
Scarring and delayed bruising – suggestive of disorders of connective tissue, e.g. Marfan's syndrome, osteogenesis imperfecta or factor XIII deficiency

---

Fig. 20.20 Investigations in haemophilia A and von Willebrand's disease.

	Haemophilia A	von Willebrand's disease
PT	Normal	Normal
APTT	↑↑	↑/normal
Factor VIII:C	↓↓	↓
vWF	Normal	↓
Platelet aggregation	Normal	Abnormal with ristocetin (an antibiotic)
Bleeding time	Normal	↑

PT = prothrombin time; APTT = activated partial thromboplastin time; vWF = von Willebrand factor

---

child should be given *Haemophilus influenzae* (Hib), meningococcal C and pneumococcal vaccines. Daily penicillin administration is recommended postsplenectomy, but compliance may be a problem. There is uncertainty about how long prophylaxis should be continued but many specialists believe it should be life-long.

BLEEDING DISORDERS

Normal blood clotting relies on the complex interaction between the vessel wall, platelets and coagulation factors (Fig. 20.18), involving not only pro-coagulant activity but also fibrinolysis. When evaluating a child with a bleeding disorder, there are some helpful features, which are shown in Figure 20.19.

Haemophilia A and B and von Willebrand's disease account for more than 90% of all patients with an inherited bleeding disorder. Laboratory screening tests help to determine the most likely causes (Fig. 20.20), whilst specialist investigation will characterise the deficiency.

In addition to the platelet count, a coagulation screen is usually performed:

- the activated partial thromboplastin time (APTT) – tests the intrinsic pathway as well as the final common pathway.
- prothrombin time (PT) – measures the extrinsic pathway and the final common pathway (factors II, V and X and the conversion of fibrinogen to fibrin).
- thrombin time and fibrinogen level – to exclude afibrinogenaemia and dysfibrinogenaemia.

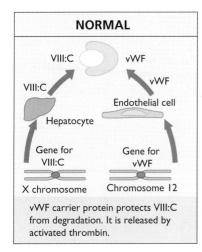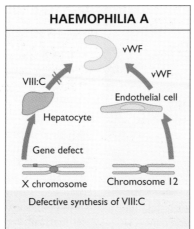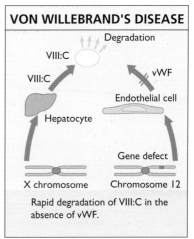

Fig. 20.21 Factor VIII synthesis – normal, haemophilia A and von Willebrand's disease.

The bleeding time is prolonged with low platelets or intrinsic platelet dysfunction in the presence of a normal platelet count. It is a difficult test to standardise, especially in children, and is only performed if specifically indicated.

Haemophilia

Haemophilia A is a sex-linked disorder which is characterised by reduced or absent factor VIII activity (Fig. 20.21). Haemophilia B (Christmas disease) is similar but is due to reduced or absent factor IX activity. The hallmark of severe disease is recurrent spontaneous bleeding into joints and muscles, leading to crippling arthritis without adequate treatment. Haemophilia A occurs in about 1 in 5000–10 000 males, whereas haemophilia B is six times less common. In about 30% there is no family history. Identifying female carriers requires a detailed family history, analysis of coagulation factors and DNA analysis. Prenatal diagnosis is available using DNA analysis.

The disorder is graded as severe, moderate or mild, depending on the factor VIII:C (or IX:C in haemophilia B) level (Fig. 20.22). The severity remains constant within a family.

Clinical features

There are usually few problems in the first year of life. It is only when the child starts to walk and falls over that abnormal bleeding is first noted. This can occur at any site but is frequently into joints and muscles. Where there is no family history, non-accidental injury may initially be suspected.

Management

Bleeding is treated by the prompt and adequate replacement with intravenous infusion of factor VIII (or IX for haemophilia B) concentrate. The quantity required depends on the site and nature of the bleed. In general, raising the circulating level to 30% of normal is sufficient to control haemorrhage. Major surgery or life-threatening bleeds require the level to be

Fig. 20.22 Severity of haemophilia.

Factor VIII:C level	Severity	Bleeding tendency
<2%	Severe	Spontaneous joint/muscle bleeds
2–10%	Moderate	Bleed after minor trauma
>10%	Mild	Bleed after surgery.

Fig. 20.23 Complications of treatment of haemophilia.

Inhibitors
5–20% develop antibodies to factor VIII which reduce or completely inhibit the effect of treatment.

Transfusion transmitted infections
Where plasma-derived factor concentrates are used, there is a risk of viral transmission. Contamination of blood products in the late 1970s and early 1980s resulted in a significant number of patients with haemophilia and other bleeding disorders becoming HIV-positive. Heat treatment and donor screening have virtually eliminated the risk of hepatitis A, B and C and HIV infection. Parvovirus may be transmitted but is rarely of clinical importance. Children in the UK are all treated with recombinant (genetically engineered) concentrates of factor VIII (haemophilia A) or IX (haemophilia B). No complications other than the development of inhibitors have been reported.

raised to 100% and then maintained at 30–50% for up to 2 weeks to prevent secondary haemorrhage. This can only be achieved by regular infusion of factor concentrate (usually 8- to 12-hourly or by continuous infusion of factor VIII) and monitoring levels by assaying plasma samples. Complications of treatment are shown in Figure 20.23.

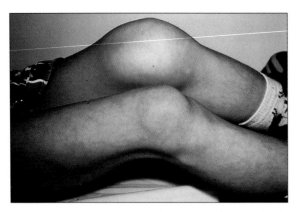

Fig. 20.24 Severe arthropathy from recurrent joint bleeds in haemophilia. The aim of modern management is to prevent this from occurring.

Repeated bleeding into the joints causes progressive arthropathy (Fig. 20.24), so prompt and adequate therapy for bleeds helps to avoid permanent damage to joints. Parents are usually taught to give replacement therapy at home. Children with good veins may go onto home therapy at 2–3 years of age. Eventually patients (from about 7 years) will administer their treatment themselves. This avoids delay and minimises inconvenience to the family. Although 'on demand' treatment (i.e. when a bleed or injury occurs) is adequate, the ideal now is to give regular 'prophylactic' therapy sufficient to raise the baseline factor VIII:C or IX:C to more than about 2%, converting 'severe' to 'moderate' haemophilia and thus reducing the likelihood of joint bleeds. Studies have shown that this results in much better joint function in adult life. The usual regimen is to give factor VIII:C three times a week, or factor IX:C twice a week.

Mild haemophilia and von Willebrand's disease are often successfully managed without the use of blood products, by using infusions of desmopressin (DDAVP), which stimulates endogenous release of factor VIII:C and von Willebrand factor. Adequate levels can be achieved to enable minor surgery and dental extraction to be undertaken.

Management of children with bleeding disorders should be supervised by a haemophilia treatment centre. These provide medical, nursing and psychosocial expertise for the children and their families. These centres are also supported by specialised laboratory facilities to undertake specific assays to diagnose and monitor therapy. Physiotherapy is needed to preserve muscle strength and avoid damage from immobilisation. Many families receive considerable support from self-help groups such as the Haemophilia Society.

Children with bleeding disorders who have no family history are often thought at presentation to be victims of non-accidental injury.

von Willebrand's disease (vWD)

The von Willebrand factor (vWF) has two major roles:

- it facilitates platelet adhesion to the damaged endothelium
- it acts as the carrier protein for factor VIII:C, protecting it from breakdown.

In von Willebrand's disease, there is usually a reduction of both factor VIII:C and vWF together with a prolonged bleeding time due to the failure of the defective vWF promoting platelet adhesion to the vessel wall. It is a heterogeneous disorder which demonstrates considerable genetic variation. The commonest subtype has an autosomal dominant inheritance. The hallmark of the disorder is mucocutaneous bleeding, often of the gums or nose or causing menorrhagia in adolescent and adult females.

Treatment depends on the type and severity of the disorder. Desmopressin (DDAVP) is used for mild disease; intermediate purity plasma-derived factor VIII concentrates or specific von Willebrand factor concentrates may be given for severe disease. The intermediate purity factor VIII concentrates are used as the newer genetically engineered factor VIII concentrate contains no vWF. Cryoprecipitate (which contains the entire factor VIII/vWF complex) is no longer used as, in contrast to the concentrates, it has not undergone viral inactivation. Whenever possible, desmopressin (DDAVP) is given rather than plasma products, to reduce the risk of viral transmission. Tranexamic acid, an antifibrinolytic agent, can be used for mucous membrane bleeding as an adjunct to therapy but should be avoided in patients with haematuria due to a risk of clot retention.

In bleeding disorders, avoid intramuscular injections, aspirin and non-steroidal anti-inflammatory drugs.

Inhibitors of coagulation

In plasma there is a balance between coagulation and 'anticoagulation' factors (see Fig. 20.18) Antithrombin and activated protein C (APC) are important, naturally occurring inhibitors of coagulation and play a central role in localising fibrin at the site of tissue damage. Any imbalance between the activators and inhibitors of coagulation or fibrinolysis (e.g. from activated protein C resistance) may predispose to thrombosis. Inherited protein C resistance has been found to be due to a point mutation in the factor V gene (factor V Leiden), which makes activated factor V resistant to breakdown by activated protein C. This mutation is very common in northern Europe, being present in about 5% of the population. While it is a risk factor for thrombosis, it is not a very strong one on its own, and there is currently much debate about who should be screened and when. In the UK, current practice is not to screen children for genetic defects which are not going to affect their medical management until they are old enough to decide for themselves. Inherited thrombophilic risk factors are unlikely to affect management of asymptomatic children until they are adolescents. More recently, a mutation has been found in the factor II (prothrombin) gene which is also a risk factor and is present in about 2% of the UK population.

Protein C and S deficiencies can be inherited or acquired. Heterozygotes for protein C and S deficiencies are at risk of thromboses beyond the second decade of life. Acquired deficiencies may follow varicella infection (due to autoantibody production), liver disease and sickle cell disease. Treatment is by replacement with fresh frozen plasma or factor concentrate with subsequent anticoagulation with warfarin.

Thrombosis in children is unusual and most often occurs in the context of some other serious condition, e.g. malignancy or cardiac disease, or in association with central venous lines. Such children should be considered for investigation for a thrombophilic risk factor.

Thrombocytopenia

Purpura from thrombocytopenia will usually develop when the platelet count falls below 20×10^9/L, with haemorrhage liable to occur if the level falls below 10×10^9/L. The causes of purpura in children are listed in Figure 20.25. While purpura may signify a platelet problem, it also occurs in infections and vascular disorders.

Immune-mediated thrombocytopenic purpura

Immune-mediated thrombocytopenic purpura (ITP) is the commonest cause of thrombocytopenia in childhood. It results from an immune-mediated destruction of circulating platelets within the reticuloendothelial system, mainly in the spleen. The reduced platelet count is accompanied by a compensatory increase in megakaryocytes within the bone marrow.

It mainly affects children between 2 and 10 years of age, with onset often 1–2 weeks after a viral infection. Affected children develop purpura and superficial bruising (see Case history 20.3). They may have epistaxis and other mucosal bleeding. Intracranial bleeding is serious but rare, occurring in 0.1–0.5%, particularly in those with a long period of severe thrombocytopenia. The most common severe bleeding results from heavy nosebleeds, but even these only occur in a minority.

In about 90% of children, the disease is acute and self-limiting. Most will require only a brief stay in hospital to confirm the diagnosis and assess its severity. There has been much debate about the need to perform a bone marrow aspiration to exclude malignant infiltration or aplasia. If the clinical features are characteristic, with no abnormality in the blood other than a low platelet count and no intention to treat, there is need to examine the bone marrow.

Treatment is controversial. The majority of children are mildly affected, as defined clinically and not by

Fig. 20.25 Causes of purpura in children.

Thrombocytopenic	
Excessive destruction	Immune ITP (commonest cause)
	Secondary – SLE, drugs, viral infections
	Alloimmune neonatal thrombocytopenia
Coagulation	Disseminated intravascular coagulation
	Haemolytic uraemic syndrome
	Thrombotic thrombocytopenic purpura
Impaired production	Leukaemia
	Aplastic anaemia
	Congenital
Sequestration	Giant haemangioma (rare)
	Wiskott–Aldrich syndrome (thrombocytopenia, eczema and immune deficiency)
Vascular disorders (non-thrombocytopenic)	
Congenital	Connective tissue disorders (osteogenesis imperfecta, Ehlers–Danlos, Marfan's syndrome)
Acquired	Meningococcal and other severe infections
Immune	Henoch–Schönlein purpura
	Connective tissue disorders – SLE
Drugs	

platelet count, and do not need any therapy. If there is bleeding, it is reasonable to give corticosteroids or a high-dose immunoglobulin infusion. Their use is confined to the treatment of bleeding and not solely a low platelet count. The main mode of action of corticosteroids appears to be inhibition of phagocytosis of sensitised platelets and the reduction of capillary fragility. Only a short course of corticosteroids (e.g. 1–2 mg/kg over 2–3 weeks) should be given and then discontinued irrespective of the platelet count, as a response after this time is unlikely. Immunoglobulin infusions often result in a more rapid rise in the platelet count. Transfused platelets are rapidly destroyed and play little role in management other than in acute life-threatening haemorrhage. The parents need immediate 24-h access to hospital treatment and the child should avoid contact sports while the count is very low.

Splenectomy is reserved for those who continue to have recurrent bleeds in spite of therapy. Most children with chronic ITP (i.e. those not remitting in the first 6 months) will remit within 3 years from the onset.

The contrast between ITP in children and in teenagers and adults is shown in Figure 20.27. If ITP in a child becomes chronic, regular screening for systemic lupus erythematosus (SLE) should be performed, as the thrombocytopenia may predate the development of autoantibodies.

CASE HISTORY 20.3

IMMUNE-MEDIATED THROMBOCYTOPENIC PURPURA (ITP)

Sean, aged 5 years, developed bruising and a skin rash over 24 h. He had had an URTI the previous week. On examination he appeared well but had a purpuric skin rash with some bruises on the trunk and legs (Fig. 20.26). There were three blood blisters on his tongue and buccal mucosa, but no fundal haemorrhages, lymphadenopathy or hepatospleno-megly. Urine was normal on dipstix. A full blood count showed Hb 11.5 g/dl with normal indices,

WBC and differential normal, platelet count 17 × 10^9/L. The platelets on the blood film were large. He was admitted to hospital, a diagnosis of ITP was made and he was discharged home. His parents were counselled and given emergency contact names and telephone numbers. They were also given literature on the condition and advised that he should avoid contact sports. Sean was reviewed within a few days. Over the next 2 weeks he continued to develop bruising and purpura but was asymptomatic. By the third week he had no new bruises, and his platelet count was 25 × 10^9/L; the following week it was 74 × 10^9/L and a week later it was 200 × 10^9/L. He was discharged from follow-up.

In immune thrombocytopenic purpura, in spite of impressive cutaneous manifestations and extremely low platelet count, the outlook is good and most will remit quickly without any intervention.

Fig. 20.26 Bruising and purpura from immune thrombocytopenic purpura.

Fig. 20.27 Contrast between ITP in children and adolescents.

Age	Children	Adolescents
Onset	Sudden	Insidious
Sex ratio, male:female	1:1	1:3
History of viral infection	Yes	No
Duration	Weeks–months	Many months–years Exclude autoimmune disorders

Disseminated intravascular coagulation

In disseminated intravascular coagulation (DIC), the coagulation pathway is activated by a trigger factor (usually endothelial disruption) leading to fibrin deposition in the microcirculation, consumption of coagulation factors and platelets. This may lead to a fulminant bleeding diathesis or may be more chronic and only detectable by deranged blood tests.

The commonest causes of activation of coagulation are severe sepsis or shock due to circulatory collapse, e.g. in meningococcal septicaemia, or extensive tissue damage from trauma or burns. Acute DIC causes bruising and bleeding. A more chronic form may present with low platelets, reduced fibrinogen and only mild bleeding.

Treatment relies on correcting the underlying cause whilst providing intensive care. Supportive care may be provided with fresh frozen plasma (to replace clotting factors) and platelets. Repeated monitoring of platelet count and coagulation profiles helps to guide therapy.

FURTHER READING

Lilleyman J S, Hann I M, Blanchette V S (eds) 1999 Paediatric haematology, 2nd edn. Churchill Livingstone, Edinburgh.
   A single volume, comprehensive textbook
Nathan D G, Orkin S H (eds) 1998 Nathan and Oski's Hematology of infancy and childhood, 5th edn. Saunders, Philadelphia.
   Comprehensive, two volume textbook

Internet

Diamond–Blackfan syndrome – www.diamondblackfan.org
Shwachman–Diamond syndrome – www.shwachman-support.org
Haemophilia – www.haemophilia.org.uk or www.wfh.org

21

Emotions and behaviour

Knowledge of children's emotions and behaviour is important in order to:

- know what constitutes the normal range
- understand common, innocent minor deviations and responses to stress, physical illness and injuries
- recognise and manage emotional and behavioural disorders.

PRINCIPLES OF NORMAL DEVELOPMENT

Normal parenting

A child's behaviour, emotional responses and personality are the end result of an interplay between genetic predisposition and environmental influences. The environment provides experience from which stems knowledge, learned behaviour or emotional responses and attitudes to oneself and the world. Personal relationships are the major environmental factor in promoting psychosocial development and the child's family is the principal source of these. Within the family, the child should be protected, nurtured, educated and civilised so that his development is supported optimally. With the rising number of single parents and divorces, the form of the family is no longer predictable, but it is possible to make statements about what constitutes competent parenting (Fig. 21.1). Beyond this, the parents' attitude towards their children and how they handle their individual children help to determine how their personalities develop.

Normal early relationships

A baby's first relationship is nearly always with his mother. He will be especially responsive to her from very soon after birth but will tolerate separations from her. However, at about 6 months, he will start to demand or seek her physical presence and show tearful *separation anxiety* if she is not there. If tired, fearful, unhappy or in pain, he will cling to her and be

Fig. 21.1 Competent parents.

- Are there when needed
- Protect their children from harm
- Love their children – provide affection, support, comfort, food and shelter
- Use their authority so that they are in charge of their children (rather than vice versa)
- Respect their children's immature status and judge it accurately
- Keep adult business (sex, marital conflict, etc.) away from their children
- Set reasonable limits of tolerance on their children's behaviour
- Establish a moderate amount of justifiable household rules
- Have their own lives and do not live through their children
- Maintain their own self-esteem and personal development

comforted by her presence as an *attachment figure*. This close attachment relationship derives from social interaction and the mother's sensitive responsiveness to the baby's needs, not from any blood tie. It need not be with the biological mother, although it usually is. Its importance lies in it being:

- a particularly close relationship within which the child's development of trust, empathy, conscience and ideals is promoted, forming a prototype for future close relationships
- the child's primary source of comfort, providing his principal method of coping with stress (fear, anxiety, pain, etc.).

This underscores the importance of having a young child's parent 'rooming in' if he has to be admitted to hospital. He would otherwise be doubly distressed both by the absence of his attachment figure and by the threat of strange surroundings or procedures and the stress of pain or illness.

If a young child is placed in strange, impersonal surroundings and separated from his mother for more than several hours, a *triphasic acute separation* reaction sets in (Fig. 21.2):

- mounting anxiety about the fact that his mother fails to reappear produces distressed, irritable tearfulness (*protest*) which is hard to comfort
- after a day or two, this turns into a withdrawn state with no play, no interest in food, and little speech or willingness for personal contact (*despair*)
- the child gradually cheers up from this but the close contact with his mother has been lost and he is relatively indifferent to her when she reappears (*detachment*).

Recreating the original closeness takes weeks and is accompanied by a phase of irritability, misbehaviour and clinging. This can sometimes be seen when children who have had to be admitted to hospital as an emergency subsequently return home.

Children who have never had the opportunity for a close, secure attachment relationship in their early years are at risk of growing up as selfish, shallow individuals who seek the affection and attention of others but otherwise have difficulty with close personal relationships and learning conformity with social rules of conduct.

The selective clinging of early attachment behaviour diminishes over time so that in the second year of life the child extends his emotional attachments to his father or other family members. By school age, the child can tolerate separations from his parents for several hours. Children vary in their ability to do this: a child who is constitutionally apprehensive, who has an exceptionally anxious mother, or who has parents who fight or utter threats of abandonment will continue to cling to his mother for protection and comfort. A series of frightening events will tend to perpetuate clinging, which may persist well into middle childhood (age 5–12 years). This interferes with the child's capacity to learn how to cope with anxiety on his own.

With entry into school, the importance of teachers and other children in shaping psychosocial development increases and their influence must be taken into account in understanding any schoolchild's development.

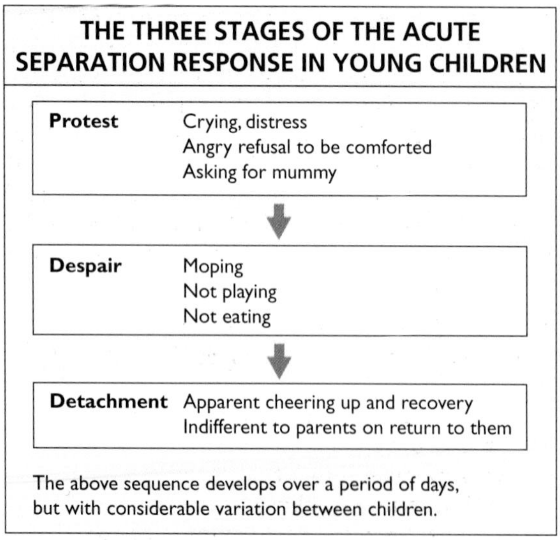

Temperament

Children differ from each other in personality from birth, just as they do in physical appearance. This individuality in behavioural style – how they go about things – is partly genetically determined. It is not fixed but changes slowly in the light of experience. It affects how other people deal with them.

A child born with a *difficult temperament* is prone to:
- predominantly negative mood – whinging, moaning, crying
- intense emotional reactions – screaming rather than whimpering, jumping for joy rather than smiling
- irregular biological functions – a lack of rhythm in sleeping, hunger or toileting
- negative initial responses to novel situations, e.g. pushing a new toy away
- protracted adjustment to new situations – taking weeks or months to settle into a new playgroup.

Such a pattern is a vulnerability factor for future emotional and behaviour problems. It may be hard for parents to maintain an affectionate relationship with a child who has a difficult temperament. Their self-confidence falters as they feel guilty that they have failed as parents. They need support to maintain a positive, loving relationship with their child who will, if this can be done, soften and become easier to handle over a period of months. If they lapse into irritable intolerance themselves, this is likely to maintain the child's grouchy and unsatisfied manner and may lead eventually to low self-esteem or the development of behaviour problems.

Self-esteem

Children develop views and make attributions about themselves. Most children experience praise and success in enough areas of their lives to develop a sense of inner self-confidence and self-worth. Those who do not are at increased risk of developing emotional and behaviour disorders which in turn may breed further shame and failure. A child who does not consider himself worthwhile and valued by others will play safe and not attempt new activities or explore new situations because of a fear of failure. This restricts his development of coping skills and knowledge of the world generally. It may also be a vulnerability factor for depression and anxiety disorders. Children who

---

THE THREE STAGES OF THE ACUTE SEPARATION RESPONSE IN YOUNG CHILDREN

Protest	Crying, distress Angry refusal to be comforted Asking for mummy

Despair	Moping Not playing Not eating

Detachment	Apparent cheering up and recovery Indifferent to parents on return to them

The above sequence develops over a period of days, but with considerable variation between children.

Fig. 21.2 The three stages of the acute separation response in young children.

lack a belief in their own worth may adopt extraordinary and problematic behaviours in order to attract the attention and acclaim of others. For instance, one child took to openly eating dog faeces because it attracted a crowd of amazed children around her. Repeated failure, academically or socially, will undermine self-esteem, as will some disorders themselves (dyspraxia, enuresis and faecal soiling in particular). The most important source of low self-esteem, though, is the child's parents, either because of their own low self-esteem or because of abuse (emotional, sexual or physical) and neglect.

Cognitive style

Below the age of about 5 years, the young child thinks in a way quite different from adults. In the term devised by Piaget, this is *pre-operational thought*, the characteristics of which are summarised in Figure 21.3. In talking with and explaining things to small children, an appreciation of this is crucial. During middle childhood the dominant mode of thought is practical and orderly (*concrete operational thought*) but tied to immediate circumstances and specific experiences rather than hypothetical possibilities or metaphors. Not until the mid-teens does the adult style of abstract thought (*formal operational thought*) begin to appear.

Coping

Children under stress use a number of mental mechanisms to handle their response or to address the source of stress itself. Many of the emotional and behavioural difficulties of childhood can be seen as misplaced and maladaptive coping. Young children tend to regress when stressed and behave as younger than they actually are. In particular, they cling, using the attachment relationship as a source of comfort. It is common for children to minimise or deny a problem as a way of cutting it down to manageable size. With increasing maturity, children learn a repertoire of coping skills so that they become more flexible in their response to adversities. Less intelligent children are slower to learn a broad repertoire and deploy it selectively, which is probably the main reason for their increased vulnerability to emotional and behavioural problems. It may also be true that the increased susceptibility of children with chronic physical illnesses to psychological problems derives from their having a narrower range of experiences, particularly with other children, from which they can learn and practice new ways of coping.

Many responses to adversity, including injury and the onset of serious illness in childhood, show a sequence of phases over a period of weeks:

- an initial impact phase of tearfulness
- subsequent 'brave' acceptance of injury with psychological denial of the seriousness of the adversity
- recoil, characterised by difficult behaviour or overt unhappiness, perhaps with some regression
- gradual adjustment and adaptation to altered circumstances.

 Children whose behaviour presents a problem are often trying to solve a problem of their own, albeit in a poorly thought out or maladaptive way.

ADVERSITIES IN THE FAMILY

Family relationships are, for most children, the source of their most powerful emotions. Similarly, parents have more effect than any one else on children's social learning and behaviour. It follows that families are generally the most potent environmental influence on a child's mental health. They are not all-powerful, since a predisposition to particular childhood emotional and behavioural problems can be inherited, but family influences interact with this so that overt disorder may or may not emerge. Not all disorders have their origin in family adversities: hyperkinetic disorder, tics and autism arise independently of them. Nevertheless, the non-genetic contribution of family interactions to emotional and behavioural disorders is often substantial and the mechanisms whereby they produce disorder are various. The following are some of the known risk factors:

- angry discord between family members
- parental mental ill health, especially maternal depression
- divorce (Figs 21.4 and 21.5) and bereavement
- intrusive overprotection
- lack of parental authority
- physical and sexual abuse
- emotional rejection or unremitting criticism
- use of violence, terror, threats of abandonment or excessive guilt as disciplinary devices

---

Fig. 21.3 The quality of preschool thought.

The child is at the centre of his world ('I'm tired so its getting dark')

Everything has a purpose ('The sea is there for us to swim in')

Inanimate objects are alive ('Naughty table hurt me') and have feelings and motives

Poor categorisation (all men are Daddies)

Use of magical thinking ('If I close my eyes, she'll go away')

Use of sequences or routines rather than a sense of time

The use of toys and other aspects of imaginative play as aids to thought (particularly in making sense of experience and social relationships)

Fig. 21.4 Reactions to parental divorce.

Preschool
Fear of further abandonment:
  intensified clinging at threatened separations
  sleep disturbances
  tearful, irritable and demanding
  desultory play

Middle childhood
Miserable at loss of father, pining for restitution
  of family
Self-blame in younger (age 6–8)
Angry blaming of one parent for divorce in older
  (age 9–12)
Loyalty conflicts
Anxiety and jealousy at parents' new partners
Educational underachievement

Adolescents
Wide variation in response
Various attempts to master the situation:
  detachment from family
  rapid maturation
  moral idealism
  critical of parents
Educational underachievement
Depression in some

Fig. 21.5 Adjustment tasks facing children of divorced parents.

1) Acknowledgement of parental separation
2) Regaining sense of direction in life activities
3) Dealing with sense of loss and rejection
4) Forgiving parents for break-up
5) Accepting permanence of divorce, relinquishing wish for the previously intact family
6) Feeling able to enter into new emotional relationships

- taunting or belittlement of the child
- inconsistent, unpredictable discipline
- using the child to fulfil the personal emotional needs of a parent
- inappropriate responsibilities or expectations for the child's level of maturity.

Many of these can be aggravated by a difficult or unrewarding child who creates an adverse environment for himself. It is wrong to always blame the parents for causing their child's problem without examining how much the child contributes to the situation himself.

Adversities may also arise outside the family. Experiences with other children are increasingly recognised as highly significant in psychosocial development. Bullying is a known adversity, a specific instance of peer rejection in which a child is actively persecuted by others. Merely being left out of things (as opposed to being driven away) is much less pernicious. Conversely, having a number of steady, good-quality peer relationships is a marker for good prognosis in an emotional or behaviour problem which has resulted from environmental influences.

PROBLEMS OF THE PRESCHOOL YEARS

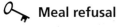 **Meal refusal**

A common scenario is a mother complaining that her child refuses to eat any or much of what she provides;

mealtimes have become a battleground. Examination reveals a healthy, well-nourished child whose height and weight are securely within normal limits on a centile growth chart, or a small and thin child with a normal growth.

An account of what goes on at a typical mealtime may reveal:

- a past history of force-feeding
- irregular meals so that the child is not predictably hungry
- unsuitable meals
- unreasonably large portions
- multiple opportunities for distraction, e.g. TV.

Most importantly, how much does the child eat between meals? A well-nourished child is getting food from somewhere. Not all parents regard sweets and crisps as having any nutritional value. Some mothers, whilst concerned about their child's apparently poor food intake, provide little variety in the child's diet. One needs to ascertain what the mother is most concerned about: nutrition or lack of discipline? The former can be dealt with by discussion of the child's growth, referring to a growth chart and commenting that he has lots of energy. If the mother remains unconvinced, ask her to complete a food diary, recording all her child's intake over a few days. Many young children prefer to eat small, frequent snacks rather than larger, infrequent meals. As long as they are offered wholesome food, children have been shown to be remarkably good at maintaining a constant energy intake when allowed a free choice. Not uncommonly, the child's refusal to eat at mealtimes is bound up with a struggle for autonomy from his parent. The parent cannot win directly, as it is impossible to force a child to eat. If the parents wish their child to have regular mealtimes, they can use other strategies as listed in Figure 21.6.

Sleep-related problems

Difficulty in settling to sleep at bedtime
This is a common problem in the toddler years. The child will not go to sleep unless his parent is present. Most instances are normal expressions of separation

---

Fig. 21.6 Strategy for meal refusal.

Mealtime history
What is the parent most concerned about?
Nutrition?
— growth chart
Discipline?
— family history
— what others say
— part of a broader problem

How much food is eaten between meals?
— food diary

Advice
Avoid confrontation at mealtimes
Develop a relaxed atmosphere
Use favourite foods as a reward
Reduce eating between meals if necessary, though
   many young children prefer small, frequent snacks

Fig. 21.7 Reasons for a child not settling at night.

Too much sleep in the late afternoon
Displaced sleep/wake cycle – not waking child in
   morning because did not settle until late on the
   previous night
Separation anxiety
Overstimulated or overwrought in evening
Kept awake by siblings or noisy neighbours or TV in
   the bedroom
Erratic parental practices: no bedtime or routine to
   cue child into sleep readiness, sudden removal
   from play to go to bed without prior warning
Use of bedroom as punishment
Dislike of darkness and silence – night light and
   playing story tapes can be helpful

---

anxiety, but there may be other obvious reasons for it which can be explored in taking a history (Fig. 21.7), supplemented if necessary by the parents keeping a prospective sleep diary. Many cases will respond to common-sense advice:

- creating a bedtime and a bedtime routine which cues the child to what is required
- telling the child to lie quietly in bed until he falls asleep, recognising that children cannot fall asleep to order (although that is what everyone tells them to do).

More refractory cases may merit a couple of nights of respite sedation (with trimeprazine) to enable parents to catch up on lost sleep themselves. Once they are feeling more on top of things, they can impose a graded pattern of lengthening periods between tucking their child up in bed and coming back after a few minutes to visit him, but leaving the room before the child falls asleep. The object is to provide the opportunity for the child to learn how to fall sleep alone, a skill he has not yet developed.

Waking at night

This is normal, but some children cry because they cannot settle themselves back to sleep without their parent's presence. This is commonly associated with difficulty settling in the evenings, which should be treated first. Some children who can settle in the evening may be unable to settle when they wake in the night because the circumstances are different – it is quieter, darker etc. The graded approach described above for evening settling can also be used in the middle of the night. Parents will find it helpful to take alternate nights on duty to share the burden. Sedative medication is less likely to be effective than with evening settling problems.

Nightmares

These are bad dreams which can be recalled by the child. They are common, rarely requiring professional attention unless they occur frequently or are stereotyped in content, indicating a morbid preoccupation. Reassuring the child will usually suffice.

Night (sleep) terrors

These are different from nightmares, occurring about $1\frac{1}{2}$ h after settling. The parents find the child sitting up in bed, eyes open, seemingly awake but obviously disorientated, confused and distressed and unresponsive to their questions and reassurances. He settles back to sleep after a few minutes and has no recollection of the episode in the morning. A night terror is a *parasomnia*, a disturbance of the structure of sleep wherein a very rapid emergence from the first period of deep slow-wave sleep produces a state of high arousal and confusion. Sleepwalking has similar origins and the two may be combined. Most night terrors need little more than reassurance directed towards the parents. If necessary, they can sometimes be stopped by keeping a record of their timing and then briefly waking the child 15 min before the terror is expected each night for about a week.

Disobedience, defiance and tantrums

Toddlers commonly and normally go through a phase of refusing to comply with parents' demands, sometimes angrily ('the terrible 2s'). This is an understandable reaction to the discovery that the world is not organised around them. They also become confused and angered by the fact that the parent who provides them with comfort when they are distressed is also the person who is making them do things they do not wish to do. This seems exceptionally unfair to them. That is one reason why children play their parents up but may be fine with others. All this can exhaust and demoralise parents, not least because many people offer advice or criticism (everyone thinks themselves

Fig. 21.8 Managing toddler disobedience.

Ensure your demand is reasonable for the
   developmental stage of the child
Tell the child what you want him to do rather than
   nagging about what you don't want him to do
Praise for compliance, especially when it is
   spontaneous (catch him doing the right thing)
Use simple incentives to reward good behaviour
Frame deals along the lines of 'If you (do this or
   that) … then we/I can do such and such' (not the
   other way round)
Avoid threats that cannot be carried out
Carry out threats that are made
Ignore defiance as much as possible

Fig. 21.9 Analysing a tantrum.

Antecedents – what happened in the minutes
   before the episode
Behaviour – exactly what the episode consisted of
Consequences – what happened as a result

Fig. 21.10 Tantrums: management strategies.

Affection and attention
Distraction
Avoiding antecedents
Ignoring:
   Effective but can be difficult
   No surrender
Time out from positive reinforcement:
   Walk away, returning when quietens down
   Separate from siblings
   Put on a 'naughty chair' for a short time
Holding
Star chart

an expert in the area of children's development and behaviour). The points listed in Figure 21.8 can be made.

Temper tantrums are ordinarily responses to frustration, especially at not being allowed to have or do something. They are common and normal in young pre-school children. If asked for advice, a sensible first move is to take a history, analysing a couple of tantrums according to the ABC paradigm (Fig. 21.9). Next, examine the child to identify potential medical or psychological factors. Medical factors include global or language delay, hearing impairment (e.g. glue ear) and medication with bronchodilators or anticonvulsants. If none are present, there are management strategies that can be adopted, some of which are shown in Figure 21.10.

The easiest course of action is to distract the child or, if this cannot be done, to let the tantrum burn itself out while the parent leaves the room, returning a few minutes later when things quieten. Obviously this should be done in a calm, neutral manner and certainly not accompanied by threats of abandonment. Tantrums which are essentially coercive (when a child is demanding something from a parent) must be met by a refusal to give in. They can often be forestalled by the simple expedient of making rules which the child can be reminded of before the situation presents itself. An alternative course is to use 'time out', which is a form of structured ignoring. The child in a tantrum is placed somewhere such as the hallway where no-one will talk to him for a short time, e.g. 1 min per year of age. During this period he is ignored completely. Parents often expect this manoeuvre to produce a contrite child, complaining if it does not do so immediately. In fact, it works according to different principles and often takes several weeks to effect a gradual improvement. It may help to ask the mother to keep records to document this.

Disobedience can be dealt with by using a star chart to reward the child for complying with parental requests. The chart needs to be where the child can see it and it must be the case that the child knows what he

has to do in order to get a star. It is probably wisest not to 'fine' the child by taking stars away once they have been earned. If the parent who is rewarding compliance by the child praises him at the same time as giving the star, there is not usually any need to tie stars in with a material reward; praise suffices.

Breath-holding attacks

Two kinds of attack can be recognised. In the commoner 'blue' variety, frustration leads to tears and holding the breath in expiration at the end of a wail of rage. This is an innocent practice which will not harm the child. It could be ignored by the parents, but would require nerves of steel. All children grow out of it before the age of 5 years.

Less common are the 'white' breath-holding attacks which are precipitated by pain or shock rather than frustration. The child slumps to the floor, pale and not breathing. A seizure may follow secondary to cerebral hypoxia (reflex anoxic seizures). Explanation and reassurance are indicated, not anticonvulsants (which do not help). Later in childhood, many of these children are prone to faints.

Aggressive behaviour

Small children can be aggressive for a host of reasons, ranging from spite to exuberance. Much aggressive behaviour is learned, either by being rewarded (often inadvertently) or by copying parents or siblings. For instance, many instances of aggressive, demanding behaviour are provoked or intensified by a parent shouting at or hitting their child. In such cases it is the

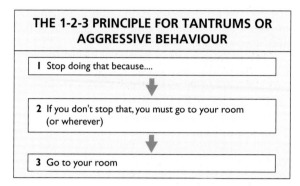

Fig. 21.11 The 1–2–3 principle for tantrums or aggressive behaviour.

parent's behaviour which needs to change. In most instances, the same principles as apply to tantrums are valid: make rules, stick to them, keep cool, don't give in and use time out if necessary. The latter can often be used on a 1–2–3 principle (Fig. 21.11). A tired or stressed child will be irritable and prone to angry outbursts, as will a child whose communication skills are compromised by deafness or a developmental language disorder so that he is frustrated and exasperated. Optimistic reassurance that the child will spontaneously grow out of a pattern of aggressive behaviour is mistaken; once established, an aggressive behavioural style is remarkably persistent over a period of years.

Autism

This developmental condition is the most severe of the pervasive developmental (autistic spectrum) disorders. It is rare, with a prevalence rate of approximately 3 per 10 000. It is commoner in boys and presents in early childhood but is a lifelong handicap. Autistic children have a triad of difficulties evident before the age of 3 years:

- *A severe language disorder*. Half will never speak at all; the others show a widespread disorder of language, with delayed and abnormal speech, poor comprehension of what is said to them, and no imaginative play. In the early years there is a tendency to echo questions, repeat instructions and to refer to themselves as 'you'.

- *A profound difficulty relating to other people*. There is extreme indifference to others and failure to meet their eye gaze in social encounters. They do not show normal attachment behaviour, do not come for comfort when hurt or distressed, do not share pleasure or draw the attention of others to things which they are interested in and do not form close relationships or make friends. They prefer their own company and share neither emotions nor play activities with others. It is as though

they do not appreciate that other people have their own thoughts and feelings.

- *Marked routines and rituals associated with a poverty of imagination*. Examples are insistence on the same foods, ways of doing things or sameness in the environment (e.g. the arrangement of furniture in the home). Some carry round odd items, such as pieces of wire, to which they become very attached. Imposing change or disrupting the child's rituals precipitates violent temper tantrums.

In addition to this triad of features, odd motor patterns such as flapping hands and walking on tiptoe are common. Autistic children seem to be in their own world, which they do not share with others. About two-thirds have a general learning disability. When describing an autistic child, it is essential to specify his level of intelligence. In addition, epileptic seizures occur in about one-quarter of autistic children, although sometimes not until adolescence.

Autism is a behavioural syndrome, most cases of which are probably genetic. Most cases have no identifiable underlying condition. It is certainly not the result of either emotional trauma or deviant parenting. Recent work suggesting a link with MMR vaccine has not been substantiated.

There is no specific treatment for autism, although new claims for curative interventions surface regularly. The parents are often keen to try these, although none have stood the test of replicated, controlled evaluation. Parents need as much support as can be provided; it is a devastating handicap to deal with. Behaviour modification is used to teach social skills and to reduce unwelcome or dangerous behaviours. An appropriate special school is probably the most important positive influence on development. In the long term, only a minority (probably less than 10%) will be able to live independently; most adults with autism will need care in special communities or to stay with their parents, attending local day centres and remaining solitary individuals with no interest in social activities or marriage.

Other developmental conditions may share some characteristics with autism. Children with severe general learning disability may have the social impairments of autism but without marked rigidity and obsessionality, so they are described as having autistic features. *Asperger's syndrome* refers to a mild form of the social impairments of autism in the presence of near-normal speech development. Such children have grave difficulties with the give-and-take of ordinary social encounters, a stilted way of speaking and narrow, strange interests which they do not share with others. Some children with developmental language disorders show a limitation of sociability and imagination. All these conditions or difficulties can be placed on a continuum which ranges from ordinary eccentricity to severe autism and may be generally referred to as autistic spectrum disorders.

Autistic children have:
- a severe language disorder
- profound difficulty relating to other people
- marked routines and rituals.

PROBLEMS OF MIDDLE CHILDHOOD

Nocturnal enuresis

Children can wet themselves by day or night, but in colloquial speech, 'enuresis' is synonymous with bed-wetting. It is quite common: about 15% of 5-year-olds and 3% of 10-year olds will wet the bed once a week or more. Boys outnumber girls by nearly 2 to 1. There is a genetically determined delay in acquiring sphincter competence, with two-thirds of children with enuresis having an affected first-degree relative. There may also be interference in learning to become dry at night. Small children need reasonable freedom from stress and a measure of parental approval in order to learn night-time continence. It is well recognised that emotional stress can interfere and cause secondary enuresis (relapse after a period of dryness). Most children with enuresis are psychologically normal and the treatment of secondary enuresis still relies mainly on the symptomatic approach described below, although any underlying stress or emotional disorder must be addressed.

Organic causes of enuresis are uncommon but include:

- urinary tract infection
- faecal retention severe enough to reduce bladder volume and cause bladder neck dysfunction
- polyuria from diabetes or chronic renal failure.

A urine sample should always be tested for glucose and protein and checked for infection.

The management of enuresis is straightforward but needs to be painstaking to succeed. After the age of 4 years, enuresis resolves spontaneously in only 5% of affected children each year. In practice, treatment is rarely undertaken before 6 years of age.

1. Explanation
The first step is to explain to both child and parent that the problem is common and beyond conscious control. The parents should stop punitive procedures, as these are counterproductive.

2. Star chart
The child earns praise and a star each morning if his bed is dry. Wet beds are treated in a matter-of-fact way and he is not blamed for them.

3. Enuresis alarm
If a child does not respond to a star chart, it may be supplemented with an enuresis alarm. This is a sensor, usually placed in the child's pants, which sounds an alarm when it becomes wet. In order to be effective, the alarm must wake the child, who gets out of bed, goes to pass urine, returns and helps to remake a wet bed before going back to sleep. It is not necessary to re-set the alarm that night. Parental help can be enlisted in the night using a baby alarm to transmit the noise of the alarm to the parents' bedroom.

The alarm method takes several weeks to achieve dryness but is effective in most cases so long as the child is motivated and has the procedure carefully explained to him. About one-third of cases relapse after a few months, in which case retreatment with the alarm usually produces lasting dryness.

4. Desmopressin
Short-term relief from bedwetting, e.g. for holidays or sleepovers, can be achieved by the use of the synthetic analogue of antidiuretic hormone, desmopressin, taken as tablets or a nasal spray. This achieves a suppressant effect rather than a lasting cure. The same is true of imipramine, which is best avoided as it also carries the risk to the child and his siblings of accidental overdose, which can be life-threatening.

Most children with enuresis are psychologically and physically normal

Faecal soiling

It is abnormal for a child to soil himself after the age of 4 years. Thereafter, soilers fall into two broad groups – those with and those without a rectum loaded with faeces. Because of this, it is important to ascertain whether there is faecal retention by abdominal palpation and by digital anorectal examination if necessary. Faeces in the rectum are always an abnormal finding. The reasons why a child's rectum should become loaded are various and commonly involve an interplay between constitutional factors and experience. Some children have a rectum that only empties occasionally, perhaps because of poor coordination with anal sphincter relaxation, and are thus more prone to developing retention. Superimposed upon this are a number of other factors:

- constipation, possibly following dehydration during an illness
- inhibition of defaecation because of pain from a fissure
- inhibition because of fear of punishment for incontinence
- anxieties about using the lavatory.

Once established, a huge bolus of hard faeces may be beyond the capacity of the child to shift. Furthermore, a rectum loaded with hard or soft faeces (both are found) dilates and habituates to distension so that the child becomes unaware of the need to empty it. The loaded rectum inhibits the anus via the rectoanal reflex and stool may seep out with sponta-neous rectal contractions beyond the child's control. Soiling occurs in the child's pants, which may then be removed and hidden out of shame.

Any reasons for faecal retention, such as an anal fissure, should be identified and treated, but the most important thing is to empty the rectum as soon as possible. The child and parents need to understand that retention is present and how it leads to incontinence.

A stool softener (docusate or lactulose) and laxative (sodium picosulphate or senna) will work in most cases, but some children will require the addition of a micro-enema if there has been no emptying within a few days. Stronger stimulant laxatives such as sodium picosulphate may be more acceptable than enemas. Once the child has an empty rectum, he can be encouraged to defaecate regularly in the lavatory, which earns stars on a star chart. Such retraining may take a number of weeks while the distended rectum shrinks to normal size. Throughout this period a regular laxative is usually needed. The stars may therefore need to be cashed in for tangible rewards such as extra pocket money in order to maintain the incentive.

In some cases, repeated soiling will have been such a humiliating experience for the child that he psychologically denies there is a problem and his cooperation is doubtful. Others find that their involuntary soiling allows them a measure of revenge against hostile parents and are reluctant to surrender a useful weapon. Such cases will need psychiatric referral.

Soiling may occur in conjunction with an empty rectum on examination for various other uncommon reasons. Some children have an urgency of defaecation for apparently constitutional reasons and can only postpone defaecation for a few minutes; they can be taken by surprise. Some children have neuropathic bowel secondary to occult spinal abnormality usually associated with urinary incontinence. Similarly, diarrhoea can overwhelm bowel control. The child may have a general learning disability with a mental age below 4 years, so that expectations of social bowel control need to be revised accordingly. Lastly, the child may defaecate intentionally as a hostile act. Such children are entrenched in distorted relationships with their parents and require psychiatric referral.

> **Most children who soil have faecal retention.**

⚡ Recurrent abdominal pain

Recurrent central abdominal pain, often sharp and colicky, affects about 10% of school-age children. The causes are considered in Chapter 12. In the vast majority of cases, no organic cause can be objectively demonstrated, yet the child is obviously in pain. Some will have an emotional cause for their pain, but in many, no aetiology, physical or psychological, can be demonstrated.

The history must attend to possible sources of stress and the child should be interviewed about school, friends and family, noting his general level of anxiety and ability to communicate. This should be an integral part of the interview and not done as an afterthought when organic causes have been excluded. A thorough physical examination is important to reassure the child and family that there is no underlying organic cause. It also provides an opportunity to gain further information about the nature of the pain and the child's reaction to it. When examining the child, it is sensible to ask him to point to where the pain is. In general, the further the pain is from the umbilicus, the more likely is organic pathology (Apley's rule).

A short interview with the child on his own can reveal sources of stress which are otherwise unrecognised by parents or which the child is wary of mentioning in front of them. Problems at school, particularly bullying and teasing, or difficulties with a teacher or classwork may only be known by the child. A report from the school may be helpful. A joint interview with both parents and the child is a good arena for explaining to the child and family how organic disease has been ruled out and, if appropriate, how tension can give rise to pain using familiar examples such as headache. It is often necessary to promote communication between family members to avoid any tendency for somatic symptoms to replace verbal communication. Learning pain coping skills such as relaxation may be helpful. Referral to child psychiatry or psychology is indicated if any identified stressors cannot be relieved by straightforward means, if there is serious family dysfunction, or if the pain impairs the child's general functioning at home or school.

Tics

A tic is a quick, sudden, coordinated movement which is apparently purposeful, recurs in the same part of the child's body and can often be reproduced by the child on request. It is not entirely involuntary in that it can be voluntarily suppressed to some extent. About 1 in 10 children develop a tic at some stage, typically around the face and head – blinking, frowning, head-flicking, sniffing, throat clearing and grunting being the commonest. They are most likely to occur when the child is inactive (watching TV or on long car journeys) and often disappear when he is actively concentrating. They may worsen with anxiety but they are not themselves an emotional reaction. In most cases, there is a family history. These simple, *transient childhood tics* clear up over the next few months, though may recur from time to time. They should be treated with reassurance in the first place.

Less commonly, the child has tics from which he is hardly ever free. They may be multiple, though there is fluctuation in the predominance of any particular tic and in overall severity. This is a chronic tic disorder which, if it includes both multiple motor tics and vocal tics such as hooting, yelping or swearing, is known as *Gilles de la Tourette's syndrome*. These conditions tend to be persistent in the medium term requiring medication (such as clonidine, haloperidol or sulpiride) and specialist supervision.

Hyperactivity

Young children are characteristically lively, some more than others, by virtue of their temperament. When their level of motor activity exceeds that regarded as normal, they may be termed 'hyperactive' by their parents. This is a judgement which depends upon the parents' standards and expectation. The term can thus incorrectly be used as a complaint about a child who is normally active in overall terms but who can be cheeky and boisterous at times. Such a child is *not* hyperactive, but the parents need advice about how to handle unwanted behaviour.

In the true *hyperkinetic disorder*, the child is undoubtedly overactive in most situations and has impaired concentration with a short attention span or distractibility. Because of the latter, the term *attention deficit hyperactivity disorder* (ADHD) has become widely used. Differences in diagnostic criteria mean that prevalence rates among prepubertal schoolchildren are variously estimated as between 10 and 50 per 1000 children, boys exceeding girls fourfold. There is a powerful genetic predisposition and the underlying problem is a dysfunction of brain neurone circuits that rely on dopamine as a neurotransmitter and which control self-monitoring and self-regulation.

Affected children have disorganised, poorly regulated and excessive activity which has been evident since early childhood. They are typically reckless and impulsive, socially disinhibited and butt into other people's conversations and play. They appear inattentive, concentrate poorly on imposed tasks, do not finish these, avoid cognitively demanding activities (though may watch TV or pursue computer games for half an hour or so), lose possessions and are generally disorganised. Typically they have short tempers and poor relationships with other children, who find them exasperating. Not uncommonly they also have developmental disorders such as dyspraxia, dyslexia and language disorders, but there is no specific association with brain damage. They do poorly in school and lose self-esteem. They usually drift into antisocial activities for a variety of reasons, not least because their behaviour drives parents, teachers and peers to use coercive management techniques which are ineffectual or breed resentment.

First-line management, particularly in pre-school children, is the active promotion of behavioural and educational progress by specific advice to parents and teachers to build concentration skills, encourage quiet self-occupation, increase self-esteem and moderate extreme behaviour. For those children in which this is insufficient, hyperactivity responds symptomatically to several types of medication, although this is usually reserved for children older than about 6 years of age. So-called stimulants such as methylphenidate or dexamphetamine channel attention and promote on-task, focused behaviour. The usual approach is not to put the child on medication until behavioural and educational progress is actively promoted by the specific measures mentioned above. It may then be necessary to continue medication for several years, discontinuing it every year or so to test whether it is still helpful. Treatment is rarely required beyond their mid-teens. Specialist supervision is mandatory.

The role of diet in the cause and management of hyperactivity is controversial. Current evidence indicates that the sort of diet which aims blindly to reduce sugar, artificial additives or colorants has no effect. A few children display an idiosyncratic behavioural reaction such as excitability or irritability to particular foods. If this seems likely, putting the child on an exclusion diet with only a few constituents may confirm this. Individual foods can be re-introduced while examining for a worsening of behaviour, so that incriminated foods can subsequently be excluded from the child's diet. This is an arduous activity, best implemented by a specialist clinic with supervision from a dietician.

Antisocial behaviour

Children steal, lie, disobey, light fires, destroy things and pick fights for various reasons:

- failure to learn when to exercise social restraint
- lack of social skills, such as the ability to negotiate a disagreement
- they may be responding to the challenges of their peers in spite of their parents' prohibitions
- they may be chronically angry and resentful
- they may find their own notions of good behaviour overwhelmed by emotion or temptation.

When serious antisocial behaviour which infringes the rights of others is the dominant feature of the clinical picture and is so severe as to represent a handicap to general functioning, a diagnosis of *conduct disorder* is made. Children with conduct disorder have not necessarily broken the law, although their behaviour excites strong social disapproval. They typically come from homes in which there is considerable discord between family members, especially between the child and his parents. A milder form, characterised by angry, defiant behaviour to authority figures such as parents and teachers, is known as *oppositional-defiant disorder (ODD)*.

Treating conduct disorder and ODD is extremely difficult, not least because parental cooperation is often minimal. It involves a combination of training techniques for parents, family therapy and behaviour therapy and is a task for a mental health professional. Medication has little part to play.

Anxiety

Pathological anxiety exists in two forms: specific and general. In phobias there is fear of a specific object or situation which is excessive and handicapping and cannot be dealt with by reassurance. Most children have a number of irrational fears (the dark, ghosts, kidnappers, dogs, spiders, bats, snakes) which are common and do not usually handicap the child's ordinary life. Some of these persist into adulthood. If they are so severe that the child's ability to lead an ordinary life is affected, then treatment by behavioural therapy may be indicated and is usually successful.

More diffuse general anxiety presents indirectly in childhood and it is rare for a child to complain directly about anxiety. Often, it is first manifest as physical complaints: nausea, headache or pain. It may take the form of hypochondriasis and the child repeatedly asks for reassurance that he is not going to die. Some children with generalised anxiety are strikingly manipulative, attempting to gain control over their parents and the world in general so that they can feel less fearful. It may be a justifiable reaction to an event or situation, or be disproportionate. If the condition follows a recognisable precipitant such as a parental illness and the parents can be directed to provide comfort and support, prognosis is good. If it arises insidiously, specialist mental health referral is indicated.

 Children rarely say they are anxious – instead they complain of aches and pains or behave manipulatively.

School refusal

During the years of compulsory school attendance, a child may be absent from school because of illness, because his parents keep him off school or because of truancy in which the child chooses to do something else rather than attend school. A few non-attenders at school suffer from *school refusal*, an inability to attend school on account of overwhelming anxiety. Such children may not complain of anxiety but of its physical concomitants or the consequences of hyperventilation. Anxiety may present as complaints of nausea, headache or otherwise not being well confined to weekday, term-time mornings, clearing up by midday. It may be rational, as when the child is being bullied. If it is disproportionate to stresses at school, it is termed school refusal, an anxiety problem with two common causes – separation anxiety persisting beyond the toddler years and anxiety provoked by some aspect of school, true school phobia. These can coexist.

School refusal based on separation anxiety is typical of children under the age of about 11 years. It may be provoked by an adverse life event such as a death in the family or a move of house. The child is unable to tolerate separation from his attachment figure without whom he cannot go anywhere, including school. Treatment is aimed at gently promoting increasing separations from the parents (e.g. staying overnight with relatives or friends) whilst arranging an early return to school.

True school phobia is seen in slightly older anxious children who are frequently uncommunicative and stubborn. Some adolescents with school refusal have a depressive disorder, but more usually there is an interaction between an anxiety disorder and long-standing personality issues such as intolerance of uncertainty. The cornerstone of treatment is an early, graded return to school at a pace the child can stand while support is provided for their parents. Any underlying emotional disorder is treated simultaneously. Close liaison with the education service (teachers, educational welfare officers, educational psychologists) is crucial.

Educational underachievement

Children who achieve less well in school than expected are sometimes brought to doctors. It is important to evaluate parents' and teachers' expectations and ensure the child is actually able to rise to them. The services of an educational psychologist are indispensable. Core medical responsibilities include testing sight and hearing and attempting to elicit the cause of underachievement according to the list in Figure 21.12.

A particular issue arises with respect to dyslexia, a difficulty in learning to read in spite of adequate intelligence and teaching. Dyslexia is a statement of a

---

Fig. 21.12 Causes of underachievement at school.

Long-standing problem
Visual problems
Hearing problems
Dyslexia
Other specific learning problems (rare)
Hyperactivity
Anti-education family background
Chaotic family background

Recent onset of problem
Preoccupations (parental divorce, bullying, etc.)
Fatigue
Depression
Rebellion against teacher, parents or 'swot' label
Unsuspected poor attendance at school
Sexual abuse
Drug abuse
Schizophrenia (rare)
Degenerative brain condition, rare but important

problem, not a complete diagnosis; otherwise competent children may find the complex task of learning to read difficult for a number of reasons, such as a developmental language disorder or visual perceptual problems. Cerebral imaging studies have shown some to have various abnormalities of brain structure but this is not a consistent finding. A number of children with dyslexia have other developmental problems such as motor dyspraxia or hyperactivity. A very small number have poorly established eye dominance, cannot follow lines of print on the page, and seem to benefit from manoeuvres such as occluding one eye for several months or wearing special coloured spectacles. The whole subject of dyslexia is controversial and there is no agreed classification. There is no medical treatment, affected children need special reading tuition from a skilled teacher. The child easily becomes demoralised and prone to develop bad classroom behaviour. Ultimately, many learn to read adequately but spelling difficulties usually supervene and persist.

ADOLESCENCE

Although a popular image of adolescence is one of angry, rebellious teenagers, alienated from their parents and embroiled in emotional turmoil, studies show that most adolescents maintain good relationships with their parents. They do, though, tend to bicker with them about minor domestic matters and what they are allowed to do. Minor psychological symptoms such as moodiness or social sensitivity are quite common (as they are in adults), but serious psychiatric problems are no more prevalent than in adult life. Family relationships are often influenced by the teenager's negotiation of their own autonomy, the emergence of their own sense of themselves and the first moves towards a personal identity. At the same time their parents may be experiencing mid-life crises of confidence in career, physical appearance or sexuality, so that parental and teenage preoccupations coincide, not always helpfully.

Cognitive style

The style of thought specifically associated with adolescence is formal operational thought (Fig. 21.13), but this is acquired at various ages by different individuals during the teenage years, and a substantial minority seem never to develop it at all. Doctors are at a disadvantage here as they have been selected by a series of examinations for excellence of their ability to manipulate abstractions and compare hypothetical predictions; they have often forgotten what it is like to think otherwise and communicate poorly with patients who still think concretely and practically (school-age children, about half of all teenagers and perhaps 1 in 5 adults). When interviewing adolescents, the skill is to avoid being patronising while being sensitive as to whether abstract and reflective thought is solidly achieved. Using practical examples (not metaphors) and checking whether you have been understood will help to avoid the common problem of being faced with an adolescent who responds to questions with a sullen 'don't know'.

Anorexia nervosa

Dieting to slim is endemic among teenage girls. Part of the reason for this is the contemporary equation between thinness and attractiveness, an assumption prevalent in advertising and fashion. Resonant with this is the finding that most teenage girls (but very few boys) overestimate their body width and depth, perceiving and judging themselves as fatter than they actually are.

Slimming through self-imposed calorie restriction is usually self-limiting because the goal is achieved or because the girl gives up; hunger wins through. In some girls, however, the slimming process takes over and there supervenes what has been called a 'relentless pursuit of thinness', typically with a phobic horror of normal body weight and shape. This is *anorexia nervosa*, and the features are:

- A distorted perception of her body which increases with weight loss.
- When body weight falls below a critical point (about 48 kg) pubertal development is halted and reversed so that menstruation ceases and the girl effectively becomes a prepubertal child. This may spare her some of the challenges of adolescence, particularly those related to sexuality.
- The discovery by a girl who has felt powerless that through self-starvation she can control her shape and development and thus increase her sense of self-worth and self-effectiveness.
- Preoccupations and dreams of food and cooking which come to dominate mental life as a response to starvation. There ensues a tremendous mental struggle not to give in and eat, which assumes prime importance in the girl's mental life. It becomes a way of pursuing a purposeful but simple life by condensing or displacing other more complex concerns so that thinness becomes the absolute standard and other issues are secondary.
- The dramatic and visible effects of self-starvation on the girl which can unite some parents in caring for their daughter and save a discordant marriage from divorce, something which she may fear is imminent.

Fig. 21.13 Formal operational thought.

The ability to form abstract thoughts
Comparing implications of hypotheses
Thinking about one's own thinking
Testing the logic that links propositions
Manipulating interactive abstract concepts

An affected girl will often deny hunger, reassure everyone that she is in the peak of health, exercise to lose weight and disagree fervently that she is too thin. She will be careless of her own emaciation and seem unconcerned that she is starving herself to death. To the bewilderment of her parents, she may cook for others and read cookery books avidly. She may well be deceitful to anyone she perceives as thwarting her in her quest. Thus she will conceal her poor eating by secretly disposing of her meals or lying about her weight. Both before and during her illness she will show obsessional, perfectionistic character traits; without these she would not have the capacity to establish herself as a persistent dieter. Indeed, she is likely to be described as having been quiet, compliant and hardworking, 'the last person to develop anorexia nervosa'. Her parents will often present as nice people who avoid conflict.

As a result of starvation, her body develops a low metabolic rate with slow-to-relax tendon reflexes, reduced peripheral circulation, bradycardia and amenorrhoea. Fine lanugo hair appears over her trunk and limbs. She does not lose pubic or axillary hair, although incompletely established puberty is delayed. Serum T3 may be low, giving rise to a false suspicion of hypothyroidism. Plasma proteins are sometimes low and ankle oedema not uncommon. Blood and urine levels of luteinising hormone and follicle-stimulating hormone are low and non-cyclical.

Some girls discover that self-restraint in carbohydrate intake can be bypassed by self-induced vomiting and that weight can be lost through diuretics. Some take laxatives in the belief that these will remove the food they have eaten. This can cause wide fluctuations in weight and metabolic abnormalities such as hypokalaemia and alkalosis. This is *bulimia*, which can occur at normal body weight or in association with low body weight as an ominous complication of anorexia nervosa. It tends to affect older rather than younger teenagers. Bulimia at normal body weight can be managed by encouraging a regular diet, monitoring this by a diary and providing individual or group psychotherapy.

The prevalence rate among teenagers for anorexia nervosa is a little less than 1%, but the incidence rate has been an increasing over the last 50 years. The peak age of onset is 14 and girls outnumber boys by about 20:1. Bulimia is commoner, although prevalence rates vary widely depending on the degree of severity. It also shows a markedly female preponderance and may also be becoming more frequent.

Management

The initial management of anorexia nervosa is to restore near-normal body weight by refeeding. If possible, this should first be done as an outpatient and will need a series of meetings with the girl and her parents in which the seriousness of the situation is explained. The girl's weight, not her eating, is monitored and a gain of about 500 g a week is required. Failure to meet this target results in admission to hospital for refeeding with no appeal or bargaining accepted. Good nursing is the key to this, but a small number of girls continue to lose weight in hospital so that tube-feeding may be required. An initial daily dietary intake of about 2000 calories is adopted, as trying to enforce large meals is usually unsuccessful. A more psychotherapeutic approach may be introduced when her weight has reached the level it was before dieting started. It is aimed at counselling the girl and her family in more constructive ways of confronting developmental demands, including handling conflict, maintaining self-esteem, personal autonomy and relationships.

The prognosis is reasonably good, but about a quarter of the most intransigent who have needed treatment in specialist units develop a chronic relapsing course. Rather less than 5% die by suicide, malnutrition or infection, though usually not until later in life. Most recover their weight permanently, although they often remain wary of eating and minor psychosexual problems affect about one-third of them.

 Girls with anorexia nervosa seldom agree that they are too thin and may deceive everyone by pretending to eat.

Chronic fatigue syndrome

Chronic fatigue syndrome (CFS) refers to persisting high levels of subjective fatigue leading to rapid exhaustion on physical or mental exertion. The term is broader and more neutral than the specific pathology or aetiology implied by myalgic encephalomyelitis (ME) or postviral fatigue syndrome, which follows an apparently viral febrile illness. There is sometimes serological evidence of recent infection with Coxsackie B or Ebstein–Barr (EBV) or a hepatitis virus. Some cases have no history or evidence of a precipitating infection and there are no specific diagnostic tests. The clinical picture is somewhat diffuse and there are no pathognomonic symptoms. Myalgia, migratory arthralgia, headache, difficulty getting off to sleep, poor concentration and irritability are virtually universal. Stomach pains, scalp tenderness, eye pain and photophobia, and tender cervical lymphadenopathy are frequently encountered. Depressive symptoms are common and there is continuing debate as to how much of the clinical picture is physical and how much psychological. Usually parents insist on there being a physical cause and there is a risk that the doctor will be pressurised into excessive unprofitable investigations. Most experienced doctors now regard the final clinical picture as resulting from both physical and psychological factors.

The majority of cases will remit spontaneously with time, but this takes months or sometimes years. Earlier recommendations of continuous rest have been shown to be unhelpful and can lead to secondary complications. The preferred approach is to adopt a gentle rehabilitative approach, possible involving physiotherapy, so that exercise tolerance is gradually increased. If too much pressure is put upon the child, tantrums or mute withdrawal can occur. Argument about how much of the condition is physical and how much psychological is unhelpful. The parents and the child need continuing support to maintain as much of a normal life as possible, including school attendance. The mood of children with depressive symptoms may respond to antidepressant medication, but this is a treatment only for depressive symptoms and it is unlikely to result in alleviation of the fatiguability.

Depression

Low mood can arise secondary to adverse circumstances or sometimes spontaneously. Depression as a clinical condition is more than sadness and misery; it extends to affect motivation, judgement, the ability to experience pleasure and provokes emotions of guilt and despair. It may disturb sleep, appetite and weight. It leads to social withdrawal, an important sign. Such a state is well recognised among adolescents, particularly girls, but occasionally affects prepubertal children. The general picture is comparable to depression in adults but there are differences (Fig. 21.14).

A diagnosis of depression depends crucially upon interviewing the adolescent on her own as well as taking a history from the parents. Teenagers will, out of loyalty, often pretend to their parents that things are all right if interviewed in their presence. It is necessary to ask about feelings directly and ask specifically about suicidal ideas and plans.

Treatment depends upon the relationship between low mood and causal circumstances. Adversity such as bullying should be reversed if possible. If this cannot be done, as in the case of impending parental divorce, then counselling support is required. If it seems as though environmental factors are an insufficient explanation, then a selective serotonin reuptake inhibitor antidepressant is indicated. Suicidal teenagers need admission to a psychiatric in-patient unit.

Deliberate self-harm

Like adults, teenagers who take overdoses do so for a variety of motives, of which suicide is only one. For a high proportion, the overdose is a way of expressing revenge, or a blind and desperate gesture which may draw attention to a predicament perceived by them as irresolvable. Issues such as bullying or abuse should be considered. Most teenagers who overdose are not clinically depressed. Episodes of deliberate self-harm must be taken seriously as they carry significant risk of recurrence.

> **Most adolescents who take an overdose are not clinically depressed.**

Drug misuse

Most teenagers are exposed to illicit drugs at some stage. A number will then experiment with them, some becoming habitual users. Usually this is for recreational purposes, but a few use them to avoid unpleasant feelings or memories. A very small number become dependent, psychologically or physically. What is taken varies with culture and opportunity but alcohol and cannabis are common; solvents, LSD, ecstasy and amphetamine derivatives a little less so; and cocaine or heroin currently least prevalent. The addictive potential of the last two is the greatest and their dangers are well known.

Abuse implies heavy misuse. The signs vary with the agent but include:

- intoxication
- unexplained absences from home or school
- mixing with known users
- high rates of spending or stealing money
- possession of the equipment required for ingestion
- medical complications associated with use.

Doctors may be asked by worried parents whether an adolescent is abusing and the question can often only be resolved by interviewing the adolescent, possibly combined with taking a urine sample for drug screening. Medical interest is predominantly focused on solitary users, who usually have other psychopathology including depression, or with the physical consequences of intoxication or injection when these threaten health. Solvent abuse (mainly glue and aerosol sniffing) is quite widespread as a group activity in some areas and is usually of no more consequence

---

Fig. 21.14 Features of depression in adolescents.

More common than adults
Apathy, boredom and an inability to enjoy oneself rather than depressed mood
Separation anxiety which reappears, having resolved in earlier life
Decline in school performance
Social withdrawal
Hypochondriacal ideas and complaints of pain in chest, abdomen and head
Irritable mood or frankly antisocial behaviour

Less common than adults
Loss of appetite and weight
Loss of sleep
Loss of libido
Slowing of thought and movement
Delusional ideas

than under-age drinking. It can occasionally give rise to cardiac dysrhythmias, bone marrow suppression or renal failure, and any of these can cause death, as may a fall when intoxicated. Cannabis and LSD use is usually not dangerous, but in occasional adolescents they trigger anxiety or psychotic disorders. Ecstasy taken at dances or raves can cause dangerous hyperthermia and dehydration.

Doctors need to ensure that any adolescent known to them who is thought to be using drugs knows the specific risks to health. Dependence is rare among teenagers and most likely to involve alcohol. The few who are using illicit drugs for respite from psychological distress need referral to a psychiatrist.

MANAGEMENT OF EMOTIONAL AND BEHAVIOURAL PROBLEMS

For most emotional and behavioural problems, there is an interplay among adversities in the family, peer group and school, and strengths or vulnerabilities in the child. Sometimes these are referred to as risk (predisposing) factors: things that do not in themselves produce a disorder but will do so when interacting with other adversities. Conversely, they are less likely to do so if there is a compensating strength (such as high intelligence, good self-esteem, secure attachment, good peer relations or an emotionally warm relationship with a parent). An environmental adversity may be acute (a life event) or chronic. It challenges the coping skills of the child, and a resulting emotional or behavioural problem results if these are overwhelmed. The problem may resolve spontaneously or persist.

With this in mind, it is possible to talk about the three Ps of causation:

- predisposition (vulnerability)
- precipitation
- perpetuation.

In clinical practice, a precipitant is what many people call the 'cause', but it is often the factors that perpetuate or maintain the problem that one has to deal with.

Assessment

It is best to interview both parents if possible. While doing so, consider the quality of their marriage and the parents' mental state. Ask open questions where possible and feel able to ask directly about feelings. Assess the attitudes of the parents to the child. Obtain examples of the problem and estimate its frequency, severity, duration and the impact it has on both the child and family.

Interview the child alone if it seems appropriate. Explain to the parents that you always like to have a few words with children on their own as you are their doctor too. Assess the extent of the child's suffering (he may be somewhat brazen and minimise this). Keep your questions very simple and specific, making sure the child understands what it is you want to know. This also applies to teenagers. Consider whether reports from school or other involved agencies might help. In many instances, it is worth asking the parents to keep a prospective record of the problem by means of a diary or chart which you can inspect in a few days time. Tell them what headings you want this under (such as 'antecedents, behaviour and consequences' for temper tantrums).

Management

Figure 21.15 shows an approach to managing a child displaying an emotional or behavioural problem. The process of making a referral to a psychiatric or psychological service is most likely to succeed if the referrer has already taken some of the history and engaged the parents and child in an attempt to alleviate the problem. Many doctors, general practitioners and paediatricians, in particular, are good generalists in child mental health issues and the psychiatrist or psychologist should be seen as a specialist extension of their expertise, rather than a completely different sort of person.

In general, the management of children's emotional and behavioural problems:

- is psychological rather than pharmacological
- does not need the child to be admitted to hospital

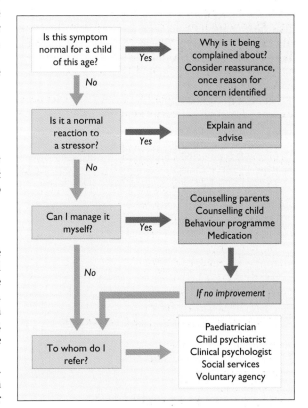

Fig. 21.15 An approach to children's psychological problems.

Fig. 21.16 Main psychological treatment interventions employed for emotional and behaviour problems.

Explanation and reassurance
Suitable for mild problems with a good prognosis arising in children from supportive families who can work out for themselves a sensible way of managing the problem until it subsides.

Counselling of child or parents
Used to modify attitudes and habits of thought. A child with a difficult temperament would be an indication for parental counselling; an adolescent who is anxiously hypochondriacal could be counselled himself.

Individual or group dynamic psychotherapy
More structured and intense extension of counselling which can help children who, for example, have emotional conflicts which are manifest as relationship difficulties with a parent. It requires a number of sessions, usually one a week, carried out in privacy. Once the mainstay of child psychiatry, it is now more sparingly used, especially with children with a distorted inner mental world.

Behaviour therapy
Uses a pragmatic approach to problems which alters the environmental factors which trigger or maintain behaviours. It is particularly effective in the management of behaviour problems in young children.

Family therapy
Has become widely used by child mental health professionals. It uses a series of interviews with the entire household to alter dysfunctional patterns of relationships between family members on the basis that many children's problems are perpetuated by the ways in which family members live with and deal with each other.

Cognitive therapy
Used by a few specialists to alter the way teenagers judge themselves in relation to a situation.

- involves parents as key participants
- may involve a variety of health and social service professionals.

Often more than one intervention is required so that treatments are combined and several professionals become involved. The main treatment interventions employed are described in Figure 21.16.

Medication plays a comparatively small role, although particular instances for which there is good evidence for efficacy are the use of stimulant drugs in hyperkinetic disorder (ADHD) and antidepressants for depressed adolescents. There is sometimes a temptation to sedate a child who is causing a problem but this is rarely effective and ethically questionable.

FURTHER READING

Hall D, Hill P, Elliman D 1999 The child surveillance handbook, 2nd edn. Radcliffe Medical Press, Oxford. *Book on young children from a general practice viewpoint*
Goodman R, Scott S 1997 Child psychiatry. Blackwell Scientific, Oxford. *Paperback textbook, mainly for trainees in psychiatry*
Spender Q, Salt N, Dawkins J, Kendrick T, Hill P 2001 Child mental health in primary care. Radcliffe Medical Press, Oxford. *Considers broad age range of mental health problems in children from a primary care viewpoint.*

22

Skin

THE NEWBORN

The skin at birth is covered with vernix caseosa. This whitish greasy coat is produced by epithelial cell breakdown and, *in utero*, protects the skin from the amniotic fluid. In the preterm infant, the skin is thin, poorly keratinised and lacks subcutaneous fat. Transepidermal water loss is markedly increased when compared with a term infant. The preterm infant is also unable to sweat until a few weeks old, whereas the term infant can sweat from birth.

Common birthmarks and rashes in the newborn period are described under the examination of the newborn infant (see Ch. 8). Some less common skin conditions presenting in the newborn period are described in this chapter.

Collodion baby

This is a rare manifestation of the inherited ichthyoses, a group of conditions in which the skin is dry and scaly. Infants are born with a taut parchment-like or collodion-like membrane (Fig. 22.1). The membrane becomes fissured and separates within a few weeks, leaving either normal or ichthyotic skin.

Epidermolysis bullosa

This is a rare group of conditions with over 20 sub-types, characterised by blistering of the skin and mucous membranes. Autosomal dominant variants tend to be milder; autosomal recessive variants may be severe and even fatal. Blisters occur spontaneously or following minor trauma (Fig. 22.2). They need to be differentiated from scalds. Management is directed to avoiding injury from even minor skin trauma and treating secondary infection. In the severe forms, the fingers and toes may become fused, and contractures of the limbs develop from repeated blistering and healing. Mucous membrane involvement may result in oral ulceration and stenosis from oesophageal erosions. Management, including maintenance of adequate nutrition, should be by a multidisciplinary team including a paediatric dermatologist, paediatrician, plastic surgeon and dietician.

Bullous impetigo

This is a blistering form of impetigo, seen particularly in the newborn (Fig. 22.3). It is most often caused by phage group II strains of *Staphylococcus aureus*.

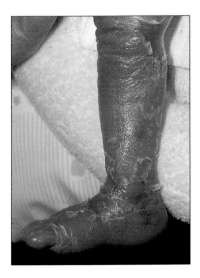

Fig. 22.1 Collodion membrane peeling in a newborn infant.

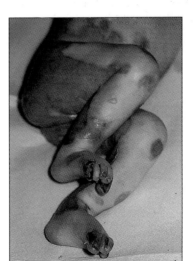

Fig. 22.2 Severe, autosomal recessive form of epidermolysis bullosa.

Treatment is with systemic antibiotics, e.g. penicillinase-resistant penicillin (see also Ch. 13).

Melanocytic naevi (moles)

Congenital moles occur in up to 3% of neonates and any that are present are usually small. Melanocytic naevi become increasingly common as children get older and the presence of large numbers in an adult may be indicative of childhood sun exposure. Prolonged exposure to sunlight should be avoided and sunscreen preparations should be applied liberally to exposed skin in bright weather and re-applied every few hours.

Congenital pigmented naevi involving extensive areas of skin (i.e. naevi more than 20 cm in diameter) are rare but disfiguring (Fig. 22.4) and carry a 4–6% lifetime risk of subsequent malignant melanoma. They require prompt referral to a paediatric dermatologist and plastic surgeon to assess the feasibility of removal. Malignant melanoma is rare before puberty except in such giant naevi. However, in adults, the incidence of malignant melanoma has increased dramatically over the past 25 years. Risk factors for melanoma include a positive family history, having a large number of melanocytic naevi, fair skin, repeated episodes of sunburn, and living in a hot climate with chronic skin exposure to the sun.

Parents should prevent their children becoming sunburnt.

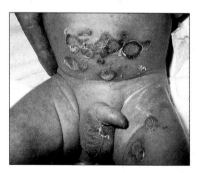
Fig. 22.3 Bullous impetigo in a newborn infant.

RASHES OF INFANCY

Napkin rashes

Napkin rashes are common, although they are much less of a problem with the widespread use of disposable nappies, as they are more absorbent. Some causes are listed in Figure 22.5. Irritant dermatitis, the most common napkin rash, may occur if nappies are not changed frequently enough or if the infant has diarrhoea. However, irritant dermatitis can occur even when the napkin area is cleaned regularly. The rash is due to the irritant effect of urine on the skin of susceptible infants. Urea-splitting organisms in faeces increase the alkalinity and likelihood of a rash.

The irritant eruption affects the convex surfaces of the buttocks, perineal region, lower abdomen and top of thighs. Characteristically, the flexures are spared, which differentiates it from other causes of napkin rash. The rash is erythematous and may have a scalded appearance. More severe forms are associated with erosions and ulcer formation. Mild cases respond to the use of a protective emollient, whereas more severe cases may require mild topical corticosteroids. While leaving the child without a napkin will accelerate resolution, it is rarely practical at home.

Candida infection may cause and often complicates napkin rashes. The rash is erythematous, includes the skin flexures and there may be satellite lesions (Fig. 22.6). Treatment is with a topical antifungal agent.

Fig. 22.5 Causes of napkin rashes.

Common	Rare
Irritant (contact) dermatitis	Acrodermatitis enteropathica (see p. 182)
Seborrhoeic dermatitis	Langerhans cell histiocytosis (Letterer–Siwe disease) (see p. 296)
Candida infection	Wiskott–Aldrich syndrome (see p. 207)
Atopic eczema	

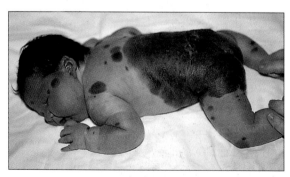
Fig. 22.4 A large (giant) congenital pigmented hairy naevus. Many other smaller naevi are also visible.

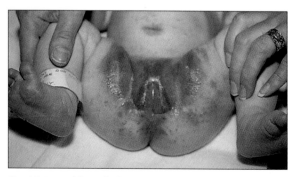
Fig. 22.6 Napkin rash due to *Candida* infection. The skin flexures are involved and there may be satellite pustules.

Infantile seborrhoeic dermatitis

This eruption of unknown cause presents in the first 2 months of life. It starts on the scalp as an erythematous scaly eruption. The scales form a thick yellow adherent layer, commonly called cradle-cap (Fig. 22.7a). The scaly rash may spread to the face, behind the ears and then extend to the flexures and napkin area (Fig. 22.7b). In contrast to atopic eczema, it is not itchy and the child is unperturbed by it. However, it is associated with an increased risk of subsequently developing atopic eczema. Mild cases will resolve with emollients. The scales on the scalp can be cleared with an ointment containing sulphur and salicylic acid

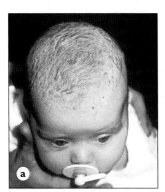

applied to the scalp daily for a few hours and then washed off. Widespread body eruption will clear with a mild topical corticosteroid, either alone or mixed with an antibacterial and antifungal agent if appropriate.

Atopic eczema

The prevalence of atopic eczema in children is 12–26%. Its onset is usually in the first year of life. It is, however, uncommon in the first 2 months, unlike infantile seborrhoeic dermatitis, which is relatively common at this age. There is often a family history of atopic disorders – eczema, asthma, allergic rhinitis (e.g. hay fever). Up to 50% of children with atopic eczema will develop asthma or hay fever. Exclusive breast-feeding may delay the onset of eczema in predisposed children but does not alter the natural history of the disorder. Atopic eczema is mainly a disease of childhood, being most severe and troublesome in the first year of life and resolving in 50% by 12 years of age, and in 75% by 16 years.

Diagnosis

The diagnosis is made clinically. If tested, most affected children have an elevated total plasma IgE level. If there is a history to suggest a particular allergic cause, skin prick and radioallergosorbent (RAST) tests may be helpful in the older child. If the disease is unusually severe, atypical or associated with unusual infections or failure to thrive, an immune deficiency disorder should be excluded.

Clinical features

Rashes may itch in many conditions (Fig. 22.8), but in atopic eczema (Fig. 22.9) itching is the main symptom at all ages and this results in scratching and exacerbation of the rash. The excoriated areas become erythematous, weeping and crusted. Distribution of the

Fig. 22.7 Infantile seborrhoeic dermatitis. (a) Cradle cap. (b) Distribution on the scalp and face, behind the ears, flexures and nappy area.

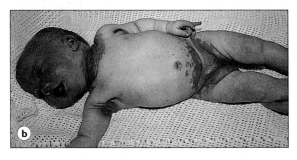

ITCHING

Fig. 22.8 Some causes of itchy rashes.

Atopic eczema
Chickenpox
Urticaria/allergic reactions
Contact dermatitis
Insect bites/papular urticaria
Scabies
Fungal infections
Pityriasis rosea

 No itch? – then it's not eczema.

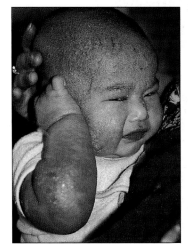

Fig. 22.9 Excoriation of the skin from scratching. Itch is the key clinical feature in eczema at all ages, leading to an 'itch–scratch–itch' cycle. It is 'the itch that rashes' in atopic eczema.

eruption tends to change with age, as indicated in Figure 22.10. Atopic skin is usually dry, and prolonged scratching and rubbing of the skin may lead to lichenification, in which there is accentuation of the normal skin markings (Fig. 22.11).

Complications

Causes of exacerbations of eczema are listed in Figure 22.12. However, flare-ups are common, often for no obvious reason. Eczematous skin can readily become infected, usually with *Staphylococcus* or *Streptococcus*. *Staph. aureus* thrives on atopic skin and releases superantigens which seem to induce and maintain eczema. Herpes simplex virus infection, although less frequent, is potentially very serious as it can spread rapidly on atopic skin, causing an extensive vesicular reaction, eczema herpeticum (see Ch. 13). Lymphadenopathy is common with active eczema and usually resolves when the skin improves.

Management

A number of treatment modalities are available.

Avoiding irritants and precipitants

It is advisable to avoid soap and biological detergents. Clothing next to the skin should be of pure cotton where possible, avoiding nylon and pure woollen garments. Nails need to be cut short to reduce skin damage from scratching, and mittens at night may be helpful in the very young. When an allergen such as cow's milk has been proven to be a precipitant, it should be avoided.

Emollients

These are the mainstay of management, moisturising and softening the skin. They should be applied liberally two or more times a day and after a bath. They include aqueous cream BP or ointments such as one containing equal parts of white soft paraffin and liquid paraffin. Ointments are preferable to creams when the skin is very dry. A daily bath using an emollient oil as a soap substitute is also beneficial.

Topical corticosteroids

These are an effective treatment for eczema, but must be used with care. Mildly potent corticosteroids, such

ECZEMA

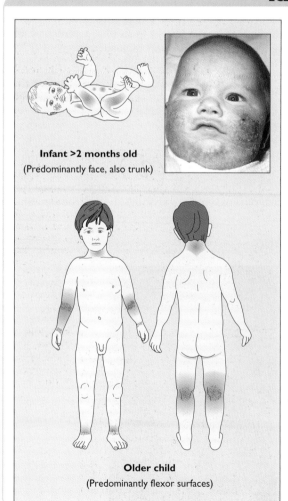

Infant >2 months old
(Predominantly face, also trunk)

Older child
(Predominantly flexor surfaces)

Fig. 22.10 Distribution of atopic eczema. The distribution of eczema tends to change with age. In infants, the face and scalp are prominently affected, although the trunk may be involved. In older children, the skin flexures (cubital and popliteal fossae) and frictional areas, such as the neck, wrists and ankles, are characteristically involved.

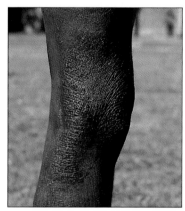

Fig. 22.11 Lichenification. Thickening of the skin with accentuation of skin creases from persistent scratching.

Fig. 22.12 Causes of exacerbation of eczema.

Bacterial infection, e.g. *Staphylococcus*, *Streptococcus*
Viral infection, e.g. herpes simplex virus
Ingestion of an allergen, e.g. egg
Contact with an irritant or allergen
Environment – heat, humidity
Change or reduction in medication
Psychological stress
Unexplained

as 1% hydrocortisone ointment, can be applied to the eczematous areas twice daily. Moderately potent topical steroids play a pivotal role in the management of acute exacerbations, but their use must be kept to a minimum and use on the face generally avoided. Excessive use of topical steroids may cause thinning of the skin as well as systemic side-effects. However, fear of these side-effects should not deter their use in controlling exacerbations.

Occlusive bandages

These are helpful over limbs when scratching and lichenification are a problem. They may be impregnated with zinc paste or zinc and tar paste. The bandages are worn overnight or for 2–3 days at a time until the skin has improved. For widespread itching in young children, wet stockinette wraps may be helpful; diluted topical steroids mixed with emollient are applied to the skin and damp wraps fashioned for trunk and limbs are then applied with overlying dry wraps or clothes.

Antibiotics or antiviral agents

Antibiotics with hydrocortisone can be applied topically for mildly infected eczema. Systemic antibiotics are required for more serious infections. Eczema herpeticum is treated with systemic aciclovir.

H_1 histamine antagonists

Itch suppression is with an antihistamine. The newer antihistamines are not sedative.

Dietary elimination

Food allergy occurs in up to 6% of infants with eczema. Food allergens include cow's milk, egg and soy. However, any food may be implicated as a cause of eczema. Dietary elimination should be considered if there is a strong suggestive history. Dietary elimination for 4–6 weeks is usually required to detect a response. This should be carried out with the advice of a dietician to ensure complete avoidance of specific food constituents and that the diet remains nutritionally adequate. A double-blind placebo-controlled food challenge is required to be fully objective, but is usually reserved for older children. Children can usually tolerate the offending foods when they are older.

Psychosocial support

In most children, eczema is mild and can be controlled with emollients and mildly potent topical steroids, and additional psychological support is not required. However, eczema can be sufficiently severe to be disrupting both to the child and to the whole family. The parents and the child need considerable advice, help and support from health professionals, other affected families or fellow sufferers. In the UK, the National Eczema Society provides support and education about the disorder.

INFECTIONS AND INFESTATIONS

Bullous impetigo has been mentioned earlier in this chapter and acute bacterial and viral infections of the skin are considered in Chapter 13.

Viral infections

Viral warts

These are caused by the human papillomavirus, of which there are nearly 80 types. Warts are common in children, usually on the fingers and soles (verrucae). Most disappear spontaneously over a few months or years and treatment is only indicated if the lesions are painful or are a cosmetic problem. They can be difficult to treat, but daily application of a proprietary salicylic acid and lactic acid paint or glutaraldehyde (10%) lotion can be used. Cryotherapy with liquid nitrogen is effective treatment but can be painful and often needs repeated application, and its use is reserved for older children.

Molluscum contagiosum

This is caused by a poxvirus. The lesions are small, skin-coloured, pearly papules with central umbilication (Fig. 22.13). They may be single but are usually multiple. Lesions are often widespread but tend to disappear spontaneously within a year. If necessary, a topical antibacterial can be applied to prevent or treat secondary bacterial infection and cryotherapy (2–3 s only) can be used in older children, away from the face, to hasten the disappearance of more chronic lesions.

Fungal infections

Ringworm

Dermatophyte fungi invade dead keratinous structures, such as the horny layer of skin, nails and hair. The term ringworm is used because of the often ringed (annular) appearance of skin lesions. A severe inflammatory pustular ringworm patch is called a kerion (Fig. 22.14).

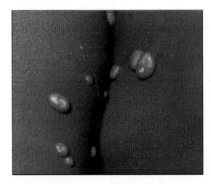

Fig. 22.13 Molluscum contagiosum on the chest and upper arm showing the pearly papules with central umbilication through which the infectious central core is eventually shed.

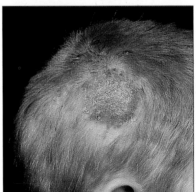

Fig. 22.14 Ringworm of the scalp showing a kerion.

Tinea capitis (scalp ringworm), often acquired from dogs and cats, causes scaling and patchy alopecia with broken hairs. Examination under filtered ultraviolet (Wood's) light shows bright greenish/yellow fluorescence of the infected hairs with some fungal species.

Rapid diagnosis can be made by microscopic examination of skin scrapings for fungal hyphae. Definitive identification of the fungus is by culture. Treatment of mild infections is with topical antifungal preparations, but more severe infections require systemic antifungal treatment for several weeks. Any animal source of infection also needs to be treated.

Parasitic infestations

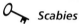 **Scabies**

Scabies is caused by an infestation with the eight-legged mite, *Sarcoptes scabiei*, which burrows down the epidermis along the stratum corneum. Severe itching occurs 2–6 weeks after infestation and is worse in warm conditions and at night.

In older children, burrows, papules and vesicles involve the skin between the fingers and toes, axillae, flexor aspects of the wrists, belt line and around the nipples, penis and buttocks. In infants and young children, the distribution often includes the palms, soles and trunk (Fig. 22.15). The presence of lesions on the soles can be helpful in making the diagnosis. The head, neck and face can be involved in babies but is uncommon.

Diagnosis is made on clinical grounds with the history of itching and characteristic lesions. Although burrows are considered pathognomonic, they may be hard to identify because of secondary infection due to scratching. Itching in other family members is a helpful clinical indicator. Confirmation can be made by microscopic examination of skin scrapings from the lesions to identify mite, eggs and mite faeces.

Complications

The skin becomes excoriated due to scratching and there may be a secondary eczematous or urticarial reaction masking the true diagnosis. Secondary bacterial infection is common, giving crusted, pustular lesions. Sometimes slowly resolving nodular lesions are visible.

Treatment

As it is spread by close bodily contact, the child and whole family should be treated whether or not they have evidence of infestation. Permethrin cream (5%) should be applied below the neck to all areas and washed off after 8–12 h. In babies, the face and scalp should be included, avoiding the eyes. Benzyl benzoate emulsion (25%) applied below the neck only (diluted according to age) and left on for 12 h is also effective but smells and has an irritant action. Malathion lotion (0.5% aqueous) is another effective preparation applied below the neck and left on for 12 h. If a child and other members of the family are itching, suspect scabies.

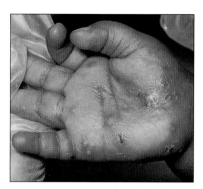

Fig. 22.15 Scabies in a young child affecting the palm.

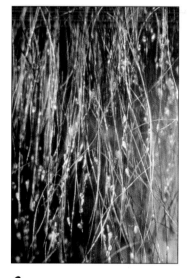

Fig. 22.16 Head lice. Profuse nits (egg capsules) are visible on these scalp hairs. Live lice were also visible on the scalp.

 Pediculosis

Pediculosis capitis (head lice infestation) is the most common form of lice infestation in children. It is widespread and troublesome among primary school children. Presentation may be itching of the scalp and nape or from identifying live lice on the scalp or nits (empty egg cases) on hairs (Fig. 22.16). Louse eggs are cemented to hair close to the scalp and the nits (small whitish oval capsules) remain attached to the hair shaft as the hair grows. There may be secondary bacterial infection leading to a misdiagnosis of impetigo. Post-occipital lymphadenopathy is common. Once infestation is confirmed by finding live lice, treatment is by applying a solution of 0.5% malathion to the hair and leaving it on overnight. The hair is then shampooed and the lice and nits removed with a fine-tooth comb. Treatment should be repeated 1 week later. Permethrin (1%) as a cream rinse would be an alternative application; it is left on for 10 min only. Flammability of alcohol-based lotions should be noted.

OTHER CHILDHOOD ERUPTIONS

Psoriasis

This familial disorder rarely presents before the age of 2 years. The guttate type (Fig. 22.17) is common in

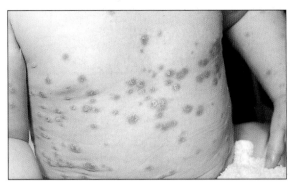

Fig. 22.17 Guttate psoriasis.

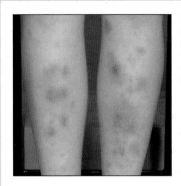

Fig. 22.18a There are discrete tender red nodules on the shins. Fever and arthralgia may be present.

Fig. 22.18b Causes.

Streptococcal infection
Primary tuberculosis
Inflammatory bowel disease
Drug reaction
Idiopathic
(Sarcoidosis, a common association in adults, is rare in children)

children and often follows a streptococcal or viral sore throat or ear infection. Lesions are small, raindrop-like, round or oval erythematous scaly patches on the trunk and upper limbs, and an attack usually resolves over 3–4 months. Chronic psoriasis with plaques or annular lesions is less common. Fine pitting of the nails may be seen in chronic disease but is unusual in children. Treatment for guttate psoriasis is with bland ointments. Coal tar preparations are useful for plaque psoriasis and scalp involvement. Dithranol preparations are very effective in resistant plaque psoriasis. Occasionally, children with chronic psoriasis develop arthritis.

Pityriasis rosea

This acute benign self-limiting condition is thought to be of viral origin. It usually begins with a single round or oval scaly macule, the herald patch, 2–5 cm in diameter, on the trunk, upper arm, neck or thigh. After a few days, numerous smaller dull pink macules develop on the trunk, upper arms and thighs. The rash tends to follow the line of the ribs posteriorly, described as the 'fir tree pattern'. Sometimes the lesions are itchy. No treatment is required and the rash resolves within 4–6 weeks.

Acne vulgaris

Acne may begin 1–2 years before the onset of puberty following androgenic stimulation of the sebaceous glands and an increased sebum excretion rate. Obstruction to the flow of sebum in the sebaceous follicle initiates the process of acne. There is a variety of lesions, initially open comedones (blackheads) or closed comedones (whiteheads) progressing to papules, pustules, nodules and cysts. Lesions occur mainly on the face, back, chest and shoulders. The more severe cystic and nodular lesions often produce scarring. Menstruation and emotional stress may be associated with exacerbations. The condition usually resolves in the late teens, although it may persist.

Topical treatment is directed at encouraging the skin to peel using a keratolytic agent, such as benzoyl peroxide, applied once or twice daily after washing. Sunshine in moderation, topical antibiotics or topical retinoids may be helpful. For more severe acne, oral

antibiotic therapy with tetracyclines (only when over 12 years old, because they may discolour the teeth in younger children) or erythromycin is indicated. The retinoid isotretinoin is reserved for severe acne in teenagers unresponsive to other treatments.

RASHES AND SYSTEMIC DISEASE

Skin rashes may be a sign of systemic disease. Examples are:

- Facial rash in systemic lupus erythematosus (SLE) or dermatomyositis.
- Purpura over the buttocks, lower limbs and elbows in Henoch–Schönlein purpura.
- Erythema nodosum (Fig. 22.18a, b).
- Erythema multiforme (Fig. 22.19a, b), which may be associated with a systemic disorder, but often no cause is identified.
- Stevens–Johnson syndrome, a severe bullous form of erythema multiforme also involving the mucous membranes (Fig. 22.20). The eye involvement may include conjunctivitis, corneal ulceration and uveitis, and ophthalmological assessment is required. It may be caused by drug sensitivity or infection, with morbidity and sometimes even mortality from infection, toxaemia or renal damage.
- Urticaria.

Urticaria

Urticaria (hives or weals) (Fig. 22.21) results from a local increase in the permeability of capillaries and

ERYTHEMA MULTIFORME

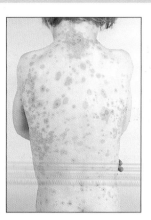

Fig. 22.19a There are target lesions with a central papule surrounded by an erythematous ring. Lesions may also be vesicular or bullous.

Fig. 22.19b Causes.

Herpes simplex infection
Mycoplasma pneumoniae infection
Other infections
Drug reaction
Idiopathic

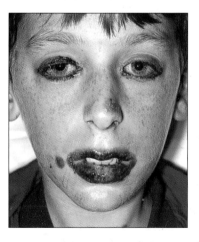

Fig. 22.20
Stevens Johnson syndrome showing severe ulceration of the mouth. (Courtesy of Dr Rob Primhak.)

URTICARIA

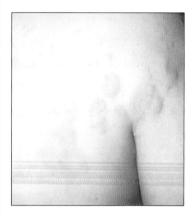

Fig. 22.21
Urticaria. There are raised pink oedematous lesions visible. Such weals may become confluent and widespread.

Fig. 22.22 Causes of urticaria.

Idiopathic (is common)

IgE-mediated
Specific food – cow's milk, nuts especially peanuts, fish
Blood products
Drugs – penicillins, cephalosporins

Pharmacological
Foods containing histamine-releasing substances, e.g. strawberries, egg white, cheese
Aspirin and other non-steroidal anti-inflammatory agents

Physical agents
Heat, cold, pressure

venules. These changes are dependent on activation of skin mast cells which contain a range of mediators including histamine. A cause may be identified, such as cow's milk allergy in infants, but most are idiopathic (Fig. 22.22). In children, urticaria is usually acute and may also involve deeper tissues to produce swelling of the lips and soft tissues around the eyes (angioedema), and even anaphylaxis. Its management is described in Figure 5.23.

Papular urticaria is a delayed hypersensitivity reaction most commonly seen on the legs, following a bite from a flea, bedbug, or animal or bird mite. Irritation, vesicles, papules and weals appear and secondary infection due to scratching is common. It may last for weeks or months and may be recurrent.

Hereditary angioedema is a rare autosomal dominant disorder caused by a deficiency of C1-esterase inhibitor. There is no urticaria, but subcutaneous swellings occur, often accompanied by abdominal pain. The trigger is usually trauma. Angioedema may cause respiratory obstruction. Treatment of a severe acute attack is with a purified preparation of the inhibitor, but replacement therapy with fresh frozen plasma can be used as a short-term measure.

FURTHER READING

Review 1998 Treating head louse infections. Drug and Therapeutics Bulletin 36: 45–46
Verbov J 1999 How to manage warts. Archives of Disease in Childhood 80: 97–99
Verbov J 2000 Handbook of paediatric dermatology. Martin Dunitz, London
Verbov J 2000 Common skin conditions in the newborn. Seminars in neonatology 5: 303–310

23

Endocrine and metabolic disorders

Features of endocrine and metabolic disorders in children are:

- Almost all diabetes mellitus is insulin-dependent.
- Hypoglycaemia must be excluded whenever children become suddenly ill.
- Congenital hypothyroidism is relatively common and is detected on routine biochemical screening (Guthrie test).
- Inborn errors of metabolism are individually rare but are considered in a wide range of differential diagnoses.

 DIABETES MELLITUS

The incidence of diabetes in children has increased steadily over the last 20 years and now affects around 2 per 1000 children by 16 years of age. This is most likely to be a result of changes in environmental risk factors. There is considerable racial and geographical variation – the condition is more common in northern countries, with the highest incidence in Finland. Almost all children are insulin-dependent (type 1 diabetes). Type 2 non-insulin-dependent diabetes due to insulin resistance is starting to occur in childhood as severe obesity becomes more common. The causes of diabetes are listed in Figure 23.1.

> **Almost all children with diabetes mellitus are insulin-dependent (type 1).**

Aetiology

Both genetic predisposition and environmental precipitants play a role. Inherited susceptibility is demonstrated by:

Fig. 23.1 Classification of diabetes according to aetiology.
(Adapted from American Diabetes Association, Report of Expert Committee on the diagnosis and classification of diabetes mellitus. *Diabetes Care* 22 (Suppl. 1), 1999.)

Type 1 Insulin-dependent
Most childhood diabetes

Type 2 Non-insulin-dependent
Usually older children, obesity-related, positive family history, not prone to ketosis

Type 3 Other specific types
Genetic defects in β-cell function (maturity-onset diabetes of the young, MODY types 1–3)
Genetic defects in insulin action
Infections, e.g. congenital rubella
Drugs, e.g. corticosteroids
Pancreatic exocrine insufficiency, e.g. cystic fibrosis
Endocrine diseases, e.g. Cushing's syndrome
Genetic/chromosomal syndromes, e.g. Down's and Turner's

Type 4 Gestational diabetes (GDM)

- an identical twin of a diabetic having a 30–50% chance of developing the disease
- the increased risk of a child developing diabetes if a parent has insulin-dependent diabetes (1 in 20–40 if the father is affected, 1 in 40–80 if it is the mother).
- the increased risk of diabetes amongst those who are HLA-DR3 or HLA-DR4 and a reduced risk with DR2 and DR5.

Molecular mimicry probably occurs between an environmental trigger and an antigen on the surface of

337

β-cells of the pancreas. Triggers which may contribute are viral infections, accounting for the more frequent presentation in spring and autumn, and diet, possibly cow's milk proteins (Fig. 23.2). This results in an autoimmune process which damages the pancreatic β-cells and leads to an absolute insulin deficiency. Markers of β-cell destruction include islet cell antibodies and antibodies to glutamic acid decarboxylase (GAD). There is an association with other autoimmune disorders such as hypothyroidism.

Clinical features

The age at presentation is shown in Figure 23.3. It is uncommon before the age of 1 year, but the incidence rises steadily during the early school years to reach a peak at 12–13 years of age. In contrast to adults, children usually present with only a few weeks of polyuria, excessive thirst (polydipsia) and weight loss; young children may also develop secondary nocturnal enuresis. Most children are diagnosed at this early stage of the illness (Fig. 23.4). Advanced diabetic

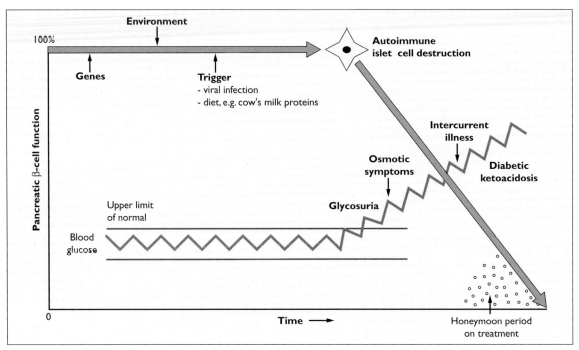

Fig. 23.2 Stages in the development of diabetes.

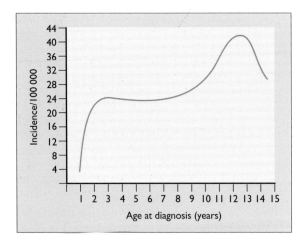

Fig. 23.3 Age at presentation. Diabetes occurs even in young children, but its incidence increases with age. (Data from Metcalfe M A, Baum J D, Incidence of insulin dependent diabetes in children aged under 15 years in the British Isles during 1988. *British Medical Journal* 1991; 302: 443–447.)

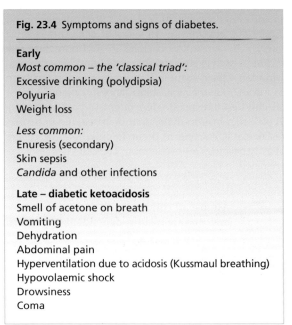

Fig. 23.4 Symptoms and signs of diabetes.

Early
Most common – the 'classical triad':
Excessive drinking (polydipsia)
Polyuria
Weight loss

Less common:
Enuresis (secondary)
Skin sepsis
Candida and other infections

Late – diabetic ketoacidosis
Smell of acetone on breath
Vomiting
Dehydration
Abdominal pain
Hyperventilation due to acidosis (Kussmaul breathing)
Hypovolaemic shock
Drowsiness
Coma

ketoacidosis has become an uncommon presentation (<10%), but requires urgent recognition and treatment. Diabetic ketoacidosis may be misdiagnosed if the hyperventilation is mistaken for pneumonia or the abdominal pain for appendicitis.

Diagnosis

The diagnosis is usually confirmed in a symptomatic child by finding a markedly raised random blood glucose (>11.1 mmol/L by the WHO definition), glycosuria and ketonuria. Where there is any doubt, a fasting blood glucose (>7.8 mmol/L) or a raised glycosylated haemoglobin (HbA_{1C}) are helpful. A diagnostic glucose tolerance test is rarely required in children.

Initial management

Diabetes in childhood is uncommon and much of the initial and routine care is delivered by specialist teams (Fig. 23.5).

The initial management will depend on the child's clinical condition. Those in advanced diabetic keto-acidosis require urgent hospital admission and treatment (see box on 'Diabetic ketoacidosis'). Most newly presenting children are alert and able to eat and drink and can be managed with subcutaneous insulin alone. Intravenous fluid is required if the child is vomiting or dehydrated. In some centres, children newly presenting with diabetes who do not require intravenous therapy are not admitted to hospital but are managed entirely at home.

An intensive educational programme is needed for the parents and child to cover:

- a basic understanding of the pathophysiology of diabetes
- injection of insulin – technique and sites
- diet – regular meals and snacks, reduced refined carbohydrate, healthy diet with no more than 30% fat intake
- matching of food intake with insulin and exercise
- 'sick-day rules' during illness to prevent ketoacidosis
- blood glucose (fingerprick) monitoring or urine testing in the very young
- the recognition and treatment of hypoglycaemia
- where to get advice 24 h a day

Fig. 23.5 The diabetes team.

Consultant paediatrician(s) with a special interest in diabetes
Paediatric diabetes specialist nurse(s)
Paediatric dietician
Clinical psychologist
Social worker
Adult diabetologist for joint adolescent clinics

- the help available from voluntary groups, i.e. local groups and, in the UK, 'Diabetes UK' (formerly the British Diabetic Association)
- the psychological impact of a lifelong condition with potentially serious short- and long-term complications.

A considerable period of time needs to be spent with the family to provide this information and psychological support. The information provided for the child must be appropriate for age and updated regularly. The specialist nurse should liaise with the school (teachers, those who prepare school meals, physical education teachers) and the primary care team.

Insulin

Insulin is made chemically identical to human insulin by recombinant DNA technology or chemical modification of pork insulin. Pork (porcine) and cow's (bovine) pancreas-derived insulin is still available, but rarely used in children. Rapid-acting insulin analogues have been developed by modifying the amino acid sequence, e.g. Lispro.

Insulin is available in short-acting (e.g. Actrapid and Humulin S), medium-acting (e.g. Insulatard and Humulin I) and long-acting (e.g. Ultratard) formulations.

A number of insulin preparations with a predetermined preparation of mixed short- and intermediate-acting insulins exist (e.g. Mixtard 30/70 and Humulin M3).

Most available insulin is human and in concentrations of 100 U/ml (U-100). It is important not to interchange insulin types or species without prior consultation with the diabetic team.

Insulin can be given by injections using a variety of syringe and needle sizes, pen-like devices and insulin-containing cartridges, as well as jet injectors that inject insulin as a fine stream into the skin.

Insulin may be injected into the subcutaneous tissue of the upper arm, the anterior and lateral aspects of the thigh, the buttocks and the abdomen. Rotation of the injection sites is essential to prevent lipohypertrophy or, more rarely, lipoatrophy. The skin should be pinched up and the insulin injected at a 45° angle. Using a long needle or an injection technique that is 'too vertical' causes a painful, bruised intramuscular injection. Shallow intradermal injections can also cause scarring and should be avoided.

In young children, insulin is usually given twice a day, before breakfast and evening meals as a mixture of short-acting (approximately 30%) and medium- or long-acting insulin (approximately 70%) (Fig. 23.6). In general, about two-thirds of the daily dose is given before breakfast and one-third before the evening meal.

Each insulin can be drawn up separately, allowing greater flexibility, or be given as a fixed mixture containing from 10 to 50% short-acting insulin. An insulin mixture with 30% short-acting is used most often.

Older children and teenagers are increasingly using a three or four injections a day regimen ('basal-bolus')

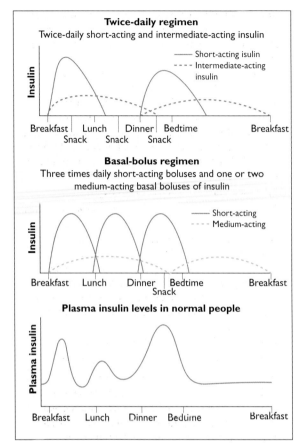

Fig. 23.6 Twice-daily and basal-bolus insulin regimens. The normal insulin profile is also shown.

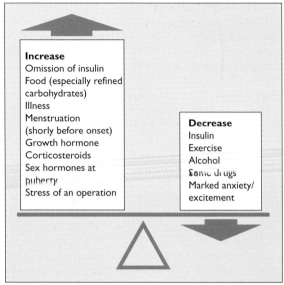

Fig. 23.7 Factors affecting blood glucose levels.

in which a short-acting insulin (often Lispro) is given before each meal and some long-acting insulin in the late evening to provide insulin overnight (and sometimes also before breakfast). This allows greater flexibility by relating the insulin more closely to food intake and exercise (Fig. 23.6).

Shortly after presentation, when some pancreatic function is preserved, insulin requirements often become minimal, the so-called 'honeymoon period'. Requirements subsequently increase to 0.5–1 or even up to 2 units/kg per day.

Diet
The diet and insulin regimen need to be matched (Fig. 23.7). The aim is to optimise metabolic control whilst maintaining normal growth. On the standard twice-daily regimen, food intake is divided into three main meals with snacks between meals and before going to bed. The snacks are required to avoid hypoglycaemia. Teenagers on a basal-bolus regimen can eat more flexibly and need not take snacks other than before planned exercise. A healthy diet is recommended, with a high complex carbohydrate and relatively low fat content (<30% of total calories). The diet should be high in fibre, which will provide a sustained release of glucose, rather than refined carbohydrate

which causes rapid swings in glucose levels. In the past, dietary carbohydrate was divided into 10 g 'portions', but this is now seldom used as it was found that few families or professionals could calculate the daily intake accurately and so compliance was poor.

Blood glucose monitoring
Regular blood glucose profiles and blood glucose measurements when a low or high level is suspected are required to adjust the insulin regimen and learn how changes in lifestyle, food and exercise affect control. A record should be kept in a diary or transferred from the memory of the blood glucose meter. The aim is to maintain blood glucose as near to normal (4–6 mmol/L) as possible. In practice, in order also to avoid hypoglycaemic episodes, this means levels of 4–10 mmol/L in children and 4–8 mmol/L in adolescents for as much of the time as possible. As children usually dislike having fingerpricks, this limits the frequency of their use. Realistic goals need to be agreed, with compromises reached about the frequency of monitoring. During changes in lifestyle (e.g. holidays) or illness, it is not unreasonable to ask for two to three tests per day. Many adolescents test less than once per week, if at all.

Urine glucose testing may be substituted in the very young or timid. Urine ketone testing is mandatory during intercurrent infections or when control is poor to try to avoid severe ketoacidosis.

The measurement of glycosylated haemoglobin (HbA$_{1C}$) is particularly helpful as a guide of overall control over the previous 6 weeks and should be checked regularly. The level is directly related to the risk of later complications, but may be misleading if the red blood cell life span is reduced, such as in sickle cell trait or if the HbA molecule is abnormal, as in thalassaemia.

Hypoglycaemia in diabetes

Most children develop well defined symptoms when their blood glucose falls below about 4 mmol/L. The symptoms are highly individual and change with age, but most complain of hunger, sweatiness, feeling faint or dizzy or of a 'wobbly feeling' in their legs. If unrecognised or untreated, hypoglycaemia may progress to seizures and coma. Parents can often detect hypoglycaemia in young children by their pallor and irritability, sometimes presenting as unreasonable behaviour. If there is any doubt, the blood glucose concentration should be checked or food given.

Treating a 'hypo' at an early stage requires the administration of easily absorbed glucose in the form of sweets (glucose tablets, e.g. Dextrosol or similar) or a sugary drink. Children should always have easy access to their hypo remedy, although young children quickly learn to complain of hypo symptoms in order to leave class or obtain sweets! Oral glucose gels (e.g. Hypostop) are easily and quickly absorbed from the buccal mucosa and so are helpful if the child is unwilling or unable to cooperate to eat. It can be administered by teachers or other helpers. Parents and school should be provided with a glucagon injection kit for the treatment of severe hypoglycaemia and taught how to administer it intramuscularly to terminate severe hypos. Severe hypoglycaemia can usually be predicted (or explained in retrospect – missed meal, heavy exercise). The aim is anticipation and prevention. Hypoglycaemia in an unconscious child brought to hospital is treated with glucose given intravenously.

Diabetic ketoacidosis

Presentation is described in Figure 23.4, essential investigations in Figure 23.8 and management in Figure 23.9.

Long-term management

The aims of long-term management are:
- normal growth and development
- maintaining as normal a home and school life as possible
- good diabetic control through knowledge and good technique
- encouraging children to become self-reliant, but with adult supervision until they are able to take responsibility
- avoidance of hypoglycaemia
- the prevention of long-term complications.

These aims are extremely difficult to achieve!

Problems in diabetic control

Good blood glucose control is particularly difficult in the following circumstances:

- Eating too many sugary foods, such as sweets taken at odd times, at parties or on the way home from school.
- Infrequent or unreliable blood glucose testing. 'Perfect' results are often invented and written down just before clinic to please the diabetes team.

- Illness – viral illnesses are common in the young and although it is usually stated that infections cause insulin requirements to increase, in practice the insulin dose required is variable, partly because of reduced food intake. The dose of insulin should be adjusted according to regular blood glucose monitoring. Insulin *must* be continued during times of illness and the urine tested for ketones. If ketosis is increasing along with a rising blood sugar, the family should know how to seek immediate advice to ensure that they increase the soluble insulin dose appropriately or seek medical help for possible intravenous therapy.

- Exercise – vigorous or prolonged planned exercise (cross-country running, long-distance hiking, skiing) requires reduction of the insulin dose and increase in dietary intake. Late hypoglycaemia may occur during the night, but may be avoided by taking an extra bedtime snack, including slow-acting carbohydrate such as cereal or bread. Less vigorous exercise such as sports lessons in school and spontaneous outdoor play can be managed with an extra snack before the exercise.

- Family disturbance such as divorce or separation.

- Inadequate family motivation, support or understanding. As children can never have a 'holiday' from their diabetes, they need a great deal of encouragement to continuously maintain good control. Educational programmes for children and families need to be arranged regularly and matched to their current level of education. Special courses and holiday camps are available; in the UK they are organised by Diabetes UK and local groups.

Management of diabetes at school

An individualised care plan should be developed by the parents, diabetes team and the school to address the specific needs of the child. This will include the child's dietary needs, requirements to have snacks at specified times and what to do if the child becomes hypoglycaemic or loses consciousness.

Puberty and adolescence

The rapid growth spurt in early puberty is governed by a complex interaction of hormonal changes, some of which involve insulin and insulin-like growth factors. Growth hormone, oestrogen and testosterone all antagonise insulin action and there is thus an increase in the insulin requirement from the usual 0.5–1.0 units/kg per day of early childhood up to 2 units/kg per day. The psychological changes accompanying adolescence may make this a time of rebellion where adherence to insulin and dietary regimens is minimal. Diabetic teenagers know that they will not become ill immediately if they cheat with their diet or miss an injection. Some will inevitably test the degree to which the rules can be broken, choosing to ignore the uncomfortable facts of diabetes provided that they 'feel OK'. This

---

DIABETIC KETOACIDOSIS

Fig. 23.8 Essential early investigations.

Blood glucose (>15 mmol/L)
Urea and electrolytes, creatinine (dehydration)
Blood gas analysis (severe metabolic acidosis)
Urinary glucose and ketones (both are present)
Evidence of a precipitating cause, e.g. infection
(blood and urine cultures performed)
Cardiac monitor for T-wave changes of
hypokalaemia
Considered salicylate level (similar presentation)
Weight

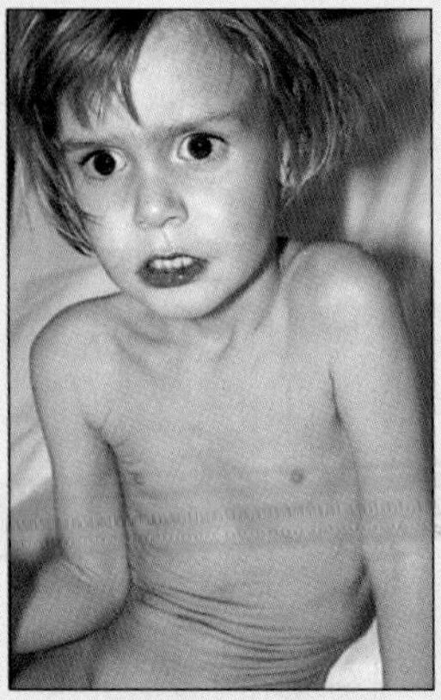

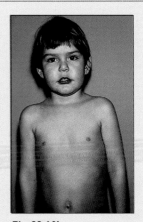

Fig. 23.10a   Fig. 23.10b

Management priorities
This regimen is initiated if the child is vomiting or has a reduced level of consciousness.
Otherwise, even if newly presenting, only subcutaneous insulin is required.

1. Fluids ➡ If in shock, intial resuscitation is with normal saline. Dehydration should then be corrected gradually over 48–72 h (see Fig. 23.10). Rapid rehydration should be avoided as it may lead to cerebral oedema. Monitor:
• fluid input and output
• electrolytes, creatinine and acid–base status regularly
• neurological state.
Insert central venous line (CVP) and urinary catheter if shocked.
A nasogastric tube is passed for acute gastric dilatation if there is vomiting or depressed consciousness.

2. Insulin ➡ Insulin infusion (0.05–0.1 units/kg per h) is started, titrating the dose according to the blood glucose. Do not give a bolus. Monitor the blood glucose regularly. Aim for gradual reduction of blood glucose of about 2 mmol/h, as rapid reduction is dangerous. Change to 4% dextrose/0.18% saline when the blood glucose has fallen to 12 mmol/L to avoid hypoglycaemia.

3. Potassium ➡ Although the initial plasma potassium is usually high, it will fall following treatment with insulin and rehydration. Potassium replacement must be instituted as soon as urine is passed. Continuous cardiac monitoring and regular plasma potassium measurements are indicated until the plasma potassium is stable.

4. Acidosis ➡ Although a metabolic acidosis is present, bicarbonate should be avoided unless the child is shocked or not responding to therapy. The acidosis will self-correct with fluid and insulin therapy.

5. Re-establish oral fluids, subcutaneous insulin and diet ➡ Do not stop the intravenous insulin infusion until after subcutaneous insulin has been given

6. Identification and treatment of an underlying cause ➡ Ketoacidosis may be precipitated by an intercurrent infection. Antibiotics may be indicated. If the child was known to have diabetes, consider the reason for the ketoacidosis

Fig. 23.9 Management priorities in diabetic ketoacidosis. **Fig. 23.10** (a) Severe dehydration and weight loss from diabetic ketoacidosis. (b) Four months later. (Courtesy of Dr Jill Challener.)

usually results in avoidance of blood testing and a tendency to work on the false assumption that feeling well equates with good control. Many teenage girls experiment with crash diets at some time, which are likely to cause major problems in diabetic control. They also learn that glycosuria can be used as an 'aid' to losing weight.

Battles with parents may concentrate on diabetic management instead of the more usual teenage concerns (Fig. 23.11). Conflict may also extend to involve the professionals of the diabetic team, because of intense anger against the disease which marks them out as different from their peers. Many parents are very protective at this time, while teenagers should be encouraged to take responsibility for their diabetes. Health education about smoking, alcohol and contraception may need to be provided. Liaison with a psychologist or child psychiatrist may be helpful. The professionals of the diabetic team may need to encourage diabetic teenagers to take better care of themselves. It is usually unhelpful to give lectures about the long-term risks to health, as these are likely to be seen as irrelevant by the teenagers. However, they may be helped if:

- there are clear short-term goals
- their efforts to improve their diabetic control, e.g. an improving or satisfactory HbA_{1C} level, are communicated promptly and enthusiastically
- there is a united team approach, with agreement between professionals of the essentials they wish to promote and clear, unambiguous guidelines for health and diabetic management
- peer group pressure is used to promote health. Activities such as holidays, etc., that allow teenagers to participate while learning about their diabetic management are encouraged. They may also benefit by being used as teachers of younger children.

 Successful long-term diabetic management depends on education and increasing self-reliance and responsibility.

Prevention of long-term complications

It has been shown that meticulous diabetic control delays or prevents diabetic retinopathy and nephropathy and slows the progression of retinopathy (American Multicentre Diabetes Control and Complications trial – DCCT). Levels of glycosylated haemoglobin above the norm are related to risk of later complications in an almost exponential fashion and so the ideal is to keep this level as close to normal as possible. In reality, this is only achieved by intensive management with three or four injections of insulin daily, four or more blood glucose estimations each day and frequent clinic check-ups. However, intensive treatment results in an increased risk of severe hypoglycaemia and weight gain. The intensive regimen is probably not suitable for young children because of the increased risk of hypoglycaemia, with its detrimental effect on the growing brain, and the unpopularity of multiple injections (including a lunchtime injection at school) and frequent blood tests.

Although long-term health problems are uncommon during childhood, there needs to be regular review for long-term complications and associated illnesses:

- *Growth and pubertal development.* Some delay in the onset of puberty may occur. Obesity is common, especially in females if their insulin dose is not reduced towards the end of puberty.
- *Blood pressure* – must be checked for evidence of hypertension.
- *Renal disease* – the detection of microalbuminuria is an early sign of nephropathy.
- *Eyes* – retinopathy or cataracts requiring treatment are rare in children but should be monitored annually after 5 years of diabetes or from the onset of puberty.

Fig. 23.11 How diabetes interferes with normal adolescence.

Aims and problems of normal adolescence	How diabetes interferes
Physical and sexual maturation	Delayed sexual maturation Invasion of privacy with frequent medical examinations
Conformity with peer group	Meals must be eaten on time Frequent injections and blood tests
Self image	Hypoglycaemic attacks show that they are different
Self esteem	Impaired body image
Independence from parents	Parental over-protection and reluctance to allow their child to be away from home Battles over diabetes
Economic independence	Loading of insurance premiums Discrimination by employers Statutory rules against becoming a pilot or driving heavy goods or public service vehicles

- *Feet* – children should be encouraged to take good care of their feet from an early age, to avoid tight shoes and treat any infections early.
- *Other associated illnesses* – thyroid disease is easily missed clinically and some centres regularly screen for hypothyroidism. Coeliac disease also occurs more frequently than in the general population, but the benefit of antibody screening and starting dietary treatment of seropositive but asymptomatic patients is disputed.

> **Good diabetes control in childhood reduces the risk of long-term complications.**

HYPOGLYCAEMIA

Hypoglycaemia is a common problem in neonates but is seen much less often beyond this period. It is often defined as a plasma glucose less than 2.6 mmol/L, although the development of clinical features will depend on whether other energy substrates can be utilised. Clinical features include:

- sweating
- pallor
- central nervous system signs of irritability, headache, seizures and coma

The neurological sequelae may be permanent if hypoglycaemia persists and include epilepsy, severe learning difficulties and microcephaly. This risk is greatest in early childhood during the period of most rapid brain growth.

Infants have high energy requirements and relatively poor reserves of glucose from gluconeogenesis and glycogenesis. They are at risk of hypoglycaemia with fasting. Infants should never be starved for more than 4 h duration, e.g. preoperatively. A blood glucose should be checked in any child who:

- becomes septicaemic or appears seriously ill
- has a prolonged seizure
- develops an altered state of consciousness.

This is often done at the bedside using glucose-sensitive strips, whose accuracy is improved by use of a reflectance meter. However, the strips only indicate that the glucose is within a low range of values and any low reading must always be confirmed by laboratory measurement.

If the cause of the hypoglycaemia is unknown, it is vital that blood is collected at the time of the hypoglycaemia and the first available urine sent for analysis so that a valuable opportunity for making the diagnosis is not missed (Fig. 23.12).

Causes

These are listed in Figure 23.13.

Ketotic hypoglycaemia is a poorly defined entity in which young children readily become hypoglycaemic following a short period of starvation, probably due to limited reserves for gluconeogenesis. The child is often short and thin and the insulin levels are low. Regular snacks and extra glucose drinks when ill will usually prevent hypoglycaemia. The condition resolves spontaneously in later life. A number of rare endocrine and metabolic disorders may present with hypoglycaemia at almost any age in childhood. Hepatomegaly would suggest the possibility of an inherited glycogen storage

---

Fig. 23.12 Tests to perform when hypoglycaemia is present.

Blood
1. Confirm hypoglycaemia with laboratory blood glucose
2. Growth hormone, cortisol, insulin, C-peptide
   Fatty acids, acetoacetate, 3-hydroxybutyrate, glycerol, branched-chain amino acids
   Glucose, lactate, pyruvate

First urine after hypoglycaemia
Dicarboxylic acids, glycine conjugates, carnitine derivatives
Consider saving blood and urine for toxicology, e.g. salicylate, sulphonylurea

---

Fig. 23.13 Causes of hypoglycaemia beyond the neonatal period.

Fasting
Insulin excess

Excess exogenous insulin, e.g. in diabetes mellitus/surreptitious
β-cell tumours/disorders – persistent hypoglycaemic hyperinsulinism of infancy (PHHI, nesidioblastosis), insulinoma
Drug-induced (sulphonylurea)
Autoimmune (insulin receptor antibodies)
Beckwith's syndrome

Without hyperinsulinaemia

Liver disease
Ketotic hyoglycaemia of childhood
Inborn errors of metabolism, e.g. glycogen storage disorders
Hormonal deficiency: GH↓, ACTH↓, Addison's disease, congenital adrenal hyperplasia

Reactive/non-fasting
Galactosaemia
Leucine sensitivity
Fructose intolerance
Maternal diabetes
Hormonal deficiency
Aspirin/alcohol poisoning

disorder, in which hypoglycaemia can be profound. Persistent hypoglycaemic hyperinsulinism of infancy (PHHI, which used to be called nesidioblastosis) is a rare problem of infancy where there is a mutation of ion channels causing dysregulation of insulin release by the islet cells of the pancreas, leading to profound non-ketotic hypoglycaemia.

Treatment

Hypoglycaemia can usually be corrected with an intravenous infusion of glucose (2–4 ml/kg of 10% dextrose). Care must be taken to avoid giving an excess volume as the solution is hypertonic. If there is delay in establishing an infusion or failure to respond, glucagon is given intramuscularly (0.5–1 mg).

Corticosteroids may also be used if there is a possibility of hypopituitarism or hypoadrenalism. The correction of hypoglycaemia must always be documented with satisfactory laboratory glucose measurements.

 Low blood glucose on Stix testing must be confirmed by laboratory measurement.

HYPOTHYROIDISM

There is minimal thyroxine transfer from the mother to the fetus, although severe maternal hypothyroidism can affect the developing brain. The fetal thyroid predominantly produces 'reverse T_3', a derivative of T_3 which is largely inactive. After birth there is a surge in the level of thyroid-stimulating hormone (TSH) which is accompanied by a marked rise in T_4 and T_3 levels. The TSH declines to the normal adult range within a week. Preterm infants may have very low levels of T_4 for the first few weeks of life whilst the TSH is within the normal range; under these circumstances, additional thyroxine is not required.

Congenital hypothyroidism

Detection of congenital hypothyroidism is important, as it is:

- relatively common, occurring in 1 in 4000 births
- one of the few preventable causes of severe learning difficulties.

Causes of congenital hypothyroidism are:
- Maldescent of the thyroid and athyrosis – the commonest cause of sporadic congenital hypothyroidism. In early fetal life, the thyroid migrates from a position at the base of the tongue (sublingual) to its normal site below the larynx. The thyroid may fail to develop completely or partially. In maldescent, the thyroid remains as a lingual mass or a thyroglossal cyst. The reason for this failure of formation or migration is not well understood.
- Dyshormonogenesis, an inborn error of thyroid hormone synthesis, in about 5% of cases, although commoner in some ethnic groups with consanguineous marriage
- Iodine deficiency, the commonest cause of congenital hypothyroidism worldwide but rare in the UK. It can be prevented by iodination of salt in the maternal diet.
- Hypothyroidism due to TSH deficiency – isolated TSH deficiency is rare (<1% of cases) and is usually associated with panhypopituitarism, which usually manifests with growth hormone and adrenocorticotrophic hormone (ACTH) deficiency before the hypothyroidism becomes evident.

The clinical features (Figs 23.14 and 23.15) are difficult to differentiate from normal in the first month of life but become more prominent with age. Fortunately, most affected infants are now identified by routine

Fig. 23.14 Clinical features of hypothyroidism.	
Congenital	**Acquired**
Failure to thrive	Short stature/growth failure
Feeding problems	Cold intolerance
Prolonged jaundice	Dry skin
Constipation	Cold peripheries
Pale, cold, mottled dry skin	Bradycardia
Coarse facies	Thin, dry hair
Large tongue	Pale, puffy eyes with loss of eyebrows
Hoarse cry	Goitre
Goitre (occasionally)	Slow-relaxing reflexes
Umbilical hernia	Constipation
Delayed development	Growth/short stature
	Delayed puberty
	Obesity
	Slipped upper femoral epiphysis
	Deterioration in school work
	Learning difficulties

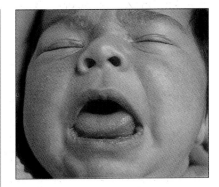

Fig. 23.15 Untreated congenital hypothyroidism.

neonatal biochemical screening (Guthrie test) for raised TSH levels in the blood (some countries also measure T_4) and treatment is usually started before 3 weeks of age. There is a slight excess of other congenital abnormalities, especially heart defects.

Early treatment is essential to prevent learning difficulties. With neonatal screening the results of long-term intellectual development have been satisfactory and intelligence should be in the normal range for the majority of children. Treatment is lifelong with oral replacement of thyroxine, titrating the dose to maintain normal growth, TSH and T_4 levels.

 Although congenital hypothyroidism is present antenatally, treatment started soon after birth results in satisfactory intellectual development.

Juvenile hypothyroidism

This is usually caused by autoimmune thyroiditis. Other autoimmune disorders, e.g. diabetes mellitus, may develop, particularly in children with Down's or Turner's syndrome. In some families, Addison's disease may also occur.

The clinical features are listed in Figure 23.14. It is commoner in females. There is growth failure accompanied by delayed bone age. A goitre is often present but this may also be physiological in pubertal girls. Treatment is with thyroxine.

HYPERTHYROIDISM

This usually results from Graves' disease (autoimmune thyroiditis secondary to the production of thyroid-stimulating immunoglobulins (TSIs)). The clinical features are similar to those in adults, although eye signs are less common (Figs 23.16 and 23.17). It is most often seen in teenage girls. The levels of thyroxine (T_4) and/or tri-iodothyronine (T_3) are elevated, TSH levels are suppressed to very low levels. Antithyroid peroxisomal antibodies may also be present which may eventually result in spontaneous resolution of the toxicosis but subsequently cause hypothyroidism.

The first line of treatment is medical, with drugs such as carbimazole or propylthiouracil which interfere with thyroid hormone synthesis. Initially, beta-blockers can be added for symptomatic relief of anxiety, tremor and tachycardia. Medical treatment is given for about 2 years, which should control the thyrotoxicosis, but the eye signs may not resolve. When medical treatment is stopped, 40–75% relapse. A second course of drugs may then be given or surgery in the form of subtotal thyroidectomy will usually result in permanent remission. Radioiodine treatment is simple and is no longer considered to result in later neoplasia. Follow-up is always required as thyroxine replacement is often needed for subsequent hypothyroidism.

Neonatal hyperthyroidism may occur in infants of mothers with Graves' disease from the transplacental transfer of TSIs. Treatment is required as it is potentially fatal but resolves spontaneously with time.

PARATHYROID DISORDERS

Hypoparathyroidism is rare in childhood. Parathormone (PTH) plays a key role in the mobilisation of calcium by osteoclasts and the excretion of phosphate in the urine. In addition to a low serum calcium, there is a raised serum phosphate and a normal alkaline phosphatase. The parathormone level is very low.

Hypoparathyroidism in infants is usually due to a congenital deficiency (DiGeorge's syndrome), associated with thymic aplasia, defective immunity, cardiac defects and facial abnormalities. In older children, hypoparathyroidism is usually an autoimmune disorder associated with Addison's disease.

In *pseudohypoparathyroidism* there is end-organ resistance to the action of parathormone. Serum calcium and phosphate levels are abnormal but the parathormone

---

Fig. 23.16 Clinical features of hyperthyroidism.

Systemic	Eye signs (uncommon in children)
Anxiety, restlessness	Exophthalmos
Increased appetite	Ophthalmoplegia
Sweating	Lid retraction
Diarrhoea	Lid lag
Weight loss	
Rapid growth in height	
Advanced bone maturity	
Tremor	
Tachycardia, wide pulse pressure	
Warm, vasodilated peripheries	
Goitre (bruit)	
Learning difficulties/behaviour problems	
Psychosis	

Fig. 23.17 Exomphalos in Graves' disease.

levels are normal or high. Other abnormalities are short stature, obesity, subcutaneous nodules, short fourth metacarpals and mild learning difficulties. There may be teeth enamel hypoplasia and calcification of the basal ganglia. A related state, in which there are the physical characteristics of pseudohypoparathyroidism but the calcium, phosphate and PTH are all normal, is called *pseudopseudohypoparathyroidism*. There may be a positive family history of both disorders in the same kindred.

Treatment of acute symptomatic hypocalcaemia is with an intravenous infusion of calcium gluconate. The 10% solution of calcium gluconate must be diluted as extravasation of the infusion will result in severe skin damage. Chronic hypocalcaemia is treated with oral calcium and high doses of vitamin D analogues, adjusting the dose to maintain the plasma calcium concentration just below the normal range. Hypercalcuria is to be avoided as it may cause nephrocalcinosis and so the urinary calcium excretion should be monitored.

ADRENAL CORTICAL INSUFFICIENCY

Congenital adrenal hyperplasia is the commonest non-iatrogenic cause of insufficient cortisol and mineralo-corticoid secretion (see Ch. 9).

Primary adrenal cortical insufficiency (Addison's disease) is rare in children. It may result from:

- an autoimmune process, sometimes in association with other autoimmune endocrine disorders, e.g. diabetes mellitus, hypothyroidism, hypoparathyroidism
- haemorrhage/infarction – neonatal, meningococcal septicaemia (usually fatal)
- adrenoleucodystrophy, a rare neurodegenerative disorder
- tuberculosis, now rare.

Adrenal insufficiency may also be secondary to hypopituitarism from hypothalamic–pituitary disease or from hypothalamic–pituitary–adrenal suppression following long-term corticosteroid therapy.

Presentation

Infants present acutely (Fig. 23.18) with a salt-losing crisis, hypotension and/or hypoglycaemia. Dehydration may follow a gastroenteritis-like illness, from which

the child recovers until the next episode. In older children, presentation is usually with chronic ill health and pigmentation (Fig. 23.19).

Diagnosis

This is made by finding hyponatraemia and hyperkalaemia, often associated with a metabolic acidosis and hypoglycaemia. The plasma cortisol is low or normal and the plasma ACTH concentration high (except in hypopituitarism). With an ACTH (Synacthen) test, plasma cortisol concentrations remain low in both primary adrenal failure and in long-standing pituitary/hypothalamic Addison's disease. A normal response excludes adrenal cortical insufficiency.

Management

An adrenal crisis requires urgent treatment with intravenous saline, glucose and hydrocortisone. Long term treatment is with glucocorticoid and mineralocorticoid replacement. The dose of glucocorticoid needs to be increased three to five-fold at times of illness or for an operation. Parents are taught how to inject intramuscular hydrocortisone in an emergency.

A MedicAlert bracelet is advisable for all children at risk of an adrenal crisis (congenital adrenal hyperplasia or Addison's disease).

CUSHING'S SYNDROME

Glucocorticoid excess in children is usually a side-effect of long-term glucocorticoid treatment (IV, oral or, more rarely, inhaled, nasal or topical) for conditions such as the nephrotic syndrome, asthma or bronchopulmonary dysplasia (Figs 23.20 and 23.21). Corticosteroids are potent growth suppressors and prolonged use in high dosage will lead to reduced adult height. This unwanted side-effect of systemic corticosteroids is markedly reduced by taking corticosteroid medication in the morning on alternate days.

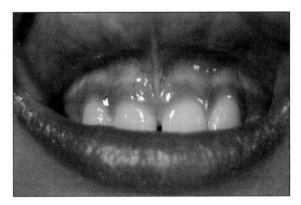

Fig. 23.19 Buccal pigmentation in adrenal cortical insufficiency (Addison's disease). This 9-year-old male presented with salt craving and pigmentation. (Courtesy of Dr Steven Robinson.)

Fig. 23.18 Features of adrenal cortical insufficiency.

Acute	Chronic
Hyponatraemia	Vomiting
Hyperkalaemia	Lethargy
Hypoglycaemia	Brown pigmentation
Dehydration	(gums, scars, skin creases)
Hypotension	Growth failure
Circulatory collapse	

Fig. 23.20 Clinical features of Cushing's syndrome.

Growth failure/short stature	Bruising
Face and trunk obesity	Carbohydrate
Red cheeks	intolerance
Hirsutism	Muscle wasting
Striae	Osteoporosis
Hypertension	Psychological problems

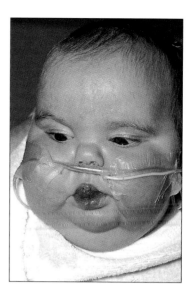

Fig. 23.21 Facial obesity from iatrogenic corticosteroid therapy for bronchopulmonary dysplasia in a preterm infant. Additional oxygen therapy is being given via nasal cannulae.

Other causes of glucocorticoid excess are rare. It may be ACTH-driven, from a pituitary adenoma, usually in older children, or from ectopic ACTH-producing tumours, but these almost never occur in children. ACTH-independent disease is usually from corticosteroid therapy, but may be from adrenocortical tumours (benign or malignant), when there may also be virilisation; these usually occur in young children. A diagnosis of Cushing's syndrome is often questioned in obese children. Most obese children are of above-average height, in contrast to children with Cushing's syndrome, who are short and have growth failure.

If Cushing's syndrome is a possibility then the normal diurnal variation of cortisol (high in the morning, low at midnight) may be shown to be lost – in Cushing's syndrome the midnight concentration is also high. The 24-h urine free cortisol is also high. After the administration of dexamethasone, there is failure to suppress the plasma 09.00 h cortisol levels. Adrenal tumours are identified on CT or MRI scan of the abdomen and a pituitary adenoma on MRI brain scan. Adrenal tumours are usually unilateral and are treated by adrenalectomy and radiotherapy if indicated. Pituitary adenomas are best treated by transsphenoidal resection, but radiotherapy can be used.

INBORN ERRORS OF METABOLISM

Many hundreds of enzyme defects have been identified, mostly with an autosomal recessive inheritance. Individually, they are rare disorders and therefore are often managed in specialist centres.

Presentation

An inborn error of metabolism may be suspected before birth from a positive family history or previous unexplained deaths in the family. In the neonatal period, these disorders must be considered whenever infants become severely ill without an adequate explanation. Other modes of presentation in the neonatal period are:

- poor feeding and failure to thrive with persistent or recurrent vomiting
- jaundice or hepatomegaly
- lethargy, convulsions or coma
- unusual smell of the body or urine.

There may be a severe metabolic acidosis, ketosis or raised plasma ammonia.

In older children, inborn errors of metabolism need to be considered as a cause of:

- unusual odour of the body or urine
- intermittent, unexplained vomiting or coma with acidosis, ketosis or raised ammonia
- children developing coarse facies, dislocated lens, abnormal hair, renal calculi and hypopigmentation
- unexplained learning difficulties, developmental delay or convulsions.

They are diagnosed by measuring the amino acid concentrations in urine and blood and organic acids in the urine. If positive, further detailed investigations are performed.

Disorders of aminoacid metabolism

Phenylketonuria

This occurs in 1 in 10 000–20 000 live births. It is either due to a deficiency of the enzyme phenylalanine-hydroxylase or in the synthesis or recycling of the biopterin cofactor for this enzyme. Untreated, it usually presents with infantile spasms and developmental delay at 6–12 months of age. There may be a musty odour due to the metabolite phenylacetic acid. Many affected children are fair-haired and blue-eyed and some develop eczema. Fortunately, most affected children are detected through the national biochemical screening programme (Guthrie test). The raised plasma phenylalanine is detected at 5–7 days of age when milk feeding has been established.

Treatment is with restriction of dietary phenylalanine, whilst ensuring there is sufficient for optimal physical and neurological growth. The blood plasma phenylalanine is monitored regularly. The recommendation is to continue the diet for at least 10 years, although it is probably best to maintain it throughout life. This is particularly important during pregnancy, when high maternal phenylalanine levels may damage the fetus.

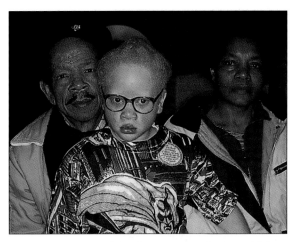

Fig. 23.22 A child with oculocutaneous albinism with her parents.

Co-factor defects are treated with a diet low in phenylalanine and high in neurotransmitter precursors.

Homocystinuria

This is due to cystathionine synthetase deficiency. Presentation is with failure to thrive and developmental delay and subluxation of the ocular lens (ectopia lentis). There is progressive learning difficulty, psychiatric disorders and convulsions. Skeletal manifestations resemble Marfan's syndrome. The complexion is usually fair with brittle hair. Thromboembolic episodes may occur at any age. Almost half respond to large doses of the coenzyme pyridoxine. Those who do not respond are treated with a low-methionine diet supplemented with cysteine.

Albinism

This is due to a defect in biosynthesis and distribution of melanin. The albinism may be oculocutaneous, ocular or partial, depending on the distribution of depigmentation in the skin and eye (Fig. 23.22). The lack of pigment in the iris, retina, eyelids and eyebrows results in failure to develop a fixation reflex. There is pendular nystagmus and photophobia, which causes a constant frowning. No treatment is available, but correction of refractive errors and tinted lenses may be helpful. In a few children, the fitting of tinted contact lenses from early infancy allows the development of normal fixation. The disorder is an important cause of severe visual impairment. The pale skin is prone to sunburn and skin cancer. In sunlight, a hat should be worn and high factor barrier cream applied to the skin.

Tyrosinaemia

Tyrosinaemia (type 1) is a rare autosomal recessive disorder of fumarylacetoacetase. Accummulation of toxic metabolites results in damage to the liver and renal tubules. Effective therapy is available with a drug called NTBC, which inhibits an enzyme required in the catabolism of tyrosine, together with a diet low in tyrosine and phenylalanine.

The organic acidaemias

These are disorders of the catabolic pathways of several essential amino acids (the branched-chain amino acids, leucine, isoleucine and valine, and odd-chain amino acids, e.g. threonine) to cause maple syrup urine disease, methylmalonic acidaemia and propionic acidaemia, among others.

Maple syrup urine disease most often presents in the neonatal period with a severe metabolic acidosis, hypoglycaemia and seizures. There is increased excretion of the branched-chain amino acids – leucine, isoleucine and valine. The urine has a characteristic maple syrup smell. If identified within 24 h, outcome with dietary manipulation may be good, but delay in diagnosis leads to learning difficulties and neurological dysfunction. There remains a high risk of early death during acute illnesses.

The management of the other organic acidaemias centres on the restriction of dietary protein. During acute decompensation, catabolism is limited by a high-carbohydrate, low-protein intake. Acidosis is corrected and hyperammonaemia treated by peritoneal dialysis or haemoperfusion. The outcome is generally poor with significant developmental delay. Some disorders respond to large doses of vitamin co-factors, e.g. vitamin B_{12}.

Urea enzyme defects

Enzyme defects have been identified for all stages of the urea cycle. They tend to cause neonatal encephalopathy from high blood ammonia but the onset may be delayed, when presentation is with coma associated with infection. Ornithine transcarbamylase deficiency is an X-linked disorder, but disorders of the other stages of the urea cycle are autosomal recessive.

Disorders of carbohydrate metabolism

Galactosaemia

This rare, recessively inherited disorder results from deficiency of the enzyme galactose-1-phosphate uridyl transferase, which is essential for galactose metabolism. The inability to mobilise glucose from galactose may result in hypoglycaemia. When lactose-containing milk feeds such as breast or infant formula are introduced, affected infants feed poorly, vomit and develop jaundice and hepatomegaly and hepatic failure (see Ch. 18). Chronic liver disease, cataracts and developmental delay are inevitable if the condition is untreated. Management is with a lactose- and galactose-free diet. Even if treated early, severe learning difficulties are common.

Glycogen storage disorders

These mostly recessively inherited disorders have specific enzyme defects which prevent mobilisation of glucose from glycogen. There is abnormal storage of glycogen. There are nine main enzyme defects, some of which are shown in Figure 23.23. The disorder may

Fig. 23.23 Some of the glycogen storage disorders.

Type	Enzyme defect	Onset	Liver	Muscle	Comments
Type I (von Gierke's)	Glucose-6-phosphatase	Infant	+++	–	See Fig. 23.24. Enlarged liver and kidneys Growth failure. Hypoglycaemia. Good prognosis
Type II (Pompe's)	Lysosomal α-glucosidase	Infant	++	+++	Hypotonia and cardiomegaly at several months. Death from heart failure
Type III (Cori's)	Amylo-1,6-glucosidase	Infant	++	+	Milder features of type I, but muscles may be affected. Good prognosis
Type V (McArdle's)	Phosphorylase	Child	–	++	Temporary weakness and cramps in muscles after exercise. Myoglobinuria in later life

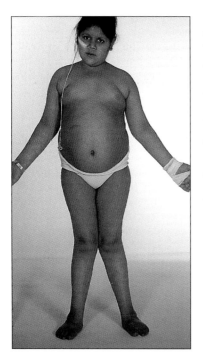

Fig. 23.24 Type I glycogen storage disease in a 12-year-old girl. There is truncal obesity with a distended abdomen from an enlarged liver; short stature and hypotrophic muscles; 'doll' facies; nasogastric feeding to maintain blood glucose levels overnight.

predominantly affect muscle (e.g. types II, V), leading to skeletal muscle weakness. In type II (Pompe's disease) there is generalised intralysosomal storage of glycogen. The heart is severely affected, leading to death from cardiomyopathy. In other types (e.g. I, III) the liver is the main organ of storage, and hepatomegaly and hypoglycaemia are prominent (Fig. 23.24). Long-term complications of type I include hyperlipidaemia, hyperuricaemia, the development of hepatic adenomas and cardiovascular disease.

Management is to maintain blood glucose by frequent feeds or by carbohydrate infusion via a nasogastric tube in infancy. In older children, glucose levels can be maintained using slow-release oligosaccharides (corn starch). In type III disorder, a high-protein diet is required to prevent growth retardation and myopathy.

HYPERLIPIDAEMIA

Hyperlipidaemia is one of the main risk factors for coronary heart disease. Identification and treatment of hyperlipidaemia in childhood may delay the onset of cardiovascular disease in later life.

Children should be screened for hyperlipidaemia if they are at increased risk – if a parent or grandparent has a history of coronary heart disease before 55 years of age or if there is a family history of a lipid disorder. At present, screening all children is not thought justifiable in view of the many uncertainties about selecting who should be treated, what treatment should be given and its effect on outcome.

If the serum cholesterol is high (>5.3 mmol/L) on random testing, fasting serum cholesterol, triglyceride and low-density lipoprotein (LDL) and high-density lipoprotein (HDL) cholesterol are measured. Secondary causes of hypercholesterolaemia should be considered, such as obesity, hypothyroidism, diabetes mellitus, nephrotic syndrome and obstructive jaundice.

Familial hypercholesterolaemia (FH)

This autosomal dominant disorder of lipoprotein metabolism is due to a defect in the LDL receptor. About 1 in 500 of the population are affected. The serum LDL cholesterol concentration is markedly raised (>3.3 mmol/L). The condition is associated with premature coronary heart disease, which occurs in half by 50 years of age in males and by 60 years in females. Skin and tendon xanthomata (Fig. 23.25) may be present, but are uncommon in childhood. Drug therapy is considered in children aged 10 years and older and depends on how high the LDL cholesterol concentration is raised, if there is a family history of premature

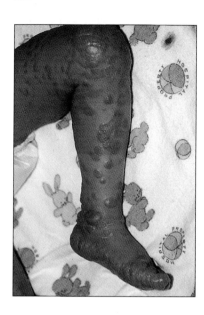

Fig. 23.25 Severe skin xanthomata. In this child it was secondary to liver failure and resolved within weeks of liver transplantation.

coronary heart disease (<55 years of age), if there is evidence of tissue lipid deposition (xanthomata or bruits) and other non-lipid risk factors, e.g. diabetes. The main drugs used are the non-systemically acting bile acid sequestrants and more recently the HMG-CoA reductase inhibitors, the statins. Although bile acid sequestrants are moderately effective, compliance remains a major problem with them. Statins have been shown to the effective in children without adverse effects on growth, maturation or endocrine function. The fibrate drug fenofibrate has also been shown to reduce LDL cholesterol and to be well tolerated by children and adolescents.

Homozygous disease is very rare and much more severe, causing xanthomata in childhood and clinical cardiovascular disease in the second decade. They require referral to a specialist centre. Response to drugs is variable depending on the gene mutation. Liver transplantation has been tried.

FURTHER READING

Brook C D G (ed) 1995 Clinical paediatric endocrinology, 3rd edn. Blackwell, Oxford
Nyhan W L, Ozand P T (eds) 1998 Atlas of metabolic diseases. Chapman & Hall Medical, London
Wales J K H, Rogol A D, Wit J M 1996 Color atlas of paediatric endocrinology and growth. Mosby, London

24

Bones and joints

CHAPTER CONTENTS

- Variations of normal posture
- Disorders of the hip, knee and feet
- Disorders of the back, spine and neck
- The painful limb
- Arthritis
- Genetic skeletal dysplasias

VARIATIONS OF NORMAL POSTURE

These are common and may be noticed by parents or on routine developmental surveillance. Most resolve without any treatment, but any that are severe, persistent, painful or asymmetrical should be referred for a specialist opinion.

Bow legs (genu varum)

This is bowing of the tibiae causing the knees to be wide apart while standing with the feet together (Fig. 24.1). It is common in toddlers and children up to 3 years of age and seldom needs treatment. Another cause of bow legs is rickets. It can be demonstrated on an X-ray of the metaphyses. Marked bow legs may also occur in Blount's disease (infantile tibia vara), an uncommon condition predominantly seen in Afro-Caribbean children. There is beaking of the proximal medial tibial epiphysis on X-ray. Orthoses (splints and special footwear) and surgical correction may be required.

Knock-knees (genu valgum)

In this condition, the feet are wide apart when standing with the knees held together (Fig. 24.2). It is seen in many children between 2 and 7 years of age and usually resolves.

Flat feet (pes planus)

Toddlers learning to walk usually have flat feet due to flatness of the medial longitudinal arch and the presence of a fat pad which subsequently disappears (Fig. 24.3). Most people develop a medial longitudinal arch; although some do not, this is rarely troublesome. An arch can usually be demonstrated on standing on tiptoe. Marked flat feet can be the presentation of a collagen disorder such as Ehlers–Danlos syndrome. Some children with flat feet develop a prominence of the navicular bone on the medial aspect of the foot which resolves, but modification of the child's shoes or an arch support may be required. This will provide

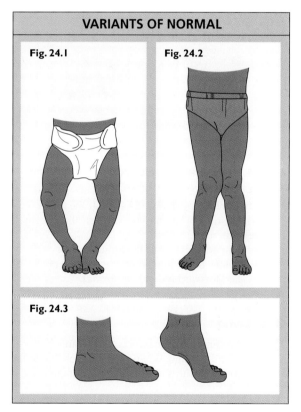

VARIANTS OF NORMAL

Fig. 24.1

Fig. 24.2

Fig. 24.3

Fig. 24.1 Bow legs.
Fig. 24.2 Knock-knees.
Fig. 24.3 Pes planus showing the flat feet of toddlers. The medial longitudinal arch appears on standing on tiptoe.

symptomatic relief but does not influence outcome. Surgery for flat feet is only indicated in symptomatic adolescents.

In-toeing

There are three main causes:

- metatarsus varus (Fig. 24.4a) – an adduction deformity of a highly mobile forefoot

353

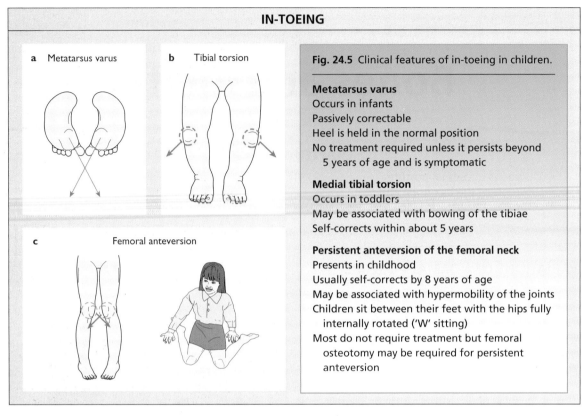

IN-TOEING

a Metatarsus varus

b Tibial torsion

c Femoral anteversion

Fig. 24.5 Clinical features of in-toeing in children.

Metatarsus varus
Occurs in infants
Passively correctable
Heel is held in the normal position
No treatment required unless it persists beyond
  5 years of age and is symptomatic

Medial tibial torsion
Occurs in toddlers
May be associated with bowing of the tibiae
Self-corrects within about 5 years

Persistent anteversion of the femoral neck
Presents in childhood
Usually self-corrects by 8 years of age
May be associated with hypermobility of the joints
Children sit between their feet with the hips fully
  internally rotated ('W' sitting)
Most do not require treatment but femoral
  osteotomy may be required for persistent
  anteversion

Fig. 24.4 In-toeing (a) at the feet, (b) lower leg, (c) hip, with 'W' sitting.

- medial tibial torsion (Fig. 24.4b) – at the lower leg, when the tibia is laterally rotated less than normal in relation to the femur
- persistent anteversion of the femoral neck (Fig. 24.4c) – at the hip, when the femoral neck is twisted forward more than normal.

Their clinical features are described in Figure 24.5.

Out-toeing

This is uncommon but may occur in infants between 6 and 12 months of age. When bilateral, it is due to lateral rotation of the hips and resolves spontaneously.

Toe walking

This is common in 1 to 3-year-old children. It may become persistent, usually from habit, but may be due to mild cerebral palsy. It may also be due to isolated tightness of the Achilles tendons. In older boys, Duchenne's muscular dystrophy should be excluded.

DISORDERS OF THE HIP, KNEE AND FEET

 Limp

Developmental dysplasia of the hip may be detected on routine examination of the newborn infant. Beyond infancy, hip disorders usually present with a limp, which may be painful or painless (Fig. 24.6). They may also present with referred pain in the knee.

Developmental dysplasia of the hip (DDH) (previously called congenital dislocation of the hip; CDH)

This is a spectrum of disorders ranging from dysplasia to subluxation through to frank dislocation of the hip. Early detection is important as it usually responds to conservative treatment; late diagnosis is usually associated with hip dysplasia which requires complex treatment often including surgery. Neonatal screening is performed as part of the routine examination of the newborn, checking if the hip can be dislocated posteriorly out of the acetabulum (Barlow's manoeuvre) or can be relocated back into the acetabulum on abduction (Ortolani's manoeuvre), as described on page 117. These tests are repeated at routine surveillance at 6 weeks of age. Thereafter, presentation of the condition may be with detection of asymmetry of skinfolds around the hip, limited abduction of the hip, shortening of the affected leg or a limp or abnormal gait.

On neonatal screening, an abnormality of the hip is detected in about 6–10 per 1000 live births. Most will resolve spontaneously. The true birth prevalence of DDH is about 1.5 per 1000 live births. Clinical neonatal screening misses some cases. This may be because of inexperience of the examiner, but in some cases it is not possible to clinically detect dislocation at this stage, e.g. where there is only a mildly shallow acetabulum. For this reason, some centres perform ultrasound

Fig. 24.6 Causes of limp.

Age	Painful limp	Painless limp
1–3 years	Septic arthritis/osteomyelitis Transient synovitis Trauma – accidental/non-accidental	Developmental dysplasia of the hip Neuromuscular, e.g. cerebral palsy Unequal leg length Juvenile idiopathic arthritis (JIA)
3–10 years	Transient synovitis Septic arthritis/osteomyelitis Trauma Juvenile idiopathic arthritis (JIA) Perthes disease (acute) Malignant disease, e.g. leukaemia	Perthes disease (chronic) Developmental dysplasia of the hip Neuromuscular disorders, e.g. Duchenne's muscular dystrophy Juvenile idiopathic arthritis (JIA)
11–16 years	Slipped upper femoral epiphysis (acute) Juvenile idiopathic arthritis (JIA) Trauma Septic arthritis/osteomyelitis Bone tumours	Slipped upper femoral epiphysis (chronic) Juvenile idiopathic arthritis (JIA) Dysplastic hip

screening on all newborn infants, which is highly specific in detecting the condition but is expensive and has a high rate of false positives.

If developmental dysplasia of the hip is suspected, a specialist orthopaedic opinion should be obtained. An ultrasound examination allows detailed assessment of the hip, quantifying the degree of dysplasia and whether there is subluxation or dislocation. This information also helps in planning management and in avoiding unnecessary treatment. If the initial ultrasound is abnormal, the infant may be placed in a positioning device, which puts the hips in abduction (e.g. Craig splint), or in a restraining device (e.g. Pavlik harness (Fig. 24.7) for several months. Progress needs to be monitored by ultrasound or X-ray. The splinting must be done expertly, as necrosis of the femoral head is a potential complication.

In most instances, a satisfactory response is obtained. If the hip has not stabilised or the condition is diagnosed late, hip abduction using traction and a further period of splinting (in a plaster hip spica) may be tried. If unsuccessful, an MRI or CT scan of the hip and/or an arthrogram will provide more detailed information of the joint. Weight-bearing on a dislocated hip should be avoided as it causes damage to the femoral head and acetabulum. Open reduction and derotation femoral osteotomy will be required if conservative measures fail.

Transient synovitis (TS, irritable hip)

This is the most common cause of acute hip pain in children. It occurs in children of 2–12 years old. It often follows or is accompanied by a viral infection. Presentation is with sudden onset of pain in the hip or a limp. There is no pain at rest, but there is decreased range of movement, particularly external rotation. The

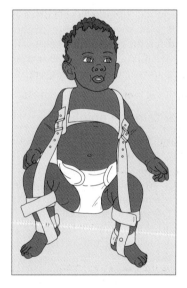

Fig. 24.7
Pavlik harness used to treat developmental dysplasia. It holds the hip abducted, allowing the hip joint to develop normally.

pain may be referred to the knee. The child is afebrile or has a mild fever and does not appear ill.

The neutrophil count and acute-phase reactants are normal or slightly raised. Blood cultures are negative and the X-ray of the joint is normal, but there may be a small joint effusion on ultrasound.

This contrasts with septic arthritis, when the child has a high fever and looks unwell, there is pain at rest and minimal or no movement of the hip. The neutrophil count and acute-phase reactants are markedly raised. If there is any suspicion of septic arthritis, the joint is aspirated under ultrasound guidance. In a small proportion of children, transient synovitis is found to be the presentation of Perthes disease or of slipped upper femoral epiphysis. Management of transient synovitis is with bed rest and skin traction. It usually improves within a few days.

Perthes disease

This is due to ischaemia of the femoral epiphysis, resulting in avascular necrosis, followed by revascularisation and reossification over 18–36 months. It mainly affects boys (male:female ratio of 5:1) of 5–10 years of age. Presentation is insidious, with the onset of a limp or hip pain. The condition may initially be mistaken for transient synovitis. It is bilateral in 10–20%. X-rays show increased density in the femoral head, which subsequently becomes fragmented and irregular (Fig. 24.8). Even if the initial X-ray is normal, a repeat may be required if clinical symptoms persist. A bone scan and MRI scan can be helpful in making the diagnosis.

In most children, the prognosis is good, particularly in those below 6 years of age with less than half the epiphysis involved. When over half the epiphysis is affected and the child is over 6 years old, deformity of the femoral head and metaphyseal damage are more likely, resulting in subsequent degenerative arthritis in adult life. If the condition is identified early and less than half the femoral head is affected, only bed rest and traction may be required. In more severe disease, the femoral head needs to be covered by the acetabulum to act as a mould for the reossifying epiphysis. This is achieved by maintaining the hip in abduction with plaster or calipers or by performing femoral or pelvic osteotomy.

Slipped upper femoral epiphysis

There is displacement of the epiphysis of the femoral head postero-inferiorly. It is most common at 10–15 years of age during the adolescent growth spurt, particularly in obese boys. Skeletal maturation may be found to be delayed. Presentation is with a limp or hip pain, which may be referred to the knee. There is restricted abduction and internal rotation of the hip. The onset may be acute, following minor trauma. In 20% it is bilateral. The diagnosis is confirmed on X-ray (Fig. 24.9), although a frog lateral view is sometimes required. Management is surgical, usually with pin fixation in situ. Severe slips may require subsequent corrective realignment osteotomy once the epiphysis has fused or, rarely, open reduction of the hip, but this carries a risk of avascular necrosis.

The painful knee

When assessing a painful knee, the hip must always be examined, as hip pain is often referred to the knee.

Osgood–Schlatter disease

This is an overuse syndrome commonly occurring in physically active males around puberty, resulting in detachment of cartilage fragments from the tibial tuberosity (traction apophysitis). There is localised tenderness and swelling over the tibial tubercle. The disease is bilateral in 25–50%. Most resolve with reduced physical activity, trying to avoid over-restriction for a disorder which is self-limiting. A knee immobiliser splint may be helpful. In some patients the disorder fails to resolve over several months; a period of immobilisation or, rarely, excision of the ossicle may then be required.

Chondromalacia patellae

In this condition there is softening of the articular cartilage of the patella. It most often affects adolescent females, causing pain when the patella is tightly apposed to the femoral condyles, as in standing up from sitting or on walking up stairs. Treatment is with rest and physiotherapy for quadriceps muscle strengthening.

Osteochondritis dissecans

Pain is caused by separation of bone and cartilage from the medial femoral condyle following avascular necrosis. Complete separation of articular fragments may result in loose body formation. Treatment is initially with rest and quadriceps exercises; sometimes arthroscopic surgery is required.

Subluxation and dislocation of the patella

Subluxation produces the feeling of instability or giving way of the knee. Treatment is with quadriceps exercises; surgery to realign the pull of the quadriceps on the patellar tendon is occasionally required.

Dislocation of the patella laterally occurs suddenly. Reduction occurs spontaneously or on gentle extension of the knee. An X-ray is required to differentiate loose bodies from bone fracture. Immobilisation, and sometimes surgery, is required.

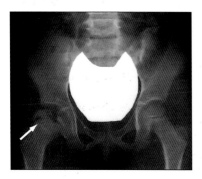

Fig. 24.8 Perthes disease, showing flattening with sclerosis and fragmentation of the right femoral capital epiphysis; the left hip is normal.

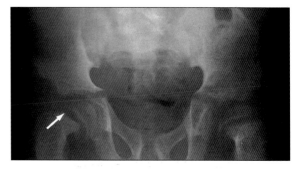

Fig. 24.9 Slipped upper femoral epiphysis of the right hip; the left hip is normal.

Injuries

Contact sports usually result in acute injuries to the knee, while non-contact sports with sustained activity tend to result in chronic injury and overuse syndromes. Sporting injuries to the menisci and ligaments are common in adolescents. MRI scans are helpful to determine the extent of damage. Management is usually conservative. In infants and young children, similar injuries are more likely to result in fractures, as their ligaments are relatively stronger than their bones.

Talipes equinovarus (clubfoot)

Positional talipes from intrauterine compression is common. The foot is of normal size and the deformity is mild and can be corrected to the neutral position with passive manipulation. Often the baby's intrauterine posture can be recreated. If the positional deformity is marked, parents can be shown passive exercises by the physiotherapist.

Talipes equinovarus is a complex abnormality (Figs 24.10 and 24.11). The entire foot is inverted and supinated

and the forefoot is adducted. The heel is rotated inwards and in plantarflexion. The affected foot is shorter and the calf muscles thinner than normal. The position of the foot is fixed and cannot be corrected completely. It is often bilateral. The birth prevalence is 0.9 per 1000 live births, with a sex ratio of males to females of 2:1. It is of multifactorial inheritance, but may also be secondary to oligohydramnios during pregnancy. It may be a feature of a malformation syndrome or of a neuromuscular disorder such as spina bifida. There is an association with developmental dysplasia of the hip (DDH).

Treatment is started promptly, while the tissues are lax, with stretching and strapping or serial plaster casts. If this corrects the disorder, treatment can be discontinued or night splints used. If the condition is severe, corrective surgery is usually necessary. As the results of corrective surgery performed at a few weeks of age have been disappointing, surgery is usually delayed to 6–9 months of age. The condition needs to be differentiated from the rare *congenital vertical talus*, where the foot is stiff and rocker-bottom in shape. Many of these infants have other malformations. The diagnosis can be confirmed on X-ray. Surgery is usually required.

Talipes calcaneovalgus

The foot is dorsiflexed and everted (Fig. 24.12). It usually results from intrauterine moulding and self-corrects. Passive foot exercises are sometimes advised. There is an association with developmental dysplasia of the hip.

Pes cavus

In pes cavus there is a high arched foot. When it presents in older children, it is often associated with neuromuscular disorders, e.g. Friedreich's ataxia and type I hereditary motor sensory neuropathy (peroneal muscular atrophy). Treatment is required if the foot becomes stiff or painful.

DISORDERS OF THE BACK, SPINE AND NECK

Back pain

Back pain is uncommon in pre-adolescent children, becoming more common during adolescence. In contrast to adults, a cause can often be identified, and the younger the child, the more likely it is that there will be significant pathology:

- *muscle spasm* or soft tissue pain from injury, often sport-related
- *poor posture* may accompany hypermobility of the joints
- *Scheuermann's disease* – an osteochondritis of the thoracic vertebrae in adolescents resulting in a fixed kyphosis; diagnosed on X-ray
- *spondylolysis/spondylolisthesis* – stress fracture of the pars interarticularis of the vertebra, typically lower

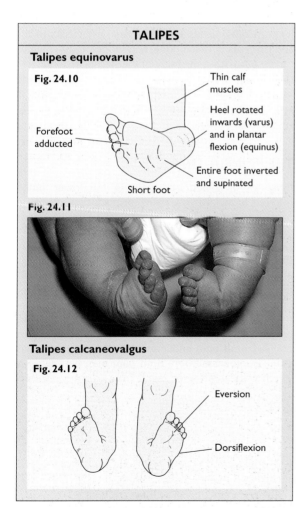

TALIPES

Talipes equinovarus

Fig. 24.10

- Thin calf muscles
- Heel rotated inwards (varus) and in plantar flexion (equinus)
- Forefoot adducted
- Entire foot inverted and supinated
- Short foot

Fig. 24.11

Talipes calcaneovalgus

Fig. 24.12

- Eversion
- Dorsiflexion

Fig. 24.10 Abnormalities in talipes equinovarus.
Fig. 24.11 Talipes equinovarus.
Fig. 24.12 Talipes calcaneovalgus.

lumbar (spondylolysis); if the affected vertebral body moves anteriorly, it produces a spondylolisthesis; diagnosis by X-ray
- *vertebral osteomyelitis/discitis* – often presents in young children with reluctance to walk or bear weight and tenderness over the affected site; while plain X-rays may show abnormalities suggesting the diagnosis, bone and CT scans are the diagnostic investigations of choice
- *tumours* – may be benign or malignant
- *spinal cord/root compression* – e.g. from a tumour or prolapsed intervertebral disc
- *idiopathic pain syndrome* – diagnosed when no physical cause is found; may be exacerbated by psychological stress.

Scoliosis

Scoliosis is a lateral curvature in the frontal plane of the spine. In structural scoliosis, there is rotation of the vertebral bodies which causes a prominence in the back from rib asymmetry. It is a cosmetic problem, but in severe cases can lead to cardiorespiratory failure from distortion of the chest.

Causes of scoliosis are:
- *Idiopathic.* The most common, either early onset (less than 5 years old) or late onset.
- *Congenital.* From a congenital defect of the spine, e.g. hemivertebra, spina bifida, VACTERL association.
- *Secondary.* To other disorders, such as neuromuscular imbalance (e.g. in cerebral palsy, muscular dystrophy, polio) or disorders of bone such as neurofibromatosis or of connective tissues such as Marfan's syndrome. It may be postural in origin such as secondary to leg length discrepancy.

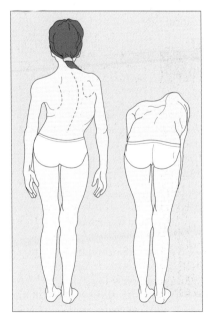

Fig. 24.13 Structural scoliosis with vertebral rotation shown by rib rotation on bending forward.

Early-onset idiopathic scoliosis usually resolves, but a few progress. Late-onset idiopathic scoliosis is the most common type (85%) and mainly affects girls of 10–14 years of age during their pubertal growth spurt.

The scoliosis can be identified on examining the child's back when bent forward (Fig. 24.13). This has been used as a screening test, but it identifies many minor degrees of curvature which resolve spontaneously and does not appear to reduce the need for surgery. For these reasons, routine screening is not currently recommended in the UK. If the scoliosis disappears on forward bending, it is postural and resolves, although leg lengths should be checked. The severity of the curvature of the spine can be determined by measuring the angle of curvature on an X-ray of the spine. Mild scoliosis usually resolves spontaneously. Treatment of severe scoliosis is with spinal braces, although their efficacy is questionable, and sometimes with specialist spinal surgery.

Torticollis

The most common cause of torticollis (wry neck) in infants is a sternomastoid tumour (congenital muscular torticollis). It occurs in the first few weeks of life and presents with a mobile, non-tender nodule, which can be felt within the body of the sternocleidomastoid muscle. There may be restriction of head turning and tilting of the head. The condition usually resolves in 2–6 months. Passive stretching is advised, but its efficacy is unproven.

THE PAINFUL LIMB

Episodes of generalised pain in the lower limbs, referred to as 'growing pains' or nocturnal idiopathic pain, are common in preschool children. The pain often wakes the child from sleep and settles with massage or comforting. It occurs less often during the day, the child is otherwise healthy and there is no evidence of musculoskeletal disease. Children with hypermobility (thumbs and little fingers can be hyperextended onto the forearms (Fig. 24.14); elbows and knees can be hyperextended beyond 10°; hands can be placed flat on the floor with legs straight) often complain of generalised limb pain and may also wake at night with pain. In older children, limb pain may be related to psychological stress or result from overprotection of

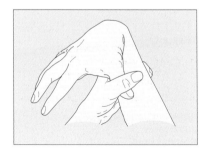

Fig. 24.14 Hypermobility syndrome, showing ability to hyperextend the thumb onto the forearm.

the limb following minor injury. The limb may be held in a splinted position and, in time, localised tenderness, swelling and alteration in colour may develop (reflex sympathetic dystrophy, complex regional pain syndrome) and eventually muscle atrophy.

Limb pain of acute onset has a number of causes. Trauma is the most common, usually accidental from sports injuries or falls, but occasionally non-accidental. Osteomyelitis and bone tumours are uncommon, but need urgent treatment.

Osteomyelitis

In osteomyelitis, there is infection of the metaphysis of long bones. The most common sites are the distal femur and proximal tibia, but any bone may be affected (Fig. 24.15). It is usually due to haematogenous spread of the pathogen, but may arise by direct spread from an infected wound. The skin is swollen directly over the affected site. Where the joint capsule is inserted distal to the epiphyseal plate, as in the hip, osteomyelitis may spread to cause septic arthritis. Most infections are caused by *Staphylococcus aureus*, but other pathogens include *Streptococcus* and *Haemophilus influenzae*. In sickle cell anaemia, there is an increased risk of staphylococcal and salmonella osteomyelitis.

Chronic infection can cause a localised abscess in the bone (Brodie's abscess) but is uncommon. Infection may be from tuberculosis, but this is rare in the UK.

Presentation
This is usually with a markedly painful, immobile limb (pseudoparesis) in a child with an acute febrile illness. Directly over the infected site there is swelling and exquisite tenderness, and it may be erythematous and warm. Moving the limb causes severe pain. There may be a sterile effusion of an adjacent joint. Presentation may be more insidious in infants, in whom swelling or reduced limb movement is the initial sign. Beyond infancy, presentation may be with back pain in a vertebral infection or with a limp or groin pain in infection of the pelvis. Occasionally, there are multiple foci (e.g. disseminated staphylococcal or *H. influenzae* infection).

Investigation
Blood cultures are usually positive and the white blood count and acute-phase reactants are raised. X-rays are initially normal, other than showing soft tissue swelling; it takes 7–10 days for subperiosteal new bone formation and localised bone rarefaction to become visible. The presence and site of infection can usually be identified on a radionuclide bone scan (Fig. 24.16).

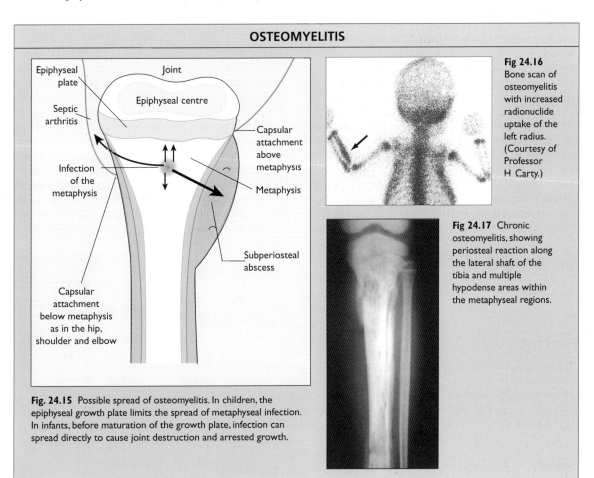

OSTEOMYELITIS

Fig 24.16 Bone scan of osteomyelitis with increased radionuclide uptake of the left radius. (Courtesy of Professor H Carty.)

Fig 24.17 Chronic osteomyelitis, showing periosteal reaction along the lateral shaft of the tibia and multiple hypodense areas within the metaphyseal regions.

Fig. 24.15 Possible spread of osteomyelitis. In children, the epiphyseal growth plate limits the spread of metaphyseal infection. In infants, before maturation of the growth plate, infection can spread directly to cause joint destruction and arrested growth.

Ultrasound may show periosteal elevation at presentation. The X-ray changes of chronic osteomyelitis are shown in Figure 24.17.

Treatment
Prompt treatment with parenteral antibiotics is required for several weeks to prevent bone necrosis, chronic infection with a discharging sinus, limb deformity and amyloidosis. Antibiotics are given intravenously until there is clinical recovery and the acute-phase reactants have returned to normal, followed by oral therapy for several weeks. Aspiration or surgical decompression of the subperiosteal space may be performed if the presentation is atypical or in immunocompromised children. Surgical drainage is performed if the condition does not respond rapidly to antibiotic therapy. The affected limb is initially rested in a splint and subsequently mobilised.

Bone tumours

Malignant tumours – osteogenic sarcoma and Ewing's tumour – are rare. They present with pain or swelling, or occasionally with a pathological fracture (see Ch. 19). Osteoid osteoma is a benign tumour affecting adolescents, especially boys, usually involving the femur or tibia. The pain is more severe at night and improves with salicylate therapy. There may be some localised tenderness. The X-ray is usually diagnostic, with a sharply demarcated radiolucent nidus of osteoid tissue surrounded by sclerotic bone. If the X-ray is normal, a CT or MRI scan is required. Treatment is by surgical removal.

ARTHRITIS

Presentation may be acute when there is a combination of pain, swelling, heat, redness and restricted movement in a joint. It must be distinguished from joint pain (arthralgia). In chronic arthritis there may be insidious onset of early morning stiffness of the joints, 'gelling' after inactivity, the development of a limp or slowness on walking. Initially, there may be only minimal evidence of joint swelling, but subsequently there may be swelling of the joint due to fluid within it (an effusion or pus or blood), inflammation and, in chronic arthritis, proliferation (thickening) of the synovium and swelling of the periarticular soft tissues. Long term, there may be bone expansion from overgrowth, which in the knee may cause leg lengthening and in the wrist advancement of bone age.

In a monoarthritis of acute onset, septic arthritis or osteomyelitis must be diagnosed and treated urgently. Other conditions which need to be considered, using the hip as an example, are listed as causes of a painful limp in Figure 24.6. The causes of polyarthritis are listed in Figure 24.18.

Septic arthritis

This is a serious infection of the joint space as it can lead to bone destruction. It is most common in children less than 2 years old. It usually results from haematogenous spread, but may also occur following a puncture wound or infected skin lesions, e.g. chickenpox. In young children, it may result from spread from adjacent osteomyelitis into joints where the capsule inserts below the epiphyseal growth plate. Beyond the neonatal period, the most common organism is *Staphylococcus aureus*, and usually only one joint is affected. *H. influenzae* was an important cause in young children prior to Hib immunisation and often affected multiple sites.

Presentation
This is usually with an erythematous, warm, acutely tender joint, with a reduced range of movement, in an acutely unwell, febrile child. Infants often hold the limb still (pseudoparesis, pseudoparalysis) and cry if it is moved. A joint effusion may be detectable in peripheral joints. Although a sympathetic joint effusion may be present in osteomyelitis, the tenderness is over the bone. The diagnosis of septic arthritis of the hip can be particularly difficult in toddlers, as the joint is well covered by subcutaneous fat (Fig. 24.19). Initial presentation may be with a limp or pain referred to the knee.

Fig. 24.18 Causes of polyarthritis.

Infection	Bacterial – septicaemia/septic arthritis, TB
	Viral – rubella, mumps, adenovirus, Coxsackie B, herpes, hepatitis, parvovirus
	Other – *Mycoplasma*, Lyme disease, rickettsia
	Reactive – gastrointestinal infection, streptococcal infection
	Rheumatic fever
Inflammatory bowel disease	Crohn's disease, ulcerative colitis
Vasculitis	Henoch–Schönlein purpura, Kawasaki's disease
Haematological disorders	Haemophilia, sickle cell disease
Malignant disorders	Leukaemia, neuroblastoma
Connective tissue disorders	Juvenile idiopathic arthritis (JIA), juvenile ankylosing spondylitis, systemic lupus erythematosus (SLE), dermatomyositis, mixed connective tissue disease (MCTD), polyarteritis nodosa (PAN)
Other	Cystic fibrosis

Investigation

There is an increased white cell count and acute-phase reactants. Ultrasound of deep joints, such as the hip, is helpful to identify an effusion. X-rays are used to exclude trauma and other bony lesions. In septic arthritis, the X-rays are initially normal, apart from widening of the joint space and soft tissue swelling. A bone scan may be helpful. Aspiration of the joint space under ultrasound guidance may reveal organisms and a positive culture in some but not all instances. A prolonged course of antibiotics, initially intravenously (e.g. flucloxacillin, which in young children is combined with a third-generation cephalosporin to cover *H. influenzae*), should be given. Washing out of the

joint or surgical drainage may be required if resolution does not occur rapidly or if the joint is deep-seated, such as the hip. The joint is initially immobilised in a functional position, but subsequently must be mobilised to prevent permanent deformity.

 Early treatment of septic arthritis is essential to prevent destruction of the articular cartilage and bone.

Juvenile idiopathic arthritis (juvenile chronic arthritis)

Juvenile idiopathic arthritis (JIA), until recently called juvenile chronic arthritis (JCA), is a group of conditions in which there is chronic arthritis lasting more than 6 weeks, presenting before 16 years of age. JIA is classified according to its onset as systemic, polyarticular (more than four joints) and pauci/oligoarticular (up to and including four joints). It is further classified according to the presence of antinuclear antibodies (ANA), HLA-B27 and rheumatoid factor and clinical examination (Fig. 24.20). Infection and other causes of arthritis must be excluded.

Systemic arthritis (Still's disease)

This usually affects young children. Clinical features are:

- acute illness, marked malaise
- high, spiking fever
- anorexia, weight loss
- salmon-pink rash at the height of the fever
- aches and pains in the joints and muscles (arthralgia/myalgia), but there is often no arthritis at presentation

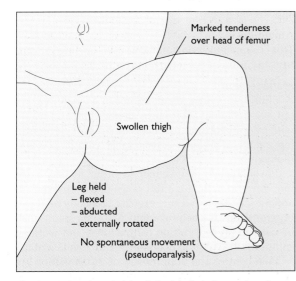

Fig. 24.19 Septic arthritis of the hip in infants, showing the characteristic posture to reduce intracapsular pressure. Any leg movement is painful and is resisted.

JUVENILE IDIOPATHIC ARTHRITIS

Fig. 24.20 Revised classification of juvenile idiopathic arthritis (proposed by the International League of Associations for Rheumatism, ILAR, 1997).

Systemic (9%)
Oligoarthritis
   Persistent (49%)
   Extended (8%)
Polyarthritis (rheumatoid factor (RF)-negative) (16%)
Polyarthritis (rheumatoid factor (RF)-positive) (3%)
Psoriatic arthritis (7%)
Enthesitis-related arthritis (7%)
Other arthritis (1%)

Percentages quoted are for the UK
(ARC/British Paediatric Rheumatology Group)

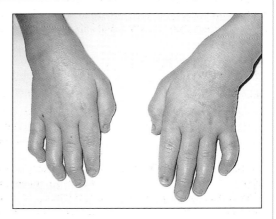

Fig. 24.21 Polyarticular juvenile idiopathic arthritis, showing swelling of the wrists, metacarpal and interphalangeal joints and early swan-neck deformities of the fingers.

- lymphadenopathy, hepatosplenomegaly and occasionally pericarditis
- anaemia, raised neutrophil and platelet count and markedly raised acute-phase reactants.

Some children recover without developing chronic arthritis, others progress to a polyarthritis.

Polyarticular

This occurs at all ages, in girls more than in boys. Any joint may be affected, but most often there is symmetrical involvement of the wrists and hands (Fig. 24.21), knees and ankles. The cervical spine and temporomandibular joint may also be affected.

A few children, usually females in the second decade, can be classified as having juvenile rheumatoid arthritis (JRA). They have a symmetrical polyarthritis, remain rheumatoid factor-positive (seropositive polyarticular) and have a pattern of disease similar to adult rheumatoid arthritis. They may have or develop subcutaneous rheumatoid nodules and over half develop chronic arthritis. Rheumatoid factor may be transiently positive acting as an acute-phase reactant, so the term 'juvenile rheumatoid arthritis' should be reserved for those children with polyarticular disease who remain rheumatoid factor positive.

Pauciarticular/oligoarthritis

This usually occurs in young children, affecting the knees and, less often, the ankles and wrists. There is an increased risk of developing eye disease, a chronic anterior uveitis, especially in females who are ANA-positive. In some of these children, further large joints become involved during the first 6 months; they are categorised as having 'extended oligoarthritis'.

Enthesitis-related arthritis (juvenile spondyloarthropathy, B27-associated arthritis)

This predominantly affects older boys, who present with a large joint arthritis, usually of the lower limbs, or a swollen digit (sausage finger). They may have the HLA-B27 tissue type and a positive family history. In addition, there may be inflammation of the insertion of tendons into bone, e.g. Achilles tendon, and of the plantar fascia (enthesitis). Subsequently there may be sacroiliac and spinal involvement. Acute symptomatic iritis may occur in these children and requires ophthalmological referral, but other complications are rare.

Juvenile psoriatic arthritis

This often involves the interphalangeal joints and may present with a sausage-shaped swelling of a digit. It may occur before the onset of skin lesions or nail pitting. For inclusion in this category, there needs to be either arthritis and psoriasis or arthritis plus two of dactylitis, nail abnormalities or a family history of psoriasis in a first-degree relative.

Other arthritis

This is used when the child's disease does not fit into any of the main defined categories or overlaps more than one category.

Complications

Chronic anterior uveitis

This is asymptomatic but can lead to severe visual impairment. Regular ophthalmological screening is indicated, especially for children with pauciarticular disease.

Flexion contractures of the joints

These occur when the joint is held in the most comfortable position, thereby minimising intra-articular pressure (Fig. 24.22). Chronic disease can lead to joint destruction and the need for joint replacement in a few children.

Growth failure

This may be generalised from anorexia, chronic disease and steroid therapy.

Amyloidosis

This is a rare but serious complication causing proteinuria and subsequent renal failure.

Management

A multidisciplinary team approach is required for optimal treatment and to provide the child and family with information and psychosocial support. Successful management requires considerable compliance and motivation.

Physiotherapy is essential in order to encourage mobility and maintain a full range of joint movement and muscle strength. Daily exercise is usually required. Hydrotherapy is a helpful adjunct. Resting splints may be used to prevent flexion contractures, and working splints for the wrists to maintain posture while writing.

Pain control and suppression of inflammation are provided by non-steroidal anti-inflammatory drugs (NSAIDs), such as naproxen or ibuprofen. Intra-articular corticosteroid therapy can be helpful in both pauciarticular and polyarticular disease. Multiple injections may be required.

Disease-modifying anti-rheumatic drugs are used for persistent active polyarthritis not controlled by

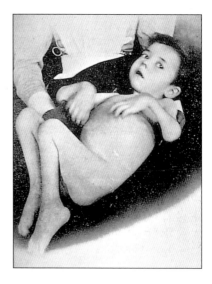

Fig. 24.22 Severe untreated polyarticular or systemic juvenile idiopathic arthritis, from Still's original description in 1897, showing severe misery, fused neck, flexion deformities and wasting of the muscles and subcutaneous tissue.

NSAIDs. Methotrexate is the drug of most benefit, but its short- and long-term side-effects need to be monitored. It can be given by subcutaneous injection if oral therapy is not tolerated. Salazopyrin can be used as a second-line agent in enthesitis-related arthritis and in children who appear to be refractory to therapy with methotrexate and steroids. Cyclosporin represents another therapeutic option. The effectiveness of previously used therapy with gold, penicillamine, hydroxychloroquine and other agents remains unproven and these agents are now seldom used. Systemic corticosteroids may be required for severe uveitis, pericarditis, severe systemic disease or immobility. They may also be needed to control polyarticular disease, using an alternate-day regimen in the lowest dose that is efficacious (see Case history 24.1). High-dose parenteral corticosteroids may be required for an acute exacerbation of joint disease. New therapies undergoing evaluation are anti-TNFα (anti-tumour necrosis factor alpha) and autologous bone marrow transplantation for severe refractory disease.

Although there have been improvements in both the physical and pharmacological management of JIA, and the overall prognosis has improved, some affected children will experience considerable problems through adolescence and into adulthood.

GENETIC SKELETAL DYSPLASIAS

These are generalised developmental disorders of bone, of which there are several hundred types. They usually result in reduced growth and abnormality of bone shape rather than impaired strength, except for osteogenesis imperfecta. The bones of the limbs and spine are often affected, resulting in short stature. Intelligence is usually normal. Improved knowledge of the molecular basis of collagen and its disorders is allowing better understanding and delineation of some of these disorders.

Achondroplasia

Inheritance is autosomal dominant, but about 50% are new mutations. Clinical features are short stature from marked shortening of the limbs, a large head, frontal bossing and depression of the nasal bridge. The hands

CASE HISTORY 24.1

SYSTEMIC-ONSET JUVENILE IDIOPATHIC ARTHRITIS

A 2-year-old boy presented with a high fever (Fig. 24.23a) and malaise. A salmon-coloured rash was present at times of fever (Fig. 24.23b). Investigation showed markedly raised acute-phase reactants. A diagnosis of systemic-onset juvenile idiopathic arthritis was made on the basis of the clinical presentation and exclusion of other disorders (Fig. 24.23c).

Shortly afterwards, he developed polyarthritic joint disease. He required high-dose alternate-day corticosteroid therapy as well as other disease-modifying drugs. He developed marked short stature. In his teens he required bilateral hip replacements. He is now at university, drives his own car and is fiercely independent.

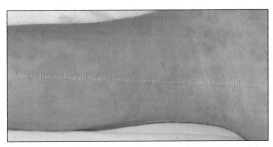

Fig. 24.23b Salmon-pink rash.

Fig. 24.23c Differential diagnosis of systemic-onset juvenile idiopathic arthritis.

Infection – bacterial/viral/protozoal (e.g. malaria), *Mycoplasma* and other (e.g. Lyme disease)
Kawasaki's disease
Rheumatic fever
Reactive arthritis – post-streptococcal, post-enteric, post-viral
Malignancy – leukaemia, neuroblastoma
Connective tissue disorders – systemic lupus erythromatous (SLE), polyarteritis nodosa (PAN)

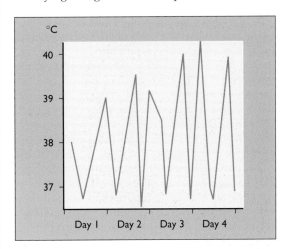

Fig. 24.23a Temperature chart.

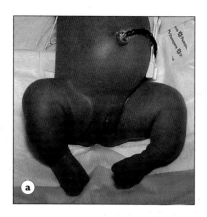
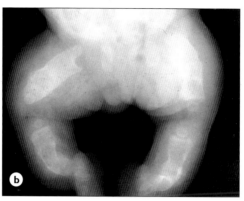

Fig. 24.24 Osteogenesis imperfecta (type II) showing (a) shortened deformed lower limbs, and (b) gross deformity of the bones of the lower limbs with multiple healing fractures.

are short and broad. A marked lumbar lordosis develops. Hydrocephalus sometimes occurs.

Thanatophoric dysplasia

This results in stillbirth. The infants have a large head, extremely short limbs and a small chest. The appearance of the bones on X-ray are characteristic. The importance of the correct diagnosis of this disorder is that, in contrast to achondroplasia, its inheritance is sporadic. It may be identified on antenatal ultrasound.

Cleidocranial dysostosis

In this autosomal dominant disorder, there is absence of part or all of the clavicles and delay in closure of the anterior fontanelle and of ossification of the skull. The child is often able to bring the shoulders together in front of the chest to touch each other as a 'party trick'. Short stature is usually present.

Arthrogryposis

This is a heterogeneous group of congenital disorders in which there is stiffness and contracture of joints. The cause is usually unknown, but there may be an association with oligohydramnios, widespread congenital anomalies or chromosomal disorders. It is usually sporadic. Marked flexion contractures of the knees, elbows and wrists, dislocation of the hips and other joints, talipes equinovarus and scoliosis are common, but the disorder may be localised to the upper or lower limbs. The skin is thin, subcutaneous tissue is reduced and there is marked muscle atrophy around the affected joints. Intelligence is usually unaffected. Management is with physiotherapy and correction of deformities, where possible, by splints, plaster casts or surgery. Walking is impaired in the more severe forms of the disorder.

Osteogenesis imperfecta (brittle bone disease)

This is a group of disorders of collagen metabolism causing bone fragility, with bowing and frequent fractures.

In the most common form (type I), which is autosomal dominant, fractures occur during childhood. Affected children also have a blue appearance to the sclerae and may develop hearing loss. The prognosis is variable. Fractures require splinting to minimise joint deformity.

There is a severe, lethal form (type II) with multiple fractures already present before birth (Fig. 24.24). Many affected infants are stillborn. Inheritance is variable but mostly autosomal dominant or due to new mutations. In other types, scleral discoloration may be minimal. Osteogenesis imperfecta is often considered in the evaluation of unexplained fractures in suspected child abuse.

Osteopetrosis (marble bone disease)

In this rare disorder, the bones are dense but brittle. The severe autosomal recessive disorder presents with failure to thrive, recurrent infection, hypocalcaemia, anaemia and thrombocytopenia. Prognosis is poor, but bone marrow transplantation can be curative. A less severe autosomal dominant form may present during childhood with fractures.

Marfan's sydrome

This is an autosomal dominant disorder of connective tissue associated with tall stature, long thin digits (arachnodactyly), hyperextensible joints, a high arched palate, dislocation (usually upwards) of the lenses of the eyes and severe myopia. The body proportions are altered, with long, thin limbs resulting in a greater distance between the pubis and soles (lower segment) than from the crown to the pubis (upper segment). The arm span, measured from the extended fingers, is greater than the height. There may be chest deformity and scoliosis. The major problems are cardiovascular, due to degeneration of the media of vessel walls resulting in a dilated, incompetent aortic root with valvular incompetence and mitral valve prolapse and regurgitation. Aneurysms of the aorta may dissect or rupture. Monitoring by echocardiography is required.

25

Neurological disorders

CHAPTER CONTENTS

- Headache
- Seizures
- Cerebral palsy
- Ataxia
- Cerebral haemorrhage

- Neural tube defects and hydrocephalus
- Neuromuscular disorders
- The neurocutaneous syndromes
- Neurodegenerative disorders

Key facts about neurological disorders in children are:

- Headaches are common in older children and adolescents.
- Febrile seizures occur in 3% of children.
- Epilepsy affects 1 in 200 children.
- Cerebral palsy usually requires multidisciplinary and multi-agency care.
- The birth prevalence of neural tube defects has markedly declined.
- Neuromuscular and neurodegenerative disorders can now be diagnosed more accurately using modern technology such as DNA analysis, MRI imaging, advanced biochemical techniques and enzyme assays.

HEADACHE

Headaches are common in children. Although infrequent in young children, their frequency increases with age. At least 95% of schoolchildren experience at least one each year, 10% have recurrent tension headaches and 6% migraine They affect females slightly more often than males. The causes of acute headache are listed in Figure 25.1. The causes of recurrent headache are considered below.

Fig. 25.1 Causes of acute headache.

Febrile illness
Migraine
Stress
Acute sinusitis
Meningitis/encephalitis
Head injury
Subarachnoid or intracerebral haemorrhage
Benign intracranial hypertension
Drugs, including alcohol

Tension headache

This is a symmetrical headache of gradual onset, often described as a tightness, a band or pressure. There are usually no other symptoms, but it may be accompanied by abdominal pain and behaviour problems. It may occur every day.

Migraine

This periodic disorder is characterised by paroxysmal headache, often unilateral, accompanied by visual or gastrointestinal disturbance. Rarely, there are unilateral sensory or motor symptoms. The visual disturbances (aura) include:

- hemianopia (loss of half the visual field)
- scotoma (small areas of visual loss)
- fortification spectra (seeing zigzag lines).

The gastrointestinal features may be:
- nausea
- vomiting
- abdominal pain.

The attacks usually last for a few hours, during which time the child prefers to lie down in a quiet, dark place. Sleep often relieves the bout.

Migraine is classified as:
- without aura (formerly called common migraine)
- with aura (formerly called classical migraine) – the headache is preceded by an aura (visual, sensory or motor); this type occurs in about 10% of sufferers (the aura may occur without a headache)
- complicated – associated with neurological phenomena such as ophthalmoplegia, hemiparesis, paraesthesiae or hemidysaesthesia (altered sensation down one side of the body). It occurs in 1–2% of cases and, rarely, results in permanent neurological deficit. Vertebrobasilar migraine may give rise to cerebellar signs, including nystagmus and vomiting with retching.

The symptoms of tension-like headache and migraine often overlap, making it difficult to separate the diagnoses, which may be part of the same pathophysiological spectrum. Half the children with recurrent headaches have an affected first- or second-degree relative. In young children, episodes of nausea, vomiting and recurrent abdominal pain may precede the development of recurrent headaches (abdominal migraine). Stressful situations at home or school may trigger headaches or make them more difficult to cope with. In some people, migraine occurs at times of relaxation, e.g. weekends. Certain foods may trigger headaches – cow's milk, cheese, chocolate, eggs, coffee and the colouring tartrazine. In some girls, headaches are related to menstruation or the oral contraceptive pill.

Raised intracranial pressure

It is the fear of a brain tumour that leads many parents to take their child with headaches to see a doctor. The cardinal feature of an intracranial space-occupying lesion is that the headache is worse when lying down (in contrast to migraine and other headaches when lying down helps) and morning vomiting is characteristic. There may be associated changes in personality and school performance. Headache from raised intracranial pressure is often accompanied by abnormal localising neurological signs:

- growth and visual fields may be affected in craniopharyngioma
- cranial nerve abnormalities in brain stem tumours
- cranial bruits may be heard in arteriovenous–venous malformations but these lesions are rare
- papilloedema, but not always present; it is also seen in benign intracranial hypertension, a syndrome of raised intracranial pressure without any space-occupying lesion or obstruction to the cerebrospinal fluid (CSF) pathways.

Other causes of headache

- *Acute sinusitis* may cause facial pain. Percussion over the affected sinus causes discomfort. Chronic sinusitis may cause 'fuzzy headedness' in the presence of chronic rhinorrhoea.
- *Temporomandibular pain* is a muscle contraction headache. Discomfort is worse on chewing. It is due to dental malocclusion.
- *Ocular headaches* are associated with refractive errors.
- *Head trauma*, even if relatively minor, may be followed by recurrent headaches, particularly in those who are already prone to them.
- *Solvent or drug abuse* in adolescents, or environmental poisoning such as from lead intoxication (very uncommon in the UK).
- *Subclinical seizures* can sometimes cause headaches.
- *Hypertension* in children only causes headaches if severe enough to cause encephalopathy. However, blood pressure should be measured in all children with headaches.

Management of headaches

The mainstay of management is a thorough history and examination with detailed explanation and advice. Investigations are rarely indicated. EEGs do not help with patient management. If there are symptoms or signs of raised intracranial pressure or growth failure, a CT or MRI scan is essential.

Children and parents should be informed that recurrent headaches are common. There are likely to be good and bad patches over months or years but they cause no long-term harm. Written information for the child and parents to take home is helpful. Children should be advised on how to live with and control the headaches, rather than allowing the headaches to dominate their lives. Steps should be taken to reduce stress due to factors such as bullying, anxiety over exams or illness in friends or family. It is usually difficult or impossible to identify specific food triggers, so exclusion diets are rarely beneficial. Relaxation and using other self-regulating techniques may be helpful.

Minor analgesics should be taken as early as possible if the child believes the headache is likely to become severe. When nausea is troublesome, older children may take anti-emetics such as metoclopramide or prochlorperazine. The latter may be used rectally. For migraine, prophylactic therapy should only be used if the above measures are unsuccessful and headaches have become troublesome and intrusive. Pizotifen, a serotonin (5-HT) antagonist, is useful but may cause sleepiness. An alternative is to use β-blockers, such as propranolol, but the dose needs to be higher than for cardiac use and may result in feelings of light-headedness or nightmares. It is contraindicated in children with asthma. For the acute disabling bout of migraine, sumatriptan, a serotonin (5-HT_1) agonist, curtails the period of vasodilatation and associated symptoms.

SEIZURES

A seizure or fit is a clinical event in which there is a sudden disturbance of neurological function in association with an abnormal or excessive neuronal discharge.

A febrile convulsion is a seizure associated with fever in the absence of another cause and not due to intracranial infection from meningitis or encephalitis.

Epilepsy is recurrent seizures other than febrile convulsions in the absence of an acute cerebral insult.

The causes of seizures are listed in Figure 25.2.

Febrile seizures (febrile convulsions)

These occur in about 3% of children, usually between 6 months and 3 years, but up to 6 years of age. There is a genetic predisposition, with 10–20% of relatives having a seizure disorder including febrile convulsions. The seizure usually occurs early in a viral infection when the temperature is rising rapidly. The seizures are usually brief, lasting 1–2 min, and are generalised

Fig. 25.2 Causes of seizures.

Epilepsy
Idiopathic (70–80%)
Secondary
Cerebral dysgenesis/malformation,
e.g. porencephalic cyst, hydrocephalus
Cerebral damage, e.g. congenital infection,
hypoxic–ischaemic encephalopathy,
intraventricular haemorrhage/ischaemia
Cerebral tumour
Neurodegenerative disorders
Neurocutaneous syndromes

Non-epileptic
Febrile convulsions
Metabolic
Hypoglycaemia
Hypocalcaemia/hypomagnesaemia
Hypo/hypernatraemia
Head trauma
Meningitis/encephalitis
Poisons/toxins

tonic or tonic–clonic. They need to be differentiated from rigors triggered by a fever and from reflex anoxic seizures. In about 15% of cases, seizures recur in the same illness. The overall risk of a further febrile convulsion is 1 in 3, and of these a further third will have three or more seizures. The recurrence risk is higher if the onset occurs before the age of 1 year and if there is a positive family history.

Febrile convulsions usually have a benign prognosis; only about 1% of children with febrile convulsions subsequently develop epilepsy. Risk factors for the subsequent development of localisation-related (partial) epilepsy are a prolonged seizure (longer than 30 min), if the seizure is focal or if seizures recur within the same illness.

Management
The immediate management of seizures is described on page 59. In caring for a child with a febrile convulsion, it is essential to be certain that the child does not have meningitis or another serious bacterial infection requiring treatment. Where this cannot be decided on clinical examination with certainty, the child will need an infection screen, including lumbar puncture for CSF examination and a urine sample to identify a urinary tract infection. A lumbar puncture should not be performed on an unconscious child; where central nervous system infection is suspected, blood cultures should be taken and antibiotics started empirically. An EEG is not indicated if the history and clinical findings are typical, as it is neither a useful guide for treatment nor a predictor of seizure recurrence or of subsequent epilepsy.

About 6% of febrile convulsions are prolonged and, as prolonged febrile convulsions may be damaging, they are best prevented. However, in 80% they occur during the first convulsion. During febrile illnesses, parents should be advised to try to keep the temperature low by removing warm clothing, by tepid sponging and giving an antipyretic, e.g. paracetamol or ibuprofen. Parents of children with an increased risk of seizure recurrence should be supplied with rectal diazepam to give for any subsequent seizure lasting longer than 5 min. Prophylactic oral anti-epileptic drugs have been used but there is no good evidence that they lower the risk of recurrence or the subsequent development of epilepsy. Parents should receive written as well as verbal advice on the first aid management of a further convulsion.

Febrile convulsions occur between 6 months and 6 years of age.

Epilepsy
The diagnosis of epilepsy is based on a detailed history, preferably from both an eyewitness of the seizures and the child's own account, as well as clinical examination and EEG findings. If available, a home video of a seizure or suspected seizure is very helpful. Epilepsy needs to be distinguished from other paroxysmal disorders. The seizure type needs to be classified as to whether it is generalised or localisation-related (partial), and any particular epilepsy syndrome identified.

Epilepsy affects 5 per 1000 school-age children, 10% of whom are severely affected. Most epilepsy is idiopathic but other causes are listed in Figure 25.2.

Generalised epilepsies
These are summarised in Figure 25.3.

- Status epilepticus, multiple seizures without recovery of consciousness in between, is described in Chapter 5.
- Absence, tonic or tonic–clonic seizure disorders may remit; identification of the epilepsy syndrome involved allows a more accurate prognosis for the individual.
- The atonic and myoclonic seizures may accompany cerebral dysgenesis or a neurodegenerative disorder and have a poor prognosis.

Localisation-related epilepsies
Localisation-related seizures (formerly known as focal or partial) are summarised in Figure 25.3.

Localisation-related seizures may arise from any of the four brain lobes. *Temporal-lobe epilepsy* is the most common, with strange feelings in the head or abdomen, unusual sensations of taste or smell, distortion of sounds or autonomic symptoms and signs. There may be psychomotor phenomena with lip-smacking, repetitive stereotyped movements such as

A CLASSIFICATION OF EPILEPSY

Generalised epilepsies

Onset in central cerebral structures

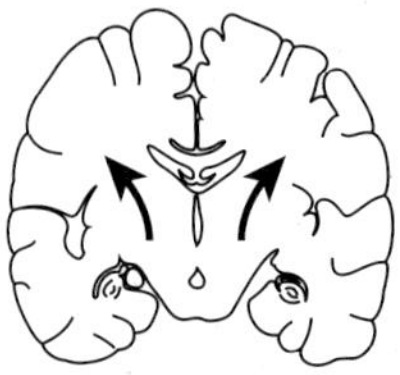

In generalised seizure disorders, there is:
- always a loss of consciousness
- no warning
- symmetrical seizure
- bilaterally synchronous seizure discharge on EEG

Absence seizures ➡ Transient loss of consciousness, with an abrupt onset and termination, unaccompanied by motor phenomena except for some flickering of the eyelids and minor alteration in muscle tone. Absences may be typical (petit mal) or atypical and can often be precipitated by hyperventilation.

Myoclonic seizures ➡ Brief, often repetitive, jerking movements of the limbs, neck or trunk

Tonic seizures ➡ Generalised increase in tone

Tonic–clonic seizures ➡ Rhythmical contraction of muscle groups following the tonic phase.
In the rigid tonic phase, children may fall to the ground, sometimes injuring themselves. They do not breathe and become cyanosed. This is followed by the clonic phase, with jerking of the limbs. Breathing is irregular, cyanosis persists and saliva may accumulate in the mouth. There may be biting of the tongue and incontinence of urine. The seizure usually lasts from a few seconds to minutes, followed by unconsciousness or deep sleep for up to several hours.

Atonic seizures ➡ Often combined with a myoclonic jerk followed by a transient loss of muscle tone causing a sudden fall to the floor or drop of the head.
Non-epileptic myoclonic movements are also seen physiologically in hiccoughs (myoclonus of the diaphragm) or on passing through stage II sleep.

Localisation-related epilepsies (partial seizures)

Onset in one of the cerebral hemispheres

Parietal
Frontal
Temporal
Occipital

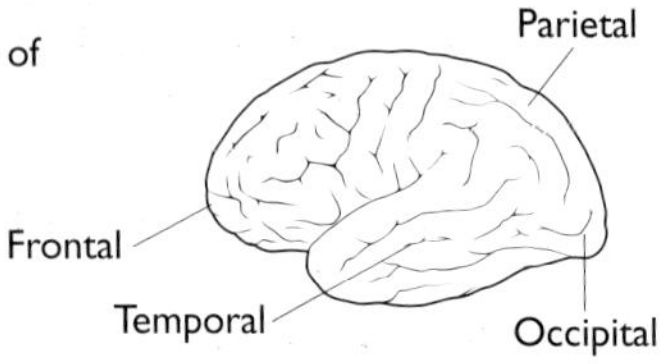

Localisation-related seizures:
- begin in a relatively small group of dysfunctional neurones in one of the cerebral hemispheres
- may be heralded by an aura which reflects the site of origin
- may or may not be associated with change in consciousness or more generalised motor jerking

Simple partial seizure ➡ The child will retain awareness with consciousness unimpaired

Complex partial seizures ➡ Altered conscious state or confusion due to the abnormal electrical discharge spreading from the originating site

Partial seizures with secondary generalisation ➡ Focal seizure manifest clinically or on an ictal EEG following by a generalised tonic–clonic seizure

Epilepsy syndromes

Generalised epilepsies

Infantile spasms
Typical (petit mal) absences
Lennox–Gestaut syndrome
Myoclonic epilepsy of adolescence (juvenile myoclonic epilepsy)

Partial epilepsies

Benign rolandic epilepsy

Fig. 25.3 Classification of epilepsy.

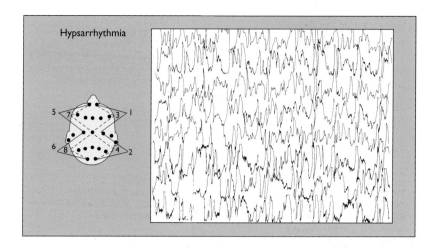

Hypsarrhythmia

Fig. 25.4 EEG of hypsarrhythmia in infantile spasms. There is a chaotic background of slow-wave activity with sharp components.

pulling at clothes, walking in a non-purposeful manner (automatisms), *déjà vu* or *'jamais vu'* phenomena (intense feelings of having, or never having, been in the same situation before) or fright. Consciousness is impaired; the child may just stop and stare as in a typical absence. The episodes usually last a few minutes. The child may not recall the seizure.

Frontal lobe epilepsy, involving the motor cortex, may lead to a simple partial seizure with clonic movements which may travel proximally up the arm (Jacksonian march). A post-ictal (Todd's) paresis may follow. Asymmetrical tonic seizures may also be seen.

Occipital epilepsies give rise to distorted vision, whilst *parietal lobe seizures* cause contralateral dysaesthesias (altered sensation), vertigo or distorted body image.

The diagnosis is suspected from the characteristic history. The EEG can be helpful in looking for abnormal electrical discharges arising most commonly from the temporal lobes, although these cannot always be demonstrated. About 60% will enter adult life seizure-free and off medication, 30% will be prone to seizures but will be controlled on medication, while the remainder will continue to have seizures in spite of medication.

Some common epilepsy syndromes

Generalised epilepsies

Infantile spasms (West syndrome)

Onset is usually between 4 and 6 months of age with violent flexor spasms of the head, trunk and limbs followed by extension of the arms (so-called 'salaam spasms'). The flexor spasms last 1–2 s and are often multiple, occurring in bursts of 20–30 spasms, frequently on waking. The spasms may occur many times a day and may be misinterpreted as colic. Social interaction is impaired, two-thirds of the children are neurologically abnormal before the onset of the seizures, and developmental progress is often then further arrested. The EEG shows hypsarrhythmia, a chaotic background of high-voltage dysrhythmic slow-wave activity with sharp components (Fig. 25.4). Treatment is with vigabatrin or corticosteroids. Their relative efficacy is not well-established from controlled studies. There is a good response in 30–40% of cases, but side-effects are common. Most infants will subsequently show loss of skills and later learning disability or epilepsy.

Typical (petit mal) absence seizures

This accounts for 1–2% of childhood epilepsy. Onset is between 4 and 12 years of age. It is rarely associated with developmental problems. Affected children momentarily stare and stop moving, although they may twitch their eyelids or a hand minimally. The episodes last only a few seconds and certainly not longer than 30 s. Afterwards the child is immediately able to continue the conversation or action which was interrupted by the seizure. Affected children have no recall of the seizure except that they may realise that they have missed something during the absence and so many look puzzled or say 'pardon' on regaining consciousness.

The episodes can be induced by hyperventilation, which is a useful test in the outpatient clinic. The EEG shows three per second spike and wave discharge, which is bilaterally synchronous during and sometimes between attacks (Fig. 25.5). The prognosis is good with 95% remission in adolescence.

Lennox–Gastaut syndrome

This affects children of 1–3 years of age who have myoclonic episodes with single jerks, atonic drop attacks or atypical absences accompanied by neurodevelopmental arrest or regression and behaviour disorder. Prognosis is poor.

Myoclonic epilepsy of adolescence (juvenile myoclonic epilepsy)

This usually presents between the ages of 10 and 20 years, with females affected twice as often as males. There may be a family history. Myoclonic seizures predominate but absences and tonic–clonic seizures also occur. They are most evident shortly after waking. Learning is unimpaired. The response to treatment is usually good.

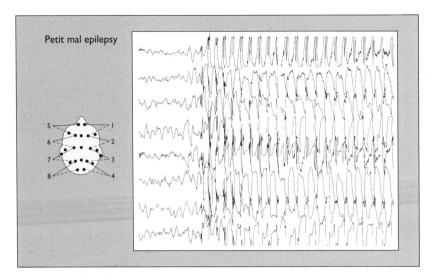

Petit mal epilepsy

Fig. 25.5 EEG in a typical absence (petit mal) seizure. There is three per second spike and wave discharge which is bilaterally synchronous during, and sometimes between, attacks.

Localisation-related epilepsies
Benign rolandic epilepsy of childhood

This is the most common benign epilepsy in childhood. It is important to recognise, as the seizures usually stop by the mid-teens and may not require treatment. Seizures often occur during sleep when they are generalised tonic–clonic; those during the day are heralded by distortion of the face and arm on one side, associated with an abnormal feeling of the tongue. Rolandic spike wave activity is seen in the centrotemporal area on the EEG.

Investigation of seizures

An EEG is indicated whenever epilepsy is suspected. If the standard EEG is normal, an abnormality may be revealed from a barbiturate-induced sleep or sleep-deprivation recording, or 24-h ambulatory monitoring.

CT or MRI brain scans may be indicated, particularly for young children (less than 5 years old) or where the seizures are drug-resistant, when a demonstrable localised brain abnormality is more likely. If there are interictal neurological signs, especially if these are focal, a brain scan should be carried out to exclude a tumour or vascular lesion which could be treatable.

In some circumstances, metabolic investigation may be required to identify the underlying disorder.

Management

Management begins with explanation, education and advice to help with adjustment to the diagnosis. A diagnosis of epilepsy does not automatically mean that the child requires anticonvulsant therapy. The decision to treat should be based on the frequency and nature of the seizures and the social or educational consequences of having further seizures. If there is no demonstrable cause for the first seizure, it is usual to wait before starting anticonvulsant therapy. There are differences of opinion about the choice of anticonvulsant therapy; a scheme for particular seizure types is shown in Figure 25.6. All anti-epileptic drugs have unwanted effects (Fig. 25.7), but these can be kept to a minimum through knowledge of how to introduce, use and modify dosages. Single drug therapy, using the minimum dose, is used where possible. Sometimes two or more anticonvulsants are required. Sugar-free preparations are used. Serum anticonvulsant levels are not routinely measured but can be useful:

- if toxicity is suspected
- to check compliance
- when high drug doses are used
- with multiple drug therapy
- in children who are severely disabled, when toxicity is difficult to recognise.

Fig. 25.6 Choice of anticonvulsants.

Seizure type	1st choice	2nd choice
Generalised epilepsies		
Tonic–clonic	Valproate, carbamazepine	Lamotrigine
Absence	Valproate	Lamotrigine, ethosuximide
Myoclonic	Valproate	Lamotrigine, clobazam, clonazepam
Partial epilepsies	Carbamazepine, valproate	Gabapentin, topiramate, lamotrigine, vigabatrin

Fig. 25.7 Some side-effects of anticonvulsants.

Drug	Side-effects
Valproate	Increased appetite and weight Transient hair loss Idiosyncratic liver failure
Carbamazepine	Lupus erythematosus syndrome Dizziness, visual disturbance
Vigabatrin	Behaviour disturbance, retinopathy Confusion, sleepiness, weight gain
Lamotrigine	Rash, behaviour disturbance, irritability
Ethosuximide	Blood dyscrasia
Topiramate	Sleepiness, anorexia
Gabapentin	Insomnia

All the above may cause drowsiness and occasional skin rashes. Liver enzyme induction, which can interfere with other medication, may occur with carbamazepine.

However, serum levels do not necessarily reflect those in the brain. In general, anticonvulsant therapy may be withdrawn slowly after 2 years free of seizures.

Seizures may be provoked by sleep, alcohol, drugs, excitement, anxiety, menstruation or too rapid withdrawal of anticonvulsant drugs. Children with photosensitive epilepsy should watch TV from a distance, in a well-lit room and with one eye covered when approaching the set. In children with intractable seizures, cure or considerable improvement can occasionally be achieved by a ketogenic diet. If seizures are localisation-related in type and are unresponsive to treatment, surgical removal of the epileptic focus may be undertaken.

The aim should be to help children with epilepsy to be as confident and independent as possible. Activities should not necessarily be limited. The risk of participation should be weighed against the benefits, taking account also the child's character, ability and seizure frequency. Some children with epilepsy and their families need psychological help to adjust to the disability. The school needs to be aware of the child's problem and teachers advised on the management of seizures. Unrecognised absences may interfere with learning, which is an indication for being vigilant about 'odd episodes' which may represent seizures, in order to achieve better seizure control. Some children require educational help for associated learning difficulties. Two-thirds of children with epilepsy go to a mainstream school; one-third attend a special school, but they often have multiple disabilities and epilepsy as part of a severe brain disorder. A few children require residential schooling where there are facilities and expertise in monitoring and treating intractable seizures.

Funny turns

There are a number of benign paroxysmal disorders which may mimic epilepsy. A detailed history, preferably from a person who has witnessed the event in question, is crucial in distinguishing epilepsy from other disorders. The causes are listed in Figure 25.8.

CEREBRAL PALSY

Cerebral palsy is a disorder of movement and posture due to a non-progressive lesion of the motor pathways in the developing brain. Although the lesion is non-progressive, the clinical manifestations evolve with cerebral maturation. It is the most common cause of motor impairment in children, affecting about 2 per 1000 live births. In addition to disorders of movement and posture, children with cerebral palsy often have other problems reflecting more widespread brain dysfunction. These include:

- associated learning impairment in about 60%
- visual impairment in 20% from errors of refraction and cortical damage
- squints in 30%
- hearing loss in 20%
- speech and language disorders (due to a combination of hearing loss, muscle incoordination and learning impairment)
- behaviour disorders
- epilepsy in 40%.

Causes
The main causes of cerebral palsy are shown in Figure 25.9. Most are antenatal in origin from cerebral dysgenesis or cerebral malformations. Only about 10% are thought to be due to hypoxic-ischaemic injury at birth and this proportion has remained relatively constant over the last decade. The rise in survival of extremely preterm infants has been accompanied by an increase in children with cerebral palsy, although the number of such children is small.

Clinical presentation
Many children who develop cerebral palsy are identified as being at risk in the neonatal period because of dysmorphic features, abnormal neurology, neonatal encephalopathy, seizures, symptomatic hypoglycaemia or a gross abnormality on cranial ultrasound.

Cerebral palsy usually presents with:
- abnormal tone and posturing in early infancy
- feeding difficulties with oromotor incoordination, slow feeding, gagging and vomiting
- delayed motor milestones
- abnormal gait once walking is achieved
- developmental delay particularly in language and social skills.

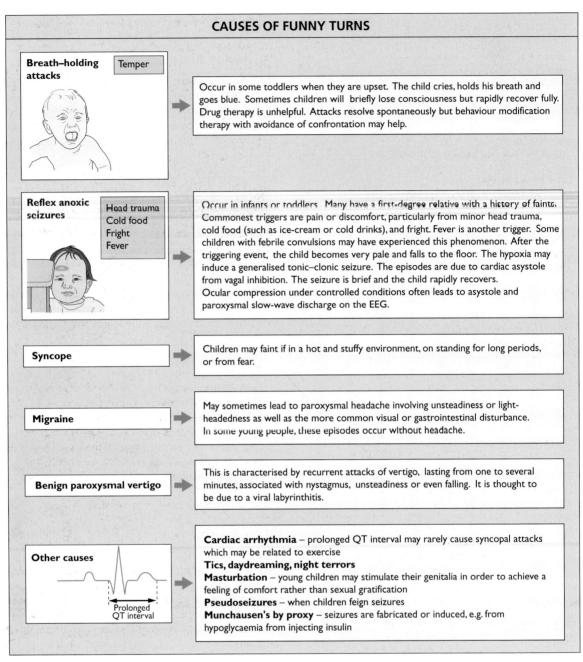

CAUSES OF FUNNY TURNS

Breath–holding attacks — Temper

Occur in some toddlers when they are upset. The child cries, holds his breath and goes blue. Sometimes children will briefly lose consciousness but rapidly recover fully. Drug therapy is unhelpful. Attacks resolve spontaneously but behaviour modification therapy with avoidance of confrontation may help.

Reflex anoxic seizures — Head trauma / Cold food / Fright / Fever

Occur in infants or toddlers. Many have a first-degree relative with a history of faints. Commonest triggers are pain or discomfort, particularly from minor head trauma, cold food (such as ice-cream or cold drinks), and fright. Fever is another trigger. Some children with febrile convulsions may have experienced this phenomenon. After the triggering event, the child becomes very pale and falls to the floor. The hypoxia may induce a generalised tonic–clonic seizure. The episodes are due to cardiac asystole from vagal inhibition. The seizure is brief and the child rapidly recovers. Ocular compression under controlled conditions often leads to asystole and paroxysmal slow-wave discharge on the EEG.

Syncope

Children may faint if in a hot and stuffy environment, on standing for long periods, or from fear.

Migraine

May sometimes lead to paroxysmal headache involving unsteadiness or light-headedness as well as the more common visual or gastrointestinal disturbance. In some young people, these episodes occur without headache.

Benign paroxysmal vertigo

This is characterised by recurrent attacks of vertigo, lasting from one to several minutes, associated with nystagmus, unsteadiness or even falling. It is thought to be due to a viral labyrinthitis.

Other causes

Cardiac arrhythmia – prolonged QT interval may rarely cause syncopal attacks which may be related to exercise
Tics, daydreaming, night terrors
Masturbation – young children may stimulate their genitalia in order to achieve a feeling of comfort rather than sexual gratification
Pseudoseizures – when children feign seizures
Munchausen's by proxy – seizures are fabricated or induced, e.g. from hypoglycaemia from injecting insulin

Prolonged QT interval

Fig. 25.8 Causes of funny turns.

Hand preference in those less than 12 months old often signifies the emergence of a hemiparesis.

Primitive reflexes facilitate the emergence of normal patterns of movements and need to disappear in order for development to progress. In cerebral palsy, they may persist and become obligatory (Fig. 25.10).

The diagnosis is made by clinical examination, with particular attention to assessment of the pattern of tone, posturing and observation of gait. There are three main clinical types of cerebral palsy, each reflecting damage to a specific motor pathway. Some children show a mixed pattern.

Spastic (70%)

In this type, there is damage to the upper motor neurone (pyramidal or corticospinal) pathway. Limb tone is abnormally increased (spasticity), with associated brisk deep tendon reflexes and extensor plantar responses. The increased limb tone may suddenly yield under pressure in a 'clasp knife' fashion. Before spasticity appears, there may be initial hypotonia particularly of the trunk. The distribution of signs may be in the form of:

• Hemiplegia – unilateral involvement of the arm and leg (Fig. 25.11). The arm is usually affected

Fig. 25.9 Causes of cerebral palsy.

Antenatal (80%)
Cerebral dysgenesis
Cerebral malformation
Congenital infection – rubella, toxoplasmosis,
 cytomegalovirus

Intrapartum (10%)
Birth asphyxia/trauma

Postnatal (10%)
Intraventricular haemorrhage/ischaemia
Meningitis/encephalitis/encephalopathy
Head trauma/non-accidental injury
Symptomatic hypoglycaemia
Hydrocephalus
Hyperbilirubinaemia

Fig. 25.10 Some primitive reflexes present at birth.
They should disappear by 6 months.

Reflex	Description
Moro	Sudden head extension causes symmetrical extension followed by flexion of all limbs
Grasp	Flexion of the fingers of the hand when an object is placed in the palm at the base of the fingers
Rooting	Turning of the head towards a stimulus near the mouth
Placing	With the infant held vertically and the dorsum of the feet brought into contact with a surface, the infant lifts first one foot, placing it on the surface, followed by the other
Atonic neck reflex	On lying supine, when the head is turned to one side, the infant adopts a 'fencing' posture, with the arm outstretched on the side to which the head is turned

CEREBRAL PALSY

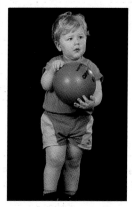

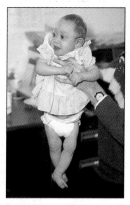

Fig. 25.11 A child with a right spastic hemiplegia. His right arm is hyperpronated.

Fig. 25.12 A child with spastic quadraplegia showing scissoring of the legs from excessive adduction of the hips, pronated forearms and 'fisted' hands. (Courtesy of Dr Diane Smyth.)

It is with functional use of the hands that motor difficulties in the arms are most apparent.

- Quadriplegia – all four limbs are affected to a fairly similar degree, often severely, although the arms may be affected more than the legs. The trunk is often involved, with extensor posturing and poor head control (Fig. 25.12). This form of cerebral palsy is often associated with seizures and moderate or severe intellectual impairment. There may have been a history of severe hypoxic–ischaemic birth injury.

Ataxic hypotonic (10%)
Signs are usually symmetrical. There is early hypotonia, poor balance and delayed motor development. Later, incoordinate movements and intention tremor may be evident, reflecting dysfunction in the cerebellum or its pathways. A genetic cause is by far the most common.

Dyskinetic (10%)
There is dyskinesia leading to constant involuntary movements (athetosis, chorea and dystonia) and poor postural control. Intellect may be relatively unimpaired. Affected children often present with floppiness and delayed motor development in infancy, with abnormal movements sometimes not appearing before 1 year of age. The signs are due to damage to the basal ganglia or their associated pathways (extrapyramidal).

Mixed pattern of the above types (10%)

Management
Parents should be given details of the diagnosis as early as possible, but prognosis is difficult during infancy until the pattern of evolving signs and the

more than the leg, with the face spared. Affected children often present at 4–12 months of age with fisting of the affected hand, a pronated flexed forearm, or tiptoe walk (toe–heel gait) on the affected side. The limb may initially be flaccid and hypotonic, but increased tone soon emerges as the predominant sign. The past medical history, including the birth history, has usually been normal.

- Diplegia – all four limbs are affected but the legs to a much greater degree than the arms, so that hand function may appear to be relatively normal.

child's developmental progress have been observed over several months or years of life. Children with cerebral palsy are likely to have a wide range of medical, psychological and social problems, making it essential to adopt a multidisciplinary approach to assessment and management. This is described in Chapter 26.

ATAXIA

In cerebellar ataxia there is an unsteady gait, difficulty in performing repetitive and alternating movements, overshooting of target-directed movement and an intention tremor which becomes more pronounced when the child puts more effort into trying to hold a posture. The gait has a wide base to provide stability to compensate for the truncal ataxia. There may be associated wobble of the head, nystagmus and a scanning dysarthria. Cerebellar ataxia may be:

- acute, from drugs including alcohol and solvent abuse
- a manifestation of postviral encephalopathy most commonly following varicella
- from a cerebellar tumour.

It may also be part of a chronic neurological condition such as ataxic cerebral palsy, ataxia telangiectasia and Friedreich's ataxia.

Ataxia telangiectasia

This disorder of DNA repair is an autosomal recessive condition. There may be mild delay in motor development in infancy and oculomotor problems (oculomotor dyspraxia), with difficulty with balance and coordination becoming evident at school age. There is subsequent deterioration, with many children requiring a wheelchair for mobility in early adolescence. Telangiectasis develops in the conjunctiva (Fig. 25.13), neck and shoulders from about 4 years of age. These children:

- have an increased susceptibility to infection, principally from an IgA surface antibody defect
- develop malignant disorders, principally acute lymphoblastic leukaemia (about 10%)

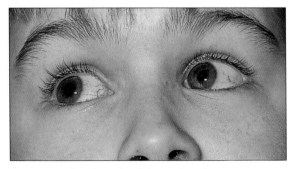

Fig. 25.13 Telangiectasia of the conjunctiva are present from about 4 years of age in ataxia telangiectasia.

- have a raised serum alphafetoprotein
- have an increased white cell sensitivity to irradiation which can be used diagnostically and to identify heterozygotes.

Friedreich's ataxia

This is the most common of the spinocerebellar degenerations. It is an autosomal recessive condition which presents with progressive clumsiness. Ataxia of the limbs and trunk, distal wasting in the legs, diminished reflexes, pes cavus and dysarthria may develop. This is similar to the hereditary motor sensory neuropathies, but in Friedreich's ataxia there is impairment of joint position and vibration sense, extensor plantars and there is often optic atrophy. The cerebellar component becomes more apparent with age, with the onset of scoliosis and cardiomyopathy. The latter often causes death at 40–50 years of age.

CEREBRAL HAEMORRHAGE

Extradural haemorrhage

This usually results from arterial or venous bleeding into the extradural space following direct head trauma. It is usually associated with a skull fracture. In young children there is often a lucid interval until the conscious level deteriorates and seizures occur due to the enlarging haematoma acting as a space-occupying lesion. There may be focal neurological signs with dilatation of the ipsilateral pupil, paresis of the contralateral limbs and a false localising uni- or bilateral VIth nerve paresis. In young children, initial presentation may be with anaemia and shock. The diagnosis is confirmed with a CT scan. Management is to correct hypovolaemia. Surgical evacuation of the haematoma and arrest of the bleeding may be required.

Subdural haematoma

This results from tearing of the veins as they cross the subdural space. In children it is seen almost exclusively in infants or toddlers due to non-accidental injury caused by shaking (see Ch. 6). Retinal haemorrhages are usually present. Subdural haematomas are occasionally seen following a fall from a considerable height.

Subarachnoid haemorrhage

Presentation is usually with acute onset of head pain, neck stiffness and occasionally fever. Retinal haemorrhage is usually present. Seizures and coma may develop. A CT scan of the head usually identifies blood in the CSF. A lumbar puncture is best avoided as haemorrhage may extend following the release of intracranial pressure. Angiography is performed to identify the aetiology, which is often an aneurysm or arteriovenous malformation. Treatment may be by interventional radiography or surgical.

NEURAL TUBE DEFECTS AND HYDROCEPHALUS

Neural tube defects

Neural tube defects result from failure of normal fusion of the neural plate to form the neural tube during the first 28 days following conception. They used to be one of the most common serious malformations detected at birth. In the 1970s, its birth prevalence in the UK was 4 per 1000 live births. This was the highest prevalence in the world, with a peak level in Ireland declining towards the south-east of England.

Since then, the birth prevalence in the UK has fallen dramatically to 0.15 per 1000 live births in 1998 (Fig. 25.14). This is mainly because of a natural decline, as well as antenatal screening.

The reason for the natural decline is uncertain but may be associated with improved maternal nutrition. It is well recognised that mothers of a fetus with a neural tube defect have a 10-fold increase in risk of having a second affected fetus. It has been shown that supplementing these mothers' diet with high doses of folic acid markedly reduces this risk. It is now recommended that women who have had a previously

NEURAL TUBE DEFECTS

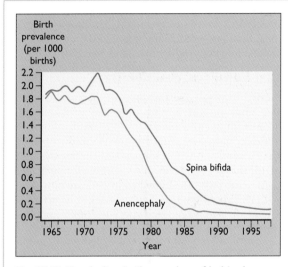

Fig. 25.14 The decline in the number of babies born with neural tube defects. This has resulted from a natural decrease together with antenatal diagnosis and termination of pregnancy.

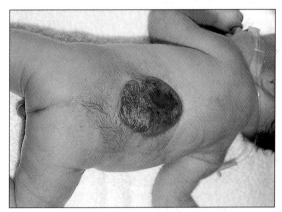

Fig. 25.16 Myelomeningocele showing the exposed neural tissue and the patulous anus from neuropathic bowel.

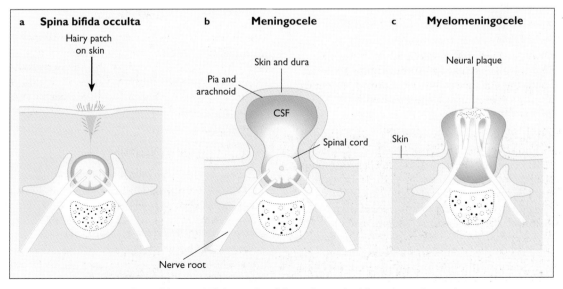

Fig. 25.15 Neural tube defects: (a) spina bifida occulta; (b) meningocele; (c) myelomeningocele.

affected infant and are planning a pregnancy should take high-dose folic acid periconceptually. Low-dose periconceptual folic acid supplementation is recommended for all pregnancies.

Anencephaly

This is failure of development of most of the cranium and brain. Affected infants are stillborn or die shortly after birth. It is detected on antenatal ultrasound screening and termination of pregnancy is usually performed.

Encephalocele

There is extrusion of brain and meninges through a midline skull defect, which can be corrected surgically. However, there are often underlying associated cerebral malformations.

Spina bifida occulta

This failure of fusion of the vertebral arch (Fig. 25.15a) is often an incidental finding on X-ray, but there may be an associated overlying skin lesion such as a tuft of hair, lipoma, birth mark or small dermal sinus, usually in the lumbar region. There may be underlying tethering of the cord (diastematomyelia) which, with growth, may cause neurological deficits of bladder function and lower limbs. The extent of the underlying lesion can be delineated using ultrasound and/or MRI scans. Neurosurgical relief of tethering is usually indicated.

Meningocele and myelomeningocele

Meningoceles (Fig. 25.15b) usually have a good prognosis following surgical repair. The main problems associated with myelomeningoceles (Figs 25.15c and 25.16) include:

- variable paralysis of the legs
- muscle imbalance which may cause dislocation of the hip and talipes
- sensory loss
- bladder denervation (neuropathic bladder)
- bowel denervation (neuropathic bowel)
- scoliosis
- hydrocephalus from the Arnold–Chiari malformation (herniation of the cerebellar tonsils through the foramen magnum), leading to disruption of CSF flow.

Physiotherapy is required to prevent joint contractures and strengthen paralysed muscles. Walking aids or a wheelchair may be required to permit mobility. With sensory loss, skin care is required to avoid the development of skin damage and ulcers.

An indwelling catheter may be required for bladder denervation, or intermittent urinary catheterisation may be performed by parents or by older children themselves. Urine samples should be checked regularly for infection. Continuous prophylactic antibiotics may be necessary. The child should be monitored for early evidence of hypertension and renal failure. Medication (such as ephedrine or oxybutinin) may

improve bladder function and improve urinary dribbling. Bowel denervation requires regular toileting, and laxatives and suppositories are likely to be necessary with a low roughage diet for lesions above L3.

Scoliosis is monitored and may require surgical treatment. Ventricular dilatation from Arnold–Chiari malformation is often present at birth and 80% of affected infants require a shunt for progressive hydrocephalus during the first few weeks of life.

Those children destined to be the most severely disabled have a spinal lesion above L3 at birth. They are unable to walk, have a scoliosis, neuropathic bladder, hydronephrosis and frequently develop hydrocephalus.

In the 1970s, follow-up studies of severely affected children showed that many had severe physical and intellectual impairment. Many had to undergo multiple operations. In adolescence and adulthood, they and their families faced many problems – psychological, sexual, finding employment and being cared for. As a consequence, many advocated a non-interventionist conservative approach, in which surgery was not performed to repair the meningeal lesion and overlying skin and supportive care only was provided. Most died from meningitis and ventriculitis, progressive hydrocephalus or renal failure. Subsequent studies have shown that with modern medical care the quality of life for severely affected children is much better than in the past. Most affected infants are now treated with closure of the lesion of the back soon after birth. Their care is managed by a specialist multidisciplinary team.

Hydrocephalus

In hydrocephalus there is increased pressure in the ventricular system. It is usually secondary to obstruction of CSF flow in the ventricular system (non-communicating) or failure of CSF reabsorption (communicating). The main causes are shown in Figure 25.17.

Fig. 25.17 Causes of hydrocephalus.

Non-communicating
(obstruction in the ventricular system)
Congenital malformation
   Aqueduct stenosis
   Atresia of the outflow foramina of the fourth
    ventricle (Dandy–Walker malformation)
Post-intracranial infection
Neoplasm or vascular malformation

Communicating (failure to reabsorb CSF)
Subarachnoid haemorrhage
Tuberculous meningitis
Arnold–Chiari malformation
Post-haemorrhagic in preterm infant

Clinical features

In infants with hydrocephalus, the head circumference is disproportionately large or its rate of growth is excessive, the sutures become separated and the scalp veins congested. The anterior fontanelle pressure, with the infant relaxed, will feel increased on palpation, and will subsequently bulge. If left untreated, the eyes deviate downwards (setting-sun sign) (Fig. 25.18). The infant subsequently develops symptoms and signs of raised intracranial pressure. Hydrocephalus may be diagnosed on antenatal ultrasound screening or in preterm infants on routine intracranial ultrasound scanning when the infant is asymptomatic. In older children, clinical features are due to raised intracranial pressure.

Management

Assessment of ventricular dilatation is with cranial ultrasound (see Ch. 9) and/or CT or MRI scan.

Treatment is required for symptomatic relief of raised intracranial pressure and to minimise the risk of neurological damage. The mainstay is the insertion of a ventricular shunt (Fig. 25.19), but endoscopic treatment is being developed. Shunt revision may be required if there is symptomatic malfunction from obstruction, infection (usually with coagulase-negative *Staphylococcus*) which is unresponsive to antibiotics, or overdrainage of fluid.

NEUROMUSCULAR DISORDERS

Any part of the lower motor pathway can be affected in a neuromuscular disorder, so that anterior horn cell disorders, peripheral neuropathies, disorders of neuromuscular transmission and primary muscle diseases can all occur. The causes of neuromuscular disorders are shown in Figure 25.20. The key clinical feature of a neuromuscular disorder is weakness, which may be progressive or static. Affected children may present with:

- floppiness
- delayed motor milestones
- muscle weakness
- unsteady/abnormal gait
- fatiguability.

Older children often show the waddling gait of proximal muscle weakness, muscle wasting, generalised hyptonia and absent or reduced deep tendon reflexes. Gower's sign is the need to turn prone when

HYDROCEPHALUS

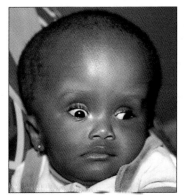

Fig. 25.18 Grossly enlarged head and downward deviation of the eyes (setting-sun sign) from untreated hydrocephalus.

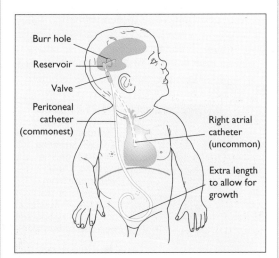

Fig. 25.19 Ventriculoperitoneal shunt for drainage of symptomatic hydrocephalus. A sufficient length of shunt tubing is left in the peritoneal cavity to allow for the child's growth. Right atrial catheters require revision with growth.

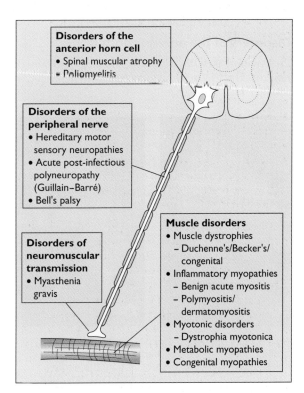

Fig. 25.20 Neuromuscular disorders.

rising from the supine: climbing 'up the legs with the hands' to gain the standing position is a later feature denoting more severe weakness (Fig. 25.21). A pattern of distal wasting and weakness, particularly in the presence of pes cavus, is usually due to one of the hereditary motor sensory neuropathies. Increasing fatiguability through the day, often with ophthalmoplegia and ptosis, suggests myasthenia gravis.

Investigations

- Serum creatine phosphokinase – markedly elevated in Duchenne's and Becker's dystrophies (the Xp21 myopathies).
- Electromyography and nerve conduction studies
- Muscle and nerve biopsies – needle muscle biopsy is usually sufficient, and modern histochemical techniques often enable a definitive diagnosis to be made.
- Recombinant DNA studies.
- Ultrasound, CT and MR imaging of muscles – allow accurate documentation of which muscles are affected.

Muscle fatiguability on repetitive nerve stimulation can be demonstrated in myasthenia gravis. The tests help in differentiating myopathic from neuropathic disorders but should be used selectively in children, as the nerve conduction studies cause a tingling sensation and electromyography requires insertion of fine needle electrodes.

Identification of the specific gene defect for a number of neuromuscular disorders allows accurate antenatal diagnosis. Genetic counselling and advice can then be offered.

Disorders of the anterior horn cell

Presentation is with weakness, wasting and absent reflexes. The features of poliomyelitis are described in Chapter 13.

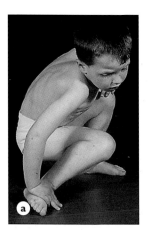 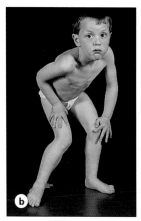

Fig. 25.21 (a,b) Gower's sign. The child needs to turn prone to rise, then uses his hands to climb up on his knees before standing, because of poor hip girdle fixation and/or proximal muscle weakness. Any child continuing to do this after 3 years of age is likely to have a neuromuscular condition.

Spinal muscular atrophy

This disorder is usually autosomal recessive and due to degeneration of the anterior horn cells, leading to progressive weakness and wasting of skeletal muscles. This is the second most common cause of neuromuscular disease in the UK after Duchenne's muscular dystrophy.

Spinal muscular atrophy type I (Werdnig–Hoffmann disease)

A very severe progressive disorder presenting in early infancy (Fig. 25.22). Diminished fetal movements are often noticed during pregnancy and there may be arthrogryposis (positional deformities of the limbs with contractures of at least two joints) at birth. Typical signs include:

- lack of antigravity power in hip flexors
- absent deep tendon reflexes
- intercostal recession
- fasciculation of the tongue.

Death is from respiratory failure by about 12 months of age. There are milder forms of the disorder with a later onset.

It is now thought that the spinal muscular atrophies and muscular dystrophies account for most of the scapuloperoneal, facioscapulohumeral or predominantly distal patterns of wasting and weakness.

Peripheral neuropathies

The hereditary motor sensory neuropathies (HMSN)

This group of disorders typically leads to symmetrical slowly progressive muscular wasting which is distal rather than proximal. Type I, formerly known as peroneal muscular atrophy (Charcot–Marie–Tooth disease), is usually dominantly inherited. Affected nerves may be hypertrophic due to demyelination followed by attempts at remyelination. Nerve biopsy typically shows 'onion bulb formation' due to these two processes. Onset is in the first decade with distal atrophy and pes cavus, the legs being affected more than

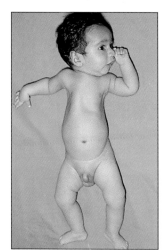

Fig. 25.22 Spinal muscular atrophy (Werdnig–Hoffmann disease) showing proximal muscle wasting, chest deformity from weakness of the intercostal muscles and thighs held abducted because of hypotonia.

the arms. Rarely, there may be distal sensory loss and the reflexes are diminished. The disease is chronic and only rarely do those affected lose the ability to walk. The presentation of Friedreich's ataxia can be similar.

Acute post-infectious polyneuropathy (Guillain–Barré syndrome)

Presentation is typically 2–3 weeks after an upper respiratory tract infection or *Campylobacter* gastroenteritis. There may be fleeting abnormal sensory symptoms in the legs, but the prominent feature is an ascending symmetrical weakness with autonomic involvement. Sensory symptoms are less striking than the paresis. Involvement of bulbar muscles leads to difficulty with chewing and swallowing and the risk of aspiration. Respiratory depression may require artificial ventilation. The maximum muscle weakness may occur only 2–4 weeks after the onset of illness. Although full recovery may be expected in 95% of cases, this may take up to 2 years.

The CSF protein is characteristically markedly raised, but this may not be seen if the lumbar puncture is done at the beginning of the illness. The CSF white cell count is not raised. Nerve conduction velocities are reduced.

Management of post-infectious polyneuropathy is supportive, particularly of respiration. Steroids have been shown to have no beneficial effect or may even delay recovery. The disorder is probably due to the formation of antibody attaching itself to protein components of myelin. Controlled trials have shown that the ventilator-dependent period can be significantly reduced by the use of immunoglobulin infusion. This is preferable to plasma exchange.

Bell's palsy

This is an isolated lower motor neurone paresis of the VIIth cranial nerve leading to facial weakness (Fig. 25.23). If symptoms of an VIIIth nerve paresis are also present, then the most likely diagnosis is a compressive lesion in the cerebellopontine angle. Although the aetiology is unclear in Bell's palsy, it is probably post-infectious. The herpes virus may invade

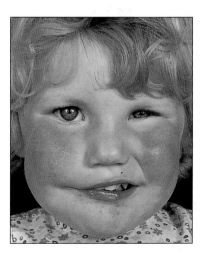

Fig. 25.23 Bell's palsy. There is right facial weakness of both the upper and lower face.

the geniculate ganglion and give painful vesicles on the tonsillar fauces and external ear, along with a facial nerve paresis. Hypertension should be excluded, as there is an association between Bell's palsy and coarctation of the aorta. Sarcoidosis should be suspected if facial weakness is bilateral.

Corticosteroids may be of value in reducing oedema in the facial canal during the first week. Recovery is complete in the majority of cases but may take some months. The main complication is conjunctival infection due to incomplete eye closure on blinking. This may require the eye to be protected with a patch or even tarsorrhaphy.

Disorders of neuromuscular transmission

Myasthenia gravis

This presents as abnormal muscle fatiguability which improves with rest or anticholinesterase drugs.

Transient neonatal myasthenia

This is described in Chapter 8.

Juvenile myasthenia

This is similar to adult autoimmune myasthenia and is due to binding of antibody to acetylcholine receptors on the post-junctional synaptic membrane. This gives a reduction of the number of functional receptors. Presentation is usually after 10 years of age. Presentation is usually with ophthalmoplegia and ptosis, loss of facial expression and difficulty chewing (Fig. 25.24). General, especially proximal, weakness may be seen.

Diagnosis is made by observing improvement following the administration of edrophonium. Treatment is with the use of anticholinesterases such as neostigmine or pyridostigmine. In the longer term, immunosuppressive therapy with prednisolone or azathioprine has been shown to be of value. Plasma exchange is used for crises. Thymectomy is performed if a thymoma is present or if the response to medical therapy is unsatisfactory.

Muscle disorders

The muscular dystrophies

This is a group of inherited disorders with muscle degeneration, often progressive.

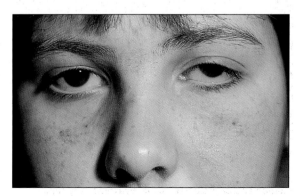

Fig. 25.24 Myasthenia gravis showing ptosis from ocular muscle fatigue which improved with edrophonium.

Duchenne's muscular dystrophy

This is the most common muscular dystrophy, affecting 1 in 4000 male infants. It is inherited as an X-linked recessive disorder, although about a third are new mutations. It results from a deletion of chromosome material on the short arm of the X chromosome (at the Xp21 site). This site is now known to code for a protein called dystrophin which maintains the integrity of the muscle cell wall. Where it is deficient, there is an influx of calcium ions, a breakdown of the calcium calmodulin complex and an excess of free radicals. These lead eventually to irreversible destruction of the muscle cells. The serum creatine phosphokinase is markedly elevated.

Children present with a waddling gait and have to mount stairs one by one. Although the average age of diagnosis remains 5.5 years, children often become symptomatic much earlier, highlighting the importance of interpreting Gower's sign correctly. There may be selective atrophy of muscle, in particular of the sternal head of the pectoralis major and brachioradialis. There is pseudohypertrophy of the calves because of replacement of muscle fibres by fat and fibrous tissue.

In the early school years, affected boys just tend to be slower and more clumsy than their peers. The progressive atrophy and weakness lead them to become non-ambulant and in need of a wheelchair by the age of about 10–14 years. Death ensues in the late teens or early 20s from respiratory failure or the associated cardiomyopathy. About a third of affected children have learning difficulties. Scoliosis is a common complication.

Management. Contractures, particularly at the ankles, should be prevented by passive stretching and the provision of night splints. Appropriate exercise helps to maintain muscle power and mobility and delays the onset of scoliosis. Walking can be prolonged with the provision of orthoses, in particular those which allow ambulation by the child leaning from side to side. Lengthening of the Achilles tendon may be required to facilitate ambulation. Attention to maintaining a good sitting posture helps to minimise the risk of scoliosis. Scoliosis is managed with a truncal brace, a moulded seat and occasionally surgical insertion of a metal rod into the spine. Later in the illness, episodes of nocturnal hypoxia secondary to weakness of the intercostal muscles may present with lassitude or irritability. Respiratory aids may be provided to improve the quality of life. As with all chronic disabling conditions, parent self-help groups are a useful continuing source of information and support for families. Affected children should be reviewed periodically at a specialist regional centre.

It may be possible to identify female carriers if they have a mildly raised creatine phosphokinase or if the gene deletion can be detected on DNA analysis. Antenatal diagnosis will then be possible.

Becker's muscular dystrophy

In Becker's dystrophy some functional dystrophin is produced. The features are similar to those of Duchenne's but clinically the disease progresses more slowly. The average age of onset is 11 years, inability to walk in the late 20s, with death in the early 40s, although this is very variable.

Congenital muscular dystrophies

This is a heterogeneous group of disorders, most with recessive inheritance, which present with muscle weakness at birth or early infancy. Typically the proximal weakness is slowly progressive with a tendency to contracture when the ability to walk is lost. Some may run a more static course. Biopsy shows dystrophic features with the reduction of specific proteins such as merosin. Central nervous involvement is evident on neuroimaging in some types and learning difficulties are sometimes seen.

The inflammatory myopathies
Benign acute myositis

This is assumed to be a postviral phenomenon as it often follows an upper respiratory tract infection and runs a self-limiting course. Pain and weakness occur in affected muscles.

Dermatomyositis

This tends to be more benign than the adult illness. It is probably due to a vasculitis. There is ascending symmetrical muscle weakness with an insidious onset over some weeks. The anterior neck flexors and trunk muscles are typically involved. Bulbar muscle involvement may lead to problems with chewing and swallowing. Post-exercise pain and aching are seen in the majority of cases and there may be tenderness of the muscles. Classically there is a violaceous hue to the eyelids with periorbital oedema (Fig. 25.25). Extensor surfaces of joints may also be affected by the rash. More rarely subcutaneous calcification may occur, leading to palpable induration. Although the erythrocyte sedimentation ratio (ESR) and creatine phosphokinase are often raised, they may be normal. Muscle biopsy reveals an inflammatory cell infiltrate. The mainstay of management is corticosteriod therapy, which usually needs to be continued for at least 2 years. If the response to therapy is poor, azathioprine or cyclosporin may be tried. Over half the children recover fully.

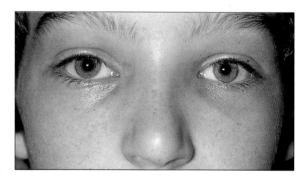

Fig. 25.25 Heliotrope rash in dermatomyositis.

Myotonic disorders

Myotonia is delayed relaxation after sustained muscle contraction. It can be identified clinically and on electromyography.

Dystrophia myotonica

This is a dominantly inherited disorder. When presentation occurs in the newborn period, there is profound hypotonia, feeding difficulty and intermittent respiratory difficulty. These infants have inherited the gene from their mother (an example of genetic imprinting). More typically, it presents with learning difficulties associated with a somewhat expressionless face (Fig. 25.26), distal wasting and myotonia. The latter usually first appears in late adolescence or the early 20s. Cataracts and, in males, baldness and testicular atrophy are common later associations. Death is usually due to an associated cardiomyopathy.

Metabolic myopathies

These present as a floppy infant or, in older children, with muscle weakness or cramps on exercise. The main causes are:

- glycogen storage disorders (see Ch. 23)
- muscle lipid disorders, affecting oxidation of fatty acids, a major source of energy for skeletal muscle, particularly during prolonged low-intensity exercise or fasting
- mitochondrial cytopathies, rare disorders which are coded as maternally inherited mitochondrial DNA.

Myopathy may be the major manifestation of a mytochondrial cytopathy, or the disorder may be multisystem with lactic acidosis and encephalopathy.

Congenital myopathies

These present at birth or in infancy with generalised hypotonia and muscle weakness. They are categorised according to the appearance of the muscle biopsy on electron microscopy. They do not show the morphological changes of muscular dystrophy. Disease types are:

- central core disease
- multicore disease
- nemaline myopathy
- congenital fibre-type disproportion.

Creatine phosphokinase levels are normal or only mildly elevated.

The 'floppy infant'

Persisting hypotonia in infants may be central or peripheral in origin (Fig. 25.27). The hypotonia can be readily felt on picking up the infant. There is marked head lag when traction is applied to the arms. If there is associated peripheral (lower motor neurone) weakness, affected infants have poor antigravity movements of the arms and legs which causes them to adopt a frog-like posture when lying supine (Fig. 25.22). When suspended prone, they slump over the examiner's hand, with their arms and legs extended under the

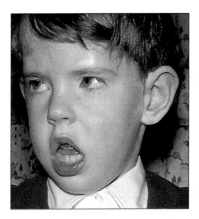

Fig. 25.26 Dystrophia myotonica in an 8-year-old who has marked facial weakness and moderately severe learning difficulties.

Fig. 25.27 Causes of the floppy infant.

Central
Cerebral
  Causes of developmental delay, e.g. Down's syndrome
  Evolving cerebral palsy
Hypothyroidism
Hypocalcaemia
Drug therapy

Peripheral
Spinal muscular atrophy
Myopathy
Myasthenia gravis

pull of gravity. With central hypotonia, the muscles are not weak and antigravity movements of the arms and legs are normal.

THE NEUROCUTANEOUS SYNDROMES

Neurofibromatosis (von Recklinghausen's disease)

This is dominantly inherited, but up to 50% are due to new mutations. It affects about 1 in 4000 live births. The cutaneous features consist of six or more café-au-lait patches (Fig. 25.28), axillary freckling and firm nodular neurofibromata which may be palpable on peripheral nerves. The cutaneous features tend to become more evident after puberty.

Neurofibromatosis type I (NF-I, peripheral) is coded on chromosome 17. Neurofibromata appear in the course of any peripheral nerve, including cranial nerves. They may look unsightly or cause neurological signs if they occur at a site where a peripheral nerve passes through a bony foramen. Visual or auditory impairment may result if there is compression of the IInd or VIIIth cranial nerve. Megalencephaly with learning difficulties and epilepsy are seen in a few cases.

Neurofibromatosis type II (NF-II, bilateral, acoustic or central) is coded for on chromosome 22. Bilateral

NEUROCUTANEOUS SYNDROMES

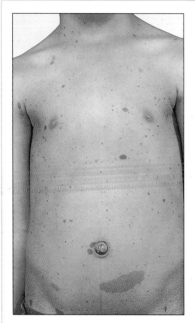

Fig. 25.28 Café-au-lait patches in neurofibromatosis.

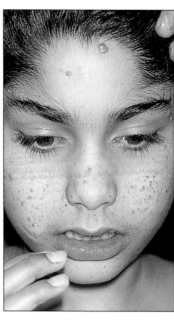

Fig. 25.29 Adenoma sebaceum in tuberous sclerosis.

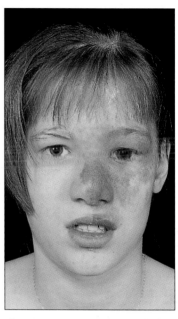

Fig. 25.30 Sturge–Weber syndrome. There is a port-wine stain in the distribution of the trigeminal nerve.

acoustic neuromata are the predominant feature and present with deafness and sometimes a cerebello-pontine angle syndrome with a facial (VII) nerve paresis and cerebellar ataxia.

There may be an overlap between the features of NF-I and NF-II. Other associations are phaeochromocytoma, pulmonary hypertension, renal artery stenosis with hypertension, and gliomatous change, particularly in central nervous system lesions. Rarely, the benign tumours undergo sarcomatous change. However, most people with the disorder carry no features other than the cutaneous stigmata.

Tuberous sclerosis

This disorder is dominantly inherited but 80% are new mutations. The cutaneous features consist of:

- depigmented 'ash leaf'-shaped patches which fluoresce under ultraviolet light (Wood's light)
- roughened patches of skin (Shagreen's patches) usually over the lumbar spine
- adenoma sebaceum (angiofibromata) in a butterfly distribution over the bridge of the nose and cheeks, which are unusual before the age of 3 years (Fig. 25.29).

Neurological features are:
- developmental delay with infantile spasms
- epilepsy – often localisation-related
- intellectual impairment.

These children have severe learning difficulties and often have autistic features to their behaviour when older. Other features are:

- fibromata beneath the nails (subungual fibromata)
- dense white areas on the retina (phakomata) from local degeneration
- rhabdomyomata of the heart which are identifiable in the early weeks on echocardiography but often resolve
- polycystic kidneys.

As with neurofibromatosis, gliomatous change can occur in the brain lesions. Many people who carry the gene have no stigmata other than the cutaneous features.

A characteristic feature on the skull X-ray is 'rail-road track calcification', usually after the first year of life. These calcified subependymal nodules can be identified earlier on CT or MRI brain scans.

Sturge–Weber syndrome

This is a sporadic disorder with a haemangiomatous facial lesion (a port-wine stain) in the distribution of the trigeminal nerve associated with a similar lesion intracranially. The ophthalmic division of the trigeminal nerve is always involved (Fig. 25.30). In the most severe form, it may present with epilepsy, learning disability and hemiplegia. Children presenting with intractable epilepsy in early infancy may benefit from hemispherectomy. For children who are less severely affected, deterioration is unusual after the age of 5 years, although there may still be seizures and learning difficulties.

NEURODEGENERATIVE DISORDERS

The cardinal feature of these disorders is developmental regression with the evolution of abnormal neurological signs. For some, the specific enzyme defect responsible has been identified. A wide variety of these inherited disorders has been described, such as the lysosomal enzyme storage disorders which include the mucopolysaccharidoses and lipid storage disorders (Fig. 25.31). The commonest lysosomal storage disorder is metachromatic leucodystrophy (a sphingolipidosis). As with all these disorders, the clinical classification depends on the age of presentation, and there are congenital, infantile, juvenile and adult forms. The commonest is the late juvenile which presents with developmental delay, hypotonia and ataxia, progressing to a severe spastic quadriplegia, and progressive dementia to a vegetative state with death within 3 or 4 years of onset. Developmental regression also occurs in subacute sclerosing panencephalitis (SSPE) following measles and in Wilson's disease.

Mucopolysaccharidoses

These are progressive multisystem disorders which may affect the neurological, ocular, cardiac and skeletal systems (Fig. 25.32). Hepatosplenomegaly is usually present. Most children present with developmental delay following a period of essentially normal growth and development up to 6–12 months of age. Developmental attainment then slows and children may show some loss of skills. It is only in the second 6 months of life that the characteristic facies begin to emerge, with coarsening of the facial features and prominent forehead due to frontal bossing (Fig. 25.33).

The characteristics of five of the varieties are shown in Figure 25.34. The diagnosis is made by identifying the enzyme defect and the excretion in the urine of the major storage substances, the glycosaminoglycans (GAGs). Treatment is supportive according to the child's needs. Successful enzyme replacement by bone marrow transplantation has been performed in these disorders but cannot reverse any established neurological abnormality.

Fig. 25.31 Lipid storage disorders.

Disorder	Enzyme defect	Clinical features
Tay–Sachs disease	Hexoseaminidase A	Autosomal recessive disorder Most common among Ashkenazi Jews Developmental regression in late infancy, exaggerated startle response to noise, visual inattention and social unresponsiveness Severe hypotonia, enlarging head Cherry red spot at the macula Death by 2–5 years Diagnosis – measurement of the specific enzyme activity Carrier detection of high-risk couples is practised. Prenatal detection is possible
Gaucher's disease	Beta-glucosidase	Occurs in 1 in 500 Ashkenazi Jews Chronic childhood form – splenomegaly, bone marrow suppression, bone involvement, normal IQ Splenectomy may alleviate hypersplenism Enzyme replacement therapy is available, but is extremely expensive Acute infantile form – splenomegaly, neurological degeneration with seizures Carrier detection and prenatal diagnosis are possible
Niemann–Pick disease	Sphingomyelinase	At 3–4 months, feeding difficulties and failure to thrive, hepatosplenomegaly, developmental delay, hypotonia and deterioration of hearing and vision Cherry red spot in macula affects 50% Death by 4 years

MUCOPOLYSACCHARIDOSES

Fig. 25.32 Clinical features of mucopolysaccharidoses.

Eyes	Corneal clouding
	Retinal degeneration
	Glaucoma
Skin	Thickened skin
	Coarse facies
Heart	Valvular lesions
	Cardiac failure
Neurology	Developmental regression
Skeletal	Thickened skull
	Broad ribs
	Claw hand
	Thoracic kyphosis
	Lumbar lordosis
Other	Hepatosplenomegaly
	Carpal tunnel syndrome
	Conductive deafness
	Umbilical and inguinal hernias

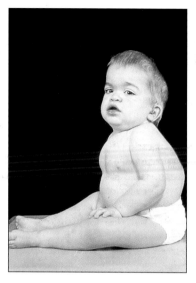

Fig. 25.33 Hurler's syndrome showing the characteristic facies and skeletal dysplasia.

Fig. 25.34 Types of mucopolysaccharidoses.

Type	Inheritance	Cornea	Heart	Brain	Skeletal
MPS I (Hurler)	AR	+++	++	+++	++
MPS II (Hunter)	X-linked	–	+	++	+
MPS III (Sanfilippo)	AR	+/–	–	+	+
MPS IV (Morquio)	AR	+	+	–	+
MPS VI (Morateaux-Lamy)	AR	+++	++	–	++

AR = autosomal recessive

FURTHER READING

Brett E M, Neville B G R 1997 Paediatric neurology, 3rd edn. Churchill Livingstone, Edinburgh. *A comprehensive textbook*
Newton R W 1995 Colour atlas of pediatric neurology. Mosby-Wolfe, London. *A well-illustrated textbook*

26

The child with special needs

The concept of special needs in a paediatric context is usually applied to children with neurodevelopmental disabilities that are long-lasting and complex. However, in a wider context, other children also have long-term needs that are greater than average, including:

- children with chronic medical conditions, e.g. cystic fibrosis, organ failure
- 'children in need', i.e. children who require additional social service input, e.g. because of child abuse or neglect
- those with emotional and behaviour problems, e.g. autistic spectrum disorder
- children with educational disorders, e.g. learning problems, attention deficit hyperactivity disorder (ADHD).

Children with all these problems require coordinated, multidisciplinary and multi-agency services. Disorders in the last four categories are considered elsewhere in the book.

Children with neurodevelopmental disabilities may have:

- an impairment – any loss or abnormality of physiological function or anatomical structure
- a disability – any restriction or lack of ability due to the impairment
- a handicap – a disadvantage from a disability which limits or prevents the fulfilment of a normal role.

However, as the term 'handicap' may give the impression of a dependent person to be pitied, it is now rarely used. The terms 'impairment' or 'disability' are used instead.

PRESENTATION

Children with special needs may present throughout childhood or adolescence. One of the aims of the child health surveillance (child health promotion) programme is the early identification of neurodevelopmental problems. Some of the more common times and modes and patterns of presentation are listed below.

Antenatal period

- suspected on family history
- identified on screening tests performed routinely, e.g. Down's syndrome identified on blood testing, spina bifida and other structural anomalies on ultrasound screening
- at increased risk, e.g. screening of Jewish couples for Tay–Sachs disease.

Perinatal period

- sequelae of birth asphyxia or neonatal encephalopathy
- preterm infants with intraventricular haemorrhage, periventricular leucomalacia or post-haemorrhagic hydrocephalus
- chromosomal abnormality or syndrome identified clinically at birth
- abnormal neurological behaviour – poor feeding, abnormal tone or movement, including a floppy infant, visual inattention, seizures.

Infancy

- delayed motor milestones, such as sitting and walking, asymmetric use of a limb, abnormally early hand preference
- visual or auditory impairment noted by parents or identified by screening
- general developmental delay – some diagnostic clinical features may only develop later, e.g. facial features in mucopolysaccharidoses or cutaneous stigmata in neurocutaneous disorders.

Preschool

- speech and language delay – specific deficit or as part of global developmental delay

- abnormal gait, e.g. tip-toeing from mild cerebral palsy or other neuromuscular conditions
- loss of skills from a neurodegenerative disorder.

School age
- clumsiness, poor dexterity, balance or coordination – may only become evident when the child mixes with peers
- specific cognitive defects – suspected if there is poor concentration and distraction which becomes more apparent when the child starts more formal learning of reading and writing
- specific learning difficulties, e.g. dyslexia, dyspraxia
- problems with hyperactivity and attention.

Any age
- following a serious illness of the central nervous system, e.g. meningitis or a head injury.

In this chapter, delay in motor development, speech and language and global development will be considered.

DELAYED MOTOR DEVELOPMENT

This may be evident during infancy or as a delay in walking. A common cause of late walking is if infants were bottom-shufflers or commando-crawlers rather than crawlers. This needs to be differentiated from common organic causes:

- cerebral palsy
- muscle weakness from a primary muscle disorder such as Duchenne's muscular dystrophy or spinal lesion such as spina bifida
- global developmental delay, e.g. from a syndrome such as Down's syndrome or unidentified cause.

Patterns of abnormal motor development which may suggest cerebral palsy are shown in Figure 26.1.

DELAYED SPEECH AND LANGUAGE DEVELOPMENT

It is necessary to distinguish between speech and language:

- Speech – the actual sounds that are made.
- Language – the underlying complex series of rules and codes governing communication. Language is divided into receptive language (language comprehension) and expressive language (facial expression, gesture, speech). A child may have a deficit in either. As in other developmental areas, receptive and expressive language go through a developmental progression.

Many language problems are suspected first by parents or primary health professionals. Assessment, diagnosis and treatment are specialist areas, the province of speech and language therapists working closely with neurodevelopmental paediatricians. Therapy may be provided by a speech and language therapist, or on their advice by a combination of parents, teachers and others caring for the child with reassessment by the therapist at intervals.

Language tests and assessment

There is considerable overlap between language development and general intellectual development. 'Performance' or 'non-verbal' intelligence tests try to disregard the language component. However, the opposite is not the case, and tests of verbal skills, especially those for the younger child, reflect general developmental skills including motor as well as language. Consequently, assessment of the verbal skills of a child with a motor disorder such as cerebral palsy is compromised and the results of verbal tests have to be interpreted with care.

Language tests are many and varied and are usually applied by speech and language therapists. Tests include:

- The symbolic toy test – assesses essential pre-language development. This test may be applied without specialist training.
- The Reynell test – for the preschool child. It has separate sections for comprehension and expression and is administered by specially trained professionals, usually speech and language therapists.

Speech and language delay

For some children this is a variant of normal, with delayed maturation of speech and language being subsequently shown to be of no long-term significance. There may be a family history of delay in language or speech which is transient. Others have speech and language delay of more worrying significance. Common causes include:

- hearing loss
- environmental deprivation – active social interaction is a prerequisite for communication skills
- oromotor impairment, e.g. cleft palate, cerebral palsy
- general developmental delay.

Once delay is identified and the child's hearing checked, a therapy programme may be initiated for the parents under the therapist's direction.

Speech and language disorders

These are more serious conditions and require specialist diagnosis and treatment (Fig. 26.2). There may be a disorder of speech and speech sounds, such as stammering (dysfluency), incomprehensible speech sounds or dysarthria. Language disorders include receptive dysphasia (inability or difficulty in comprehending language) and expressive dysphasia (inability or difficulty in producing speech while knowing what is

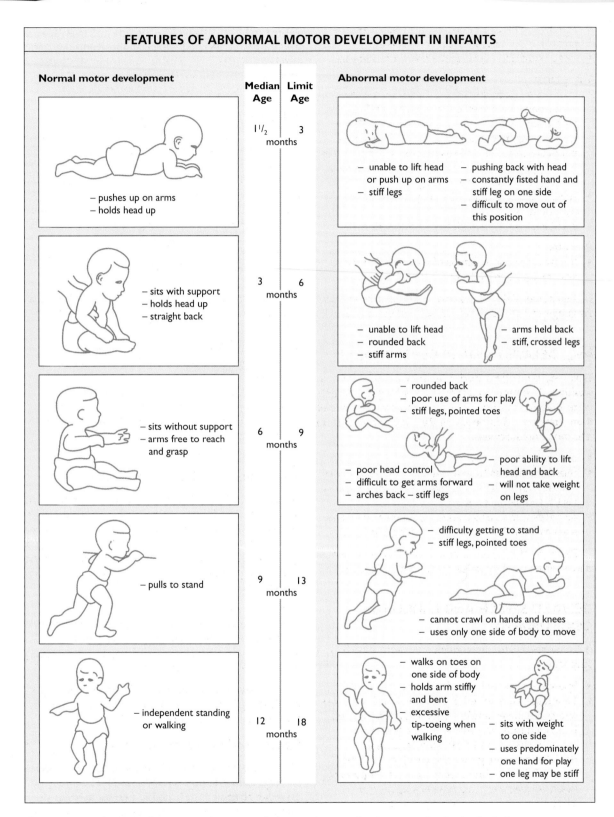

Fig. 26.1 Normal motor milestones and patterns of abnormal motor development. Cerebral palsy is the commonest cause of the developmental problems shown. (Adapted from Pathways Awareness Foundation, 123 North Wacker Drive, Chicago, IL. Tel. 800-326-8154, Internet: www.pathwaysawareness.org)

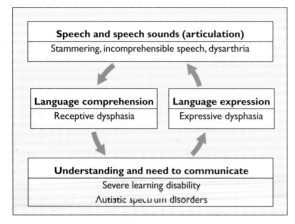

Fig. 26.2 The structure of speech and language and the classification of some language deficits.

wanted to be said). Intensive therapy and even special schooling may be needed. Social and communication disorders within the autistic spectrum are separate from speech and language disorders.

GLOBAL DEVELOPMENTAL DELAY

This implies developmental delay in all skill areas, but predominantly in language, fine motor and social skills. Gross motor skills are usually delayed, but this can be variable. The condition is usually associated with learning disability, although the latter may not become clear until a year or two after global developmental delay is recognised. Common causes and investigations to be considered for global developmental delay are listed in Figure 26.3.

Fig. 26.3 Causes and investigation of global developmental delay and learning difficulties. Many of these conditions also cause cerebral palsy; it is the timing, site and severity of the brain injury that determine whether the child has cerebral palsy, global developmental delay or severe learning difficulties.

Cause	Investigations (chosen selectively)
Genetic	
Chromosomal disorders, syndromes, e.g. Down's syndrome, fragile X, Duchenne's muscular dystrophy	Chromosomes including fragile X
Metabolic, e.g. phenylketonuria	See below
Brain – structural anomalies, e.g. hydrocephalus, microcephaly	Cranial ultrasound in newborn, CT/MRI brain scan
Antenatal	
Teratogens, e.g. alcohol and drug abuse	
Congenital infection, e.g. rubella, CMV, toxoplasmosis	Urine for viral culture; viral serology
Congenital malformations, e.g. hypothyroidism	Thyroid function tests
Perinatal	
Extreme prematurity, e.g. intraventricular haemorrhage, periventricular leucomalacia	Cranial ultrasound in newborn, CT/MRI brain scan
Hypoxic–ischaemic injury, e.g. birth asphyxia	CT/MRI brain scan
Metabolic, e.g. hypoglycaemia, hyperbilirubinaemia	See below
Postnatal	
Head trauma, e.g. accidental, non-accidental	CT/MRI brain scan; EEG may be indicated
Anoxia, e.g. suffocation, near-drowning	CT/MRI brain scan; EEG may be indicated
Infection, e.g. post-meningitis or encephalitis	CT/MRI brain scan; EEG may be indicated
Metabolic, e.g. hypoglycaemia	Urine – amino and organic acids; muco- and oligosaccharide screen; reducing substances
	Blood – pH and lactate and ammonia; plasma urea and electrolytes, calcium, liver function tests; white blood cell enzymes; very long-chain fatty acids (VLCFAs) for specific motor deficit; maternal amino acids for raised phenylalanine
Unknown (about 25%)	EEG, creatinine phosphokinase (in boys with learning difficulties), blood lead, copper, nerve conduction and electromyography, nerve and muscle biopsy

Specific features to note on examination are:

- growth, including head circumference for brain growth
- dysmorphic features, e.g. Down's or Williams' syndromes
- skin for neurocutaneous syndromes, e.g. tuberous sclerosis
- neurology for posture, gait, tone, reflexes; also fundi, vision and hearing.

LEARNING DISABILITY

This term is now preferred to 'mental retardation' or 'mental handicap'. It can be classified as mild, moderate, severe or profound.

One way in which cognitive function can be assessed objectively is by an IQ test, but this has the disadvantage that it is affected by cultural background and linguistic skills, does not test all skill areas and does not necessarily reflect an individual child's ultimate potential. It can be classified:

- moderate learning disability (IQ of 50–70)
- severe (IQ of 20–50) – this enables a person to learn minimal self-care skills and acquire minimal speech and language; supervision is required
- profound (IQ of 0–20) – this is associated with virtually no language or self-help skills and the need for full lifelong supervision.

Severe or profound learning disability is usually apparent as marked global developmental delay from infancy. When less severe, learning disability affects mainly language and social skills; mild learning disabilities may only become apparent when attending school.

The prevalence of severe learning disability is about 4 per 1000 children. Most have an organic cause and it does not vary according to parental social class, in contrast to moderate learning disability, in which children of lower socioeconomic parents are over-represented.

Common causes of moderate and severe learning disability are listed in Figure 26.3. Choice of investigation is determined by the history and clinical findings, although in about 25% no cause can be identified. Investigations are not necessarily all done at once.

THE MULTIDISCIPLINARY CHILD DEVELOPMENT SERVICE

The current approach to assessing a child with special needs is to define functional skills and therefore to identify what is difficult for the child as well as what he can do. This often requires assessment by a team of professionals. Functional skills can be categorised according to:

- mobility
- hand function
- vision

- hearing
- language and communication
- behaviour, social and emotional skills
- physical health
- self-care, including continence
- learning.

Once the child's abilities and difficulties are identified, it is possible to formulate a plan to help the child develop to his full potential. Child development services have been established to coordinate the needs of these children. The service is delivered by multidisciplinary child development teams who focus their effort on providing support to the preschool child with moderate or severe difficulties but who may also have resources to support children with milder problems. There is an increasing effort to monitor needs and provide multidisciplinary support up to school-leaving age. Members of the child development team are predominantly health professionals but close liaison is established with social services, local education authorities and voluntary agencies (Fig. 26.4) who may be represented on the child development team. In England and Wales, social services departments are required (by the 1989 Children Act) to maintain a register of children with disabilities and special needs in order to facilitate the provision of their care.

The multidisciplinary child development service may be organised in a number of different ways. It may be based in the community or hospital, but preferably should work flexibly across both. The professionals constituting the child development team can vary, but those usually included are listed in Figures 26.5. The paediatrician provides medical assessment, investigation, diagnosis and continuing medical management and helps coordinate the input of therapists and other health professionals. Many teams nominate a specific key worker for the family, usually a team member, to help families gain access to the resources their child needs and to resolve anxieties that may arise. Families should be provided at an early

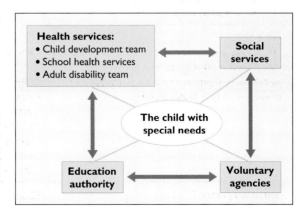

Fig. 26.4 Children with special needs are supported by the integrated input of health and social services, local education authorities and voluntary agencies.

Fig. 26.5 Child development team members.

Paediatricians
Have special medical expertise in neurodevelopmental problems and management of complex disability.

Physiotherapists
Assess patterns of movement and help development of balance and mobility skills and the prevention of muscle contractures and abnormal posture. Assist with mobility aids.

Occupational therapists
Assess fine motor and independent skills, particularly feeding, dressing and toileting. Provide aids to improve hand and manipulative skills and advise on appropriate seating and mobility aids including wheelchairs. Also advise on how to adapt houses to make them more suitable for a disabled person.

Speech and language therapists
Assess speech, language and other aspects of communication. Advise parents on how to encourage language development. This could include using an alternative means of communication such as the Makaton sign language and Bliss symbols boards, which are suitable for children with severe learning difficulties (Fig. 26.6), or communication aids such as voice synthesisers. In conjunction with occupational therapists, psychologists and dietitians, speech and language therapists may help children with feeding difficulties.

Psychologists
Perform detailed developmental assessments using standardised tests, which help parents and teachers to identify learning problems. They also advise on ways to modify disordered behaviour, often with behaviour modification programmes. Educational psychologists assess cognitive skills and advise on appropriate educational support to meet the child's needs.

Social workers
Act as advocates for the child and individual family and advise and help secure resources, e.g. allowances, day nursery placements, housing, respite care, voluntary agencies. Social workers can also help parents to formulate questions they may have about their child's problems and, as with other team members, offer practical and emotional support. Social services have statutory duties, e.g. to maintain a register of children with special needs.

Community nurses/specialist health visitors
Help to coordiante care between professionals in the community (home, nursery, school) and hospital, enabling as much care as possible to be carried out in community settings. Also provide psychological support for the family. Deliver nursing care, e.g. gastrostomies, continence. May advise parents on the play they can incorporate into everyday activities to help children attain further developmental progress (e.g. Portage scheme).

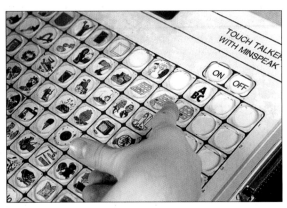

Fig. 26.6 A touch pad communication system using symbols. This child with dystonic posturing can still press the desired key.

stage with information on available financial benefits, voluntary support agencies and respite care.

There is a change in the emphasis of care and support needed as the child with a disability grows older. Preschool children are predominantly supported by the health-led multidisciplinary child development team, with educational psychologists playing a role in assessment and provision of support. For school-age children, the key input is likely to be from the education authority, with pediatricians and therapists working in the schools. By contrast, social services become the key agency for school-leavers and young adults. Young adults with learning or physical disabilities are supported by community-based learning disability teams. However, there is a need for all three statutory services – health, education and social services – to be available to a greater or lesser extent at all stages of the child's life, with an emphasis on providing coordinated care. Attention is also needed to avoid a proliferation of professionals and overlap of activity whilst still ensuring the child's needs are met.

PARENTAL REACTION TO DISABILITY

The confirmation that their child has a disability, together with the associated diagnosis, may come as the culmination of months of parental concern about their child's development or may be sudden, as with the diagnosis of a chromosomal abnormality in the immediate postnatal period. Either way, the parents are likely to feel great distress, with their expectations of having a normal child shattered. The initial interview, when the diagnosis is discussed, is extremely important and difficult for all, and has to be handled with the utmost sensitivity in order that the relationship between the parents, doctors and other professionals can remain constructive. This requires honesty and trust on all sides. The importance of seeing both parents together and the need to present the facts truthfully and as early as possible, but in an unhurried manner, have been discussed in Chapter 4.

Some of the greatest resentment arises if doctors are subsequently seen to have withheld information on the grounds that the family were not 'ready to receive it'. Because of anxiety, parents are often not able to assimilate information given at the initial meeting and further meetings are required. It is often helpful to have an advocate for the parents present, such as their social worker, health visitor or a relative, who will help them in subsequent, more private, discussions and in formulating questions they may wish to ask later.

Some disabilities, e.g. cerebral palsy, may become apparent only gradually over the first months of life. Considerable experience and clinical judgement are needed in the early recognition of disabilities and in determining their likely prognosis. The parents' initial reaction to the news that their child may have a disabling condition is usually grief accompanied by anger, guilt, despair or denial. Realisation and acceptance often follow, with psychological adaptation to the new circumstances when parents start to plan and organise for the future. The father, mother and other family members may all react differently to the news about the disability. Parents may find counselling and support helpful during this period. The grief parents feel may be centred on the image of the perfect child they were expecting, now replaced by the idea of a disabled child, possibly further aggravated by their perception of a particular disability.

Doctors, too, may harbour prejudices about particular disabilities. Doctors can learn how to deal with these emotions by listening to families of children with these disabilities, by reading literature on the subject and by networking with colleagues who have experience in this field.

Often no curative treatment is available, but health professionals have much to offer children with special needs and their families. They can explain how the child is progressing and what services are available, thus allowing the families to develop a realistic but positive approach to helping their child reach optimum potential, even when the disability is severe.

CONTINUING MEDICAL CARE

Many children with special needs have active medical problems which require investigation, treatment and review (Fig. 26.7). Good interprofessional communication is vital for well coordinated care. This will be assisted by all professionals keeping entries in the child's Personal Child Health Record up-to-date.

SPECIAL PROBLEMS OF CONSENT

Rarely, parents of children with a handicap will not consent to life-saving operative procedures. For example, they may decline the repair of duodenal atresia in Down's syndrome. In an emergency, doctors are legally entitled to intervene in the best interests of the child without the consent of parents but, where there is more time, legal advice should be obtained about seeking a judgement in court.

The question may arise as to whether it is lawful for doctors to withhold life-saving treatment from a child with severe disabilities. In the UK it has been found to be 'not unlawful' to allow a child to die where severe disabilities exist and where suffering would be avoided.

In the UK, children may give consent to a medical procedure if their understanding of the situation appears adequate. Where a person is incapable of understanding the issues involved but is over 16 years, and when the treatment is controversial, e.g. sterilisation, leave of the court should be sought. If the treatment is not controversial, doctors can proceed with the agreement (but not the consent) of the parents or the person's usual caretakers provided it can be defended as being in the child's best interests. The Human Rights Act has relatively recently become law in the UK. The central tenet of this legislation is the right to life. It is not yet known what bearing this will have on medical issues of this sort. It clearly remains crucial to ensure that everyone involved in the care of an individual child, including parents, doctors, nurses and therapists, is in agreement with any management plan. The development of local hospital ethical committees which may assist with making such decisions is foreseen.

EDUCATION

In England and Wales, the 1981 and 1993 Education Acts were devised to provide adequate rights and safeguards for children with disabilities and learning difficulties, and to ensure their right to integration into mainstream school whenever possible. Education authorities have a duty to identify children whose special educational needs will require additional resources.

Initial recognition that a child may have special educational needs may come at the preschool stage by the child presenting with specific or global developmental delay or with specific medical problems, or may only become evident when the child is of school age. Recognition leads to formal notification to the local education authority. Notification at the preschool age is generally from a health professional,

Fig. 26.7 Medical problems commonly encountered by children with special needs.

Microcephaly

This reflects failure of the brain to grow and is accompanied by problems with cognitive skills.

Visual and hearing impairment

Function needs to be regularly reviewed, as minimising any impairment will help to optimise the child's progress. Assessment in children with disabilities can be difficult.

Epilepsy

Seizures are common in children with neurodevelopmental problems. They may be difficult to control and manipulation of anticonvulsant therapy may be necessary.

Orthopaedic problems

Regular physiotherapy, adequate seating and the provision of appropriate aids are required to optimise posture and mobility (Fig. 26.8a,b,c) and prevent or reduce skeletal deformity. Muscle contractures should be minimised by encouraging movement and weight-bearing. Drug therapy (with baclofen or dantrolene) is sometimes used when muscle spasticity causes distress, compromises function and makes care difficult. Postural deformity can be minimised by physiotherapy, footwear, callipers, orthoses and serial splinting. Botulinum toxin injection into dynamic muscle contractures may improve function and so delay or avoid the need for surgical intervention. Fixed ankle deformities from muscle contractures may require surgery to slide or elongate the Achilles tendon. Regular hip joint surveillance, looking particularly for subluxation from tight adductor muscles, allows early detection and intervention to prevent hip dislocation. Increasing kyphoscoliosis may require serial bracing or surgical insertion of a spinal rod to allow more comfortable positioning of the child and protect respiratory function.

Behaviour

Many children with central nervous system abnormalities have behaviour disorders. They may be a part of the disorder or environmentally determined. The clinical psychology or child psychiatry service can help parents by analysing the situation and advising on appropriate behaviour management. Parents and siblings of a child with special needs may have behavioural needs in their own right as a consequence of their predicament.

Feeding and gastrointestinal problems

These are often associated with cerebral palsy, particularly spastic and dyskinetic quadriplegia, and may be from oromotor incoordination, gastro-oesophageal reflux or both. This may result in food inhalation and chest infections, oesophageal pain and poor weight gain. Calorie intake may be increased with advice from the dietician, speech and language therapist and occupational therapist about food texture and feeding position, particularly of the head and trunk. If the child's food intake is inadequate because of impaired oromotor function or vomiting, or if oral feeding is complicated by significant risk of inhalation, insertion of a gastrostomy tube needs early consideration.

Chest infections

These are common in non-ambulant children. Aspiration pneumonia and wheezing may be secondary to oromotor incoordination and gastro-oesophageal reflux.

Bladder and bowel function

Problems arise from delay in acquiring continence, from an unstable bladder, vesicoureteric reflux or a neurogenic bladder or bowel. Children with a neurogenic bladder require regular renal function tests, radiological monitoring of the kidneys and urinary tract and pressure monitoring of the bladder. Intermittent urinary catheterisation, drugs to improve bladder function or surgical intervention may be required.

Constipation and faecal incontinence

This is a common problem in children with cerebral palsy or a neurogenic bowel. Attention needs to be paid to optimising the diet and regular toileting. Laxatives and enemas may be required.

often the involved paediatrician. Notification of a school-age child is by an education professional, generally only after involvement of the educational psychologist supporting the particular school. Notification results in a more detailed assessment of the child's education needs. Parents can also request such an assessment. A 'Statement of Special Educational Needs' may follow assessment, with the statement identifying the extra help the child should receive. Although children are integrated into mainstream school where practicable, special schools or units are usually more suitable for children with severe learning difficulties and sometimes for those with severe physical, sensory, communication or behaviour problems. Many special educational placements will have a need for therapy input (physiotherapy, occupational and speech/language therapy) as well as specialised teaching resources. Support for the behavioural needs of a child may come from a clinical or educational psychologist.

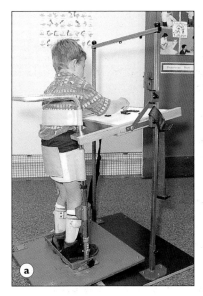
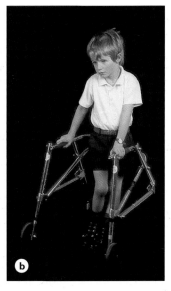
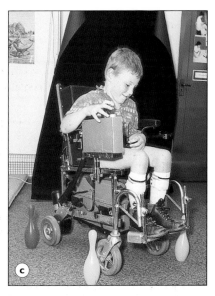

Fig. 26.8 (a) A standing frame assisting a boy with cerebral palsy to be upright. (b) A boy with athetoid cerebral palsy is able to walk with the help of a frame. (c) A 6-year-old boy with four-limb spasticity is able to steer this electric wheelchair. (Reproduced from Newton R, *Color Atlas of Pediatric Neurology*, Mosby–Wolfe, London, 1995.)

RIGHTS OF DISABLED CHILDREN

Irrespective of their disability, the aspirations and rights of children as affirmed by the United Nations Convention on the Rights of the Child need to be respected. Technological advances to improve mobility, communication and emotional expression are helping to enable disabled people to better achieve their full potential, rather than being held back by their disability. However, this requires adequate resources and skilled assistance. Prominent public figures who function effectively despite disabilities help to make the public appreciate what can be achieved and serve as an inspiration to those with disabilities.

YOUNG ADULTS

Young adults with physical and mental disability have their own special needs for medical support, therapy, assistance with social problems (housing, employment, mobility, finance, leisure, etc.) and sexual and genetic counselling. Unfortunately this service is still poorly developed compared with the multidisciplinary services available for young children with complex disabilities. Careful planning of issues and needs arising from the transition to adulthood is needed. Recent legislation in the UK aims to ensure that such planning does actually take place.

FURTHER READING

Hall D, Hill P, Elliman D 1999 The child surveillance handbook. Radcliffe Medical Press, Oxford. *A practical handbook*
Harvey D, Miles M, Smyth D 1995 Community child health and paediatrics. Butterworth-Heinemann, Oxford.
   A comprehensive textbook

Appendix

GROWTH CHARTS

These are examples of growth charts used in the UK (Fig. A.1a, b).

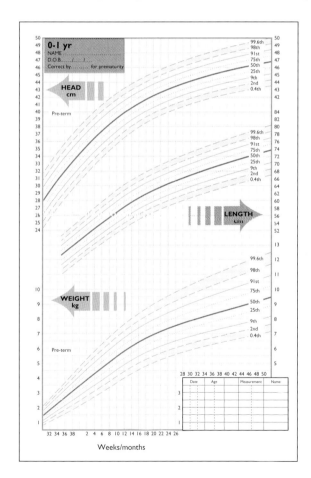

Fig. A.1a Growth chart for female infants in the first year of life. It includes measurements of weight, length and head circumference. This nine centile UK growth chart shows the 0.4 and 99.6 centile lines. The interval between each pair of centile lines is the same (–2/3 standard deviation). (Chart © Child Growth Foundation.)

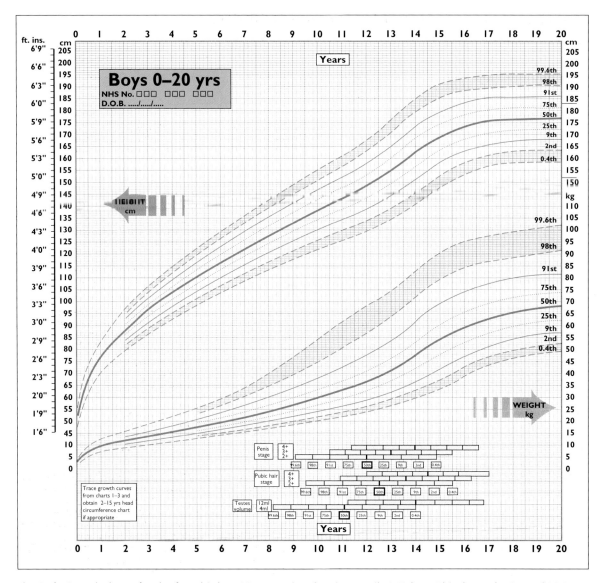

Fig. A.1b Growth chart of males from birth to 20 years using the nine centile UK chart. This shows the 0.4 and 99.6 centile lines. The interval between each pair of centile lines is the same (2/3 standard deviation). (Chart © Child Growth Foundation.)

GESTATIONAL AGE ASSESSMENT OF NEWBORN INFANTS

(a) External appearance.

External sign	0	1	2	3	4
Oedema	Obvious oedema of hands and feet; pitting over tibia	No obvious oedema of hands and feet; pitting over tibia	No oedema		
Skin texture	Very thin gelatinous	Thin and smooth	Smooth; medium thickness. Rash or superficial peeling	Slight thickening. Superficial cracking and peeling especially of hands and feet	Thick and parchment-like; superficial or deep cracking
Skin colour	Dark red	Uniformly pink	Pale pink; variable over body	Pale; only pink over ears, lips, palms, or soles	
Skin opacity (trunk)	Numerous veins and venules clearly seen, especially over abdomen	Veins and tributaries seen	A few large vessels clearly seen over abdomen	A few large vessels seen indistinctly over abdomen	No blood vessels seen
Lanugo (over back)	No lanugo	Abundant; long and thick over whole back	Hair thinning especially over lower back	Small amount of lanugo and bald area	At least half of back devoid of lanugo
Plantar creases	No skin creases	Faint red marks over anterior half of sole	Definite red marks over > anterior half of sole; indentations over < anterior 1/3	Indentations over >anterior 1/3 of sole of foot	Definite deep indentations over >anterior 1/3 of sole
Nipple formation	Nipple barely visible; no areola	Nipple well defined; areola smooth and flat, diameter <0.75 cm	Areola stippled, edge not raised, diameter <0.75 cm	Areola stippled, edge raised, diameter >0.75 cm	
Breast size	No breast tissue palpable	Breast tissue on one or both sides, <0.5 cm diameter	Breast tissue both sides; one or both 0.5–1.0 cm	Breast tissue both sides; one or both >1 cm	

(b) Neurological examination.

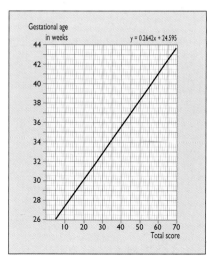

Neurological sign	Score					
	0	1	2	3	4	5
Posture						
Square window	90°	60°	45°	30°	0°	
Ankle dorsiflexion	90°	75°	45°	20°	0°	
Arm recoil	180°	90-180°	<90°			
Leg recoil	180°	90-180°	<90°			
Popliteal angle	180°	160°	130°	110°	90°	<90°
Heel to ear						
Scarf sign						
Head lag						
Ventral suspension						

Fig. A.2 Scoring system for assessment of gestational age in newborn infants (Dubowitz examination). This is a method of assessing gestational age according to external appearance (a) and neurological examination (b). The infant's gestational age (± 2 weeks) is determined from the total score using a conversion graph (c). (Adapted from Dubowitz L M S, Dubowitz V, Goldber C, Clinical assessment of gestational age in the newborn infant. *Journal of Pediatrics* 1970; 77: 1–10.)

(c) Graph for reading gestational age from total score.

$y = 0.2642x + 24.595$

BLOOD PRESSURE CHART

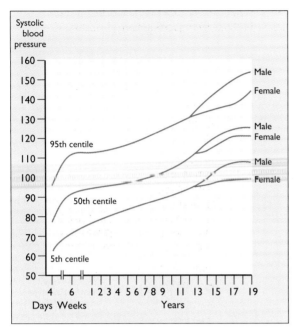

Fig. A.3 Systolic blood pressure according to age. Blood pressure charts are also available according to height. (Data from de Swiet M, Fayers P, Shinebourne E A, Blood pressure in a population of infants in the first year of life: the Brompton Study. *Pediatrics* 1980; 65: 1028–1035 and de Man S A et al, Blood pressure in childhood: pooled findings of six European studies. *Journal of Hypertension* 1991; 1(9): 109–114.)

PEAK FLOW CHART

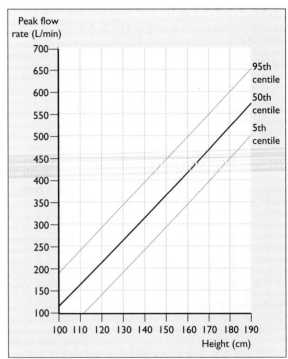

Fig. A.4 The normal range of peak flow measurements according to height. (Reproduced with permission from Godfrey S, Kamburoff P L, Nairn J R, Spirometry, lung volumes and airway resistance in normal children aged 5 to 18 years. *British Journal of Diseases of the Chest* 1970; 64: 15–24.)

NORMAL RANGES: HAEMATOLOGY

Age	Hb (g/dl)	MCV (fl)	WBC (×10⁹/L)	Platelets (×10⁹/L)
Birth	14.5–21.5	100–135	10–26	150–450 at all ages
2 weeks	13.4–19.8	88–120	6–21	
2 months	9.4–13.0	84–105	6–18	
1 year	11.3–14.1	71–85	6–17.5	
2–6 years	11.5–13.5	75–87	5–17	
6–12 years	11.5–15.5	77–95	4.5–14.5	
12–18 years				
Male	13.0–16.0	78–95	4.5–13	
Female	12.0–16.0	78–95	4.5–13	

NORMAL RANGES: CLINICAL CHEMISTRY

As the normal range for tests varies between laboratories, this must be checked with the local laboratory. (Values adapted with permission from Addy D P, *Investigations in Paediatrics*, WB Saunders, London, 1994 and other sources).

Test		Normal range (plasma or serum)	
Alanine aminotransferase (ALT)		<40 U/L	
Albumin	Neonate*	25–35 g/L	
	Child	35–55 g/L	
Alkaline phosphatase (ALP)	Neonate*	150–700 U/L	
	1 month–1 year	250–1000 U/L	
	2–9 years	250–850 U/L	
	Years	Females	Males
	10–11	250–950 U/L	250–730 U/L
	14–15	170–460 U/L	170–970 U/L
	>18	60–250 U/L	50–200 U/L
Ammonia	Neonate	<100 µmol/L	
	Infant/child	<40 µmol/L	
Amylase	Neonate	<50 IU/L	
	1–3 months	<100 IU/L	
	>1 year	<130 IU/L	
Aspartate aminotransferase (AST)		<50 U/L	
Blood gas (arterial, not preterm)	pH	7.35–7.45L (Hydrogen ion 35–44 nmol/L)	
	P_{O_2}	11–14 kPa (82–105 mmHg)	
	P_{CO_2}	4.5–6 kPa (32–45 mmHg)	
	Bicarbonate	18–25 mmol/L	
	Base excess	–3 to +3 mmol/L	
Calcium (total)	24–48 h	1.8–3.0 mmol/L	
	>1 week	2.15–2.60 mmol/L	
Calcium (ionised)	24–48 h	1.00–1.17 mmol/L	
	>1 week	1.18–1.32 mmol/L	
Chloride		96–110 mmol/L	
Creatine kinase	Infant/child	60–300 U/L	
Creatinine	Infant*	20–65 µmol/L	
	1–10 years	20–80 µmol/L	
Creatinine clearance	1–3 months	27–69 ml/min/1.73 m²	
	3–6 months	61–84 ml/min/1.73 m²	
	6–12 months	77–126 ml/min/1.73 m²	
	>2 years	110–200 ml/min/1.73 m²	
C-reactive protein		<10 mg/L	
Ferritin	Child	15–150 µg/L	
Gammaglutamyl transferase (GGT)	1–12 months	<80 U/L	
Glucose	1 day	2.2–3.3 mmol/L	
	>1 day	2.6–5.5 mmol/L	
	Child	3.0–6.0 mmol/L	
Glycosylated haemoglobin (HbA$_{IC}$)	5–16 years	3–6%	
17-Hydroxyprogesterone (17-OHP)	>2 days	0.7–12 nmol/L	
	Child	0.4–4 nmol/L	

CLINICAL CHEMISTRY *(continued)*

Test	Normal range (plasma or serum)	
Iron	Infant	5–25 μmol/L
	Child	10–30 μmol/L
Lactate (fasting)		0.5–2.0 mmol/L
Magnesium		0.6–1.0 mmol/L
Osmolality		275–295 mosm/kg
Phosphate	Neonate*	1.4–2.6 mmol/L
	Infant	1.3–2.1 mmol/L
	Child	1.0–1.8 mmol/L
Potassium	Infant	3.5–6.0 mmol/L
	Child	3.3–5.0 mmol/L
Protein (total)	Neonate*	54–70 g/L
	Infant	59–70 g/L
	Child	60–80 g/L
Pyruvate		40–70 μmol/L
Sodium		133–145 mmol/L
Thyroid-stimulating hormone (TSH)	>1 week	0.3–4.5 mU/L
Thyroxine (T_4, total)	Child	85–180 nmol/L
Urea	Neonate*	1.0–5.0 mmol/L
	Infant	2.5–8.0 mmol/L
	Child	2.5–6.5 mmol/L
Urate		120–350 μmol/L

*Depends on gestational age

Index

401